Good Design Practices for GMP Pharmaceutical Facilities

DRUGS AND THE PHARMACEUTICAL SCIENCES

Executive Editor

James Swarbrick
PharmaceuTech, Inc.
Pinehurst, North Carolina

Advisory Board

DRUGS AND THE PHARMACEUTICAL SCIENCES
A Series of Textbooks and Monographs

1. Pharmacokinetics, *Milo Gibaldi and Donald Perrier*
2. Good Manufacturing Practices for Pharmaceuticals: A Plan for Total Quality Control, *Sidney H. Willig, Murray M. Tuckerman, and William S. Hitchings IV*
3. Microencapsulation, *edited by J. R. Nixon*
4. Drug Metabolism: Chemical and Biochemical Aspects, *Bernard Testa and Peter Jenner*
5. New Drugs: Discovery and Development, *edited by Alan A. Rubin*
6. Sustained and Controlled Release Drug Delivery Systems, *edited by Joseph R. Robinson*
7. Modern Pharmaceutics, *edited by Gilbert S. Banker and Christopher T. Rhodes*
8. Prescription Drugs in Short Supply: Case Histories, *Michael A. Schwartz*
9. Activated Charcoal: Antidotal and Other Medical Uses, *David O. Cooney*
10. Concepts in Drug Metabolism (in two parts), *edited by Peter Jenner and Bernard Testa*
11. Pharmaceutical Analysis: Modern Methods (in two parts), *edited by James W. Munson*
12. Techniques of Solubilization of Drugs, *edited by Samuel H. Yalkowsky*
13. Orphan Drugs, *edited by Fred E. Karch*
14. Novel Drug Delivery Systems: Fundamentals, Developmental Concepts, Biomedical Assessments, *Yie W. Chien*
15. Pharmacokinetics: Second Edition, Revised and Expanded, *Milo Gibaldi and Donald Perrier*
16. Good Manufacturing Practices for Pharmaceuticals: A Plan for Total Quality Control, Second Edition, Revised and Expanded, *Sidney H. Willig, Murray M. Tuckerman, and William S. Hitchings IV*
17. Formulation of Veterinary Dosage Forms, *edited by Jack Blodinger*
18. Dermatological Formulations: Percutaneous Absorption, *Brian W. Barry*
19. The Clinical Research Process in the Pharmaceutical Industry, *edited by Gary M. Matoren*
20. Microencapsulation and Related Drug Processes, *Patrick B. Deasy*
21. Drugs and Nutrients: The Interactive Effects, *edited by Daphne A. Roe and T. Colin Campbell*
22. Biotechnology of Industrial Antibiotics, *Erick J. Vandamme*
23. Pharmaceutical Process Validation, *edited by Bernard T. Loftus and Robert A. Nash*

Good Design Practices for GMP Pharmaceutical Facilities

Andrew A. Signore
IPS
Lafayette Hill, Pennsylvania, U.S.A.

Terry Jacobs
Jacobs/Wyper Architects
Philadelphia, Pennsylvania, U.S.A.

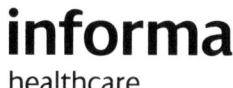

Informa Healthcare USA, Inc.
52 Vanderbilt Avenue
New York, NY 10017

© 2009 by Informa Healthcare USA, Inc. (Original copyright 2005 by Taylor & Francis Group, LLC)
Informa Healthcare is an Informa business

No claim to original U.S. Government works
Printed in India by Replika Press Pvt. Ltd.
10 9 8 7 6 5

International Standard Book Number-10: 0-8247-5463-8 (Hardcover)
International Standard Book Number-13: 978-0-8247-5463-1 (Hardcover)

Visit the Informa Web site at
www.informa.com

and the Informa Healthcare Web site at
www.informahealthcare.com

Contributors

James P. Agalloco
Bruce F. Alexander
Todd Allshouse
David Barr
Michael Bergey
Eric Bohn
Jack C. Chu
Robert Del Ciello
Stuart Dearden
Phil DeSantis
David Eherts
Jon F. Hofmeister
Terry Jacobs
Dave Kerr
William Kesack
David Lonza
Daniel Mariani
Art Meisch
Joseph Milligan
Miguel Montalvo
George Petroka
Denise Proulx
Andrew A. Signore
Charles Sullivan
Ed Tannebaum
William B. Wiederseim
George Wiker
Julian Wilkins
Peter Wilson
Gary V. Zoccolante

Advisors

Peter T. Bigelow
Robert E. Chew
Jim Dougherty
John Dubeck
A.J. (Skip) Dyer
Anthony Felicia
Robert J. Hoernlein
Thomas Jeatran
Sterling Kline
Larry Kranking
Brian Lange
James Laser
Stanley F. Newberger
George Petroka
Joseph X. Phillips
Wulfran D. Polonius
Denise Proulx
Hank Rahe
Eric Sipe
Teri C. Soli
Ashok Soni

Contents

Preface

Ask any busy pharmaceutical facility professional about their work and invariably you will hear, among a series of everyday challenges, such responses as "there's just too little time for me to do a good job," "new regulations keep coming but budgets aren't increasing," and "I simply do not have a enough experienced staff to achieve stated objectives." Designing a modern, compliant pharmaceutical facility is a daunting task within an increasingly complex and demanding business environment.

Successful pharmaceutical facilities are continually challenged to respond to evolving developments in technology and external regulation. This book aims to help the facility professional provide facility services that deliver faster, better, and more valued products to market. We herein provide useful tools in the form of relevant materials, practical advice, lessons learned, and insights into prevailing practices.

Good Design Practices (GDPs) provide a set of essential references for planning and delivering business-aligned, capital projects. GDPs, which include Good Manufacturing Practices (GMPs), form an essential aspect of project delivery and, when applied properly, help organizations deliver facilities that "perform and conform" to the growing body of regulatory requirements and business imperatives.

Webster defines "design" as "intentional functionality." GDPs offer a framework and a mindset to achieve acceptable functionality while meeting stringent tests of "fitness for purpose" in pharmaceutical facilities. Imaginative and effective application of GDPs can also achieve prudent risk management for manufacturing operations. GDPs also incorporate non-pharma specific public statutes, including environmental, occupational, safety, health, and local business code issues.

Pharma manufacturing facilities are increasingly considered strategic assets. Whether the firm meets its production requirements through fully integrated in-house manufacturing operations or obtains goods and services through external, third-party sources, pharma manufacturing facilities occupy a growing strategic role for the enterprise, where the bar is being raised for global compliance and competitive achievement.

GDPs also offer a framework for quality assurance to ensure that products are consistently produced and controlled by application of appropriate standards to their intended use as required by marketing authorization. GMP issues are also clearly a part of a quality program and form essential elements of facility planning. GDPs and, in turn, GMPs raise the importance of documentation and the process by which facilities are designed, built, and validated to demonstrate their ability to meet intended functionality and to confirm that what has been done is in accordance with what was planned. In addition to including GMPs, GDPs also help projects align with business objectives as captured in design standards and procedures, and assist the firm to achieve speed to market, flexible capacity, and conformance to other standards of care at acceptable cost and risk. Facilities professionals can increase their contributions through prudent application of GDPs where techniques provide additional tools to deliver valuable services.

It was not our intent to definitively and comprehensively treat all aspects of underlying engineering and science upon which good design practices are built. This book, however, does gather current practice and offers a convenient source of information provided by practicing professionals who are experts in their respective fields. Our contributors also encourage a strong awareness of the vital role that manufacturing plays in the modern firm and how prudent application of GDPs can increase the impact that each facility can have on the success of the firm and society as a whole through delivery of safer, cost-effective medicinal products.

Our approach encouraged each author (i.e., chapter expert) to frame their materials in the context of why the information was relevant to good design practices; how cost, schedule, and related project management issues are affected; and how historical insights and emerging trends can be highlighted for possible future development.

The successful application of scientific and engineering principles to the task of "practical design" remains a lifelong professional challenge. Incorporating affordable innovation into business-aligned facility solutions at acceptable risk is a worthy goal. We trust this book will prove helpful to those who set out on the wonderful "facilities" journey and will put to good use the wisdom inherent in "good design practices."

Andrew A. Signore, PE
Terry Jacobs, AIA

Acknowledgments

We had a wonderful journey compiling this book. The many rich opportunities to discuss, challenge, and interact with our group of contributing experts were exciting and immensely enriching. We truly thank our authors and advisors for their involvement and the deep insights given into the evolving practices of our profession. We are indebted to the openness and generosity of the team who persevered to see this project through, all the while remaining committed to their full time professional endeavors (day jobs).

On the production side we owe a deep debt of gratitude to a few dedicated individuals who helped produce the work. Our sincerest thanks are due on the administrative side to Jackie Bachowski, Terry Kane, and Rose Ottaviano who provided many hours of able support in compiling the text and helping to corral our book team. Gracious acknowledgments are warmly due Kim Goodman, Joanne Melero, and Shannah Schodle for their professional assistance, especially in gathering and producing the images, graphics, and other special touches. Thanks also to Lynne Stankus, our web master, who provided invaluable support in creating and maintaining our web site that helped the book team stay in touch. And of course, we would be remiss without thanking our dear wives and life sponsors, Annemarie and Sally, for their understanding and loving support through the many hours of intellectual separation required to prepare this work.

A.A.S.
T.J.

1
Pharmaceutical Industry Profile

Leader:	Andrew A. Signore
Advisor:	Wulfran D. Polonius

INTRODUCTION

The pharmaceutical industry is a major global economic force, which increasingly relies on the safe and efficient production of technically advanced products. This environment challenges the facilities professional who is charged to plan, design, construct, validate, and operate complex manufacturing facilities that meet world-class pharmaceutical standards. The facilities professional must master the many dynamic, interacting industry forces and understand how they influence pharmaceutical manufacturing facilities, and must apply prudently good design practices in response to these challenges.

The pharmaceutical industry is an economic entity comprised of multi-product, multi-market companies. The industry's operating environment is complex because of economic, political, technical, and social influences within a growing global environment for product development and delivery. The pharma industry has grown in the last several decades and has become quite complex, promising to deliver valuable products that enhance the quality of life to an expanding global population that demands greater access and more affordable choices. The role of the facilities professional is increasingly important to the industry as it addresses sourcing and manufacturing delivery objectives.

Pharmaceutical manufacturing facilities are charged with meeting two significant objectives: They must perform and conform. Facilities deliver increasingly complex and valuable products configured in evolving, technically complicated dosage forms and therapies. Facilities must also comply with ever-changing and demanding regulatory overview from the world's statutory bodies. These two fundamental challenges are addressed by facility professional's keen appreciation of the dynamic forces shaping the industry and by prudent facility designs that contribute to the enterprise's strategic long-term viability.

This chapter presents a broad overview of strategic industry driving forces to develop a solid informational framework for the facility professional's guidance. Key issues and concepts covered include speed to market, performance and conformance, cost of goods, risk management, and supply chain, as well as other issues that bear on facilities planning, design, delivery, and operation.

PROFILE—A LOOK BACK

The modern pharmaceutical industry has its roots in the chemical industry, which grew rapidly in the late 1800s when manufacturing chemists would compound specialty formulas that appeared to have "medicinal" effects. A few leading pharmaceutical companies trace their roots back to Europe (for example, Merck, Bayer, and Schering) where advances in organic chemistry in the late 19th century developed processes that delivered complicated molecules through efficient, large-scale chemical operations. A steady refinement of pharma production followed in the 20th century where product "finishing" often borrowed processes from allied food and candy industries.

Pharma Industry Dynamics

	1980s	1990s	2000s
Vision	Pharmaceutical	Health Care	Patient-Centered
Mission	Safety and Efficacy	Cost Effectiveness	Value/Health Outcomes
Culture	Product Management	Disease/ Brand Management	Health Management
Performance Indicators	Top-Line/Sales Focused	Bottom-Line/ Product Focused	ROI/Team Focused
Systems	Operational	Decision Support	Knowledge Management

The modern pharmaceutical industry took shape in the mid-20th century as a result of global development in advanced research techniques and clean/sterile production technologies. International pharmaceutical organizations were forming to manufacture drug products, mostly as many small-scale facilities located around the globe, in response to marketing opportunities and regionally preferred dosage forms. With the close of World War II and the general world prosperity that followed, a growing availability of medical care spawned increased demand for pharmaceuticals, especially in Western Europe, Japan, and the United States, which is the largest single market. Combined with growing productivity in research and development, powerful new medications were developed and sold around the world. Good Manufacturing Practices (GMP)—regulatory-driven, quality control guidelines—were developed by the pharma-focused regulatory bodies that grew significantly in the 1960s.

With the growth of worldwide "harmonized" regulatory groups, a body of coordinated GMP policy is developing, providing an expanded "tool book" of guidance

Pharma Industry Development

Year	1900	1940	1960	1990	2000 +
Focus	Manufacturing Chemists	Prescription (Rx)	Prescription (Rx)	Rx, Over the Counter Generics	Outsource Supply Chain
Scope	Local	Local	International	Global	Global

for facilities professionals that emphasize quality control, and forming the framework for planning and delivering modern GMP manufacturing facilities. As a result of several tragedies in the 20th century, including thalidomide in the 1960s and a series of lesser yet still devastating injuries to the public, the regulatory bar has been raised for safe, effective medicinal products from today's pharma manufacturing facilities.

Editor's Note

New Prescription for Drug Makers: Update the Plants
The pharma industry has opportunities to improve current manufacturing processes/techniques. The FDA has concluded that the industry needs to adopt manufacturing innovations, partly to raise quality standards. The agency is overhauling its elaborate regulations for the first time in 25 years. After years of neglect, the industry focus is on manufacturing, with the FDA as the catalyst. (*Reported by the Wall Street Journal, Sept. 3, 2003*)

THE CURRENT SITUATION
The global pharmaceutical market is growing in impact to the world's well-being and economic activity. The total retail market is estimated to be approaching $1 trillion, with the U.S. market as the largest single consumer marketplace. Recent industry mergers and consolidations have focused economic power in multi-national, research-driven entities. Market share is concentrated in fewer, larger global enterprises. Previously, the largest pharmaceutical company had only a few percent market share, typically concentrated in a few medical specialty areas. Today, several firms have over 5% share and Pfizer, which recently acquired Warner-Lambert and Pharmacia, has over 11% worldwide market share. However, in comparison to other industries (e.g., auto, computer, energy) the pharma industry is still widely diverse with one-half of the world's market share held by approximately ten firms. There are hundreds of significant, smaller, specialty pharmaceutical firms competing for the remaining half of the market.

Manufacturing requirements for the modern pharmaceutical industry are increasingly complex and subject to imperatives of cost, value, safety, and complexity. Modern pharmaceutical industries must respond to these strategic manufacturing drivers within an evolving compliance framework. Over the last ten years, significant consolidation of manufacturing power and redirection has yielded fewer, yet larger and more complex, pharmaceutical manufacturing facilities around the world. These new "centers of technical excellence" operations are being strategically located to exploit market presence and favorable tax incentives, as well as to deliver economies of scale in manufacturing.

The U.S. pharmaceutical market is the world's largest and fastest growing. Global companies increasingly source the United States and other larger world markets (Europe and Japan) from several strategic, tax-advantaged locations, including Singapore, Puerto Rico, and Ireland. Independent contract manufacturers emerged in the 1990s and present a viable source of manufacturing for "Big Pharma," as well as resolving some elements of risk management and better leveraged capital deployment for enhanced marketing and R&D initiatives. Contract manufacturers initially provided bulk pharma manufacturing of chemicals and ingredients, but now have developed new finishing capabilities, as well as bulk bio and related specialties and novel dosage forms including soft shell capsules. Today's pharma manufacturing supply chain is considerably more complicated, especially to regulators who see many varied sources of supply spreading to new product providers and to new plant locations, such as India and central Europe. GMPs still rule and Good Design Practices (GDPs) are vital, regardless of the origin of the source material. Globalization of guidance (harmonization) takes on new importance in such a diverse environment.

A LOOK AHEAD

The future of the global pharmaceutical industry is certain to be dynamic and highly responsive to marketing and regulatory forces. Expectations for efficient and effective manufacturing facilities will also rise in response to requirements for flexibility, safety, value, and speed to market. Conforming and performing to the many economic and regulatory requirements is clearly *the* manufacturing objective of the future. Whether the firm manufactures their products in a vertical, direct way, or procures and integrates production sources from third parties or from various facilities within their company's internal supply chain, the manufacture of highly technical, potentially potent, innovative new products will demand the very best from facilities professionals.

The future market place appears ripe for additional consolidations where firms will continue to combine in order to gain financial leverage and global marketing presence. These corporate combinations will yield powerful new economic entities seeking greater efficiencies and technical excellence from their "value-added" production facilities. Manufacturing professionals will be challenged to deliver a prudent blend of value, cost effectiveness, safety, and quality from future facilities that support the development, manufacture, and distribution of new products.

In the future, we will likely see a diverse manufacturing environment comprised of small- to mid-sized specialty and novel manufacturers, as well as fully integrated, globally sourced, research-intensive firms that handle a portion of their own manufacturing while outsourcing the rest. GDPs will apply to all manufacturers as they respond to the dual forces of business performance and conformance to globally harmonized guidelines that address an increasingly safety- and quality-conscious community.

The cost of future facilities (capital and operations costs both) will certainly rise in response to the complicated technologies and requirements placed on documentation, safety, and demonstration for "fitness for purpose." Many new products will be "potent" and require special manufacturing handling (containment), necessitating application of closed processing schemes and borrowing "clean manufacturing" techniques from other industries.

Global demographics appear to strongly favor the increased use of prescription medicines to manage and/or eliminate disease. As life expectancies increase, cost-effective prescription products will be a popular political topic, with forces seeking to capitate drug consumer costs and influence the vote of a graying public who are intensely interested in the cost of and access to health care.

With the "graying" of the world, future production volumes will rise. Business margins will be tighter for commodity products and will stress research-intense firms to fund discovery and development of novel blockbusters. The manufacturing scene is likely to see a growing contract supply business for commodity bulk and lower-margin finished products where economies of scale and technology expertise provide competitive advantages to certain specialty manufactures. Use of tax-favored regions for manufacturing high value products will likely accelerate in order to gain maximum leverage from value-added activities to the global markets, tempered perhaps by local political instability.

What does this mean for the facility professional? We are likely to see a dynamic, challenging environment where manufacturing and supply chain activities increase in strategic importance within the firm. Given a scarcity of capital and the need for prudent allocation, future "expensive" facilities will be thoroughly scrutinized as corporate expectations rise for efficient output and for consistency of high quality products. Future manufacturing plants will be expected to run smoothly with minimal disruptions and high confidence levels to eliminate possibilities of product recall.

Evolving GMP are likely to spread throughout the entire "quality scheme," and will include personnel training to raise and maintain competencies of staff, consultants, and suppliers as well as mastery of technology and equipment. From the facilities standpoint, there's a strong case for further integration of the supply chain, including closer cooperation and seamless merging of technology skill sets between vendors, equipment manufacturers, custom fabricators of systems, and the architects/engineers/builders who design and implement the facility. This teamwork will be essential to squeeze additional value out of deployed capital and to advance the safe output of various processing schemes while maintaining an acceptable cost profile and speed of delivery.

The current pharma facility and manufacturing "service supply chain" are fractured with opportunities to be more valuable. Competitive bidding and low contractor profit margins do not support innovation in R&D, and tend to reduce synergies between entities in the "supply" market place. Future manufacturing programs will likely be more reliant on the integration of supplier's skill sets and delivery abilities. Regulators are also seeing the value (and necessity) of working closer with the industry to guide technology advancement, process analytical technology, documentation, computer control, and the application of sound yet prudent science while balancing risks to the public.

STRATEGIC ISSUES: POLITICAL/SOCIAL

The graying of America (and the world) is a significant force in public policy. Development of affordable drugs is a popular topic and is forging powerful strategic dimensions for the pharmaceutical industry. Insurers are very active in managing health care and influencing drug availability and affordability policies. These market pressures will be consistently translated into the need for value and efficiency in manufacturing. There are many "value" issues confronting a manufacturing firm and "cost of goods" will increase in importance as every dollar of sales is stretched to cover expenses for innovation, R&D, and marketing. The "cost" profile for a firm is clearly a strategic issue as costs rise due to compliance and safety, as well as complexity of bulk and finished goods processing schemes.

Growth in Number of People Over 65 (in Millions)

Every day several thousand Americans celebrate their 65th birthdays. Some 1.4 million Americans are in their nineties, and another 64,000 are 100 or older: Year 2030 estimated population—70 million.

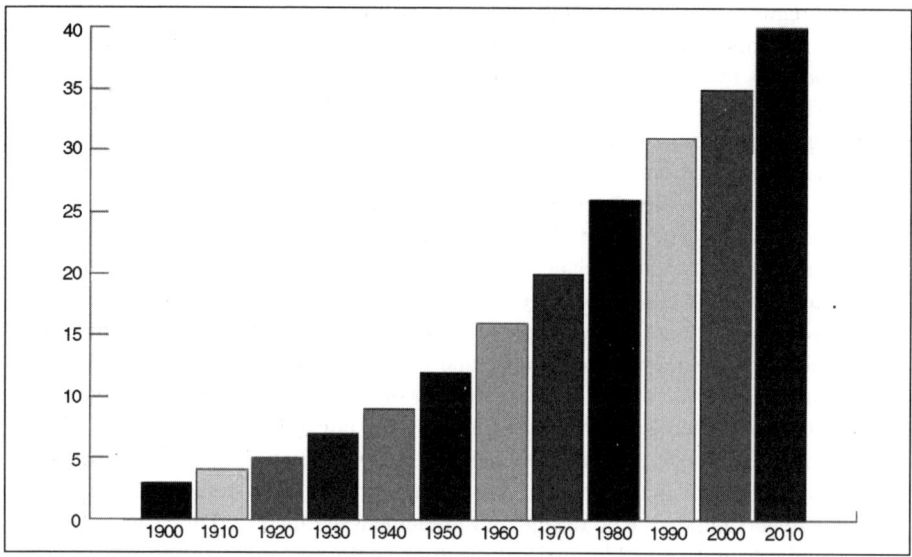

Source: National Academy on an Aging Society.

Pharmaceuticals' Share of Gross Domestic Product in Industrialized Countries

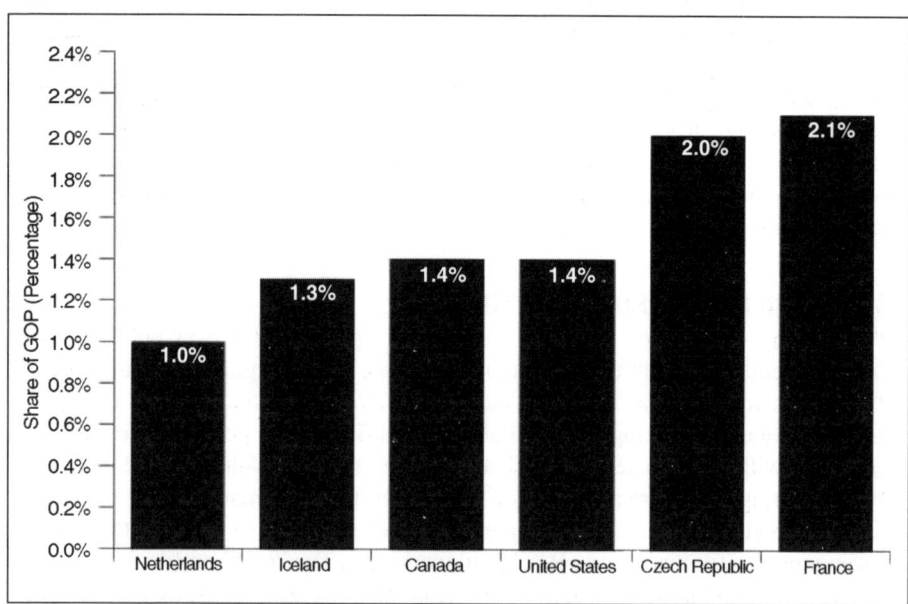

Source: CE CD, *DE CD Health Data*, CD ROM, 2002.

Market Share vs. Dollar Volume

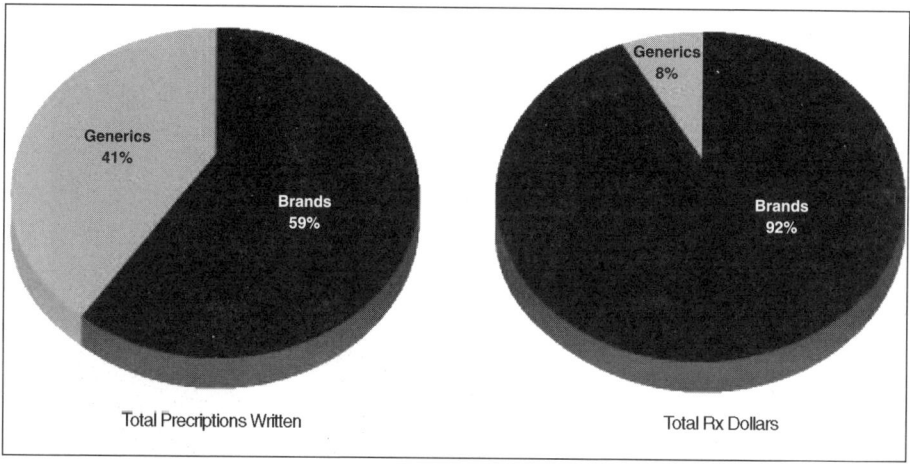

Source: IMS Health and Gruntal Co.

REGULATORY ISSUES

The pharmaceutical industry is strongly regulated with many legal requirements to comply with global GMPs, as well as safety, health, and environmental regulations promulgated by federal, state, and local authorities. Strict regulatory issues have been a reality for many years. Of late, there has been significant globalization of the industry and an associated interest on the part of regulators to harmonize the rules and regulations applying to medicinal products. The primary health care regulators (FDA, MCA, JIT, and WHO) are cooperating more than ever to rationalize rules and improve risks and safety profiles among a fractured supply chain market place where suppliers, contract manufacturers, and integrated firms are producing a growing list of products delivered in varying dosage forms to a wide group of globally based consumers. There is constant dialogue between industry and government regarding the prudent balance of public safety and economic activity generated by the relatively profitable pharmaceutical industry.

Regulatory driven manufacturing requirements are presented as Good Manufacturing Practices (GMPs) and cover various issues, including facilities design,

Product Pipeline

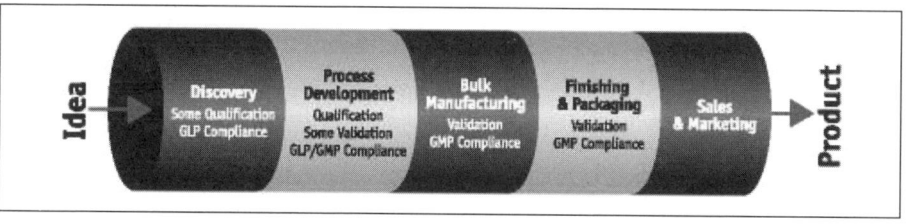

Cost of Developing a New Drug Over Time

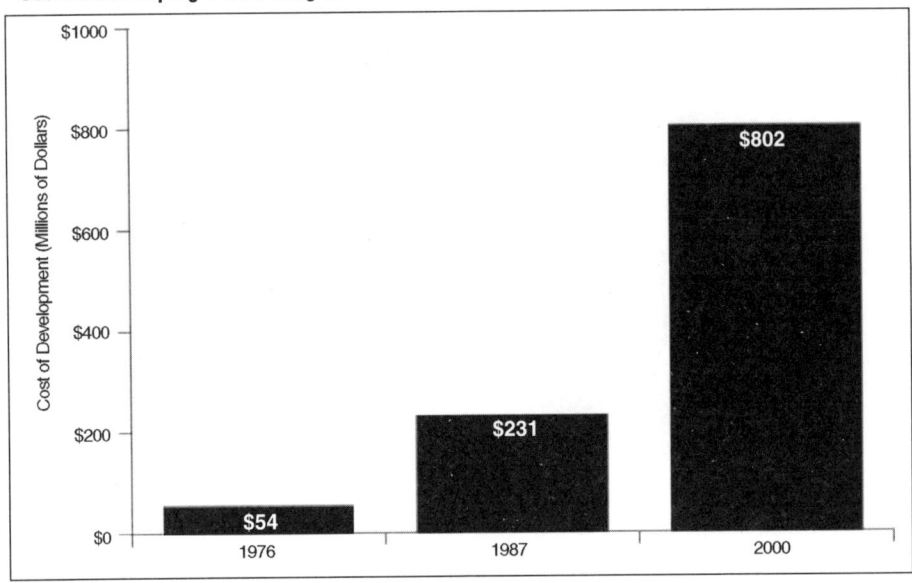

Source: DiMasi, et al., *J. Health Ecco.* 1991 10.107–142 and Tufts Center for the Study of Drug Development, 2001.

Effective Patent Life for Drugs Lags Behind Other Products

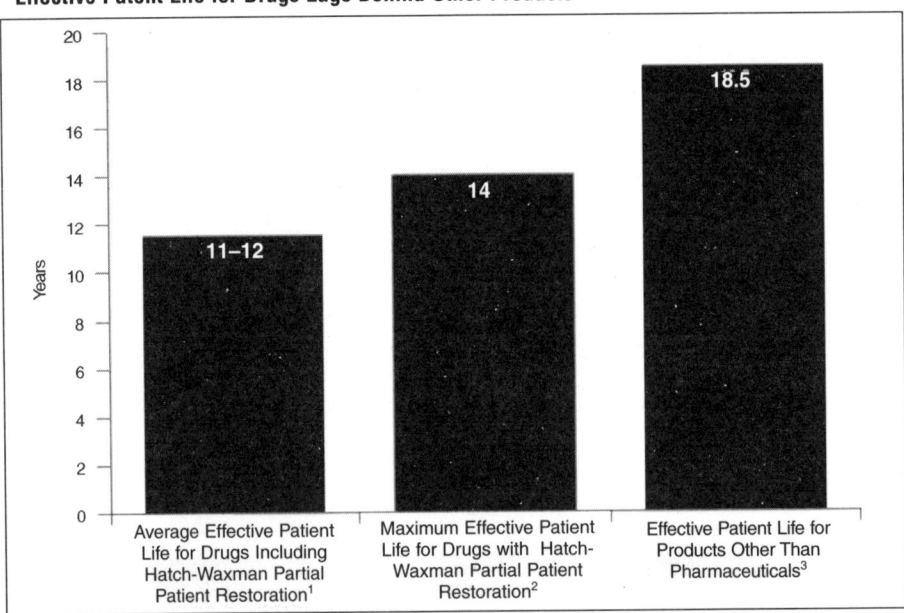

Source: Grabowski, H., and Vernon, J., Longer Patents for Increased Generic Competition in the US; The Waxman-Hatch Act After One Decade. *PharmacoEconomics.* Vol 10. Suppl. 2, pp. 110–123, 1996. Drug Price Competition and Patent Term Restoration Act of 1984, 35 U.S.C. &156(c)(3); American Intellectual Property Law Association, Testimony of Michael K. Kirk on H.R. 400 Before House Subcommittee on Courts and Intellectual Property. February 26, 1997.

product delivery, and validation issues. GMPs are interpretive and demand consistent evaluation as technologies and control mechanisms evolve and are applied. Prudent application of Good Design Practices (GDPs) includes consistent response to GMPs. GDPs also include compliance with applicable safety, health, and environmental regulations as well as statutes, codes, and ordinances applying to the manufacturing plant.

Editor's Note

Loss of patent protection typically results in dramatic market shifts. Generic wholesalers and distributors are able to achieve a 90% switch from branded drugs to generics within the first weeks of a generic launch. (*Reported by Generic Line, Sept., 2003*)

SOURCING AND SUPPLY ISSUES

Over the last few years, there has been a growing use of third-party contract manufacturers and a robust integration of various sources of raw material, finished goods, and distribution. Manufacturing is today outsourced more than ever before. Partners

Pharmaceutical Supply Chain

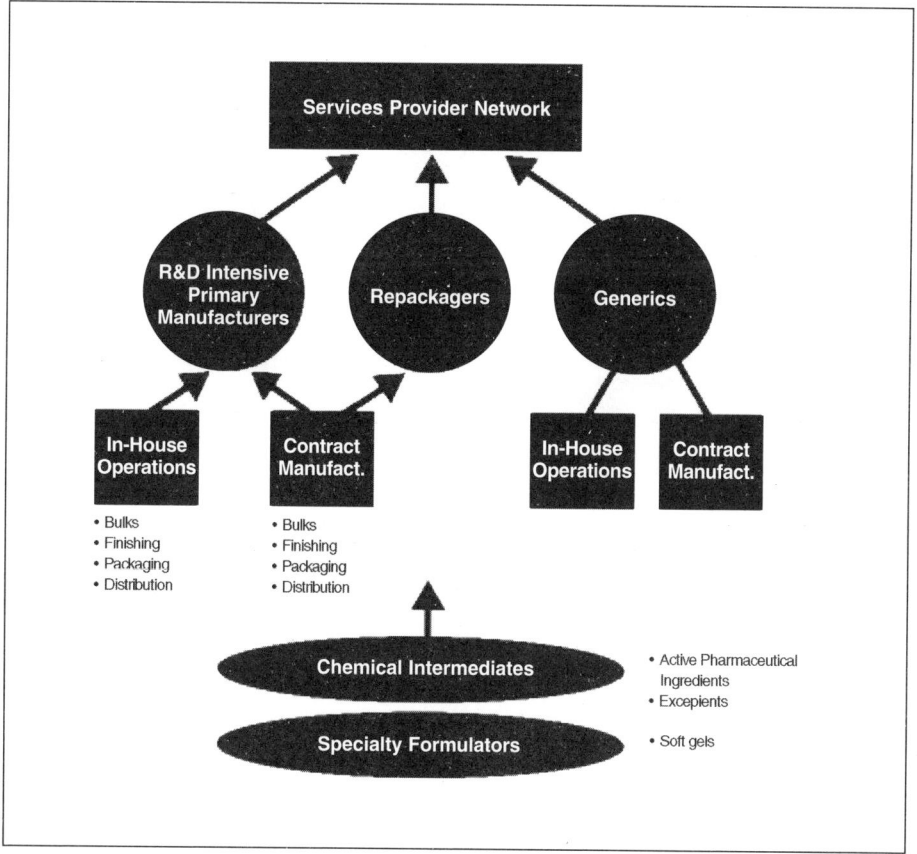

work closely to comply with applicable GMPs as they offer to improve a product's cost, speed of production, and performance. Outsourcing is now a considerable force within the industry as firms transfer technology yet remain responsible for the end product's "fitness for purpose of use." Various strategic imperatives are at work here, including use of capital, balance sheet financing, flexibility, and cost structures.

Future GMP-driven manufacturing facilities, regardless of who operates them, need to comply with applicable GMPs. Whether bulk, finished, or medical device, the governing regulatory factor is the use and the claim of the product by the originator. Future facilities will also incorporate GDPs to be economically viable, as well as "in conformance."

Originators of New Drug Applications (NDAs), remain responsible for the entire product supply chain on through to the consumer. While certain manufacturing functions can be delegated (or outsourced), the originator holds final market accountability. Facility professionals are now working for a diversity of owners and manufacturers. The necessary skill sets, tools, and procedures will vary and will challenge designers to prudently apply judgment and experience to new facilities that must be economically viable and align with business strategies.

Typical Pharma Industry Facility Services Supply Chain

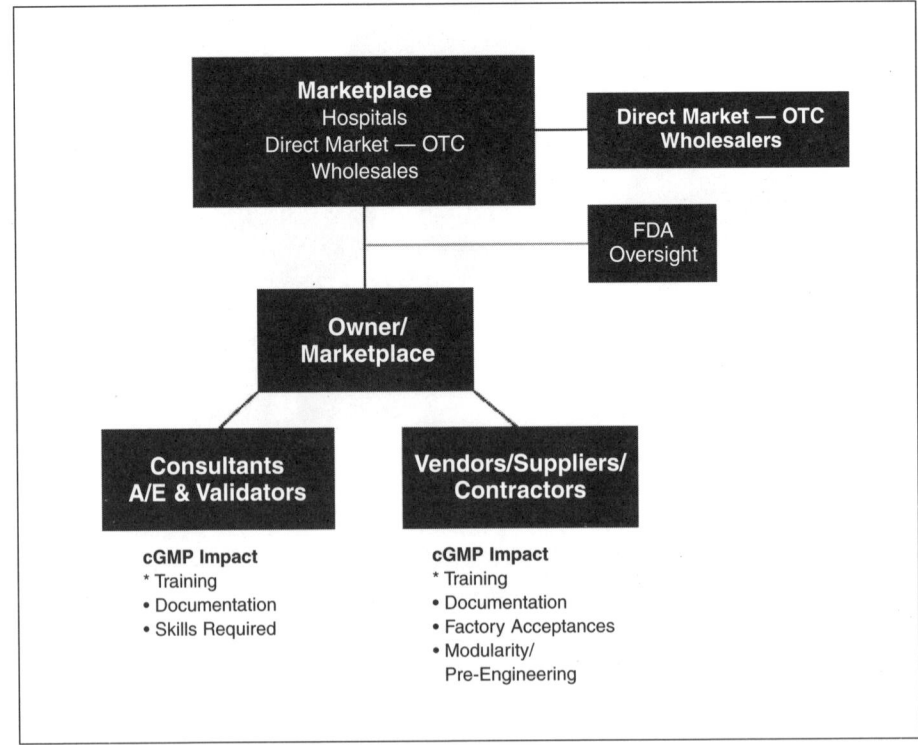

Generics' Share of U.S. Prescription Drug Market (1984–2005)

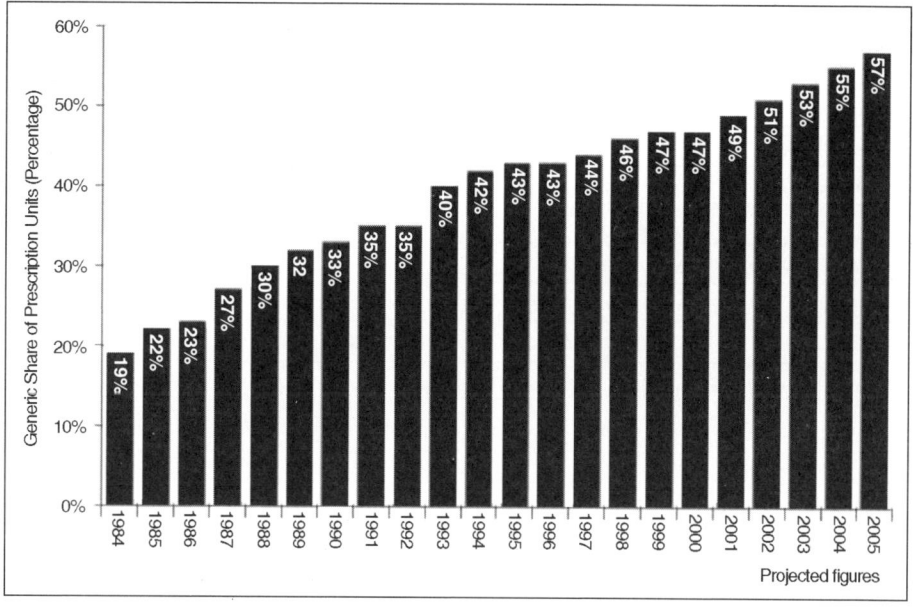

Note: Generics' share of countable units, such as tablets.
Source: Insights 2003, PhRMA.

Editor's Note

President Bush signed the Prescription Drug and Medicare Modernization Act of 2003 on December 8, 2003. The law, which is expected to cost over $500 billion over 10 years, provides for a federally sponsored prescription drug benefit for the more than 40 million senior citizens enrolled in Medicare. The law includes no price controls and should boost overall industry revenues, adn profits to a lesser extent. (*Reported in Value Line, Jan. 23, 2004*)

MARKETING ISSUES

The global pharmaceutical industry is driven by successful marketing and distribution. Many products are now being promoted directly to the consumer. Insurers are also powerful market forces by placing limitations on price reimbursements and access. Successful market competition relies heavily on novel therapeutic indications and attractive economics. Rising consumer participation in sales decisions is raising the bar for innovative therapies delivered in attractively packaged presentations. Such packaging preferences have an influence on future manufacturing and supply chain activities.

Speed to market is a widely heralded competitive advantage. Seizing early market share is considered an essential economic objective. GDPs can assist the facility professional to design and deliver and start-up new/upgraded facilities in less time.

Global Pharmaceutical Sales by Region

World Audited Market	2003 Sales (US$B)	% Global Sales (US$)	% Growth Year-over-Year (Constant $)
North America	$229.5	49%	+11%
Europe (EU)	115.4	25	+8
Rest of Europe	14.3	3	+14
Japan	52.4	11	+3
Asia (excluding Japan), Africa and Australia	37.3	8	+12
Latin America	17.4	4	+6
TOTAL	$466.3	100%	+9%

Source: IMS *World Review,* 2004.

Expanding Markets

From 1989 to 2001, the worldwide pharmaceutical market increased from $117.8 to $351.8 billion, representing a compound annual growth of nearly 10%. The US market grew at a compounded rate of 14.6% over the same period, increasing from roughly $33 billion to $172 billion.

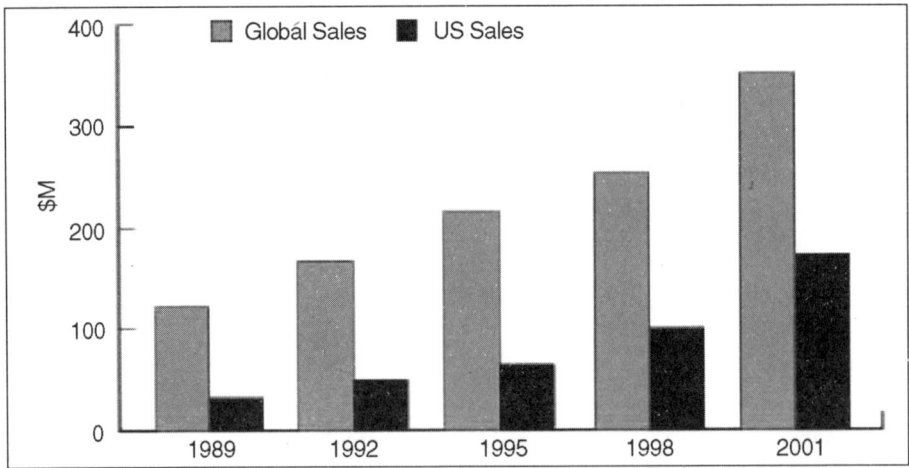

Source: IMS Worldwide Rental and Provider Perspective.

LEGAL ISSUES

The modern pharmaceutical industry operates within a highly active legal environment. Product liability actions are enormously influential on company policy and operations. Costs to position and defend class actions and private law suites are formidable. Legal action originating from regulators is also trending upward.

Evolving trends in public awareness and readiness to bring legal action place extraordinary pressures on the modern pharma organization to carefully

Blockbuster Drugs

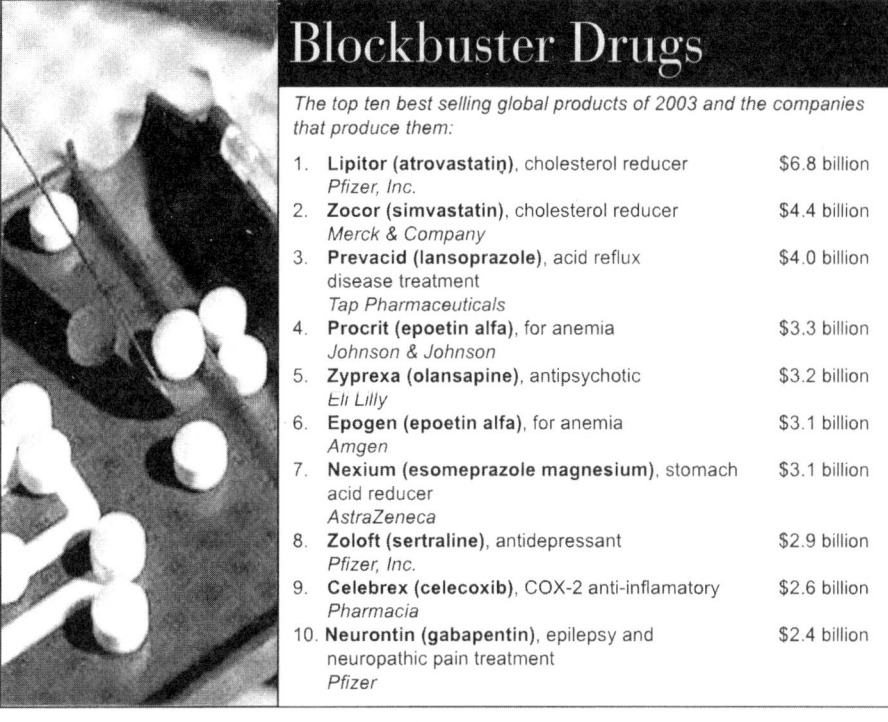

Blockbuster Drugs

The top ten best selling global products of 2003 and the companies that produce them:

1. **Lipitor (atrovastatin)**, cholesterol reducer $6.8 billion
   Pfizer, Inc.
2. **Zocor (simvastatin)**, cholesterol reducer $4.4 billion
   Merck & Company
3. **Prevacid (lansoprazole)**, acid reflux $4.0 billion
   disease treatment
   Tap Pharmaceuticals
4. **Procrit (epoetin alfa)**, for anemia $3.3 billion
   Johnson & Johnson
5. **Zyprexa (olansapine)**, antipsychotic $3.2 billion
   Eli Lilly
6. **Epogen (epoetin alfa)**, for anemia $3.1 billion
   Amgen
7. **Nexium (esomeprazole magnesium)**, stomach $3.1 billion
   acid reducer
   AstraZeneca
8. **Zoloft (sertraline)**, antidepressant $2.9 billion
   Pfizer, Inc.
9. **Celebrex (celecoxib)**, COX-2 anti-inflamatory $2.6 billion
   Pharmacia
10. **Neurontin (gabapentin)**, epilepsy and $2.4 billion
    neuropathic pain treatment
    Pfizer

Source: Med Ad News, May 2004.

Top Ten Pharmaceutical Companies by U.S. Prescription Sales

	Company	2003 Sales (US$ Billions)	Percent Growth Year-Over-Year
1	Pfizer	29.2	9.7
2	GlaxoSmithKline	18.6	4.6
3	Johnson & Johnson	15.2	14.0
4	Merck and Co.	14.1	9.1
5	AstraZeneca	10.4	-5.8
6	Bristol-Myers Squibb	9.6	6.6
7	Novartis	9.5	23.8
8	Amgen	7.7	34.7
9	Wyeth	7.6	4.9
10	Lilly	7.5	11.7
	Total	**129.4**	**9.6**

Wholesale prices, sales include prescription products only.
Source: National Sales Perspectives, 2004.

Key Country Drug Purchases—Retail Pharmacies: 12 Months to November 2004

	12 Months November 2004 US$ Millions	12 Months November 2003 US$ Millions	% Growth US$	% Growth At Constant Exchange*
Selected World	345,064	309,728	11	7
North America	183,773	168,974	8	8
United States	173,824	160,167	8	8
Canada	9,949	8,357	19	10
Europe (Leading 5)	86,115	73,475	17	6
Germany	25,092	21,723	16	4
France	21,035	17,978	17	6
Italy	14,409	12,495	15	4
United Kingdom	15,429	12,728	21	8
Spain	10,179	8,550	19	7
Japan (*Including Hospital)	56,758	51,470	10	2
Latin America (Leading 3)	13,179	11,644	13	2
Mexico	6,441	6,097	6	11
Brazil	4,954	4,060	23	23
Argentina	1,784	1,507	18	18
Australia/New Zealand	5,229	4,164	26	10

*Constant exchange takes out the effect of fluctuating exchange rates.
Source: 2004 IMS Health, Inc.

Key Types of Drug Purchases—Retail Pharmacies: 12 Months to December 2003

Therapeutic Category				
1 Cardiovascular	67,894	60,108	13	7
2 Central Nervous System	64,283	56,197	14	11
3 Allmentary/Metabolism	49,260	45,738	8	3
4 Respiratory	29,885	27,490	9	4
5 Anti-Infectives	27,784	26,335	5	1
6 Musculo-Skeletal	22,472	19,291	16	12
7 Genlto Urinary	18,469	17,205	7	4
8 Cytostatics	16,959	14,388	18	12
9 Dematologicals	10,101	9,441	7	9
10 Blood Agents	12,515	10,480	19	13
11 Sensor Organs	6,977	6,269	11	6
12 Diagnostic Agents	6,327	5,611	13	7
13 Hormones	5,540	4,896	13	8
14 Miscellaneous	4,089	3,956	3	(1)
15 Hospital Solutions	1,999	1,887	6	(2)
16 Parasitology	500	434	15	11

*Constant exchange takes out the effect of fluctuating exchange rates.
Source: 2005 IMS Health, Inc.

Product Innovation Exclusivity Profile

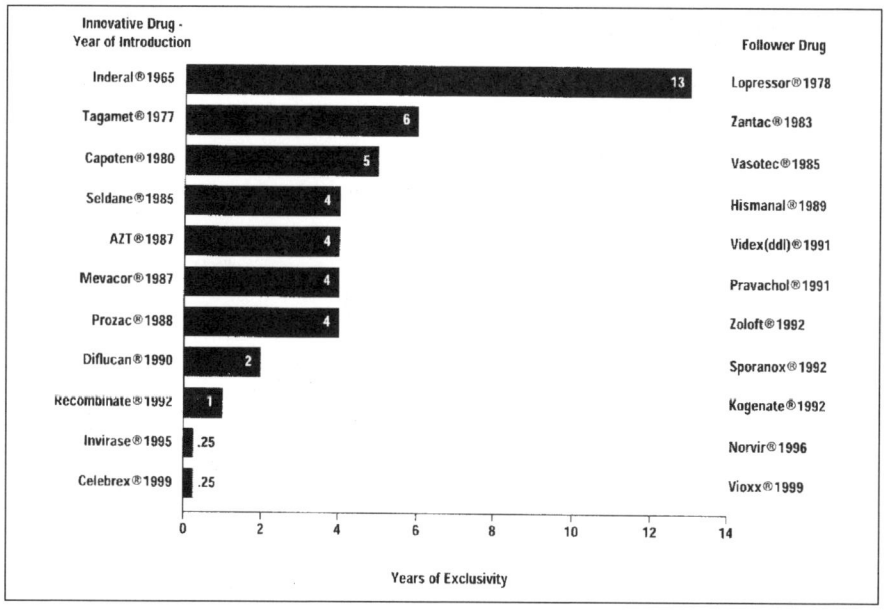

Sources: *PhRMA, 2000;* The Wilkerson Group, 1995.

craft marketing strategies to deliver compliant products that meet expectations for efficacy and safety. Highly publicized regulatory-based legal actions are very costly in terms of remediation and reputation. Consent decree actions cause deep disruption in an organization in terms of fines, lost production, and cost compliance.

Product recalls arising from GMP failures, coupled with the associated legal defense, offer considerable incentives for organizations to produce products in consistent, compliant fashion. A prudent balance of risk management and cost positioning is essential. Extreme fines and costs of product rework can easily overshadow any apparent cost savings sought from hurried, lower spending on capital facility and system upgrade projects.

Editor's Note

According to an industry consultant David Moskowitz, "Investors will pay for good compliance and punish noncompliance." As an example, "the consent decree Abbott was forced to sign is likely to be a benchmark for judging the effects of compliance on company stock values. . . . Abbott was fined $100 million in 1999 for GMP problems . . . that was followed by over $400 million in fines, (an) additional $600 million in fines related to practices for Lupron and Ross Nutraceuticals. The company lost $21 billion in market capitalization alone in 1999 because of GMP problems. Drug makers put their business seriously at risk if they cut corners in GMP compliance." (Reported in Drug GMP Report, December, 2003)

Compound Success Rates by Stages

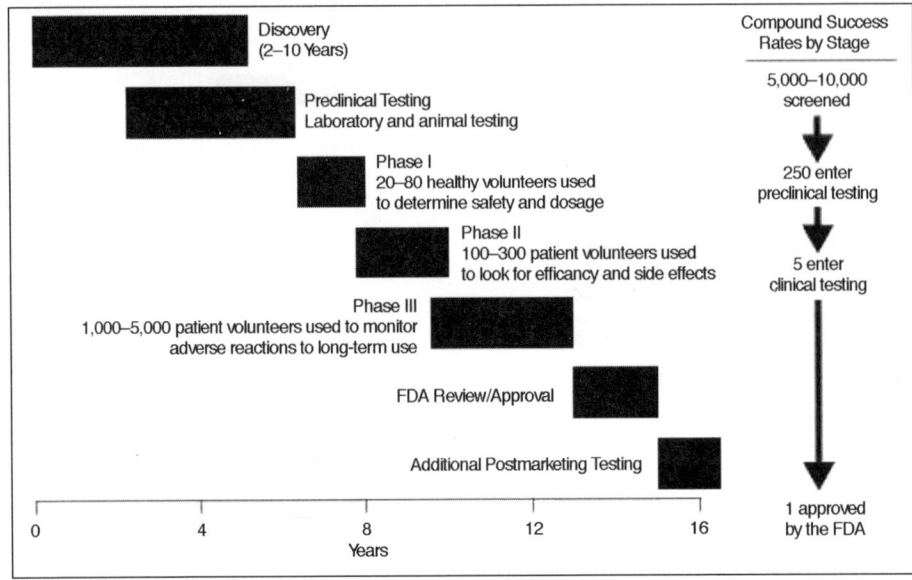

Source: PhRMA, based on data from Center for the Study of Drug Development, Tufts University, 1995.

FINANCIAL ISSUES

Pharmaceutical companies generally enjoy a solid reputation for financial stability with long-term investor yields well above average for research-intensive companies. Maintaining a "growth" reputation industry places pressures on pharma organizations to outperform their peers. Such competitiveness typically drives the entire firm to excel. High investor expectations are the rule and premiums are placed on achievement.

Editor's Note

In 2003, the pharma industry lagged most industries in reported profits. Increases were reported for many industrial sectors. Business Week (Feb.23,2004) reported that corporate scoreboards for all industries rose 76% for 2003 profits over 2002, with 47 of 60 industry groups showing increasing profits. The pharma industry reported that profits decreased 17% in 2003.

The global financial environment rewards companies for well spent capital and prudent investing in R&D and marketing. Manufacturing capital outlays typically compete for capital deployment. The capital intensity of the pharma industry, however, is relatively low. Typically, pharma firms invest 5–10% of manufacturing sales for capital outlays, in comparison to 15–40% investments by infotech, semiconductors, and other capital-intensive industries like mining and chemicals.

Achieving efficiencies in capital deployment and delivering acceptable "cost of goods" is an important economic activity for the industry as competition increases and gross margins are directed toward R&D and marketing. Applying GDPs can help an organization obtain more leverage for their outlays through better risk management and efficient product delivery derived from excellent facilities that perform (deliver in an aligned way) and conform to evolving regulatory initiatives.

TECHNOLOGY/R&D ISSUES
The pharma industry depends on innovation and technology for the development and delivery of capital products and services. For over 100 years, the industry has distinguished itself for the successful commercial application of science and medicine. The industry spends heavily on research and development to identify and produce new entities. Historically, the industry outspends virtually all others in the percentage of sales dollars invested in R&D.

However, the industry has not enjoyed the same reputation for innovation in manufacturing. Production processes have historically been adaptations of technologies used in other industries, including bulk chemical, food, and confectionary, and other process industries. Of late, various developments in production demands

U.S. Pharmaceutical Investment in Research and Development
Every five years since 1980, U.S. pharmaceutical companies have practically doubled spending on R&D. In 2003, companies invested $33.2 billion to discover and develop new medicines. Research-based companies pour back $1 out of every $5 in domestic sales into R&D, a higher percentage than any other industry.

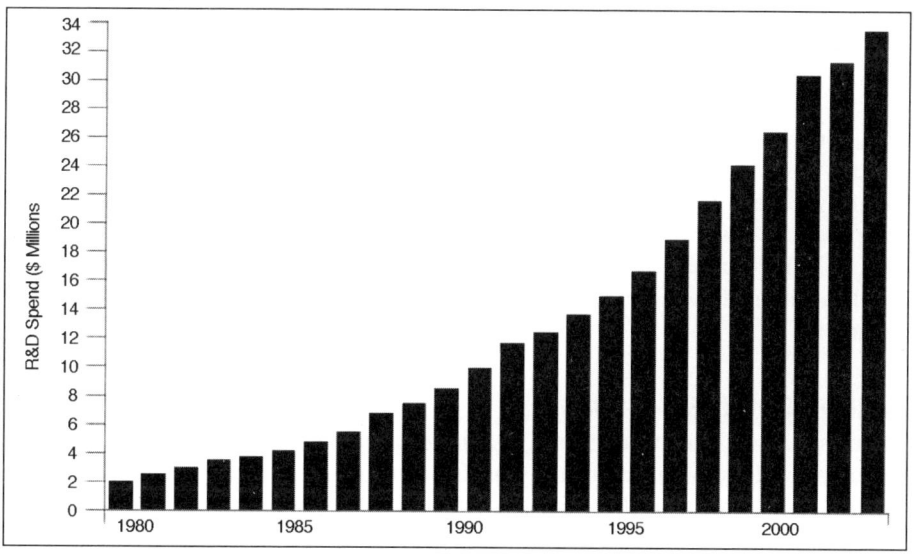

Note: Year 2002 sales = $31.9 billion; year 2003 sales = $33.2 billion.
Source: PhRMA Industry Survey.

have led to a heightened importance of innovative procedures for biopharma, contained-production, and oral dosage formulas. These deliveries have in turn led to heightened interest in new solutions and approaches to capture competitive advantages from cleaner, better, faster, safer, less costly, manufacturing processes and facilities.

New Product Approvals Over Time

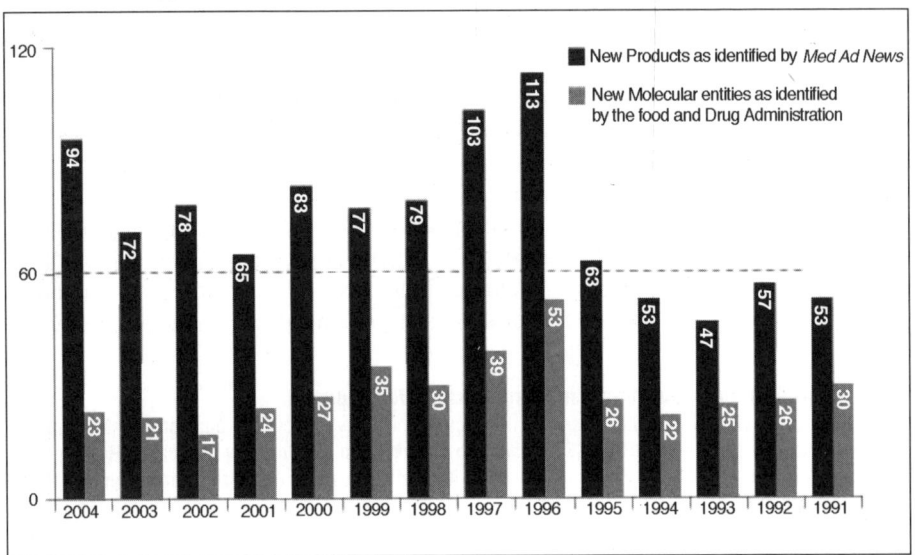

Successful R&D programs include timely commercialization for market entry. Compliant facilities are needed to support these objectives. Increased regulatory scheduling can lengthen the program. Identifying the best time and required assets to introduce new products are a key strategic activities. Technically challenging production processes demand increased efforts from well-positioned facilities and/or new alliances/partnerships to bring products to market.

PROJECT DELIVERY ISSUES

Pharmaceutical manufacturing facilities are complicated and occupy an increasing share of an enterprise's strategic horizon. The total cycle of events to deliver a pharmaceutical facility typically includes traditional elements of planning, design, construction, qualification, validation, and operation. The growing complexities of the modern "supply chain" have made facilities planning more important and challenging to the firm. Integrating output from various product

Top Ten Pharmaceutical Companies by R&D Expenditure*

Company	Estimated R&D expenditure 2003	% Higher than 2002	Estimated R&D as % of sales, 2004
Pfizer	$7.50 billion	6%	15%
Sanofi-Aventis	$5.19 billion	8%	16%
GlaxoSmithKline	$4.83 billion	5%	16%
Novartis	$3.96 billion	5%	14%
AstraZeneca	$3.78 billion	7%	18%
Roche	$3.77 billion	6%	16.5%
Eli Lilly % Co.	$2.64 billion	12%	19%
Bristol-Myers Squibb	$2.43 billion	6%	11%
Wyeth	$2.42 billion	15%	14%
Amgen	$1.88 billion	15%	20%

*Not all R&D expenditures are devoted to pharmaceuticals.
Source: *Contract Pharma*, July/August 2003.

R&D as Sales Percent

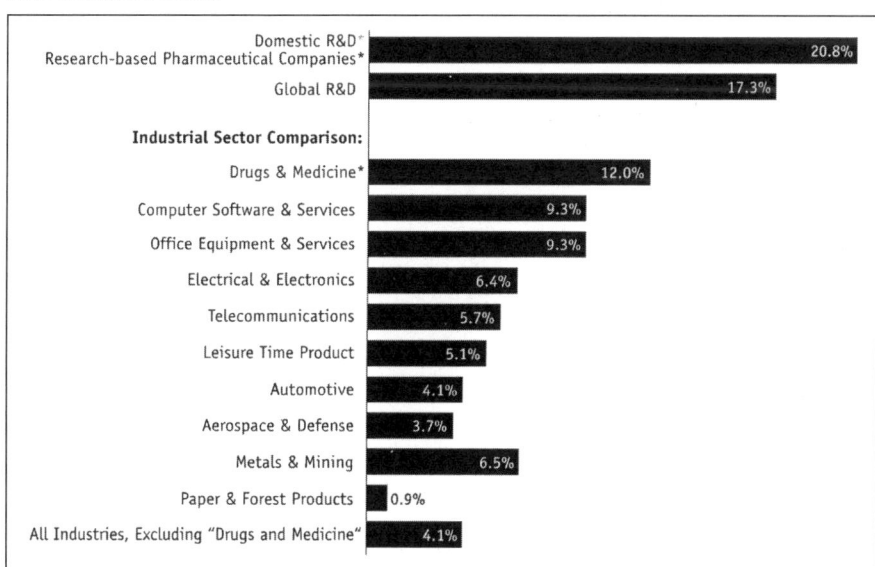

*"Research-based Pharmaceutical Companies" based on ethical pharmaceuticals sales and ethical pharmaceutical R&D only as tabulated by PhRMA "Drugs and Medicine" category based on total R&D and sales from companies classified within the "Drugs and Medicine" sector as tabulated by Standard & Poor's Compustat, a divsion of McGraw-Hill.
Source: *PhRMA, 2000* based on data from PhRMA Annual Survey and Standard & Poor's Compustat, a division of McGraw-Hill.

Technology—Process Equipment and Facility Trends

- Multi-purpose/Multi-step process equipment
- Contained vessel charging/sampling
- Barrier techniques
- Transport bins/closed systems
- HVAC/once-thru flows
- Dedicated processing areas and equipment systems
- Larger storage spaces – WIP – Goods

suppliers, originating either from internal or external forces, through contract sourcing has grown in urgency.

The choice of a project delivery method influences the skill sets required for project success. Capital facilities delivery methods rely on divergent team members bringing various skills and values to the endeavor. Equipment technology expertise now resides largely within sophisticated vendors. Architecture/engineering firms maintain process and critical utilities skills for manufacturing plants, incorporating specialty processing systems, and GMP operation. Pharma project delivery requires effective collaboration of specialty construction contractors and managers with expertise in the regulated environment. Design/build teams can integrate specialty projects in imaginative ways, sometimes concurrent with ongoing GMP operations to expand, alter, or add grass roots production capacity.

Typical Project Cycle

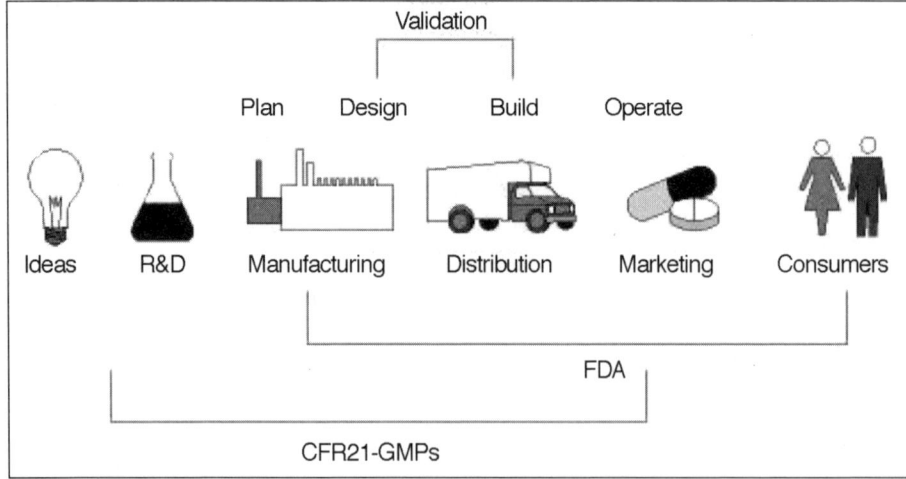

Delivering modern pharmaceutical manufacturing facilities typically takes between six months and three years, and can cost hundreds of millions of dollars when considering the buildings, facilities, complicated equipment, and sub-systems

Typical Pharmaceutical Manufacturing Facility Cost Profile

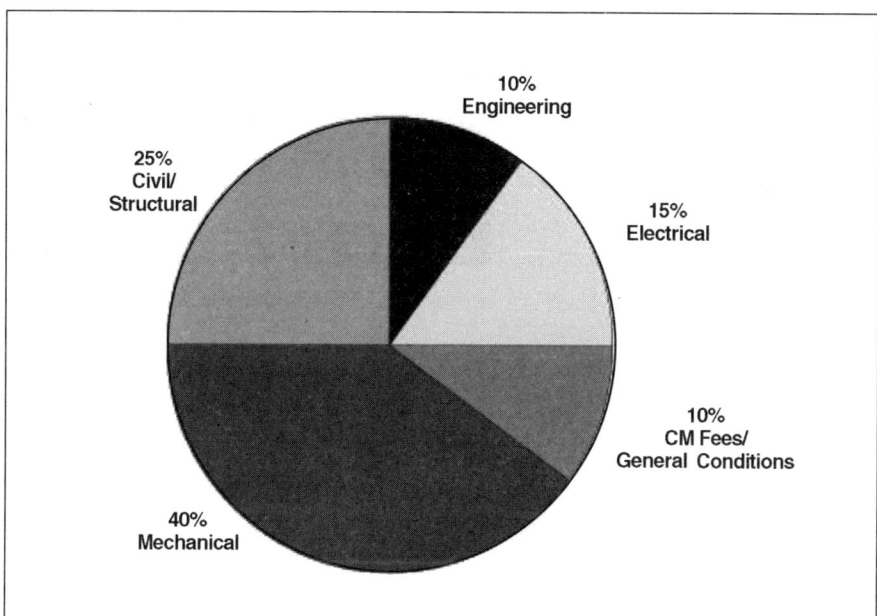

necessary to achieve the intended production output and quality. Outside technical consultants are increasingly deployed in response to demands for expertise in validation, high purity materials, process applications, and automation.

Incorporating innovative project delivery schemes may also include use of "turnkey" sub-unit assemblies, modular systems, and pre-engineering approaches to unit operations with the intended benefits of lower costs or shorter installation cycles. Facilities professionals are challenged with the integration of many delivery options. Timing and budgeting processes for new facilities are complicated by issues flowing from partners and alliances, as well as market entry dates dependent on R&D and regulatory approvals. Anticipating launch dates and production requirements for sample production and market entry have an impact on capital deployment. Funding approvals are typically phased, with each organization requiring multiple management decisions coordinated with marketing and regulatory affairs.

GDPs offer solid techniques for the pharmaceutical industry to achieve the powerful objective of maximizing efficiency of deployed capital, while maintaining an acceptable conformance profile and aligning output capabilities to the business' evolving objectives. The facilities professional plays a key role in assessing the capabilities of existing assets, and defining opportunities to rationalize the manufacturing base of the organization in light of forecasted demand, evolving technology, and regulatory developments.

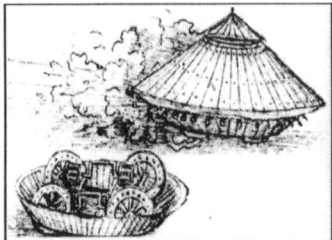

Any fool can make things bigger and more complex... It takes a touch of genuis — and a lot of courage to move in the opposite direction.

Albert Einstein

2
Current Good Manufacturing Practices

Author: Robert Del Ciello

Advisor: Peter T. Bigelow

INTRODUCTION

The need to meet the current Good Manufacturing Practices (cGMP) regulations is paramount in the pharmaceutical industry. Facilities that effectively incorporate the GMP requirements are easily licensed and thus bring the project on stream in a timely fashion. The incorporation of the GMP requirements into Good Design Practices (GDP) at the onset of the project ensures that this aspect of regulatory requirements is met. Facility designs that do not adequately or that poorly address cGMP requirements, face more regulatory scrutiny and possibly will not be licensed without significant changes.

The question of good cGMP design, and thus the use of GDP, is implicit and explicit to every facility and equipment design project. Does the design meet GMP regulations? Will the design, once realized, be acceptable to the Food and Drug Administration (FDA) inspectors? One would expect that such questions would be easy to answer, but needs only to review the regulations, especially 21 CFR Part 211 Subparts C and D,, to ascertain the agency's requirements and expectations. Unfortunately, these sections, while delineating requirements, do not provide solutions to the various design challenges present in a facility or equipment that fall under these regulations. The facilities and equipment necessary for each dosage form have special challenges. While the intent of the GMP regulations is the same, the method of achieving these requirements can be quite different. The FDA's approach toward the written regulations has been to indicate the requirements that a manufacturer must meet, not the method(s) to achieve these results. Basically, the FDA tells a manufacturer what must be done, but not how to do it. This fact has led to a variety of interpretive solutions to achieve the desired results relative to facility design. Utilizing this approach enables technologies to develop that can more effectively achieve the desired goals and objectives set forth by the agency. If the FDA instructed manufacturers on how to perform an operation, developing technologies would be impaired. Thus, the importance of the small "c" in cGMP: The "current" in current Good Manufacturing Practices allows solutions to technical issues to vary and also allows the expectations and regulatory requirements to change with technology without the need to revise the actual regulations. Therefore, a review of the development of the printed regulations as well as the Agency's evolving expectations is of interest.

Looking back in recent history, the impact that the regulations have had on design solutions has steadily grown. The GMP regulations have always impacted the physical facility in which drug products have been manufactured, and this impact has increased over the past 25 years. Prior to the mid 1970s, minimal attention was provided to process, personnel, and waste flow patterns. While efficient facility arrangements were sought, there was very little link to GMP design. In the mid-1970s, the FDA issued proposed changes to the regulations. These changes more definitively delineated requirements for facilities design and equipment. In addition to the changes in 21 CFR 210 and 211, the Agency also proposed Section 212 for the manufacture of large volume parenteral products. These proposed regulations, for the first time, indicated specifics for various facility and support systems. For example, these proposed regulations were the first to provide specific engineering solutions to design challenges; e.g., 316L stainless steel for the construction of water for injection systems. Although the 21 CFR 212 proposed regulations were never adopted by the agency; however, the revisions to 21 CFR 210 and 211 were.

The use of the proposed Section 212 regulations by inspectors during the late 1970s is indicative of the "c" in cGMP regulations. While this new section was out for comments by the industry, inspectors reviewing large (and small) volume parenteral manufacturing facilities utilized the specific sections on "c"requirements for facilities and equipment. So while this section was never incorporated into the regulations, the specific requirements were used as a yard stick by inspectors, thus changing what was acceptable practice in the industry. This situation developed because the specific comments by inspectors can be traced back to an applicable Section in 21 CFR Part 211.

A review of the Preamble or Director's Comments to the mid-1970s changes provides insight into the thinking of the agency. The proposed changes, which were adopted with some modification, placed stricter requirements on facility and equipment design. To fully understand the revised regulations, it is necessary to review the Commissioner's answers to the questions that were raised by industry.

The following is an excerpt from the Commissioner's remarks to the questions received:

130. A number of comments indicated that the requirement in 211.42(c) that "operations shall be performed in specifically defined areas of adequate size" was unnecessarily restrictive on the flexibility of plant space use.

The requirement relates to several different types of operations that are enumerated in the proposal; however, the comments seemed to relate mainly to storage areas. It is the Commissioner's belief that a significant type of control over products is a physical one, which precludes mixups by physically placing an article in an area clearly identified as to status. The extent of the physical separation imposed in a particular situation can vary from locked, walled-off areas to simple designation of an area for a single purpose by means of a sign. The degree of physical control will vary depending on the other controls in use by a firm. If a firm has effective controls, whatever they may be, that would increase their confidence that mixups will not occur, then the degree of physical control may be less than in another firm where no other controls exist.

These remarks provide the depth needed to fully understand the intent of the regulations. It is highly recommended that the preamble to the regulations be reviewed to achieve a better understanding of the regulations. Over the ensuing years, as technology has improved and provided more efficient solutions to design challenges, the methods of achieving compliance with the regulations have changed while the intent of the regulation has remained the same.

A significant issue in complying with the regulations—whether U.S. FDA, EU (European Union), or any other nation's regulations—is the decision that the designer needs to make concerning the balance between physical facility solutions and procedural solutions to operational challenges.

As indicated previously, regulatory requirements can be met utilizing differing solutions. These solutions can consist of the arrangement of the physical facility or the establishment of operational procedures. The choice of either type of solution is usually dependent upon the nature of the operations. For example, a cGMP development operation usually requires flexibility to adequately perform its intended function. Such facilities usually have layouts that allow for different flow patterns for personnel, materials and equipment since the unit operations required by each product under development varies. In order to meet the requirements of the regulations for no cross contamination of products and to prevent the mixing of various components or product intermediates, the procedures used during the operations delineate the guards against such results rather than the solution being in the physical facility. A large-scale manufacturing facility usually does not require the same level of flexibility as a small one. The facility is usually dedicated to products requiring the same unit operations and thus the physical facility arrangement can control flow patterns.

The following diagrams illustrate this concept.

Assume we are designing a tablet operation and the main unit operations are:

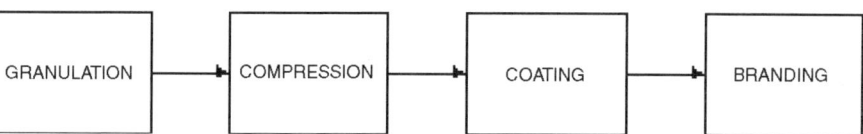

If this were a manufacturing operation where the unit operations did not vary, the layout could look very similar to the following flow diagram:

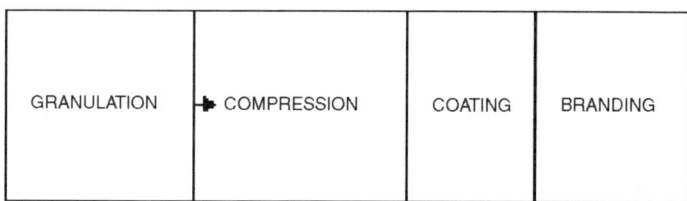

Flow from one unit operations to the other is very restricted and the physical facility assists in eliminating mix ups and cross contamination.

The production facility could handle another product that was not coated with the following flow scheme:

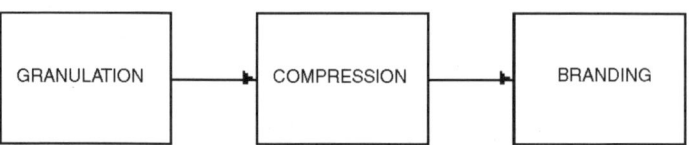

Another production line could be provided as follows:

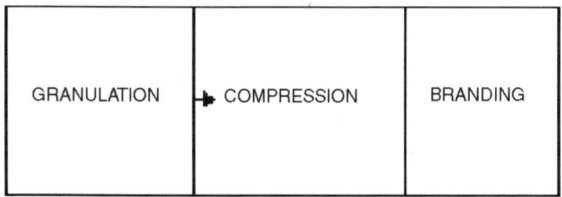

Again the physical facility controls flow patterns.

However, if the facility were a small manufacturing operation or a development/clinical manufacturing operation, both of these products could be handled by a layout that provides greater flexibility such as:

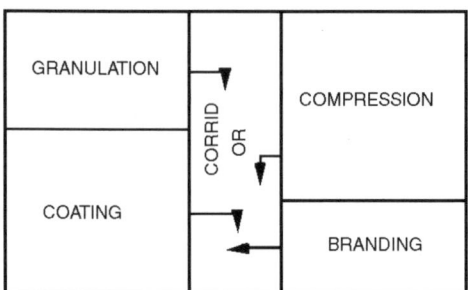

Under this arrangement, the physical facility provides operational flexibility. Operating procedures would be in place to ensure that products and intermediates are not mixed and cross contamination has been prevented.

The balance between the use of physical barriers or procedural barriers needs to be discussed with the operating unit and the quality unit prior to finalization of the conceptual design.

The ability of the designer to meet the regulatory requirements delineated in the cGMP regulations is totally dependent on the designer utilizing the GDP discussed in this text. As mentioned in the opening paragraph, a well-designed facility that addresses the regulatory requirements will provide the operating unit with an entity that is easily licensed, easily maintained, and efficiently operated.

Later in this text specific design practices are discussed that provide the tools for the designer to meet the GMP regulations. In addition the ISPE Baseline Guides provide tools and methodologies for the designer to meet the GMP regulations.

REGULATORY ISSUES

U.S. Food and Drug Administration (FDA)

When designing a manufacturing facility that produces pharmaceutical products, whether generated from a chemical or biological synthesis route, the FDA's cGMPs regulations provide minimal guidance. The cGMPs outline facility requirements and the requirements for the documentation of manufacturing procedures. The FDA's approach toward the written regulations has been to indicate the results that a manufacturing process must attain, not the method(s) to achieve these results. Basically, the FDA tells a manufacturer *what* must be done, but not *how* to do it. This fact has led to a variety of interpretive solutions to achieve the desired results relative to facility design. Utilizing this approach enables technologies to develop processes that can more effectively achieve the desired goals and objectives set forth by the Agency.

The FDA issues regulations in the Code of Federal Register (CFR) 21. The applicable regulations that include facility and equipment requirements can be found in the following:

Number	Title
21 CFR 210	Current Good Manufacturing Practices in Manufacturing, Processing, Packaging, or Holding of Drugs, General
21 CFR 211	Current Good Manufacturing Practices for Finished Pharmaceuticals
21 CFR 600	Biologics Products, General
21 CFR 820	Quality Systems Regulations

The applicable sections of the regulations for finished pharmaceuticals are found in 21 CFR 211, Subpart C—Buildings and Facilities and 21 CFR, 211 Subpart D—Equipment. A review of several of the pertinent paragraphs will illustrate this point.

Paragraph 211.42 delineates the features for the design and construction of facilities:

§ 211.42 *Design and construction features.*

(a) Any building or buildings used in the manufacture, processing, packing, or holding of a drug product shall be of suitable size, construction, and location to facilitate cleaning, maintenance, and proper operations.

(b) Any such building shall have adequate space for the orderly placement of equipment and materials to prevent mixups between different components, drug product containers, closures, labeling, in-process materials, or drug products, and to prevent contamination. The flow of components, drug product containers, closures, labeling, in-process materials, and drug products through the building or buildings shall be designed to prevent contamination.

(c) Operations shall be performed within specifically defined areas of adequate size. There shall be separate or defined areas for the firm's operations to prevent contamination or mixups as follows:

(1) Receipt, identification, storage, and withholding from use of components, drug product containers, closures, and labeling, pending the appropriate sampling, testing, or examination by the quality control unit before release for manufacturing or packaging;

(2) Holding rejected components, drug product containers, closures, and labeling before disposition;

(3) Storage of released components, drug product containers, closures, and labeling;

(4) Storage of in-process materials;

(5) Manufacturing and processing operations;

(6) Packaging and labeling operations;

(7) Quarantine storage before release of drug products;

(8) Storage of drug products after release;

(9) Control and laboratory operations;

(10) Aseptic processing, which includes as appropriate:

(i) Floors, walls, and ceilings of smooth, hard surfaces that are easily cleanable;

(ii) Temperature and humidity controls;

(iii) An air supply filtered through high-efficiency particulate air filters under positive pressure, regardless of whether flow is laminar or nonlaminar;

(iv) A system for monitoring environmental conditions;

(v) A system for cleaning and disinfecting the room and equipment to produce aseptic conditions;

(vi) A system for maintaining any equipment used to control the aseptic conditions.

(d) Operations relating to the manufacture, processing, and packing of penicillin shall be performed in facilities separate from those used for other drug products for human use. [43 FR 45077, Sept. 29, 1978, as amended at 60 FR 4091, Jan. 20, 1995]

The paragraph on lighting states:

§ 211.44 *Lighting.*

Adequate lighting shall be provided in all areas.

On ventilation systems:

§ 211.46 *Ventilation, air filtration, air heating and cooling.*

(a) Adequate ventilation shall be provided.

(b) Equipment for adequate control over air pressure, micro-organisms, dust, humidity, and temperature shall be provided when appropriate for the manufacture, processing, packing, or holding of a drug product.

(c) Air filtration systems, including prefilters and particulate matter air filters, shall be used when appropriate on air supplies to production areas. If air is recirculated to production areas, measures shall be taken to control recirculation of dust from production. In areas where air contamination occurs during production, there shall be adequate exhaust systems or other systems adequate to control contaminants.

(d) Air-handling systems for the manufacture, processing, and packing of penicillin shall be completely separate from those for other drug products for human use.

The regulations dealing with equipment requirements are written in a similar fashion. For example:

§ 211.63 *Equipment design, size, and location.*

Equipment used in the manufacture, processing, packing, or holding of a drug product shall be of appropriate design, adequate size, and suitably located to facilitate operations for its intended use and for its cleaning and maintenance.

§ 211.65 *Equipment construction.*

(a) Equipment shall be constructed so that surfaces that contact components, in-process materials, or drug products shall not be reactive, additive, or absorptive so as to alter the safety, identity, strength, quality, or purity of the drug product beyond the official or other established requirements.

(b) Any substances required for operation, such as lubricants or coolants, shall not come into contact with components, drug product containers, closures, in-process materials, or drug products so as to alter the safety, identity, strength, quality, or purity of the drug product beyond the official or other established requirements.

The requirements in these paragraphs can be satisfied utilizing various systems. The example provided in the chapter Introduction to this chapter discusses an approach to meeting paragraph 211.42 Design and construction features. To design a pharmaceutical facility, a designer must be thoroughly knowledgeable of industry practices and systems that have been approved by the FDA. This knowledge is obtained through education and experience. There are numerous courses sponsored by universities and professional and educational associations that can introduce an individual to the requirements of facility design. (Note: the full text of 21 CFR 210 and 211 as well as the preamble can be obtained at www.FDA.gov.)

European Union GMPs

The majority of manufacturing facilities located in the United States also need to meet European (EU) and local country requirements. For example, the United Kingdom GMPs are described in a publications know as the "Orange Book" due to the color of the book's cover. A review of the EU GMPs and the UK GMPs indicates that the facility and equipment requirements in these regulations are consistent. Other countries within the EU also have specific requirements but again these are consistent with the requirements indicated in the EU regulations. Therefore, a discussion of the EU regulations is in order.

The EU has issued nine volumes constituting *The Rules Governing Medicinal Products in the European Union.* Of interest to the designer is Volume 4—Good Manufacturing Practices, Medicinal Products for Human and Veterinary Use. The document consists of a general section followed by product specific sections call annexes. Each of these sections contains requirements for facilities and equipment. The EU regulations are slightly more prescriptive than the FDA's cGMPs; however, these regulations still allow the designer a good deal of flexibility when designing a pharmaceutical plant.

Within Volume 4, Chapter 3: Premises and Equipment, covers the general requirements for these items in a similar fashion as Subparts C and D of 21 CFR 211. For example, the first paragraph of this chapter states:

Principle
Premises and equipment must be located, designed, constructed, adapted and maintained to suit the operations to be carried out. Their layout and design must aim to minimize the risk of errors and permit effective cleaning and maintenance in order to avoid cross-contamination, build up of dust and dirt and, in general, any adverse effect on the quality of products.

A reading of other requirements indicates more detail than the FDA's regulations but they are still are general in nature, allowing flexibility for the designer in providing adequate solutions to fit the specific requirements of the facility being designed.

Where the EU regulations become more prescriptive is in the annexes section. There are 14 annexes included in the regulations covering various dosage forms as follows:

Annex Number	*Title*
1	Manufacture of sterile medicinal products
2	Manufacture of biological medicinal products for human use
3	Manufacture of radiopharmaceuticals
4	Manufacturer of veterinary medicinal products other than immunologicals

5	Manufacture of immunologicals veterinary medicinal products
6	Manufacture of medicinal gases
7	Manufacture of herbal medicinal products
8	Sampling of starting and packaging materials
9	Manufacture of liquids, creams and ointments
10	Manufacture of pressurized metered dose aerosol preparations for inhalation
11	Computerized Systems
12	Use of ionizing radiation in the manufacture of medicinal products
13	Manufacture of investigational medicinal products
14	Manufacture of products derived from human blood or human plasma

The designer is required to perform a thorough review of the annex applicable to the type of manufacturing entity being designed. These annexes provide more detailed requirements than those presented in the FDA's regulations. However, these annexes do include much of the same information that the FDA provides in its guidance documents. These annexes are not in conflict with the expectations of the FDA concerning facilities and equipment. There are additional requirements in the EU regulations for the operational aspects of the licensed facility, but these usually do not impact the design.

A good example of the additional details provided in the annexes is in the annex 1 covering sterile products. The annex contains specific information on the environmental classification of various operating areas (class A, B, C, and D). For example, the annex indicates that class A is to be employed for high risk operations such as filling stopper bowls, open containers, and making aspect connections. This is consistent with FDA expectations. The annex proceeds to provide detailed functional requirements for particulates in each of the four environmental classifications as well as recommended microbial limits to be utilized for the monitoring program in each of these areas.

While this information is more specific than found in the FDA's regulations, it is consistent with the FDA's guidance documents and is currently being utilized in the industry as the baseline standards.

Harmonization

In the early 1990s, an international effort was begun to harmonize the requirements for pharmaceutical manufacturing and licensing among the United States, Japan, and the European Union. The focus of the International Conference on

Harmonization (ICH) program is the technical requirements for pharmaceutical products containing new drugs. Since the majority of new drugs are developed in the United States, Western Europe, and Japan, it was agreed that the scope of this activity would be confined to registration in these three geographical regions.

As stated in the mission statement:

> The International Conference on Harmonization of Technical Requirements for Registration of Pharmaceuticals for Human Use (ICH) is a unique project that brings together the regulatory authorities of Europe, Japan, and the United States and experts from the pharmaceutical industry in the three regions to discuss scientific and technical aspects of product registration.

> The purpose is to make recommendations on ways to achieve greater harmonisation in the interpretation and application of technical guidelines and requirements for product registration in order to reduce or obviate the need to duplicate the testing carried out during the research and development of new medicines. The objective of such harmonisation is a more economical use of human, animal and material resources, and the elimination of unnecessary delay in the global development and availability of new medicines whilst maintaining safeguards on quality, safety and efficacy, and regulatory obligations to protect public health.

The harmonization effort has resulted in several standards in the areas of quality, safety, and efficacy. Of interest is Q7A—Good Manufacturing Practice Guide for Active Pharmaceutical Ingredients. This document provides a template for other GMP guide documents will follow. A review of this document finds that the terminology and structure are very similar to the FDA's cGMP requirements in 21 CFR 211 and the EU GMP Vol 4. Similar harmonization efforts are underway for aseptic manufacturing and non-sterile manufacturing.

Validation

An important regulatory issue affecting the design of a pharmaceutical facility is validation. The FDA requires that all processes producing drug substances be validated. The FDA's definition for process validation, as stated in the Guideline on General Principals for Validation, is:

> Establishing documented evidence which provides a high degree of assurance that a specific process will consistently produce a product meeting its predetermined specifications and quality attributes.

This statement not only requires that manufacturing processes be validated, but the facility systems that support production as well. For example, an aseptic processing operation requires a "clean" room. Consequently, the heating, ventilating, and air-conditioning (HVAC) system must be validated in order to ensure that the process is truly aseptic. Furthermore, all critical utility systems (e.g., water, steam, compressed air) need to be tested to ensure proper operation. The nature of the testing that takes place during validation varies depending upon the system or piece of equipment. Certain systems are "validated" and others are "qualified." The difference is whether or not a challenge test is conducted. Sterilization systems and procedures undergo a specific challenge to determine their adequacy. Support utilities and HVAC systems are not specifically challenged but are determined to be operating within acceptable criteria and, therefore, are qualified. Industry and the FDA have generally agreed regarding which systems fall into each category. In general, those systems that directly affect the product are challenged, while those that support the operation are qualified. The entire documentation and testing effort is generally known as *validation*. (Details of this program are discussed elsewhere in this text).

The requirement for validation is delineated in 21 CFR 210 and 211 for finished drug products and 21 CFR 820 for medical devices. (The guideline mentioned above provides the specific paragraph references for validation. A complete text of the guideline can be obtained at the FDA's web site.) The requirement for validation is included in the EU regulations in Volume 4, Chapter 5: Production, Sections 5.21 through 5.24.

The above regulatory requirements ensure that a designer, in addition to a knowledge of design, must also have knowledge of how the facility is to operate and how it is to be validated. These activities have a direct impact on the facility and equipment design. The owner needs to define the approach to validation at the beginning of the project. A useful tool in conveying this information is the Validation Master Plan. (VMP) This document delineates the validation program that will be utilized and is usually developed in conjunction with the design basis of the facility. Both documents require the use of User Requirement Specifications (URS) as their foundation. These two documents are discussed elsewhere in this text.

APPROACH TO GMP DESIGN

General

The non-specific requirements delineated in the regulations require a disciplined approach to the design of pharmaceutical manufacturing facilities, thus GDP. As discussed inthe ISPG Baseline Guides, the foundation of this approach is the manufacturing process(es) and the product(s) that will be produced, tested, or held in the facility under design. The majority of design decisions and design criteria should be based on the critical quality attributes of the product.

A designer must have knowledge of how the facility is to operate and how it is to be validated. The company define its approach to validation at the beginning of the project. The Validation Master Plan (VMP), the document which delineates the validation program that will be utilized, is developed in conjunction with the design basis of the facility.

During the development of the design basis, the manufacturing process and facility requirements are defined. These are developed through discussions with the end user, including the manufacturing, QA/QC, engineering, and the validation groups. Items addressed during this phase are:

- Establishing goals and objectives
- Preparing user Requirements Specifications (URS), process, and operational flow diagrams
- Developing system design criteria
- Developing the facility conceptual design

Goals and Objectives

Goals and objectives of the manufacturing unit depend upon the following:

- Corporate philosophies
- Operating philosophies
- Regulatory requirements

A corporate philosophy, such as the requirement to maintain a minimum level of finished goods inventory, will directly affect the size of the warehouse and production equipment output rates. Corporations have requirements concerning capital investment. Prior to the commitment of funds, the investment must meet certain criteria for return on investment (ROI) and the time period within which an investment pays for itself (payback period). The inclusion of systems such as energy management and production automation, may be dependent upon their payback period. A period of two to five years for such systems is common in the industry.

An operating philosophy that encompasses the presence or absence of in-process material quarantine areas during the manufacturing operation will affect the physical size and layout of the new facility.

The cGMPs regulations place restrictions on the design of the facility. For example" Are entry and exit gowning areas required? How will material control be dealt with in a batching operation?

An understanding of these factors is essential in designing a compliant manufacturing facility.

User Requirements Specifications, Process Flow, and Operational Flow Diagrams

In order to fully understand the expectations of the user of the manufacturing facility, it is necessary to develop the User Requirements Specifications (URS). These documents delineate the requirements and expectations of the end user of the facility, equipment, and system. The designer needs to understand that the objective is to deliver a design for a licensed operation, not just a design of a building filled with equipment. The manner in which the facility, equipment, and systems are to be utilized forms the foundation for manufacturing operation. These documents also are utilized as the starting point in the validation effort.

A constructive technique to assist in the understanding of all aspects of the manufacturing process is the preparation of process flow diagram (PFD) and operational flow diagram (OFD).

PFDs depict each unit operational step of the manufacturing process. In analyzing the overall production scheme, the operation can be broken down into its basic elements.

These elements are arranged in a facility OFD that depicts the inter-relationships between the manufacturing process steps and other operating departments (QA, Production, In-Process Testing, etc.). In this manner, the designer can incorporate the entire operation into the layout of the facility without inadvertently neglecting some component or preventing required interactions.

System Design Criteria

System design criteria must be established for each production and support system required by the manufacturing process. The products being manufactured form the focus for establishing design criteria. An analysis of the manufacturing process being conducted in each room/area must be completed to identify all systems that can impact the quality of the product and/or the efficiency of operations. The PFD and OFD, along with the URS, should form the basis for this analysis.

Facility Conceptual Design

The activities leading to this point have resulted in the development of a design basis for the facility. Alternative concepts can exist that will satisfy the requirements developed. These concepts need to be explored and decisions made as to which are to be used.

The conceptual designs of the manufacturing process are developed during the creation of the PFD. The concepts for the support utilities are derived when the quantity of the utility is known and a decision concerning the segregation of process and building utilities is reached. Once the manufacturing process and support utility conceptual designs are completed, the facility layout is developed.

The engineering and validation disciplines should be involved at this phase of the project to develop the approach to validation of the facility and to prepare the Commissioning Plan (CP) and the VMP.

Normally at the end of this project phase, a report is issued delineating the facility requirements and presenting the concepts that were investigated, including drawings that indicate the schematic design of the facility. This report is used for the Design Development phase of the project. At this point in time, the first draft of the VMP should be issued and the first meeting with the FDA arranged.

Prior to the meeting with the FDA, the project team should conduct a cGMP audit of the project. The purpose of this audit is to determine whether the design of the facility meets cGMP requirements and accepted industry practices. The audit should be conducted by personnel who are familiar with cGMP design practices and who are not directly involved in the project.

The meeting with the FDA includes a review of the conceptual design of the facility and the VMP. While the FDA will not approve the design, the agency will indicate areas of concern both in the facility design and validation plan. By addressing the agency's concerns early in the design process, re-work of design effort or corrective actions after construction is completed can be eliminated. Such a review will assist in the expeditious certification of the facility after construction is completed.

Summary

The above outlines a disciplined approach to the design of a GMP facility. Input is provided by a multi-disciplined team consisting of facilities professionals with backgrounds in manufacturing, quality, engineering, and validation. The approach includes a sanity check of the GMP review (design qualification) at the appropriate time in the design cycle as well as the inclusion of the commissioning and validation requirements. In this manner, the regulatory requirements will be met. A well-designed facility is by definition one that meets regulatory needs. The important issue is to fully understand the manufacturing process and commissioning and validation requirements. An experienced designer can then provide a proper design.

This approach can be utilized on any type of facility, realizing that different manufacturing facilities have specific compliance issues that must be addressed. Elsewhere in this text, specific solutions to each of these issues will be discussed. Following are highlights of the compliance issues on inspectors' lists for specific dosage forms.

Aseptic and Biotech Facilities Issues

While the type of products handled in an aseptic facility and a biotech facility can be widely different, there are several areas of commonality. Both of these facility types require the use of environmentally classified clean rooms, protection of the product from the environment and personnel, and the need for clean and/or aseptic support systems and utilities.

The issues that are of interest to regulatory inspectors are:

- Material, personnel, and equipment flow patterns
- Integrity of the manufacturing equipment/systems in respect to aseptic operations
- Maintenance of the clean space (environmental monitoring)
- Integrity of a classified space around exposed product
- Integrity of the clean spaces within which manufacturing operations occur
- Integrity of cleaning and sterilization processes
- Integrity of the clean support utilities
- Containment of operations that handle environmentally hazardous organisms

The various regulatory agencies have provided guidance around the environmental classification within which various operations are to occur. This guidance also includes specific design criteria for the various clean room classifications. It is ncumbent upon the designer to understand these regulations and guidance and to be able to provide a design that can be constructed and tested to demonstrate that the environmental conditions are met.

In addition, cleaning and sterilization processes, and the equipment and systems that support these processes, come under extensive scrutiny during inspections. Again, the key to a successful design is one that can be easily constructed and tested to demonstrate proper operations. The testing requirements, both from a commissioning and validation perspective, must be well understood by the designer in order for all regulatory requirements to be met.

Oral/Solid Dose Facilities

Solid dose manufacturing facilities present some unique challenges to the designer from a compliance perspective. Although the regulations appear less stringent for this type of operation versus a facility and equipment perspective regulatory expectations, in fact are just as stringent.

The need for facilities and equipment that are easily cleaned and maintained are as important for oral and solid dose manufacturing facilities as for aseptic and biotech facilities. While the bioburden aspects significant in the aseptic/biotech facilities are not as stringent in oral/solid dose facilities, it has become common practice of late to have monitoring programs that measure background environmental bioburden profiles for these operations. This results in facility finishes that are designed to be easily cleaned (e.g., minimum ledges or corners) and that can stand up to mild disinfective solutions.

Cross contamination is a significant issue. Inspectors are concerned with the potential for cross contamination due to personnel traffic as well as the HVAC systems and dust control systems. Therefore, the layout of the operations, as well as the HVAC systems, must be designed to minimize or eliminate the potential for cross contamination. A later chapter in this text concerning the design of these facilities addresses various approaches to solving this challenge).

Active Pharmaceutical Ingredients (API) Facilities

From a facility and equipment perspective, API operations pose a challenge different from other dosage forms. With other dosage forms, the final active ingredient is present at the onset of production activities. In API facilities, the active molecule is being developed through the various manufacturing steps. The question raised for such operations is: When are full GMPs applicable? Accepted practice is that full GMPs are applicable at the point in time when the active molecule is formed. This point in the process is the milestone used for validation purposes.

The designer needs to determine what effect this concept has on the design of the equipment and facilities. It is recommended that the design practices for piping and instrumentation in the areas of drainability and cleanability be consistent through the operations; i.e., there is no difference in piping, equipment, and instrumentation design from initial steps to final steps in the manufacturing process.

The concept of final formation of the molecule usually can affect the architectural finishes and HVAC systems of the operations. As the active ingredient becomes purified, the environment in which it is handled is usually upgraded to be in line with traditional pharmaceutical operations. (Details of how this is achieved are included in the appropriate chapter within this text.)

REGULATORY TRENDS

Since the late 1970s, regulations have become more stringent over time. The main impetus for this is not that the regulators are devising new rules but rather technology has improved our ability to address key issues in the regulatory world. Thus, the concept of the term "current" in current Good Manufacturing Practices is a reality. As new technologies come into play, they change the nature of what is industry practice and thus change what is current from a regulatory expectation perspective.

For example, the improvement of measurement and control devices in HVAC systems has resulted in the expectation of a robust area-differential pressure control in operations where classified environments are required. The use of barrier technology in the recent past may very well result in revisions in the early twenty-first century in expectations for the parenteral industry from a facility and equipment perspective. This trend should be expected and should be welcomed. New technologies help us ensure product quality and integrity.

A recent trend to enforcement of cGMPs is the *quality system approach*. This approach is delineated in the Quality System Regulations in 21 CFR Part 820. While these regulations are directly applicable to the device industry, the quality system approach is very easily transferred to other dosage form manufacturing operations. In effect, the regulatory agencies are stating that the manufacturing operation is a system whose elements must be robust and efficient and enable the manufacturing to control product quality, identify deviations, and react in a timely fashion to correct of deviations and continue the process.

In the early 2000s, the U.S. FDA is taking a "risk assessment" approach to enforcement of the regulations. This means that the agency will target those products that reflect the greatest threat to the safety of public health. Sterile dosage forms will be high on the list, with oral/solid dosage forms near the bottom. This does not necessarily result in numerous inspections and enforcement activities for manufacturers of sterile products and none for oral/solid dose manufacturers, but the trend will be to focus on sterile products.

Both of these approaches will have a major impact on the manner in which pharmaceutical industry companies operate. The effect on facility and equipment design is yet to be determined; however, this effect should be minimal to nonexistent. Equipment and facilities, while playing a major role, need to be of the appropriate quality level for the products being manufactured no matter the regulatory enforcement posture.

Editor's Note: _____

FDA has announced new GMP initiatives indicating their commitment to "efficient risk management" in GMP enforcement. On August 20, 2003 the Agency said "best practices in manufacturing technologies and methods have undergone significant progress in other industries . . . but hasn't been the subject of as much attention in the pharma industry. . . . The Agency wants to make sure that its regulations are encouraging such progress." . . . the implication being that regulations may have, in fact, inhibited technological innovation. (*Drug GMP Report 9/03*)

CONCLUSIONS

The nature of the cGMP regulations are such that there is no "cookbook" approach to the design of pharmaceutical manufacturing operations. The regulations, for the most part, describe what needs to be accomplished rather than how to accomplish the requirement. Therefore, a disciplined approach is required to ensure that the intent of the regulations is met as well as the business goals for the operation. Input needs to be received from the various operating functions within the pharmaceutical plant to ensure all requirements are met. New technologies will be constantly developed to provide the designer with additional tools to meet the regulations. It is imperative for the designer to keep abreast of new developments in the industry.

In order to ensure that the facility will meet the regulatory requirements, the designer needs to understand the following list of issues.

- Regulatory agency(ies) that will have jurisdiction over the operation
- Understanding of the agency's expectations and requirements
- Understanding the project's goals and objectives
- Preparing User Requirements Specifications (URS), and Process and Operational Flow diagrams
- Developing system design criteria
- [a] Developing the facility conceptual design
- Corporate philosophies
- Operating philosophies
- Knowledge of the manufacturing process
- Understanding of the material, personnel, and equipment flow patterns within the operation
- Understanding of the commissioning, qualification, and validation approach that will be utilized for the new facility
- Business objectives of the operations

These issues form the basis for a well-designed facility that meets corporate and regulatory objectives. Without such a foundation, the resulting facility design can be fraught with flaws, thus causing project delivery and budgetary problems.

Remember, there are many ways to achieve compliance in facility design, whether through the building of physical restraints or through the development of procedural restraints. The balance between the two is dependent upon the operating firm's philosophy and budget. It is the responsibility of the designer to achieve the desired balanced.

BIBLIOGRAPHY

Code of Federal Regulations, Title 21, Parts 1-211; 600–680, 820, April 2003.

Guidelines on Sterile Drug Products Produced by Aseptic Processing, Center for Drugs and Biologics, FDA, 1987.

Guidelines on General Principles of Process Validation, Center for Drugs and Biologics, FDA, 1987.

The Rules Governing Medicinal Products in the European Union, Volume 4, Good Manufacturing Practices, 1997 edition.

ICS Harmonized Tripartite Guideline—Good Manufacturing Practice Guide for Active Pharmaceutical Ingedients, November, 2000.

Rules and Guidance for Pharmaceutical Manufacturers and Distributors 1997, Medicines Control Agency.

3
Facility Planning

Author: William B. Wiederseim

Advisors: Anthony Felicia
Sterling Kline

WHY FACILITIES PLANNING IS IMPORTANT

Facilities planning is one of the most important endeavors in which one can engage in the pharmaceutical industry. Without quality facilities, there would be no life-saving or life-enhancing drugs. Facilities also greatly impact the financial performance of the enterprise, and represent the vision of the company—architecturally, it speaks volumes about the leadership of the company and its commitment to its employees and the manufacturing of world-class drug products. The facility supports the mission of the company by providing the spaces and services needed to support the mission.

A facility also represents the company to the health care community:

• The payers (insurance companies)
• The providers (doctors and health care workers)
• The patients
• Governments and regulatory agencies

Facilities are a direct reflection of the facility planner and reflect excellence or mediocrity equally well. The facility will reflect the planner's value and performance for at least twenty years—a facility that will enhance or save lives on an industrial scale with the precious resources of the company.

Editor's Note

The project manager (PM) for pharma facility projects occupies a critical role in project delivery. Especially for planning activities, the PM is the central figure in orchestrating the many inputs, issues views, and objectives into a coherent project plan, destined for delivery in a challenging environment.

It is beyond the scope of this book to discuss in detail the many aspects of project management and how the PM leads the endeavor. One useful reference is the Project Management Institute (PMI) that has developed a professional certification program, including a body-of-knowledge-based test leading to Project Management Professional (PMP) certification. The knowledge requirements of the PMP program reflect many vital areas that are revelant to delivering a pharma project and are worthwhile to consider when reviewing good design practice issues for pharma facilities.

THE PLANNING PROCESS

Facilities represent a large capital cost and fixed investment for the company. A wise facility planner knows that *"the only number my CEO remembers is the first one we give him."* (Walter Hetrick, PE—Hoffmann-La Roche; Facility 2001, November 1992)

Many people believe the planning process is better understood if presented graphically over time. We believe facilities planning must consider the:

- Strategic goals of the corporation
- Business case for action
- Options on "what to do"
- Packaging of the planning process to be communicated to all relevant members of the organization

One may consider the following process map as indicative of the planning phases over time.

Editor's Note _____

In managing a facility, a Master Plan should be developed and updated to create a blueprint for the future.

DEVELOPING A FACILITY PROJECT PLAN FROM A BUSINESS CASE
The Business Case

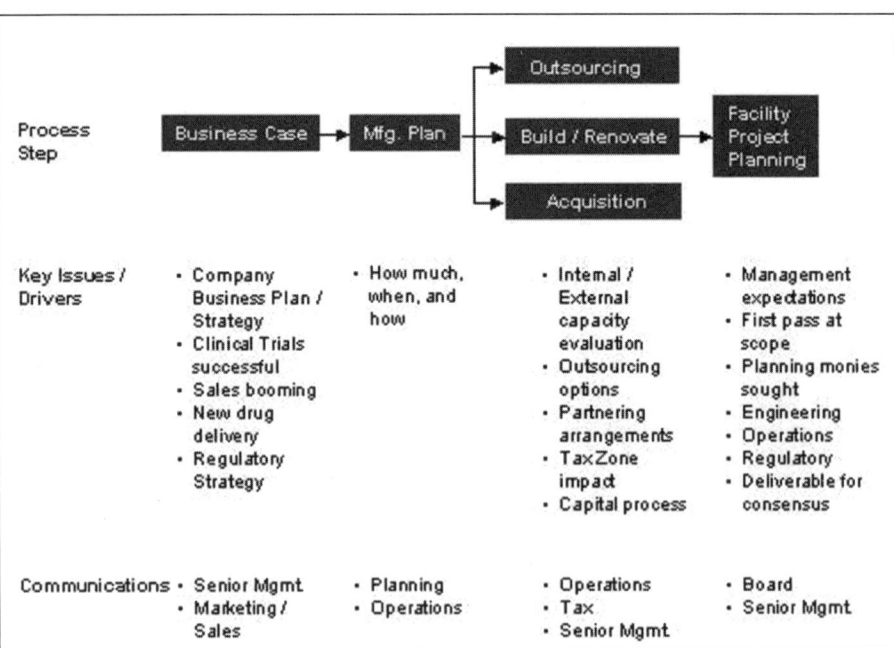

The Business Case

There must be a reason to plan a facility, meaning there must be a compelling event or anticipated compelling event. Within the pharmaceutical and biotechnology business, this compelling event is usually one of four things:

1. Clinical trials have been successful and management believes that a commercial business may be possible.
2. Sales of existing drugs have exceeded the capacity of the facility and an expansion is possible.
3. A project is created to enhance compliance, whether it is for the FDA, EPA, or other regulatory agency.
4. A product is created to enhance the efficiency (performance) and continuous improvement of the facility.

Launching a new product is the riskiest type of planning because of the many variables. The two biggest variables are when the product will be approved and how well it will sell. Management guidance will be necessary regarding how much risk is taken; i.e., what, when, and how much you should spend. There are no right or wrong answers, no rules of thumb, but in general, manufacturing does not want to be in the position of holding up the success of the organization. One way to plan is to create revenue and time scenarios such as the following example:

Benchmark Facility Construction Timeline (Without Validation)

Fill/finish:	1 year
R&D:	2 years
Parenteral:	3 years
Biologic:	4 years

Creating "what if" scenarios that consider the relationship between time and money is a good planning tool. Using this type of tool in conjunction with your own capital planning process is highly useful in preparing your management teams and framing decisions with discipline.

Manufacturing Planning

New information and technology to enhance manufacturing is wonderful but incredibly difficult. One must be careful not to build your own prison. (Carl Wheeldon— Warner-Lambert/Bristol-Myers Squibb, June 1997)

In many industries, and to a certain extent the pharma/bio industry, manufacturing must often compete for projects. This is certainly the case in the high capitalization industries such as automotive and steel.

Competing internally for manufacturing projects keeps organizations sharp and competitive. Pharmaceutical and biotechnology manufacturing are driven by different standards:

- Active Pharmaceutical Ingredients (API) are driven by centers of existing excellence (people / assets with relevant training). There is a significant difference between facilities projects for chemical innovation and biologic innovation.
- Tax Zones / Incentives usually has greater impact on secondary facilities because the products are more easily transferable. Chemically derived drug products in solids are perhaps the most transferable.
- Manufacturing planning must consider the alternatives available to manufacturing. Concluding a capital project without considering alternatives is becoming less acceptable. This is clearly the case with all the available facilities on the market, and with outsourcing is growing by more than 20% per year.

To be successful today, the facilities planner must consider:

- Outsourcing: The possibility of using third-party manufacturing or packaging resources
- Existing facility acquisition: The possibility of acquiring an existing facility

Developing Scope From a Facility Project Plan

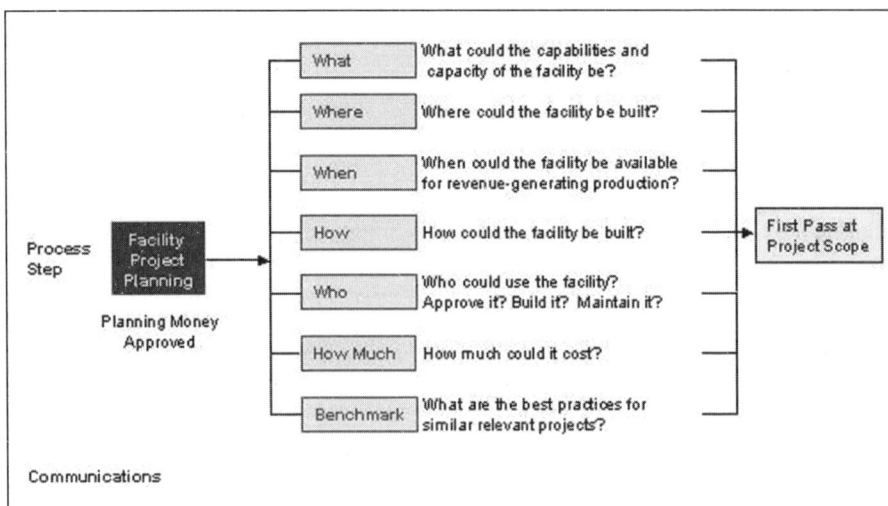

The First Pass at Project Scope

It seems that only pharmaceutical companies who are outsourcing have an idea of what the real cost of goods is. (Susan O'Donnell, Analyst—PharmaBioSource, Inc., March 2003)

The first pass at a project scope should consider the alternatives to manufacturing the new drug:

Renovation Costs Relative to Age of Facility

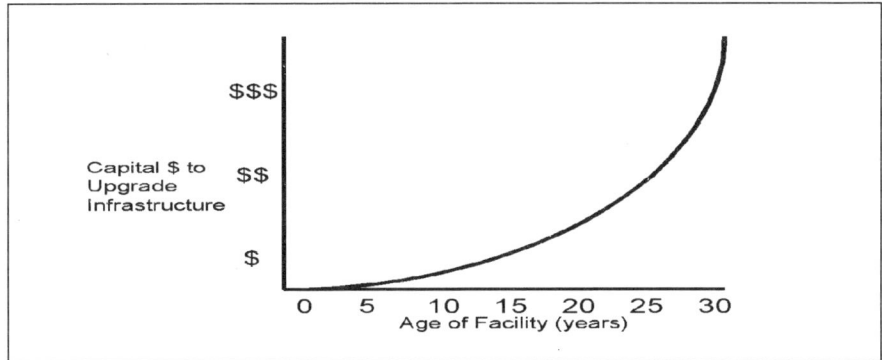

- *Outsourcing:* Outsourcing has enjoyed considerable success in the last several years, fueled by the excess capacity being generated by mergers. In addition, many corporations desire to conserve capital for drug innovation in lieu of manufacturing and prefer outsourcing. Outsourcing also has the certainty of a defined price (cost of goods sold, or COGS) at the expense of control.
- *Build new:* In many cases, a new facility is more than additional capacity but an opportunity to enhance or change the culture, performance and the compliance of an organization. New facilities are the most capital-intensive way to build capacity and calculating anticipated COGS is difficult to assess.
- *Renovate the existing facilities:* Many projects desire to renovate rather than build new as there is present value in existing facilities and afford a lower project (capital) cost. At the same time, facility renovation is very challenging from a planning perspective

Developing a Board-Level Presentation from Project Scope

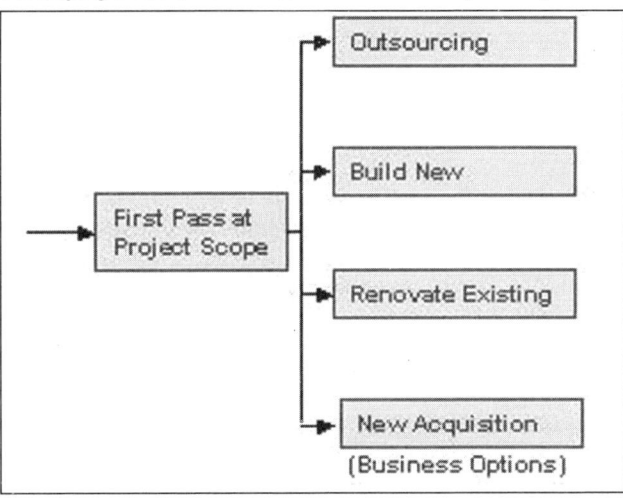

because it usually disrupts existing commercial operations and reuses existing technical infrastructure in a new way. Renovation is also capital intensive and calculating COGS is also difficult.

One of the biggest oversights is the planning for capital dollars for older facilities. Older facilities can continue to function optimally with an updated infrastructure. There is a trend in facilities to recycle "old space" into new updated space for new functions.

- New acquisition: Mergers have generated a large number of facilities either as real estate or as an on-going concern that may dramatically reduce capital investment yet maintain control. Control of the production staff and response to customer needs and regulatory situations are the more significant challenges to outsourcing. Of the 6,000 regulated facilities in the world, we estimate 20% are available for acquisition.

Facilities Planning Scope Development

Early sharing of the project is essential to project approval. This process is called "dusting." (Ed Thiele—Cardinal Health, Hoffmann-La Roche, Facility 2001, November 1992)

Facilities planning scope is the communication vehicle used to brief the stakeholders on how the capacity requirements will be achieved and subsequently the project goals. The communication must be formal; i.e., presentations, adherence to corporate standards, etc. It can also include informal communication; i.e., casual conversation, informal e-mail updates, etc. The creative facilities planner must always answer the question "what's in it for the stakeholder?" Communication of the project tailored to each stakeholder is key to project approval. All methods of communication—forman and informal—are required for project approval. When the formal management presentation is made, the project should be a "fait accompli," because the project planners have created approval momentum informally and inclusively.

Senior Management-Level Presentation

The best projects are the ones where the science is engineered. (Tony Felicia—AstraZeneca, July 2003)

Making a high level presentation for the first time can be an intimidating experience because the confidence in the outcome may be uncertain. Senior management are stakeholders and are financially evaluated on five criteria:

- Earnings/share
- Price of the stock
- Sales volume, cost metrics
- Regulatory compliance
- Successful launch (acquisition of new products)

When making recommendations to a CEO or to senior management, the facilities planner is presenting to the shareholders of the company. Having a project that is financially justifiable and in regulatory compliance is essential. There are three keys for successful senior management-level presentations:

- Pre-sell: The senior management-level presentation should be a fait accompli. The presenter should have had contact with the CEO and other senior management prior to a formal meeting. All dissenting opinions must be understood and resolved before the meeting. Deal-busting questions raised late in the game is a sign that the facilities planner is unprepared.
- Be concise: A one hour meeting with twenty slides should be plenty to accomplish the goals. A good agenda could be:
  Business case for action (*why?*)
  Selected alternate (*what?*)
  How much
  Selected resources (*how?*)
  Key milestones (*when?*)
  Actions (*who?*)
  Measure of success
- Be prepared for issues that have nothing to do with your area of expertise, such as:
  What is the competition doing (benchmarking)?
  How to recoup from planning/cost/schedule mishaps?
  Why does it cost so much and how can the costs be cut?
  Why do you think this product will make it to market?
  Do you trust the forecast?

Developing a Senior-Management Level Presentation From Project Scope

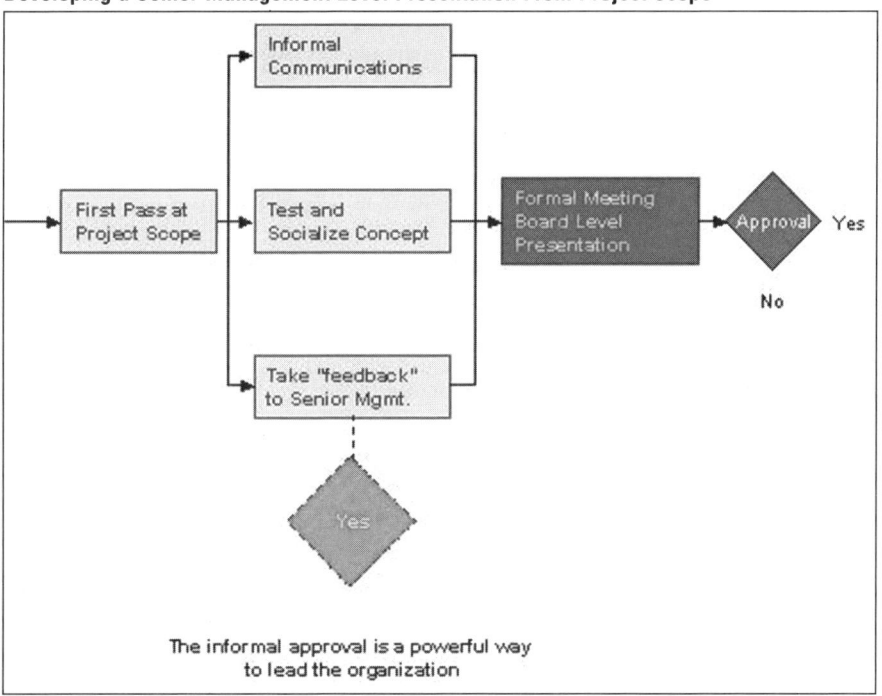

The informal approval is a powerful way
to lead the organization

BUSINESS DEVELOPMENT ORGANIZATIONS

There are many useful worldwide resources serving the pharmaceutical and biotechnology industries that may be consulted when considering facility planning. They range from the university level to the state level to the national level and the international level.

On a national and international level one of the most comprehensive biotechnology resources is the Biotechnology Industry Organization (Bio), (www.bio.org). The organization focuses on biotechnology information, advocacy and business support. Bio represents more than 1,000 biotechnology companies, academic institutions, biotechnology centers, and related organizations in all 50 U.S. states and 33 other nations. It has an extensive member list complete with company profiles as well as updates on research and policy issues affecting the industry. The Bio website also has a listing of upcoming conferences and events all around the world on various industry topics.

Almost every state has a biotechnology association and website that highlights its biotechnology resources and objectives. Because of the economic advantages of a growing and thriving biotech industry many states have created incentives with the objective of attracting companies to their state. These incentives are often in the form of tax advantages, financial resources, strong government relations, business networking, etc.

Various universities and institutions have biotechnology centers, which often have a particular focus and objective and may be useful to investigate for a company with a similar focus and objective.

TAX ZONE BUSINESS DEVELOPMENT ORGANIZATIONS

The international locations with the most advantageous tax zones for pharmaceutical and biotechnology development and manufacturing are Ireland, Puerto Rico and Singapore. The primary attraction for companies locating their business in these areas is largely the tax advantage, which can be as low as 2%.

- Ireland: IDA Ireland (www.ida.ie)
- Puerto Rico: Puerto Rican Industrial Development Company (www.pridco.com)
- Singapore: Singapore Economic Development Board (www.sedb.com)

Ireland targets the following sectors for investment in Ireland:

- Chemicals, pharmaceuticals, and health care
- E-commerce
- Information and communications technology
- Software
- Internationally traded services, including financial services, customer contact centers, and shared services centers

Puerto Rico targets the following sectors for investment in Puerto Rico:

- Pharmaceutical
- Medical devices
- Biotechnology

- Electronics
- Call center

Singapore focuses on the following industries for investment in Singapore:

- Biomedical sciences
- Electronics
- Chemicals
- Engineering

Tax Zones often concentrate their efforts and resources in the following areas with the objective of creating an optimal environment that will be attractive to companies looking to relocate their business or some aspect of it:

- Economy: Government economic policies
- Taxation: Corporate tax rates that can range from . . .
- Workforce: Educated and skilled workforce
- Competitive costs: Operating costs
- Infrastructure: Land, telecommunications, logistics, etc.

SECURITY

In a recent survey of 14 parenteral site acquisition candidates, my client rejected the best candidate because the site could not be secured. (William B. Wiederseim— PharmaBioSource, Inc., May 2003)

Providing a safe and secure work environment requires a combination of physical security measures, administrative controls, and personal ownership. Since the 9/11 attack, security concerns for terrorism have increased. The degree of success for any program is dependent upon the partnership between management and staff. Management must be committed to providing the necessary resources to identify and control security risks to an acceptable level. Staff must be willing to take ownership of the security program and ensure compliance with the requirements. The following information is provided to assist engineers, facility managers and security professionals in facility design, building modifications, or physical security improvements.

Designing a Secure Facility

Projecting a positive corporate image to the community at large is an important factor in the design of any facility. The challenge is to build a secure facility that is aesthetically pleasing to the neighbors, community, and local elected officials.

1. Perimeter barrier protection
   a. Landscape
      1. Large rocks
      2. Berm
   b. Fence
      1. Height: May be limited by local ordinances
      2. Type: Standard cyclone versus ornamental types
2. Manned guard stations at entrances/exits

    a. Material of construction: Prefab unit, brick, or block need for bullet or explosion proof glass

    b. Distance from roadway: Need to avoid incurring liability by allowing incoming traffic to back-up onto the public road

    c. Need for gates: Remote-controlled gates or a type of hydraulic arm gate

    d. Need for barrier protection: Bollards, anti-ram barriers, etc.

3. Building location

    a. Proximity to public roads should be considered

    b. Distance from property lines should be considered

4. Parking lots

    a. Consider ground, above, or below grade parking options

    b. Should be at least 100 feet from nearest building

    c. For lots closer than 100 feet, should consider restricting parking close to building during elevated Homeland Security alerts

    d. Need to balance security and ADA requirements

5. Lighting considerations

    a. Facility entrances

    b. Building entrances

    c. Walkways

    d. Parking Lots: Security needs often conflict with local ordinances

    e. Property/Perimeter: Consider local light pollution ordinances

    f. Effective use of "off-hours" lighting cycles

Building Design

1. Materials of construction

    a. A threat and vulnerability assessment along with a risk analysis should be conducted to determine the most appropriate material of construction and the need for security walls

2. Windows

    a. Natural daylight can improve worker productivity and reduce energy cost but presents significant security challenges

    b. The size, location, and use of glazing material should be considered

    c. Public view should be considered

    d. Appropriate design of external/internal vehicle or pedestrian traffic patterns

3. HVAC

    a. Air intakes should be designed and situated to protect from sabotage

    b. Consider the need for filtration (supply and discharge)

    c. Units should be located in a restricted access area

4. Infrastructure protection (electrical, water, steam, natural, and specialty gases)

    a. Consider redundant systems for critical operations

    b. Consider emergency generators/UPS systems

    c. Limit access to mechanical rooms

5. Entrances

    a. Should be 100 feet from roadway

    b. Minimum number necessary to meet Life Safety Code and local ordinances

    c. Minimum size necessary to meet ADA requirements

    d. Consider the need for bollards or anti-ram devices

6. Lobby

    a. Entrance should be at least 100 feet from roadway

b. Consider the use of glazing on all windows and glass doors

c. Consider the need for bollards or anti-ram devices

d. Consider the need for optical or barrier arm turnstiles

e. Consider the need for a dedicated HVAC system

f. Consider the use of glazed glass to protect reception staff

g. Need to meet ADA requirements

h. Should consider installation of restrooms

7. Auditorium/training/meeting rooms

  a. Consider constructing a freestanding building

  b. Consider isolation from critical areas

  c. Consideration should be given regarding the general public's use of facilities

  d. Consider the location/installation of restrooms

  e. Consider team areas for internal use

8. Loading dock

  a. Consider locating away from critical areas

  b. Consider constructing a guard post

  c. Consider a dedicated HVAC system

  d. Consider isolation from critical infrastructure piping/systems

  e. Consider installation of fire suppression systems and/or smoke detection systems

  f. Consider need to secure entrance to the loading dock area

  g. Consider the location/installation of restrooms for use by delivery/service personnel

  h. Consider a buffer zone between dock and building

9. Mailroom

  a. Consider constructing a freestanding building

  b. Consider isolation from critical areas

  c. Consider a dedicated HVAC system

  d. Consider isolation from critical infrastructure piping/systems

  e. Consider screening equipment

10. 24/7 Manned control room

  a. Consider monitoring all access control systems

  b. Consider monitoring all internal radio communications

  c. Consider monitoring and recording (1:1) all CCTV data

  d. Consider monitoring all building operations systems

  e. Consider monitoring all life safety systems

  f. Consider recording all incoming calls to the control room

  g. Consider isolation from critical areas

  h. Consider a dedicated HVAC system

  i. Consider emergency power needs (generator/UPS system)

  j. Consider installation of restroom and kitchen facilities

  k. Should be ADA compliant

  l. Consider the use of remote technology as appropriate

Surveillance Systems

1. Consider the use of CCTV

  a. Strategically placed to cover potential exposures and vulnerabilities (critical areas, lobby, corridors, loading docks, building entrances, mechanical equipment areas, parking lots, grounds, perimeter fence line, etc.)

  b. Consider equipment that is capable of high resolution, low light/night vision

    c. Consider digital equipment with 1:1 recording capabilities

    d. Consider PTZ (pan, tilt, zoom) equipment

    e. Consider the use of passive/disguised units

2. Break glass detectors

    a. Consider usage on all ground level windows and other areas that could be vulnerable

    b. Consider the use of passive/disguised units

3. Motion/sound detectors

    a. Consider usage on all critical areas where other means of surveillance is not feasible

    b. Consider the use of passive/disguised units

Access Control

1. Control systems

    a. Key

    b. Key pad

    c. Photo ID

    d. Photo ID plus proximity card reader

    e. Photo ID plus proximity card reader plus keypad

    f. Photo ID plus proximity card reader plus biometrics

    g. Time sensitive photo ID system for visitors and service providers

    h. Consider flexibility in system capability

    i. Must consider life safety codes versus security

2. Hardware

    a. Basic lock system

    b. Removable core lock system

    c. Local keypad lock system

    d. Centralized electromagnetic lock system

3. Access control points

    a. Perimeter vehicle/pedestrian gates

    b. Lobby

    c. Loading docks

    d. Computer rooms

    e. Mechanical equipment rooms

    f. Elevators

    g. Building roof (egress and ingress)

    h. Mailrooms

    i. Laboratories

    j. Vivarium

    k. Procedure rooms

    l. Other areas deemed to critical to business

Personnel Security

1. Background checks

    a. Consider employees

    b. Consider contract staff

    c. Consider construction (pre-approved list of authorized individuals)

     d. Consider outside service providers (pre-approved list of authorized individuals)
2. Visitors
     a. Consider need for temporary photo ID system
     b. Consider need for escort policy
3. Individual responsibilities and accountabilities
     a. Need to develop and implement a security policy
     b. Policy needs management endorsement and approval
     c. Needs to be communicated to all individuals captured by program
4. Workplace violence
     a. Need to develop, implement, and communicate a workplace violence policy

CASE STUDY

AstraZeneca's corporate move to Delaware was the most significant event for Delaware in the 1990s. (Governor Tom Carper—State of Delaware, April 1999)

AstraZeneca: Corporate Move to Delaware (R&D)—*Tony Felicia*

- The recent merger between Astra and Zeneca created a need for a more consolidated U.S. process. Numerous factors were critical to the site selection process and included the following:
- Amount of asset already owned by the legacy companies prior to the merger
- Ability to expand an existing site or purchase a Greenfield site
- State, county, or local tax incentives
- Community support by business, education, scientific, and non-profit leaders
- Support by top political leaders to maintain the economic vitality of a location
- Quality of life for employees such as distance to work, education, adequate housing, cost of living, roads/traffic, etc
- And lastly, any issues key to the senior executive team such as building the right culture for the newly merged company

The logical site for the new North American Headquarters of AstraZeneca was the Blue Ball Triangle, adjacent to the existing Zeneca site on Route 202 north of Wilmington. But the community believed that this great economic development opportunity should be balanced by meeting a longstanding need for open space and an improved transportation system. Addressing the concerns of the community was vital, since company executives had said that they would only go where they felt welcome.

In response, the state committed to a purchase of 220 acres of land—roughly 86 acres for AstraZeneca with the remaining acreage for open space and parkland.

Delaware officials vowed they would "leave no stone unturned." For a month, a multi-agency, inter-governmental team worked 12 hours a day, 7 days a week to put together a proposal that would demonstrate to AstraZeneca executives every benefit of doing business in Delaware.

A Research and Development Tax Credit was considered a key component of the proposal. The General Assembly introduced and passed legislation, and the governor signed it into law—in just 10 days. Since other states have taken as long as 3 years to pass similar legislation, this was a clear statement to AstraZeneca of the responsiveness of "smarter, quicker, more flexible" Delaware.

The financial package presented to AstraZeneca was valued at more than $400 million. DEDO researchers conducted a massive comparative analysis of the cost of doing business in Delaware vs. Pennsylvania and identified more than $300 million in potential savings. The state offered an $18.7 million package of land grant assistance. DelDOT committed to accelerating $79 million in improvements along Route 202.

The AstraZeneca merger was completed in April of 1999. C. G. Johansson, AstraZeneca CEO, personally contacted both Delaware Governor Carper and Pennsylvania Governor Tom Ridge, and a decision was publicly announced on April 29, 1999: AstraZeneca would be headquartered in Delaware.

It's easy to see what AstraZeneca gets by choosing Delaware, but what does Delaware receive in return? For starters, the potential of 6,500 jobs in an industry with typical salaries in the $50,000+ range. At full employment, it is estimated that AstraZeneca will generate $50 million a year in state and local taxes. The road improvements will ease congestion on Route 202. Delaware is preserving one of its most endangered mature forests, a treasured piece of an old duPont estate; restoring three historic buildings; and taking control of land to link the greenways belt from the Delaware River to the Brandywine River. In addition, a recreational park will be created for all residents to enjoy.

But the greatest benefit will be seen in years to come. AstraZeneca remains the northern anchor of a burgeoning biotechnology corridor along Route 141 that is expected to provide thousands of high-paying jobs in the future. The loss of Zeneca would have been a crushing blow to Delaware's economic growth. The gain of AstraZeneca gives Delaware a jump-start to the future.

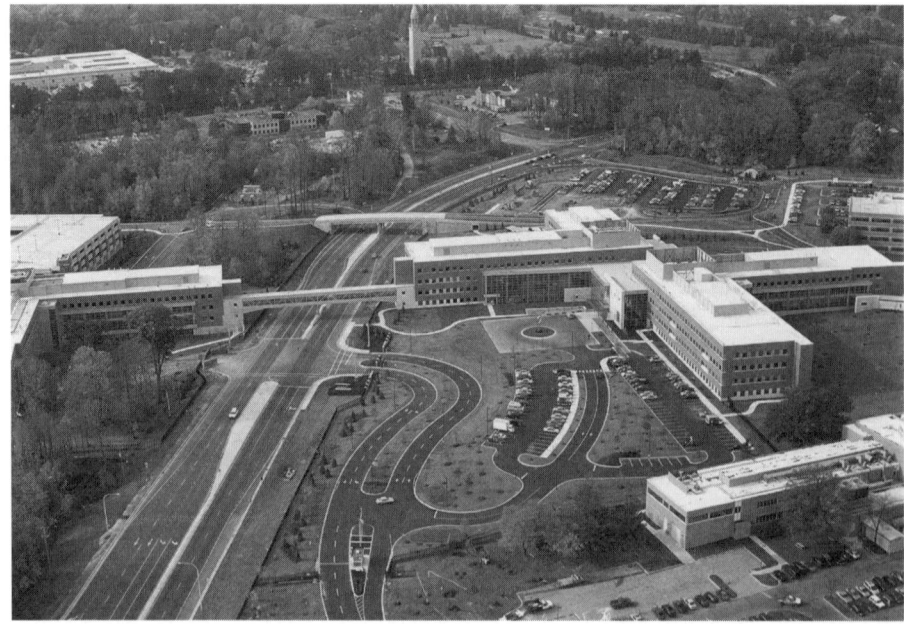

4
Architecture

Author: Terry Jacobs

INTRODUCTION

Architectural design integrates the process flows, equipment flows, personnel flows, and mechanical systems into an operating cGMP pharmaceutical manufacturing facility.

The architect must clearly understand the people, product, and process flows of the facility, as well as the manufacturing goals, to make the two-dimensional flow diagrams into a three-dimensional building that works efficiently, meets cGMPs and other compliance issues, embodies Good Design Practices, and creates a positive workplace for the employees, as well as, creating an efficient facility whose output is a regulated product.

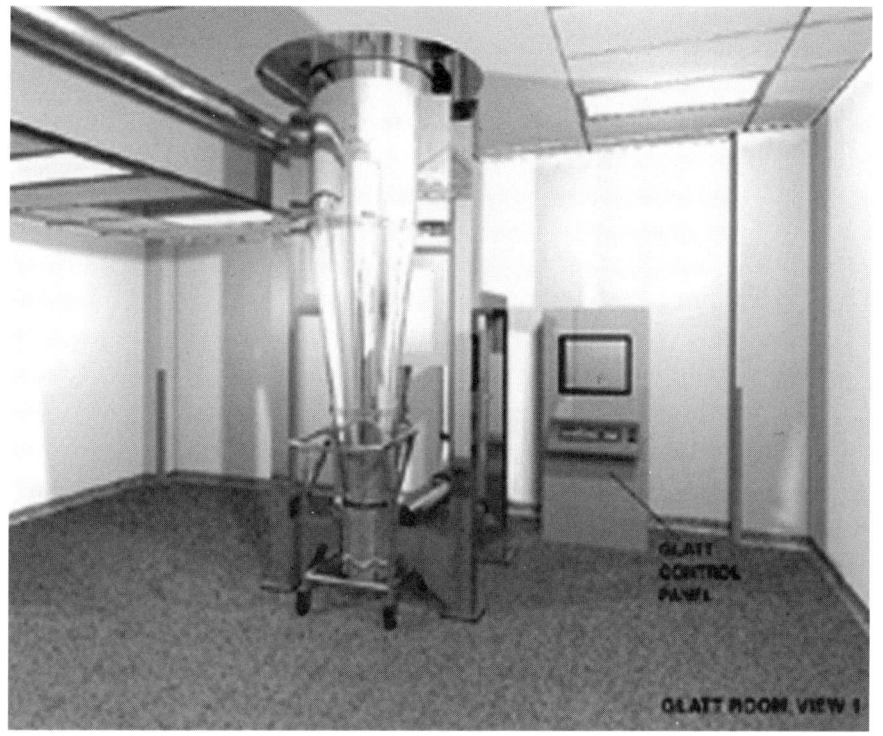

Design Process

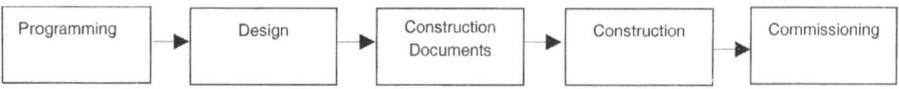

The history of pharmaceutical manufacturing facility design has been one of an increasing compliance driven requirement, as well as an understanding of how to integrate the process and mechanical systems into the facility. Many older facilities have grown over time, resulting in a confusing mixture of small rooms with circulation (hallways and corridors) that is unclear. This is a challenge from a functional, aesthetic and building code perspective in the renovation of an older facility.

The following is a photograph of a current cGMP facility:

View of a Typical cGMP Corridor

![View of a Typical cGMP Corridor]

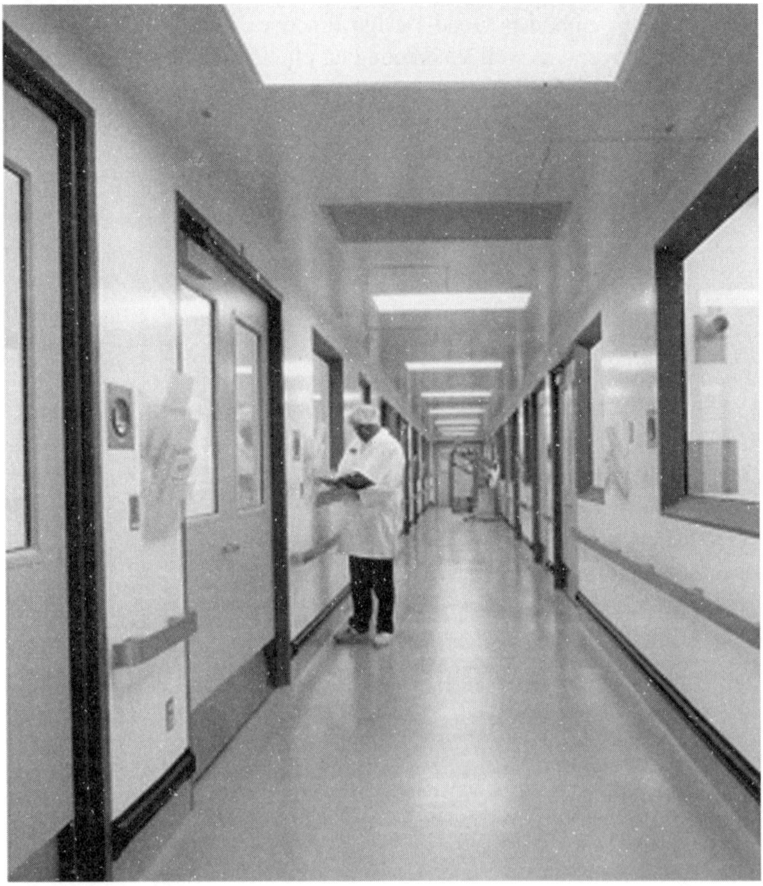

Pharmaceutical manufacturing facilities differ from assembly-line type manu-facturing facilities in that a "car manufacturing" facility is typical a more linear process. Pharmaceutical facilities have traditionally been designed around "batch" processes, which are not linear.

A pharmaceutical facility manufactures in discrete "batches" that may vary in size and in length of batch run. This requirement suggests a facility of rooms where different batches are made, rather than a linear, assembly-line type facility. Therefore the architecture of a pharmaceutical facility is not linear in the sense of an auto plant or manufacturing line of widgets. There is currently a trend toward more continuous processing which affects the layout. There have been plants designed, using vertical flow, such as the SmithKline French facility built in Milan, Italy in the 1980s, which utilized gravity for processing and stacked functions in a vertical manner.

Batch Facility Diagram

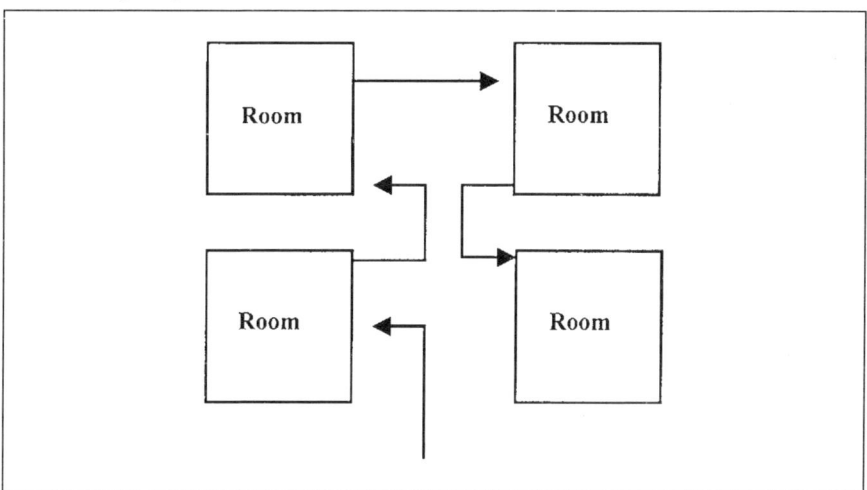

KEY CONCEPTS AND PRINCIPLES

There are several major types of pharmaceutical manufacturing facilities, which include: Oral Solid Dosage Facilities (refer to Chapter 10), Sterile Facilities (Chapter 11), and API Bulk Facility (Chapter 12).

The Society for Life Sciences Professionals (ISPE) has written several guides co-sponsored by the FDA, for the design of Oral Solid Dosage (1), Sterile Facilities (2), and API/Bulk Facilities (3).

Each facility type has common and unique aspects from an architectural per-spective. The ISPE guides have established several *key concepts* that have gained industry acceptance, including three levels of protection for facilities (3):

- Level 1: An area of general housekeeping and maintenance.
- Level 2: An area in which steps are being taken to project the exposed product and materials, which will become part of the product from contamination.

- Level 3: An area in which specific environmental conditions or materials, which become part of the product, are defined, controlled, and monitored to prevent contamination.

Other industry guides or nomenclature refer to white, gray and black areas.

- Level 1 would be equivalent to a Black Zone.
- Level 2 would be equivalent to a Grey Zone
- Level 3 would be equivalent to a White ZoneOne

The following matric compares those areas:

Level 1 (ISPE)	Level 2 (ISPE)	Level 3 (ISPE)
An area of general house-keeping and maintenance.	An area in which steps are being taken to protect the exposed product and materials, which will become part of the product from contamination.	An area in which specific environmental conditions are defined, controlled and monitored, to prevent contamination, or materials, which become part of the product.
Black Zone	**Grey Zone**	**White Zone**

A common nomenclature is to define a GMP area as any area that is used to manufacture, package or process a product or ingredient.

The ISPE Guides also established a methodology for evaluating process alternatives, which has an impact on the design layouts:

- Red Area: An area that requires specific attention.
- Yellow Area: An area that must be considered as an impact to design.
- Green Area: An area where problems usually do not occur.

Key concepts from the ISPE Guides include the identification of product protection factors such as facility flexibility: Is the facility a single product facility with no flexibility? In this type of facility, foreign contamination is the primary concern. The facility may have multiple products in dedicated equipment, where contamination between areas of the facility is a concern or the facility has multiple products in multi-use equipment, where cross contamination is the principal concern.

Understanding Product, People, and Material Flow

The key to designing a pharmaceutical manufacturing facility is to understand the product, people, and material flow issues of the facilities. In Chapter 1 we learned what the facility drivers were and that a certain output is required for the facility in terms of product. Product and material flow provide the foundation for detailed facility design (Ref. 4, p. 22).

The ISPE Oral Solid Dosage Guide (1) highlights the following key architectural concepts in terms of product flow design guidelines:

- Provide logical, direct, and sequential flow, minimizing the potential for confusion
- Minimize the moving distance; that is, the distance material has to move

• Provide adequate protection against contamination
• Provide adequate staging and access
• Provide the proper level of protection

The code of Federal Regulation CFR Title 21, subpart C Building and Facilities 211.42 outlines design issues in a general manner. For instance:

(b) Any such building shall have adequate space for the orderly placement of equipment and materials to prevent mix-ups between different components, drug product containers, closures, labeling, in-process materials, or drug products, and to prevent cross contamination. The flow of components, drug product containers, closures, labeling, in process materials and drug products through the building or buildings shall be designed to prevent cross contamination (4). The designer's challenges are to take this general requirement and create a facility which meets this general guide.

The general flow of materials in a facility does not change dramatically for different facility types. The designer's challenge is to create a design that meets these general criteria.

The following is a general flow chart of how a facility flow is created.

Diagram of Facility Flow

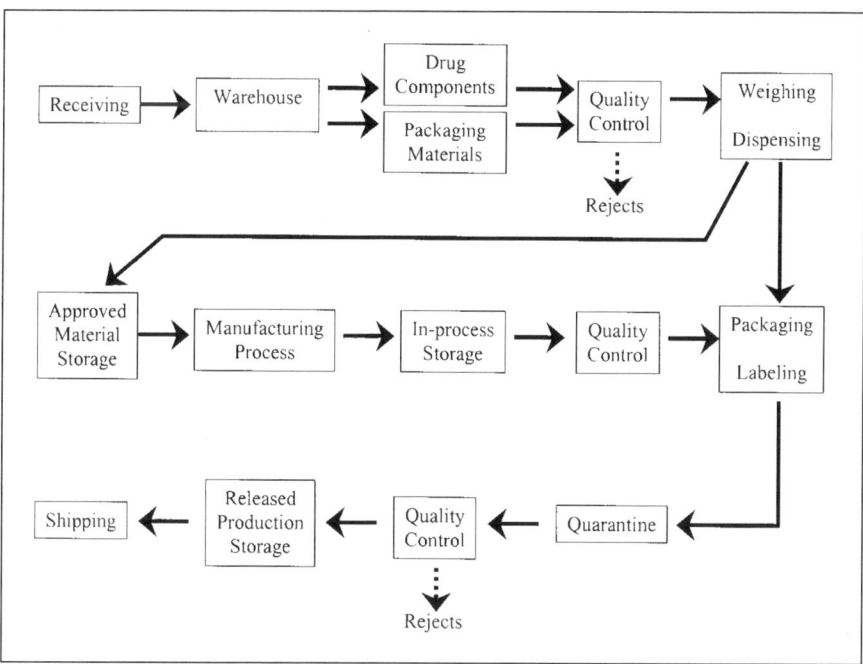

Different facility types such as Solid Dose Manufacturing, Sterile Facilities, and Bulk Facilities will have modifications to this basic flow diagram. The designer needs to understand the flow diagram before proceeding with the design. The architect/engineer should create a flow diagram at the initiation of the project that is specific for the project they are designing, and in more detail for each sub-component of the general flow.

There is discussion in the industry about exactly which product and material flows need to be "one way"; that is, where product does not cross paths. This has been referred to as "clean" and "dirty" corridors. Using "clean" and "dirty" terminology" is not recommended.

The ISPE Guide states that product flow need not be one way. One- way flow is where people or equipment move in only one direction and paths do not cross or are minimized. This increases the gross square footage of the facility, which increases the cost, but may have functional benefits. The designer and owner need to weigh the options before making a decision. The goal is to demonstrate control of the product.

Two Way Flow-Diagram

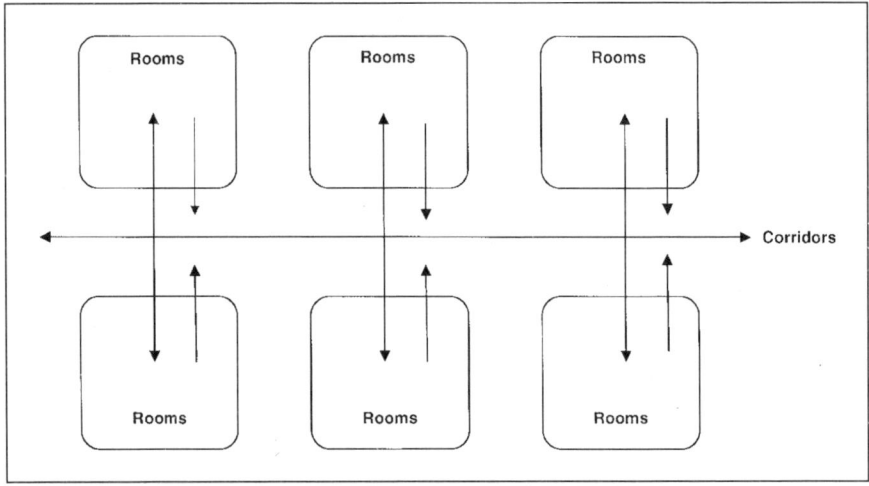

This may be achieved via one way or two way flows. The cGMPs do not specify exactly how to achieve this. The designer may work from the layout if desired, or may use operational procedures.

This may be a solution that works best for your facility, but it is not a requirement. The *requirement* is to *prevent product mix up* and to ensure *control*. You may address these issues through air control, and operating procedures. *Your philosophy may be, however, that the facility design is the best place to ensure that this critical design goal is met.* (This was discussed more fully in Chapter 2.) This approach, a **key concept**, is to utilize the physical design to ensure that mix-ups are less likely to occur.

The design of facilities that handle "potent compounds" may be affected in by which circulation scheme is chosen. (The layout of potent compound facilities is discussed in Chapter 16). Potent compounds require minimizing the chance of cross contamination in the layout of the facility.

One Way Diagram

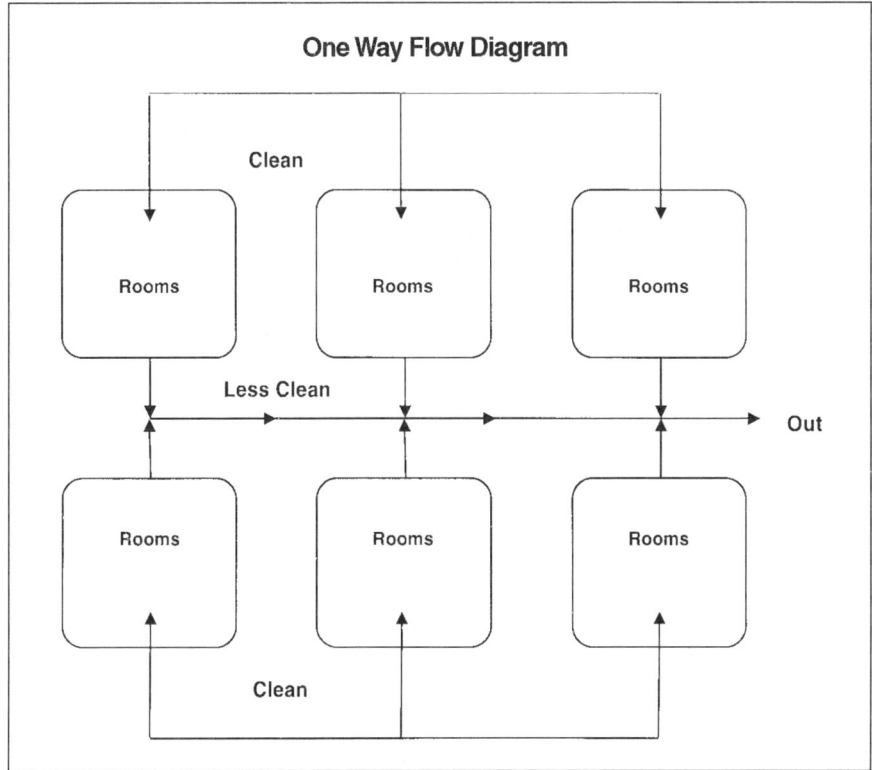

FACILITY DESIGN
Functional Areas of a Pharmaceutical Manufacturing Facility

From the generic flow diagram, there are certain areas that are common to all pharmaceutical manufacturing facilities. The following generic areas typically found in a pharmaceutical facility are briefly discussed. Each has its own design considerations as well as HVAC (heating, ventilation and air conditioning), plumbing, electrical, and finish requirements.

Shipping/Receiving Areas

Shipping/receiving areas are areas where incoming and outgoing materials for the facility are received and shipped. These areas are generally Black Areas or Level One Areas in terms of finishes.

Separate shipping/receiving areas are not a requirement (Ref. 1, p. 27), but may be utilized to prevent mix up between incoming and outgoing goods. By this we mean a physically separated shipping area and receiving area.

The components of a shipping/receiving area are the number of loading docks required, whether the trucks may or should be visible from the street, and providing security to the facility from people utilizing the loading dock. It is common to include a trucker's lavatory in the area, so that no breech of the facility is required by outside personnel.

Adequate space for staging incoming or outgoing materials is required, and can be verified by testing the layout with the number of pallets that may be anticipated in the facility. The shipping/receiving area will also contain a sampling area or weigh booth, where incoming materials may be tested. There is an increase of the use of containment booths with Hepa® Filtration for sampling booths. These booths may be pre-manufactured or custom engineered.

A Weigh Room

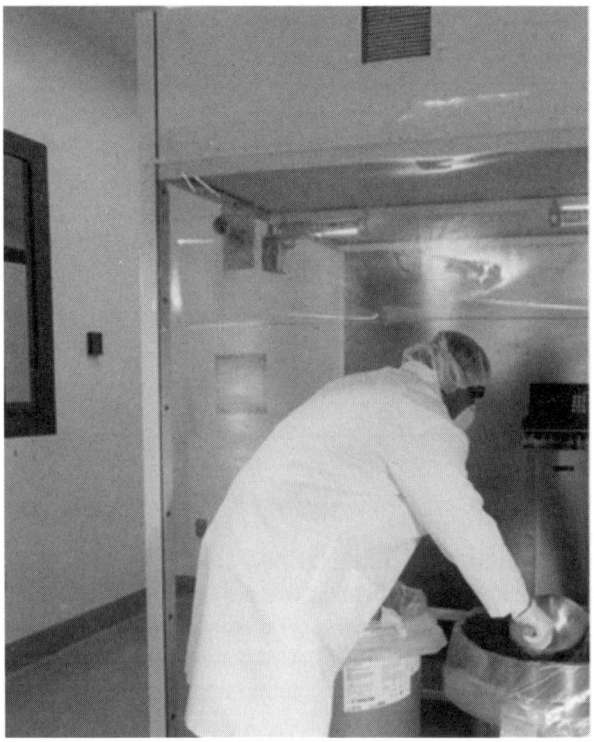

Facilities that handle narcotics require a separate vault for which requirements are specified by the Drug Enforcement Agency (Federal DEA) (4).

Warehouse

The 21 CFR Part 211.42 Design and Construction States: *(c) (1) Receipt, identification, storage and withholding from use of components, drug product containers, closures and labeling, pending the appropriate sampling, testing or examination by the quality control unit before release for manufacturing or packaging.* As mentioned, there may be products that require special storage conditions, much as temperature and humidity control, as well as regulated products, such as narcotics that will require a vault designed to DEA Standards (4).

KEY CONCEPT: Design a facility that controls materials and prevents mix-ups (1).

Each warehouse will have a quarantine area where incoming raw materials and components are stored before being released for production or packaging. This may be an area separated from other areas with walls or open fencing or by other methods such as delineation on the floor. These are just examples of the design; however, a separate area may make it easier to avoid any mix ups because of physical separation.

Warehouse Layouts

The size and capacity of the warehouse are driven by the number of pallet spaces that are required for storage of all materials. A pallet (either wood, fiberglass, or metal, usually stainless steel or aluminum) is typically 40 inches x 48 inches. The pallet is the base component of the storage system. Other material-handling containers such as bins and totes may be utilized, which will affect the warehouse racking system.

KEY CONCEPTS: Allow space for upper and lower sprinkler heads in the rack; locate them so they are not sheared off when pallet racks are installed.

The height of the building may also impact whether in-rack sprinklers are required. The architect should coordinate the sprinkler and ductwork with future racking plans to ensure that the clear heights are maintained.

There are many approaches to warehouse layout. Some facilities rely on the architectural design to dedicate certain physical areas using partitions, or wire mesh, and/or coding and tracking of materials. Again, the physical design can be as simple as outlines on the floor or mesh partitions.

How to Layout a Warehouse: The key driver is to determine the racking system to be utilized and the aisle widths required.

From the aisle widths and spacing of the pallets, a planning module may be established to create a structural grid. The height of the warehouse will be determined by forklift capabilities. It is important to be aware that the building height may be governed by the local zoning codes, and height limitations as well as clearances for sprinklers from the top of pallets may be governed by your insurance carrier and the NFPA (National Fire Protection Association). The following codes should be considered:

- NFPA 230: Standard for the Fire Protection of Storage
- NFPA 30: Flammable and Combustible Liquids Code
- NFPA 13: Installation of Sprinkler Systems

Airlocks

Airlocks are a physical solution to segregate and separate different functional areas, and to control airflow and pressurization. They may have manual or automated inter-locked doors.

Weighing and Dispensing Areas

Weighting and dispensing areas are those areas where the incoming product is weighed and dispensed. Recent trends in sampling and dispensing areas have been to utilize pre-manufactured down flow booths, which have self contained Hepa® Filtered fans, and which can be designed to limit the exposure limits OEL (occupational exposure limits) to the user of the booth. (Refer to Chapter 16 for detailed discussion on containment facilities.) There are a number of manufacturers that make these booths.

Staging Areas

Staging areas are those areas where the material is staged for batches. It is important to create a design layout of staging areas and anticipate the number of pallets, drums, and so forth that may be in the area to allow adequate space. This staging area requirement needs to be determined with the process engineering department depending on the batch requirements.

Manufacturing Operations

The manufacturing areas are driven by the selection of the process equipment that is required to manufacture the product, and the space needed for maintenance of the process equipment.

The room or area requirements are built around the requirements of the process equipment. The layout of the room is determined by the size of equipment and the flow of product between the rooms. The rooms then become the building blocks for the facility. The process equipment must be laid out in the room, with associated staging and personnel requirements, as well as all utility and access space for maintenance requirements. Manufacturing operations may be organized vertically also, depending on the equipment.

Oral Solid Dosage Facility: The following are the unit operators that typically occur in an OSD (Oral Solid Dosage) facility. Blending Areas, Milling Areas, Granulation Areas, Tablet Compression and Capsule Filing Areas, and Coating Areas.

Aseptic Facilities: Aseptic facilities will have areas for formulation, filling, lyophilization, sealing, capping, inspection and storage. Facilities may be multi-product or single product facilities, which will effect the layout and organization.

Packaging Areas and Labeling Areas: The packaging area is where the product in its final form, is packaged for distribution. The packaging area is laid out to accommodate width and length of the packaging line. There are two types of packaging areas, Primary and Secondary Packaging.

> *KEY CONCEPTS:* Understand the packaging line philosophy; provide adequate staging for materials and finished product; provide visual connection between the packaging lines; provide adequate storage space for packaging materials.

Primary Packaging Area: This is an area where the product may be exposed, such as in a tableting facility. These areas are generally open areas where automated packaging lines (equipment) are located.

Secondary Packaging Area: This is an area where the product is not exposed, and is in its final vial, bottle, etc., but may be packaged for shipment. This is referred to as a "closed system." These areas are generally open areas where secondary packaging may occur in an automated form or by hand, depending on the scale of the facility.

Architectural layouts need to consider the space required for each line, as well as the space required for the cartons of packaging materials, as well as the finished goods.

There is a trend for separating packaging lines to minimize mix-up and confusion of batches, by separating packaging lines with full or one-half height partitions. This is not a requirement, however, but is recommended as a good design practice. It is architecturally important to keep these areas as open as possible. This can be achieved by using partitions with glass to the ceiling, and creating views to the outside if possible.

Packaging Line with Partitions

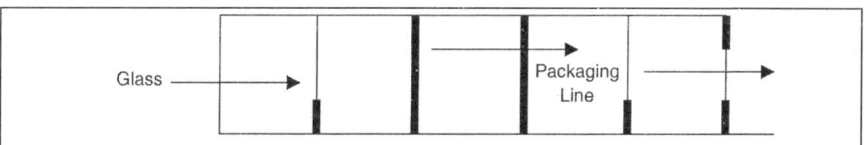

Labeling Areas: These are rooms where labels are stored and prepared for the packaging lines. These rooms should be secured. *A packaging area may be very simple, from a manual line, to a very complex automated packaging line* (3). Lighting is extremely critical in these areas, as the operators are performing tasks that, although extremely repetitive, are critical.

> *KEY CONCEPT:* Provide views to the exterior with natural light.

Potent Compounds

An API or drug substance is usually defined by an OEL/OEG of less than 20 μg/m3/8 hours. Utilizing potent compounds in facilities have special layout requirements and design considerations, and are further described in Chapter 16.

Potent Compound Suite

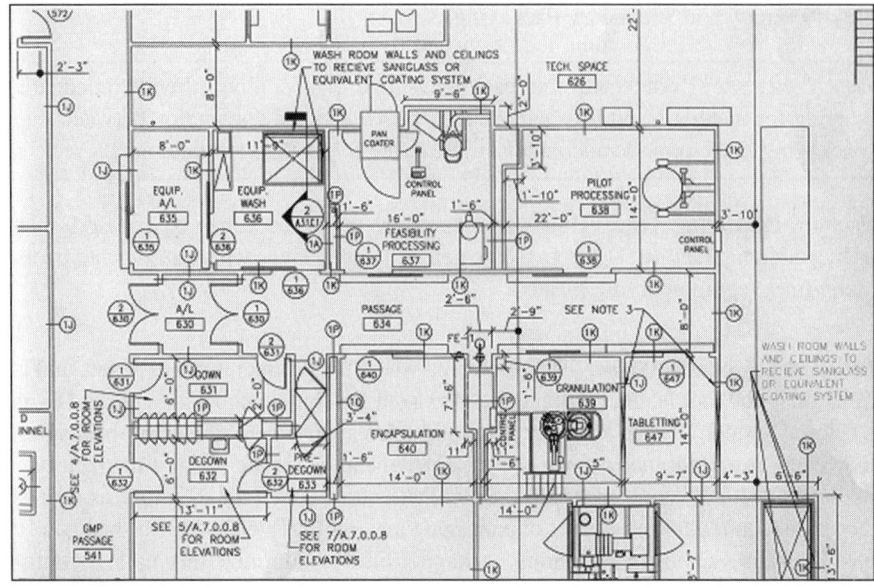

Support Areas

Lockers/Gowning Rooms/Changing Rooms

Locker rooms are designed to accommodate the needs of employees and the "gowning philosophy" of the facility. There may be several levels of gowning in a facility. Employees should progress from factory change to clean change in a logical progression. A changing/locker room is to support the changing for employees. The architectural design of the area can reinforce the garment and changing philosophy of the facility, with step over benches, and clear and logical progression. The following is a bubble diagram of the flow from street clothes through the facility:

Growing Diagram

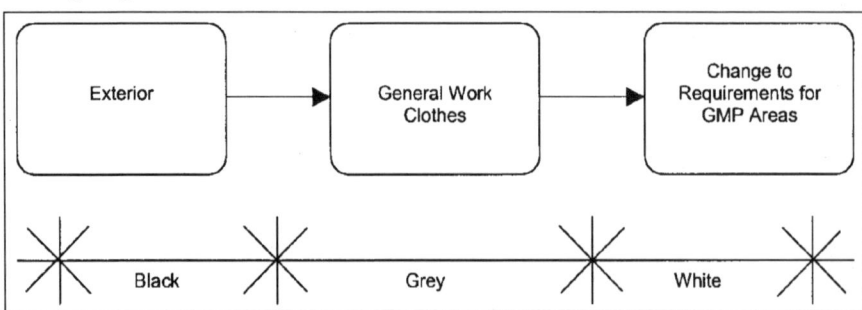

There may be a changing area between the Level 1 area (black) and then from the (grey) Level 2 areas to the (white) Level 3 or GMP areas. The GMP areas are the areas with the strictest gowning requirements.

The ISPE Guide states: *Gowning may be required to protect the product, operator or the environment.* The design of an area for gowning for potent compounds or sterile facilities differs from that of a solid dosage facility. There is generally a degowning area in potent compounds/sterile facilities, as well as air showers for decontamination. Gowning is also required for laboratory areas, where generally safety glasses and lab coats are required. To prevent cross contamination, strict procedures must be established for personnel traffic from these restricted areas (such as toilet, and cafeteria and break areas).

The Quality Control Laboratory should be located in a central area, easily accessible to the plant but also accessible to the laboratory personnel from the main entrance. Typical laboratory layout needs to allow for multiple HPLCs (High Pressure Liquid Chromatography) and other bench-top testing equipment. Unlike research laboratories, the design layout is unlikely to change dramatically from month to month, because procedures are fully established.

DETAILS: IMPLICATIONS FOR PERFORMANCE IN THE DESIGN OF THE FACILITY

There are several critical and generally recognized phases in the design of a pharmaceutical facility that are both contractual and procedural.

The phases generally organize the design from problem seeking to problem solving and then construction, commissioning and validation. It is critical to include the commissioning and validation teams as part of the early design teams.

Phases in the Design Process

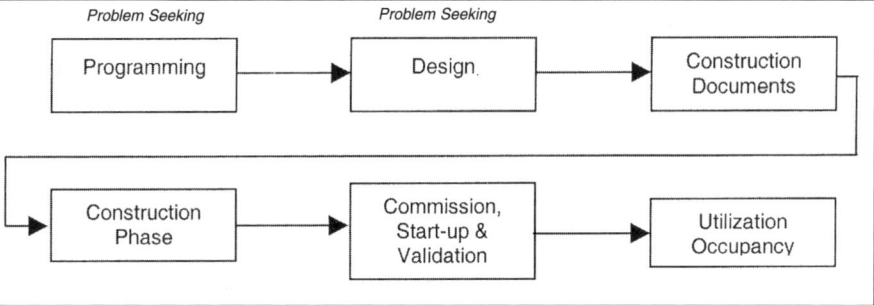

Programming Phases

The programming phase is the "problem-seeking" phase. During this phase, the design criteria for the facility, not the solutions, are defined. Since manufacturing facilities are process driven, the process diagrams need to be defined. The next task is to create a space program, which lists the spaces and requirements for each space in the facility. Interviewing the facility users by functional department based on their needs to meet the facility output, creates a functional space program. The following is an example of a typical space program.

The equipment layout determines the space for that equipment required for production. A layout is required to adequately understand that actual space required:

Typical Space Program

The space program may be customized to add spaces to capture other requirements.

				2002			2005									
NO	SPACE	Size		NSF	Per	No	NSF	Per	No	NSF	Ceiling Height	Floor	Wall	Wall Type	Clg	Rating	Bench Info
4,000	R & D Pilot Plant & Processing Area XP																
4,001	High Shear Mixer/Granulator Room No. 1	16	×17	272	0	1.0	272	0	0.0	0	10'4"	Epoxy	Epoxy Paint CMU	FULL CMU	Epoxy Paint GYP.	CL I DIV I	—
4,002	High Shear Mixer/Granulator Room No. 2	16	×17	272	0	1.0	272	0	0.0	0	10'4"	Epoxy	Epoxy Paint CMU	FULL CMU	Epoxy Paint GYP.	CL I DIV I	—
4,003	Liquid Preparation Room	6	×13	78	0	1.0	156	0	0.0	0	14'0"	Epoxy	Epoxy Paint CMU	FULL CMU	Epoxy Paint GYP.	CL I DIV I	—
4,004	Fluid Bed Room No. 1	12	×18	216	0	1.0	216	0	0.0	0	18'0"	Epoxy	Epoxy Paint CMU	FULL CMU	Epoxy Paint GYP.	CL I DIV I	—
4,005	Fluid Bed Room No. 2	12	×18	216	0	1.0	216	0	0.0	0	18'0"	Epoxy	Epoxy Paint CMU	FULL CMU	Epoxy Paint GYP.	CL I DIV I	—
4,006	XP Airlock	8	×11	88	0	1.0	88	0	0.0	0	9'0"	Epoxy	Epoxy Paint CMU	FULL CMU	Epoxy Paint GYP.	CL I DIV I	—
4,007	Tray Dryer Room	12	×15	180	0	1.0	180	0	0.0	0	9'0"	Epoxy	Epoxy Paint CMU	FULL CMU	Epoxy Paint GYP.	CL I DIV I	—
4,008	Tray Dryer Room	12	×15	180	0	1.0	180	0	0.0	0	9'0"	Epoxy	Epoxy Paint CMU	FULL CMU	Epoxy Paint GYP.	CL I DIV I	—
	Subtotal				0	9.0	1.580	0	0.0	0							

> *KEY CONCEPT:* The space program is calculated in terms of Net Square Feet (NSF), which is the space inside the room.

NSF Space Inside a Room

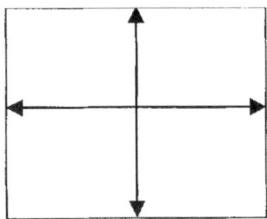

Gross Square Feet (GFS) is generally the total square footage of the building to the exterior wall. There are different definitions that vary slightly (refer to BOMA guidelines, Building Owners and Management Association). GSF as the total size of your building to the outside of the exterior wall.

KEY CONCEPT: Gross Square Feet (GSF) is the total square feet calculated to the outside of the wall.

Gross Square Feet (GSF)

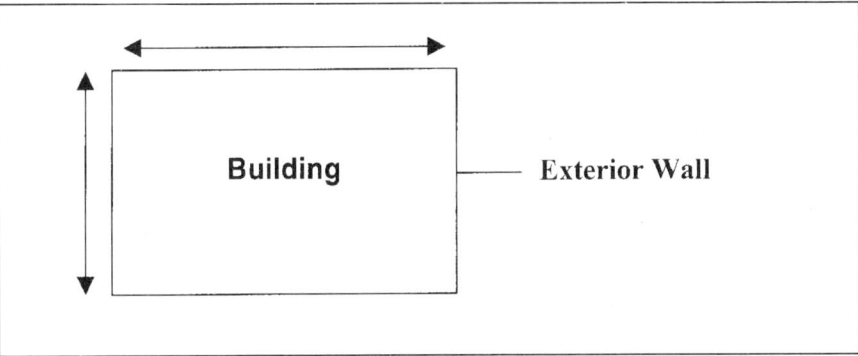

The ratio of Net Square Feet/Gross Square Feet (NSF/GSF) = Building Efficiency. This is a useful tool when you are trying to determine how big your facility is from your space program.

Layout

Allow and understand clearances that the equipment requires for operation, servicing and removal from the space.

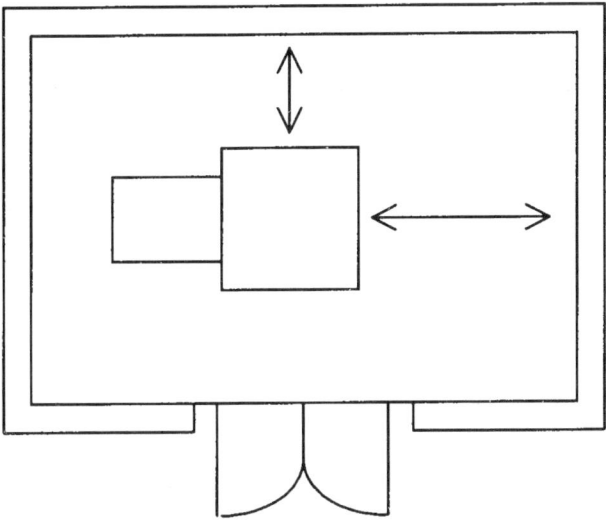

Example:

You must create a space program with the following summary of the key areas in the facility:

Space or Area	NSF	Less Efficient	Middle	Most Efficient	GFS (Less Efficient)	GFS (Middle)	GFS (Most Efficient)
Warehouse	30,000	80%	85%	90%	37,500	35,294	33,333
Shipping Receiving	5,000	65%	75%	80%	7,692	6,667	6,250
Manufacturing	40,000	50%	55%	60%	80,000	72,727	66,667
Packaging	20,000	55%	60%	65%	36,364	33,333	30,769
Quality Control Laboratory	5,000	50%	55%	60%	10,000	9,091	8,333
Office Support	15,000	55%	60%	65%	27,273	25,000	23,077
Total NSF	115,000						
Total Facility Size (GSF)					198,829	182,112	168,429

NSF = Net square feet; GSF = gross square feet..

Conclusion:

The facility of 115,000 NSF may range in size from 168,429 to 198,829 GSF before you test the layout.

When you have established the GSF (gross square feet) of the building, you can then apply a range of costs per functional area and begin to understand what the costs of the facility are.

Lab Card

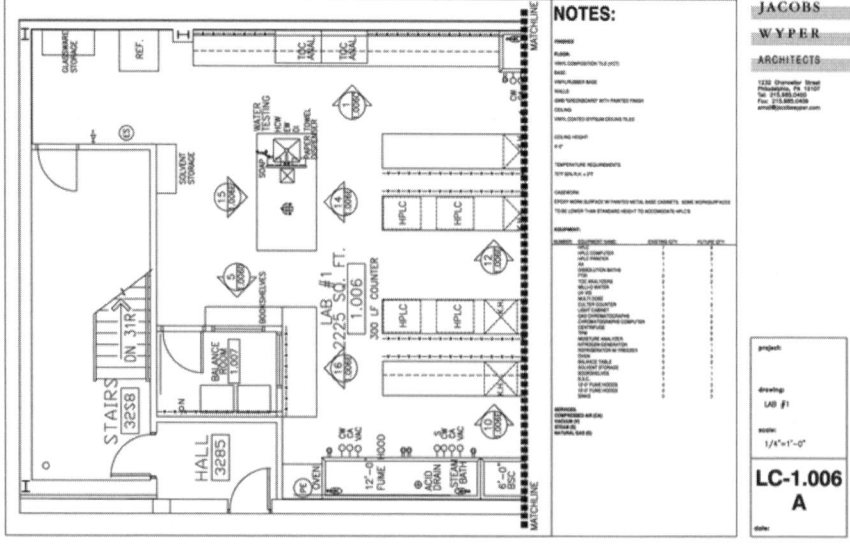

Programming Phase: Lab Cards

The next step for the architect in the programming phase is to create *lab cards*, which are defined as room layouts for each important functional area. Lab cards contain all the important data about the room for finishes, ceiling heights, equipment layout and all the MEP requirements. This is done before the actual facility design is started. A typical lab card format is illustrated below. The lab card is critical in the design of pharmaceutical manufacturing facilities because it captures all the users' needs and the engineering criteria at a very early date.

Zoning Codes and Building Codes

Zoning and building codes impact the form, design, layout, and construction of a pharmaceutical facility.

Zoning Codes

The zoning codes should be viewed as the "macro codes." They cover the allowable use, amount of site coverage, building height, and parking requirements. (Refer to Chapter 15 for details.)

KEY CONCEPTS:

• *Allowed Use:* Each code has zoned its township's land into areas for different uses, such as residential, commercial, manufacturing, and R&D. In evaluating a site, the first issue to determine is if the manufacturing use that you are proposing is permitted by the zoning code.

• *Height and Area Limitations:* The zoning codes determine the area and height limitations on the site. This may be through a variety of methods, but they typically determine the building footprint and the required (minimum) and the total coverage (maximum) of building and parking, which is the impervious surface of both the building and parking areas. The height limitations are important as to the total height of the building and whether penthouses and other appurtenances are allowed. Some height restrictions may vary from the set back toward the center of the plant site.

• *Hazardous Materials:* Many zoning codes have language that references the codes used for storage and other functions of hazardous materials. It is important to be aware of these sections of the codes.

Building Codes

The building codes form the physical characteristics of your project.

KEY CONCEPTS:

• *Use Group Classification:* The use groups define the area limitations and construction type depending on use. The following areas are typical use groups in a facility:
B—Business for Office and Laboratory Areas
F—Manufacturing
S—Storage and Warehouse
H—1-5 for Hazardous Materials

Continued

The use group determines the height of the building, number of stories, and area allowed for each construction type.

- *Types of Construction:* Types of construction such as Type 1, non-combustible protected, and Type 2 protected and unprotected, determines how the building is to be constructed. The more fire protection you use, the larger areas you are allowed to build. You need to balance the construction costs with the type of construction.
- *Hazardous Areas:* Hazardous areas are determined by the amount of hazardous materials present and if there is a chanced of deflagration.

The primary purpose of Building Codes is to govern the Life/Safety Issues in construction. The Code section in Chapter 18 fully covers this area, but there are several key areas that effect the design and layout of the facility. Most municipalities have adopted National Codes, but they may also have local supplements that take precedence as well as the issues of the legal code official and fire marshall.

Designing the Facility

The Programming Phase has determined the project requirements for the flow of people, product, and materials. The Building and Zoning Codes have determined general area and size requirements. Now, the architectural design organizes the facility into a two- and three-dimensional layout, and tests the criteria based on the program. Several steps can be generally described:

Establish a Planning/Structural Module for the Layout

This model may work with various functional areas of your facility. Try to create a structural grid that will work for all areas of your facility; that is, use a base size, such as 30'-0" × 40'-0". This needs to work with your layout, as well as and in determining what is the most efficient structural grid in terms of tons of steel utilized.

Establish a Planning Module
The module size will vary.

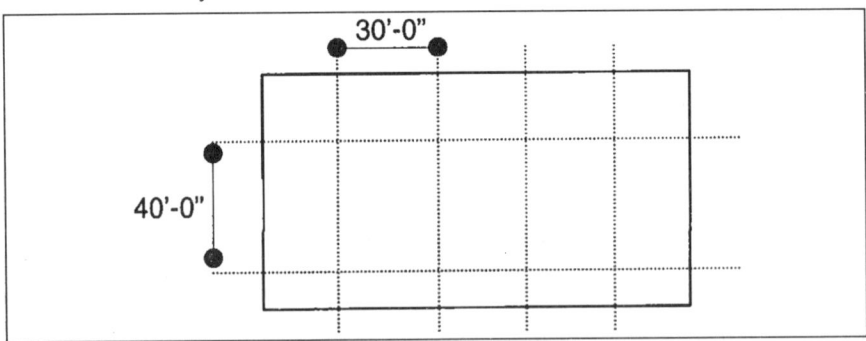

Create block plans of functional areas in GSF or bubble diagrams in actual GSF illustrated below, of the areas:

Bubble Diagram or Block Diagram to Scale

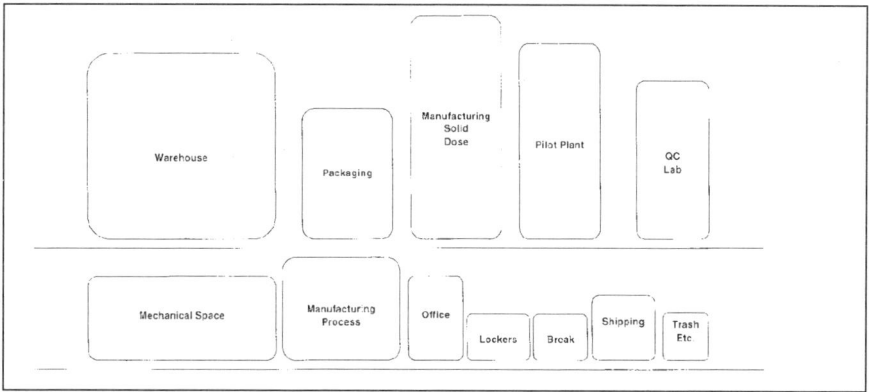

MANUFACTURING BUILDING COMPONENTS
Determine a mechanical distribution requirement for your facility:

Roof Mounted Equipment
Least desirable, lowest cost, but roof mounted equipment is functional.

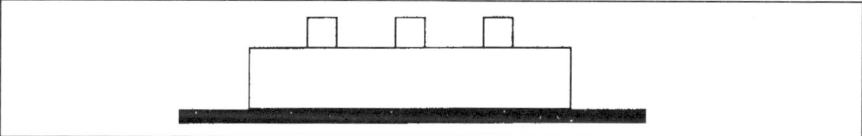

Penthouse
Penthouse is defined as an enclosed space on or partially below the roof of the building, where mechanical equipment is enclosed.

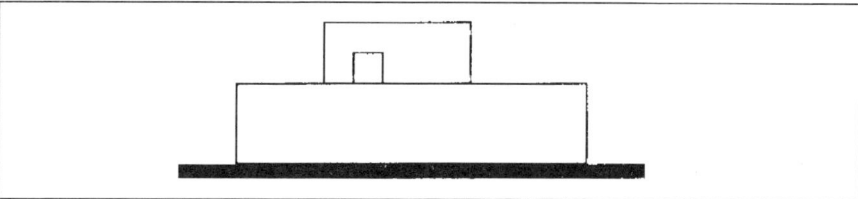

Interstitial
Interstitial is a mechanical access floor completely above the manufacturing area that allows access from above.

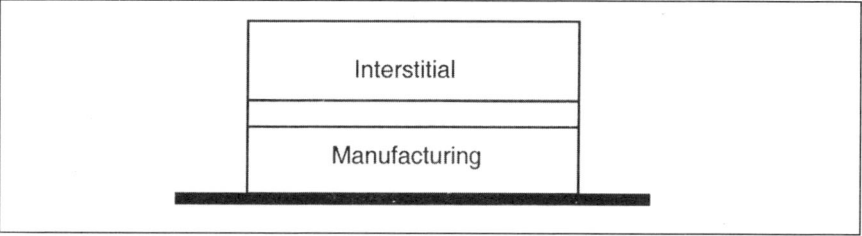

Walkable Ceilings
Walkable ceilings allow "walking" on all the ceilings to a manufacturing area and access from. Above.

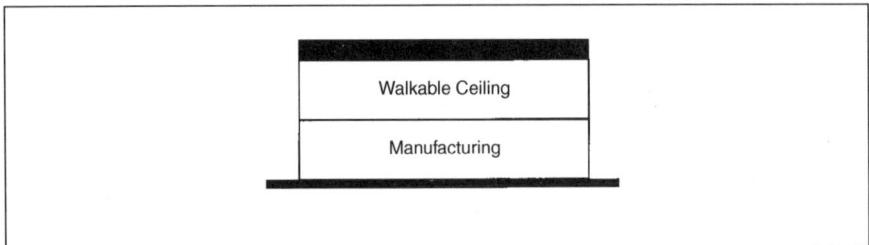

    The integration and allowing of adequate space for the MEP (mechanical, electrical and plumbing). Systems is critical in the design, and may be modified in the future.

DESIGNING THE FACILITY
After understanding the block plan process flow and mechanical concept, the designer will create a concept for the circulation and growth of the facility.

    For instance the diagram below illustrates a concept for the main organization of the facility along a "center spine."

ORGANIZATION
Using the general process flow diagram, we now want to organize the functional areas to test the adjacencies and product flow. The following is an example of a bubble diagram that tests the block area requirements and circulation. From your circulation, add our block plans to test your design.

Circulation Diagram

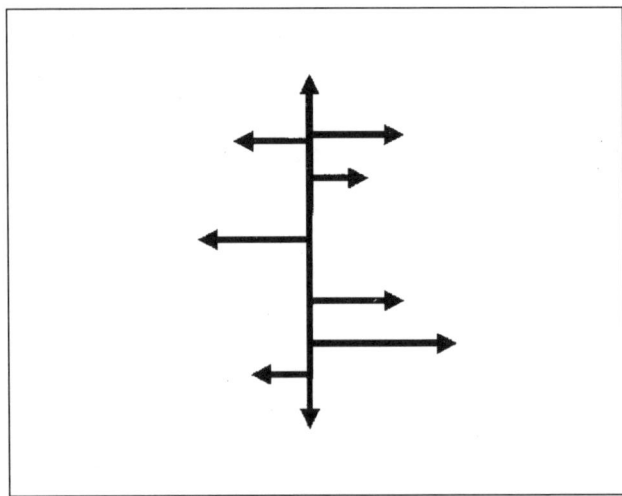

Vertical Concept

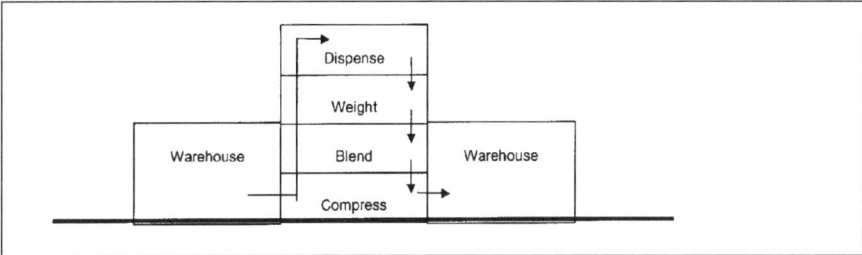

Vertical Concept

In the 1970s, SmithKline French developed a vertical solid dosage facility in Milan, Italy, designed by Willie Lhoest: "This building has four upper floors and a ground floor designed to maximize the use of growing feeding procedures and product starting in the dispensary and finishing in the packaging area" (5).

The use of gravity should be considered in areas such as compression and encapsulation.

Establish a concept for the facility:

• Linear
• U shaped
• L shaped

Establish the Circulation

Using the above diagram, we now look at the "circulation"; that is, the corridors as "streets" to access the functional area of the facility. The circulation-only as a diagram may look as follows:

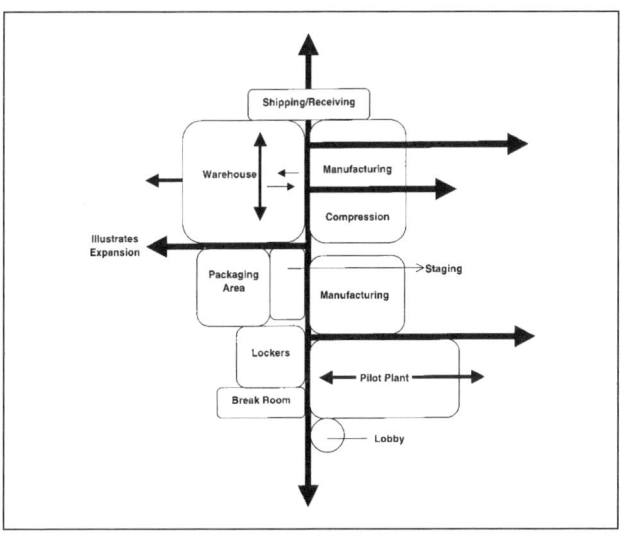

Using this diagram, the facility should be tested for the ability to expand the functional areas, as well as to consider how areas could be renovated in the future.

Locate your break rooms on outside walls from the block plan and established circulation. The program can be "test fit" into the facility (that is, the initial layout of rooms and staging areas) based on the approved program and flow diagrams may be completed.

The floor plan and building section can now be tested against the criteria established during the programming phase, to confirm that the product and process flows work, and that a mechanical concept, if established, works for the facility as well.

It is important that MEP engineering create "mechanical concepts" at this early phase.

> KEY CONCEPTS: Determine at an early phase the amount of space required for the air handling units, compressed air systems, water systems, electrical systems, and so forth. The engineer should create schematic layouts of this equipment at the early phases, so the adequate space is provided and a destruction concept established.

What Will the Facility Look Like?

The image of the facility, both from the exterior and interior, needs to be discussed at the earliest phase. The cost of the building exterior should be identified so that the designer can present options. Manufacturing facilities should present a clean and crisp exterior that reflects the "clean" nature of the operation.

This may be achieved via a variety of materials—from metal panel to brick or other masonry—to create an exterior that may be part of a campus or as a stand-alone building.

DESIGN DETAILS AND MATERIAL FINISHES

The detailing and material finish selections in the design of pharmaceutical manufacturing facilities are critical to the final building success. There are no specifically approved cGMP materials; rather, there are materials in use that have become the current standards. The FDA does not certify or endorse a certain caulk or paint product.

Considerations in the selection of finishes for pharmaceutical facilities should include the following. For instance, the ISPE Oral Solid Dosage Guide identifies:

- Durability
- Cleanability
- Functionality
- Maintainability
- Cost effectiveness

The finishes selected should also be based on the functional areas of the facility. The ISPE Guides have established suggested levels of finishes for different functional areas. The purpose of this is to help prevent the escalation in costs of facilities trying to anticipate what may be approved and accepted. This may be used as a base reference to select materials appropriate to your facility's needs and budgets. The following is a matrix of finishes we recommend for different functional areas, with links to these products.

AstraZeneca Manufacturing Dining Facility

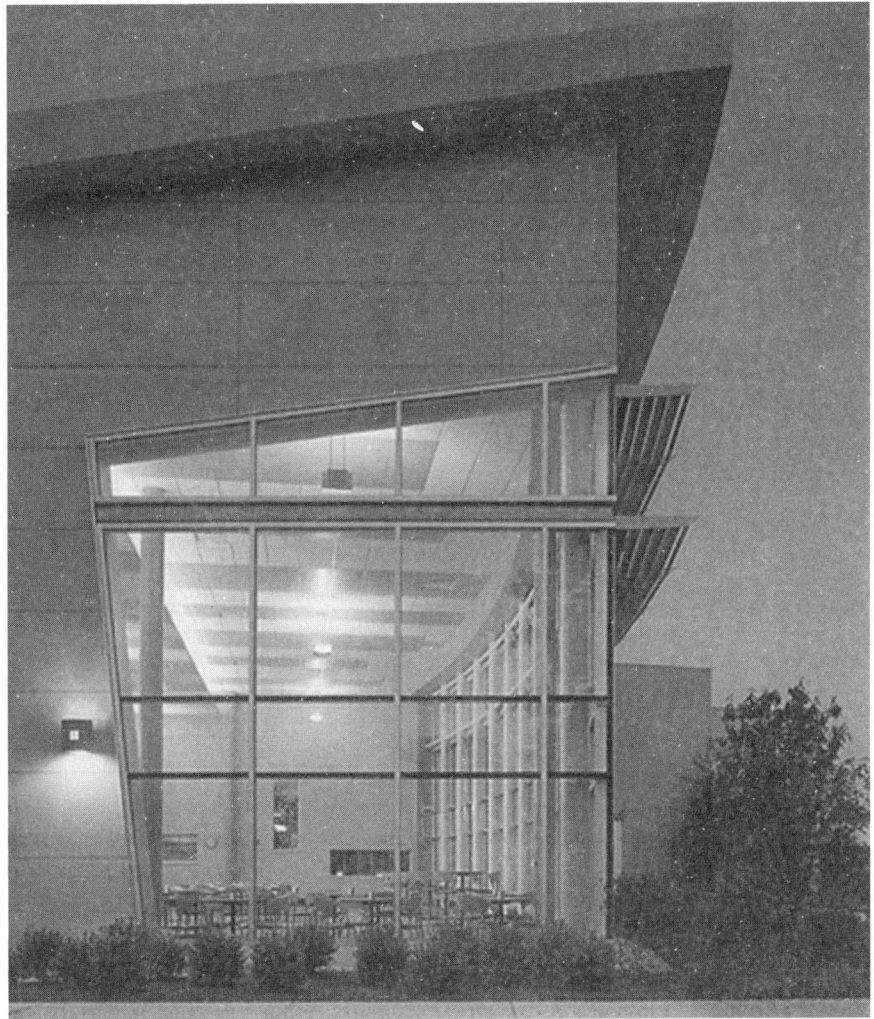

Architects: Jacobs/Wyper Architects, LLP.

Area	Walls	Floors	Base	Ceiling	Details/Lesson Learned
Shipping Area	CMU or gypsum wall or equivalent area needs to withstand abuse. Epoxy paint on walls is not required.	Concrete with sealer, or painted are minimum area needs to withstand forklift traffic. (Note: If you do more than seal the concrete select a material that can withstand fork lift traffic.)	Vinyl base is adequate.	Ceiling is not required but is recommended; a 2x4 lay-in ceiling with standard acoustical tile is acceptable.	Roll up exterior doors Dock levels Ballard to protect covers
Warehouse	CMU with block filler and semi-gloss paint Use gypsum wall in traffic area	Concrete with sealer, or painted are minimum area needs to withstand forklift traffic. (Note: If you do more than seal the concrete select a material that can withstand fork lift traffic	Vinyl base is adequate.	Ceiling not required but should be considered for GMP warehouse. Recast of AC and humidity control.	Coordinate sprinklers, ductwork, and lighting.
Packaging Area	CMU with epoxy paint Impact-resistant gypsum wall with epoxy paint	VCT (vinyl) composition tile is acceptable. Seamless vinyl can be used.	Vinyl base.	2x4 acoustical ceiling Acoustic quality	Use glass walls between packaging area to create openness. Ensure foot candles are adequate. Create ceiling height in proportion to the space.
Manufacturing Area	CMU with epoxy paint (not allowed in England) Impact-resistant drywall with epoxy paint Prefabricated metal wall panels Seamless vinyl	Epoxy terrazzo Board cast epoxy Seamless vinyl	Epoxy terrazzo Board cast epoxy Seamless vinyl Utilize finish detail for sterile facilities.	Vinyl coated gypsum panels in ceiling grid For sterile facility, utilize flush ceiling (drywall, metal).	Utilize cove details on floor, wall, and ceiling intersections for sterile facilities. (Nice to have for solid dose but not required.)

Detailing of Pharmaceutical Facilities

Architectural details are required where dissimilar materials meet. Since details are what you actually see, it is important to spend time and attention in developing these details. There are no FDA approved details, only details that have been developed that help meet the goals of cleanability, durability, maintainability, and cost. Following are some typical details that are utilized in a pharmaceutical facility.

There is a **trend** to utilize high impact drywall in facilities.

KEY CONCEPT: Know where a room will be washed down with a hose verses wiped down. A wall that needs to withstand a hose is more expensive and needs to utilize different materials than a "wipe down."

Details

The following are typical door and interior window details.

(Non-GMP) Standard Window Frame

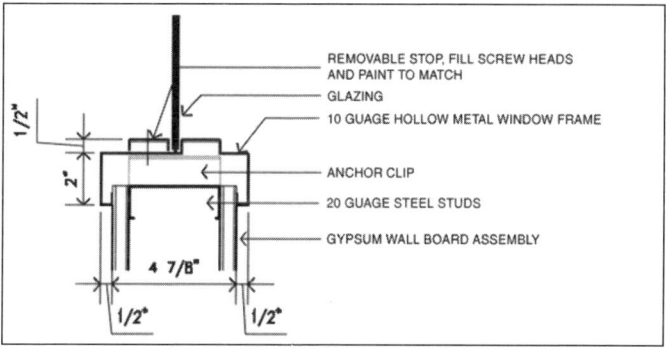

Sloping Sill, Single Glazed GMP Window for Oral Solid Dosage (OSD) Areas

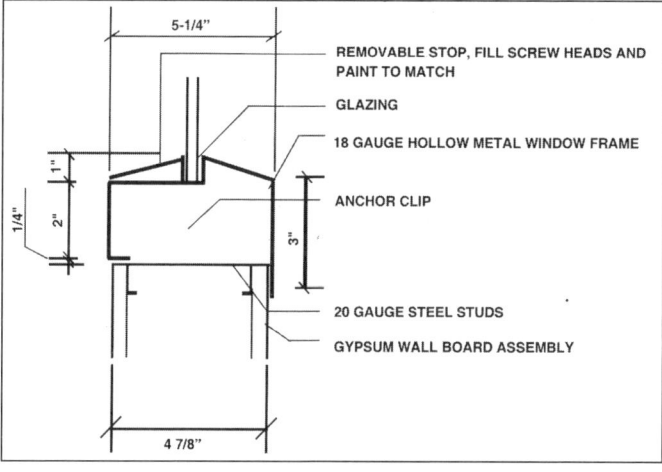

Flush, Double Glazed Window

This detail is used for sterile facilities where no ledge is designed.

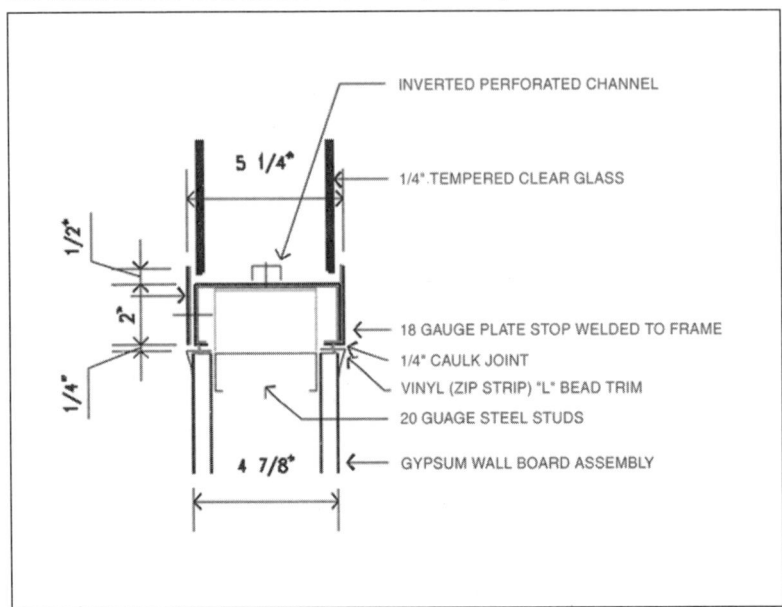

INVERTED PERFORATED CHANNEL

5 1/4"

1/4" TEMPERED CLEAR GLASS

1/2"

2"

18 GAUGE PLATE STOP WELDED TO FRAME

1/4" CAULK JOINT

VINYL (ZIP STRIP) "L" BEAD TRIM

20 GUAGE STEEL STUDS

1/4"

4 7/8"

GYPSUM WALL BOARD ASSEMBLY

Flush Window Detail

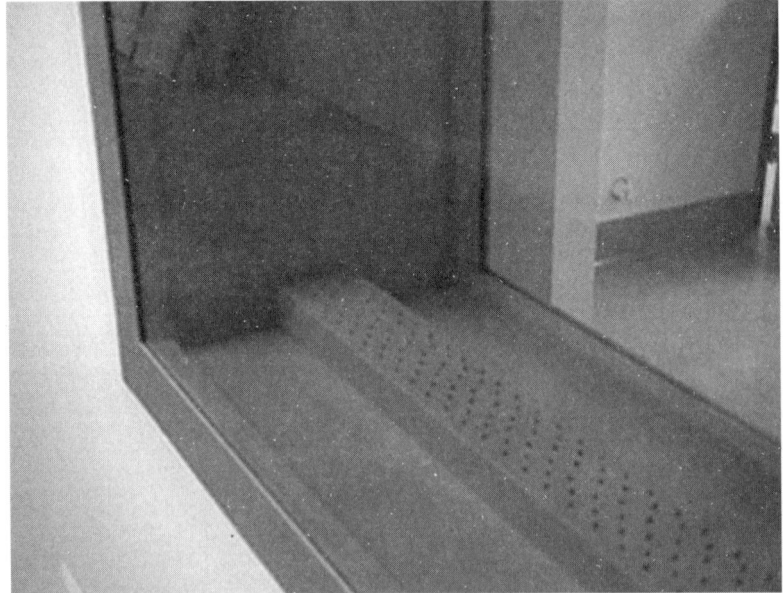

(Non-GMP) Standard Door Frame

This standard doorframe has a small ledge.

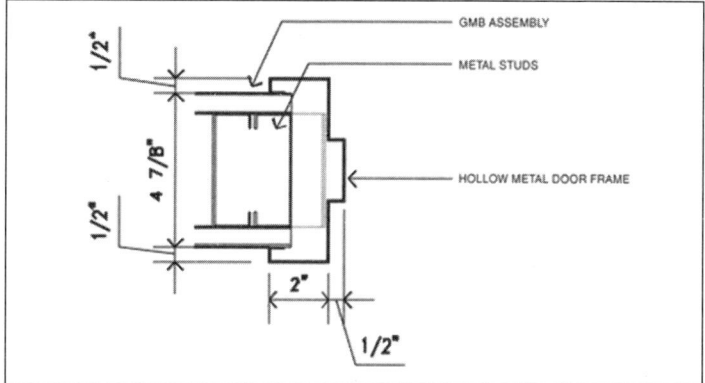

Flush Door Frame

This door detail is utilized where a flush condition is desired.

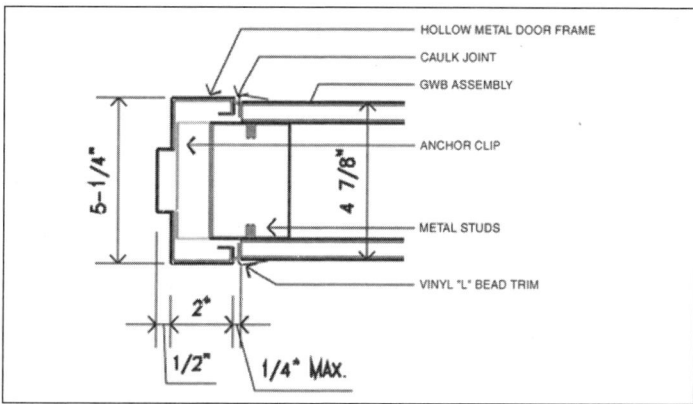

Flush Base Detail with Epoxy Flooring

Achieving a flush base detail is difficult with drywall. This detail is more typically used for sterile facilities.

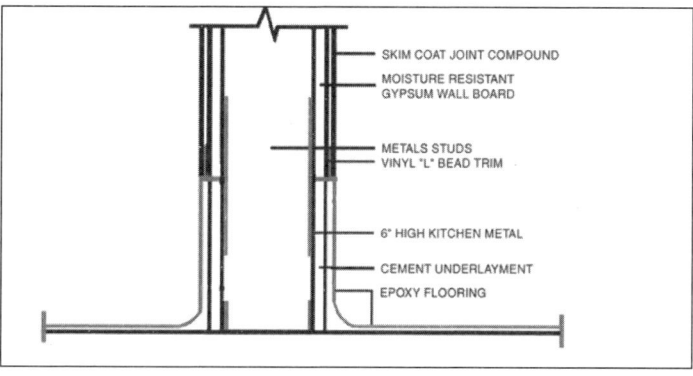

Semi-Flush Base Detail
This detail is less difficult to construct, and leaves a very small ledge where the epoxy meets the way.

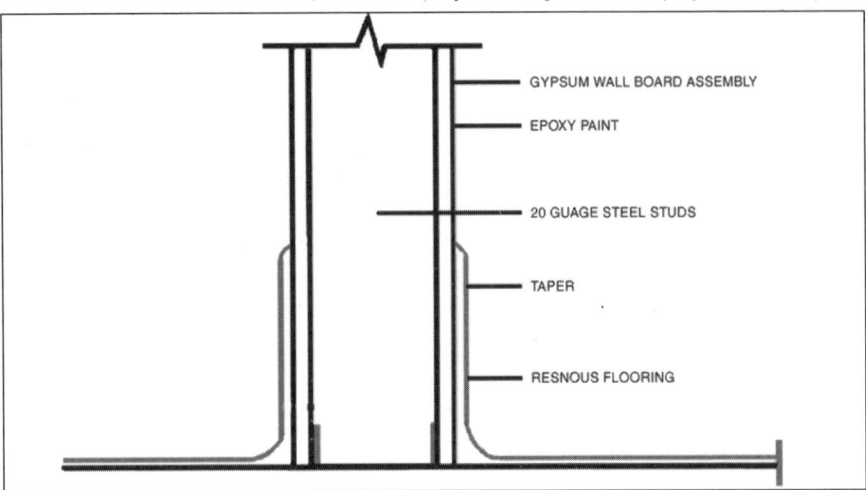

GYPSUM WALL BOARD ASSEMBLY

EPOXY PAINT

20 GUAGE STEEL STUDS

TAPER

RESNOUS FLOORING

Wall Bumper Detail
Wall bumpers are critical to maintain walls in good condition from impact from carts, panels, etc.

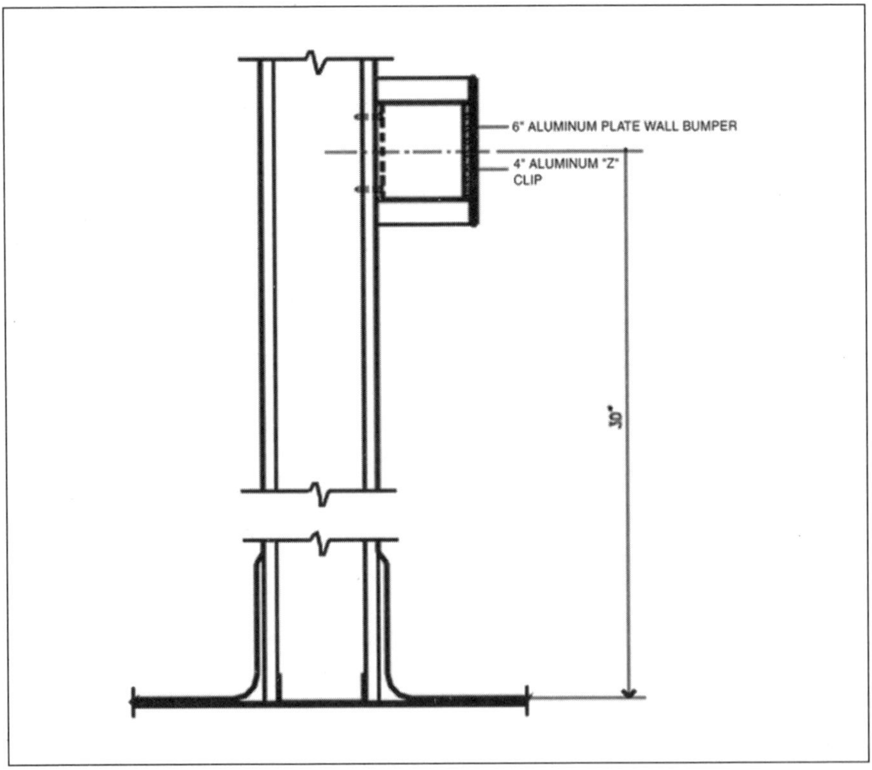

6" ALUMINUM PLATE WALL BUMPER

4" ALUMINUM "Z" CLIP

30"

Service Panel

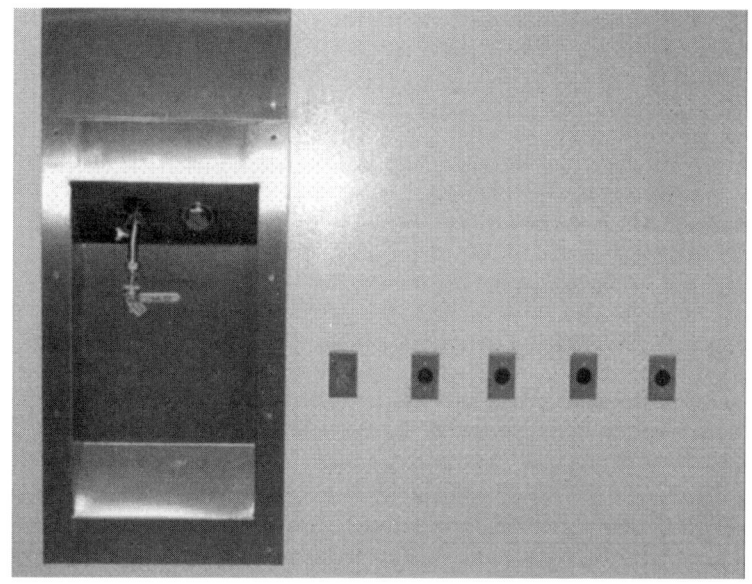

Interior Glass Windows and Skylights

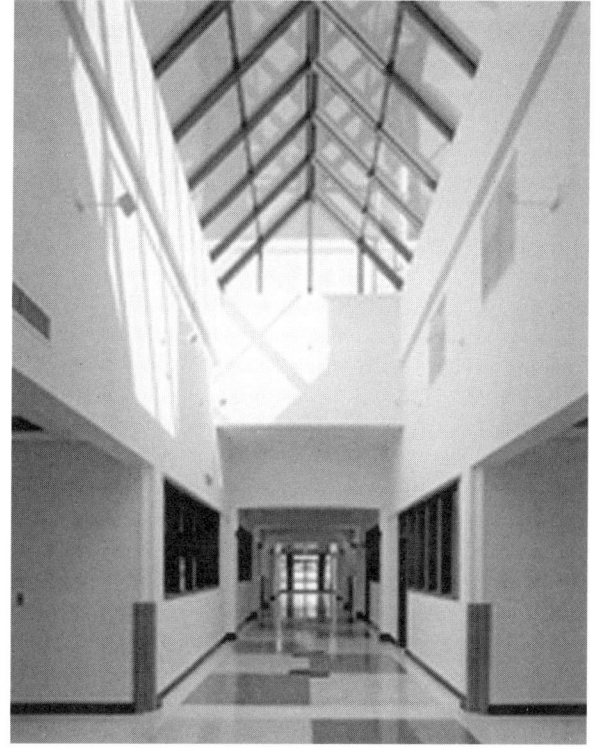

Design Opportunities

The following are several key concepts in design opportunities for a pharmaceutical manufacturing facility.

KEY CONCEPTS:

- Utilize interior glass windows in manufacturing spaces for visual control and safety, as well as aesthetics to provide visual openness in the facility.
- Introduce natural light into the facility in the packaging lines, and where possible break rooms.
- Use color and floor pattern in main corridors for way finding, and to differentiaate functional areas.
- Provide well-designed and detailed amenity areas, such as break rooms, locker rooms, and cafeterias.
- Utilize color and pattern in floor materials, such as vinyl tile.
  - Walkable ceilings and interstitial spaces help create flexibility for mechanical modification and service.
  - Create crisp, modern building facades that reflect a well designed building.
  - Organize utilities in utility panels.

AstraZaneca Cafeteria

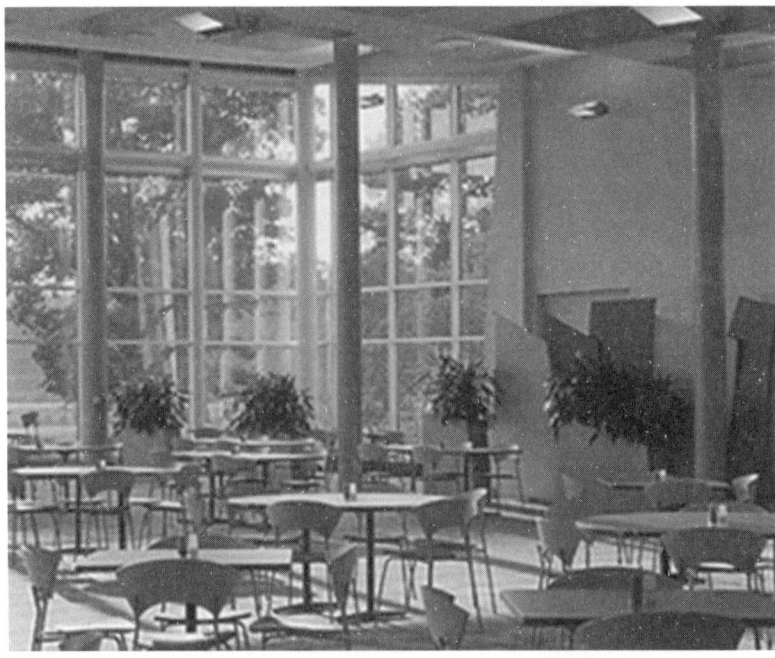

Architects: Jacobs/Wyper Architects, LLP.

Good cGMP Design Features Include:
- Clear layouts
- Appropriate detailing and finishes
- Adequate room sizes and staging areas
- Presentation drawings that illustrate flows for people, product and equipment.

Flexibility:
- Able to adapt to different uses
- Able to bring new services to the rooms
- Ease off clean up
- Modulations

TRENDS

Sustainable Design and Leadership in Energy and Environmental Design (LEED) Building Certification

There is a trend globally to design facilities around sustainable design principles, that minimize the use of natural resources in the design, construction, and maintenance of buildings. The goals are to minimize the energy uses of buildings and to use materials that are renewable and sustainable. LEED is a program sponsored by the United States Green Building Council (USGBC), and awards points (a minimum of 26 points for a certified award) for meeting these criteria. Major corporations, universities, and pharmaceutical companies are embracing these goals.

Pre-Project Review by the FDA

A recent trend has been for pre-design completion review of the facility plans with the FDA. This architectural review can show the circulation for people, equipment, and product, and demonstrate the hierarchy of finishes by utilizing colored block plans, as well as the approach for MEP system design and overall compliance.

Security

Post 9/11 concerns have raised security to a higher level starting with the site layout of a facility, access to the site via a guard booth, and ensuring a secure perimeter. A trend is to have an increase in the utilization of card access to most areas of the facility. Possible contamination of critical facilities by terrorists should be considered in the design of facilities for critical products such as vaccines.

Potent Compound Facilities

There has been a trend in the utilization of potent compounds in facilities, which changes the design requirements and requires special consideration (see Chapter 16).

Process Analytical Technology (PAT)
This may impact the design of facilities in that batch processing may give way to more continuous processing, which may effect design layouts.

3-Dimensional Design
There is a trend to utilize 3-dimensional design and animation to experience the facility and demonstrate to the user what the facility will look like early in the design. "Fly throughs and walk throughs" are useful to communicate to the user and management what the facility will look like and to make design changers. The documentation of facilities will serve as a new generator of AutoCAD or other programs, which will change the way projects are documented.

AstraZeneca Dining Center
The use of natural light, interior windows, color, and floor pattern, can enhance a building with minimal construction cost.

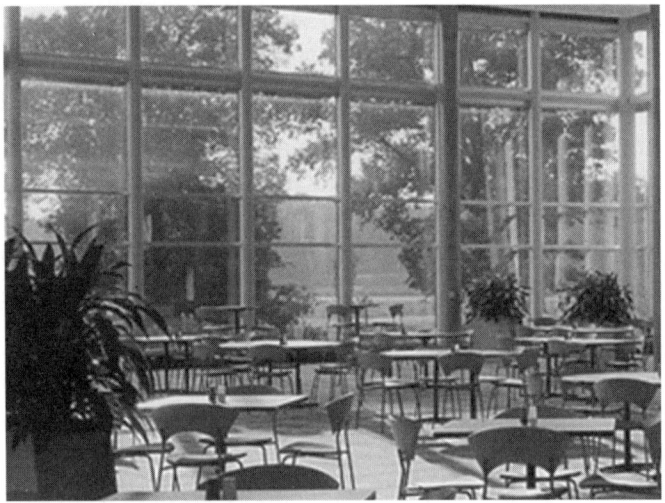

Architects: Jacobs/Wyper Architects, LLP.

Better Design of Amenities
There is a trend to improve the "amenity" spaces for the manufacturing employee, by designing cafeteria and support spaces that are attractive, as well as introducing more glass and natural light into facilities.

Summary
The architect designs a pharmaceutical cGMP manufacturing facility around the process and the engineering systems required to support the process. Attention to details such as utility panels, functional flows, and personnel needs will create an efficient, safe, and attractive facility and a productive work environment.

PROJECT MANAGEMENT ISSUES AND COSTS

Project Approach

Manufacturing facilities are process-driven project types. Therefore, the design team is typically lead by the engineer, so that the architect builds the facility around the process requirements.

Project Delivery

There are three standard types of project delivery with variations for pharmaceutical manufacturing facilities.

Type of Project Delivery	Comments
1. Design, bid, build, commission, validate	• Takes longest • Possibly lowest price • Adversarial

2. Construction management (cm)
  • With guaranteed price (at risk)
  • Target budget (not at risk)
	• CM on board early
	• Faster
	• Less adversarial

3. Design/build* • Signing contract for design and construction	• Faster • As competitive as CM • Single point

*Also referred to as EPC. Engineering procurement, and construction.

Costs

The following are benchwork costs for the design of pharmaceutical manufacturing facilities:

Facility Type	Cost Range		
	Lower	Middle	Higher
Solid dose	$200	$300	$600
Sterile	$400	$600	$1000
Pilot plant	$200	$300	$500

*In millions of dollars.

These costs can vary widely depending on factors such as site, process, location, and redundancy, and the percentage of expensive spaces (manufacturing) in the facility in relation to with less expensive spaces, such as warehousing.

Project Management

Web based project management allows project documentation—from drawings to letters and memos—to be posted to a secure web site accessible by permission to appropriate team members.

REFERENCES

1. ISPE Baseline Guide for Oral Solid Dosage Facilities

2. ISPE Baseline Guide for API Facilities

3. ISPE Baseline Guide for Sterile Facilities

4. Graham, Design of Pharmaceutical Production Facilities

5. Code of Federal Regulations: CFR 21

5

Mechanical Utilities

Authors: Jack C. Chu

Jon F. Hofmeister

INTRODUCTION

Under the Food, Drug, and Cosmetic Act, a drug is deemed to be adulterated unless the methods used in its manufacture, processing, packaging, holding, and the utilized facilities and controls, conform to current Good Manufacturing Practices (cGMP). These require the drug to meet the safety requirements of the Act, contain the proper strength and identity, and meet the quality and purity characteristics that it is represented to have. A properly designed and constructed manufacturing facility and its associated utilities support these practices.

The product and associated manufacturing processes present design criteria that must be satisfied by the facility utility system design. Individual design disciplines must offer solutions for their portion of the design challenge. These must integrate into a complete and coordinated design facilitating the operations of the user, the operations and maintenance groups, the company culture, and the construction process.

This chapter discusses engineering criteria, and system and component design solutions for process and facility requirements outlined elsewhere in this text, as well as overall system design concepts applicable to the pharmaceutical manufacturing environment. It is stressed that the purpose of this discussion is to indicate typical design considerations, and that only a careful consideration of specific design and process requirements will dictate specific design solutions.

After discussion of several separate design concepts, the balance of this chapter will cover mechanical systems design including heating, ventilating, and air conditioning (HVAC); instrumentation and control, process and piping; and fire protection systems.

WHY IS THE DESIGN OF FACILITY UTILITY SYSTEMS SO IMPORTANT?

Very simply, among all of the facility design discipline impacts, beside the actual manufacturing process systems, facility utility systems have the greatest impact on the quality and consistency of the manufactured product and the safety of the manufacturing personnel. Facility utility systems, as a whole, can make up as much as

40% of the "bricks-and-mortar" capital cost of the manufacturing facility. These issues make the proper design of these systems extremely important.

KEY CONCEPTS: The facility utility systems discussed in this chapter are primarily mechanical systems and include HVAC systems and associated controls and instrumentation, plumbing and piping systems, and fire protection systems. Some specific concepts follow.

EXISTING FACILITIES

Quite often manufacturing facilities are built as supplemental to or phased replacements for existing facilities. These existing facilities have their own unique operations flow not to be disrupted by construction of the new facility. An integral part of programming and designing these projects is developing a series of phasing strategies dealing not only with movement, but also with issues of safety and the prevention of product contamination or adulteration during facility construction and changeover periods.

Existing buildings have in-place and operational utility systems designed with their own sometimes unrecognizable logic. Expediency rather than flexibility and appropriateness often dictate the layout of these systems, and the possibility of future expansion is seldom a design determinant. Since many of these systems are built and modified over a matter of years, seldom are they thoroughly documented. A complete survey of these existing systems by a multi-disciplinary architectural and engineering team is essential to orderly planning and integration. The results of this survey, along with process flow diagrams, form the basis of phasing and construction diagrams.

Device and Systems Finishes

Of all the architectural systems in a pharmaceutical manufacturing facility, the interior finishes and colors are most uniquely identified with this specific building type. Particularly in the process areas, finishes are selected for their durability, resistance to cracking and microbial growth, and cleanability. Exposed engineering system devices and terminal equipment must also be selected to support these criteria.

Reliability

Each system must be studied to identify probable modes of failure and the reliabilities and redundancies that should be provided to eliminate critical single point failures. The cost of such redundancy or availability must be justified by the critical nature of the operations and the risk and consequence of failure. This includes not only potential production loss due to a process equipment failure, but potential facility damage due to freezing upon heating system failure. Reliability can be provided by redundancy or the provision of extra equipment or systems. Reliability can also be provided by availability; for example, upon the failure of one piece of four manifolded pieces of equipment, 75% of full capacity remains available. Availability often can provide the required reliable capacity without the capital expenditure of a redundant piece of equipment. The activities during a failure must also be closely controlled. Careful analysis of the failure sequence will minimize productivity loss and facility damage and maximize personnel safety.

Maintainability

Reliable system operation is achieved only when good design and construction is combined with competent maintenance. Each system should be reviewed for maintainability, ideally by the group that will be responsible for maintenance of that system. System components, as far as possible, should be located in a position where routine preventive maintenance can be easily performed with minimal impact to facility and process operations. System shutdowns and testing and sampling methods should also be carefully designed to minimize interruption to productivity.

Commissioning and Validation

Commissioning and validation of utility systems is extremely important. Commissioning, as defined in the ASHRAE Guideline 1-1996, is: *The process of ensuring that systems are designed, installed, functionally tested, and capable of being operated and maintained to perform in conformity with the design intent . . . commissioning begins with planning and includes design, construction, start-up, acceptance and training, and can be applied throughout the life of the building.*

Validation is a documented program that provides a high degree of assurance that a specific process, method, or system will consistently produce a result that meets pre-determined acceptance criteria.

In the pharmaceutical manufacturing arena, these two concepts are extremely critical and because engineering systems can have such a large impact on product quality, it is even more important that these concepts be understood.

MECHANICAL SYSTEMS
Overview

In general, mechanical systems provide for heat transfer (both process and facility); air flow and filtration leading to maintenance of cleanliness; provision of water and gases for product and process requirements; and drainage and disposal of wastes.

Utility and services systems are provided to accommodate the facility and processes. These requirements are determined primarily by the products manufactured, the processes utilized, and established machinery and user criteria, as well as operational and maintenance factors and economic and scheduling requirements. Many of the specific requirements are very different depending upon whether the utility is product contact or non-product contact.

The following sections discuss the various mechanical service disciplines including Heating, Ventilation, and Air Conditioning System (HVAC),; Process and Piping Systems, and Fire Protection Systems, and how these relate to the process requirements outlined elsewhere in this text.

HEATING, VENTILATING, AND AIR CONDITIONING SYSTEMS

Overview

The heating, ventilating, and air conditioning or HVAC discipline serves a critical role in the manufacture of pharmaceutical products. Through the current Good Manufacturing Practices and guidelines, the Food and Drug Administration has set strict facility requirements for the manufacturing environment that the HVAC systems support.

System Design Criteria

Specific facility and process criteria define the system solutions that are provided. These criteria are defined as follows.

Temperature and Moisture

Space and process temperature and moisture (or relative humidity) conditions are generally determined by the product or process performed. Personnel comfort is also important, though secondary to the product requirements. In general, most product or processes can be performed within temperature and relative humidity conditions comparable to human comfort and system control parameters. On occasion, products or processes are sensitive to moisture and may even attract moisture hydroscopically. If product or process requirements are significantly outside of these parameters, an independent enclosed process environment is often provided.

Generally, process operators may be gowned at levels from laboratory coats to full coveralls with head, face, hand, and shoe covers. This level of gowning requires lower space temperature and relative humidity conditions than a standard occupied space to increase personnel comfort and reduce shedding of contaminants. Uncomfortable operators are also more prone to commit errors. Depending on specific gowning conditions, temperature setpoints generally range between 65° and 70°F, and relative humidity setpoints between 40% and 50%, depending on temperature setpoint.

Independent of gowning requirements, relative humidity ranges must be carefully selected. Continuous relative humidity levels below 15% can cause static electricity discharge and health concerns and levels above 60% can be the source of microbial growth and corrosion.

Areas may be designated to operate at a range of controlled temperature and relative humidity to provide flexibility. These must be designed for operation at full load conditions at either end of the operating range.

Allowable space and system control tolerances must also be identified, as well as the impact of these tolerance requirements on the systems design.

Proper outdoor ambient design conditions must be determined in order to select the proper conditioning equipment. Equipment is designed to meet the indoor design criteria based on outdoor conditions and the capacity of the equipment. If outdoor conditions are chosen too conservatively, the equipment will be oversized, costing more than required and possibly requiring more energy for operation. If conditions are not chosen conservatively enough, space or process conditions may not be met under certain circumstances. An assessment must be made as to the possible risks of not making space or process conditions and the effects on productivity.

Air Cleanliness

The level of acceptable airborne contamination within the space must be identified, whether supporting product quality or employee safety.

Environmental cleanliness is determined by several factors:

- The quality of air introduced into the space
- The quantity of air introduced into the space
- The effectiveness of air distribution through the space
- The effectiveness of the removal of the air contaminant

Removal of the contaminant as close to its source is always the most effective method of contamination control—whether it is central filtration at an air handling unit before supply to the facility, or dust collection at a point source of contamination within a space.

Cleanroom design takes contamination control to its highest level. Federal Standard 209 historically had been the document governing cleanroom design. This standard has been replaced by the ISO 14644 and 14698 global cleanroom standards.

Previously, cleanroom cleanliness was categorized by cleanliness classes, which were qualified by the quantity of 0.5 micron or larger particles per cubic foot of air within a specific area. Particulate control is crucial because particles entering the product may contaminate it physically or through microorganisms associated with the particle. Standard categories of cleanliness were Classes 100,000, 10,000, 1,000, 100, 10, and 1. As an example, the FDA Guideline on Sterile Drug Products Produced by Aseptic Processing recommends a minimum of Class 100 when measured not more than 1 foot from the sterile open product work site; that is, no more than 0.5 micron can occupy any cubic foot of air within the space at any time.

The ISO standards have been an outgrowth of these classes but have expanded the classifications to ISO 1 through 9 and widened the range of particulate sizes to 0.1 micron through 5 microns. A rough comparison of the ISO and Federal Standard 209E is as follows:

ISO	Federal Standard 209E
1	—
2	—
3	1
4	10
5	100
6	1,000
7	10,000
8	100,000
9	1,000,000

This table does not reflect the complexity of the ISO cleanroom standards. These should be considered thoroughly before embarking on a cleanroom design.

Air must also have low microbial levels. The above guidelines also recommend a maximum allowable level of colony-forming unit (CFU) per given volume of air. Particulate filtration can eliminate the majority of microbial contamination. In areas with high background microbial levels (such as facilities surrounded by large amounts of farmland); however, other methods may also be employed such as carbon bed prefiltration.

Pressurization

Space relative pressurization will be determined primarily by requirements of the product, but also by characteristics of the product that may adversely effect personnel. Space containment and isolation techniques, in general, can protect the product, the operator, or both. Where product contamination control is required, the space relative pressurization must be designed to assure that the movement of exfiltrated air is from the clean to the less clean areas. In some cases, especially when dealing with hazardous products (e.g., high potency compounds), this relative pressurization and resultant air movement is sometimes reversed to contain the hazard and protect personnel. In these cases, product contamination can be controlled by the use of special laminar flow hoods or personal isolation suits, and/or positive and negative pressurization utilizing airlocks. Some operations may require flexibility for either positive or negative pressurization, depending on the application. A pressure differential of at least 0.05 inches water gage with all doors closed is preferable between spaces with a pressure differential requirement. See the Isolation and Containment section for more discussion on this topic.

Typical Space Pressurization Configuration

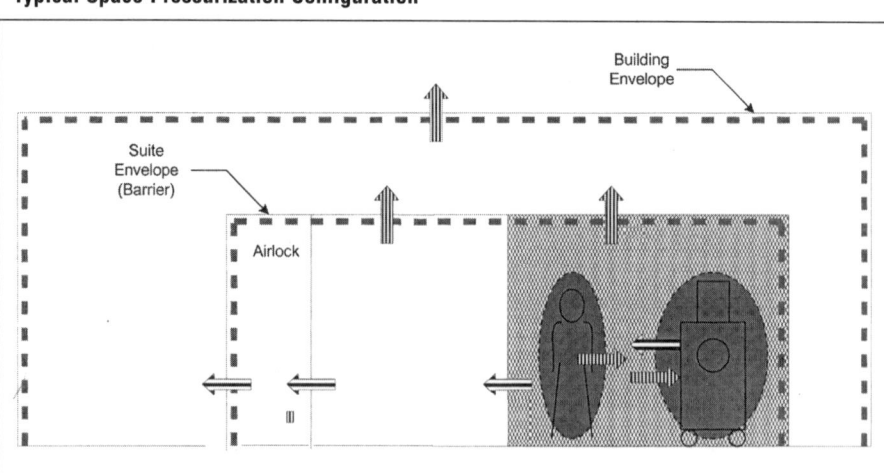

Note: All components may not be required.

Building Intake and Exhaust

Careful attention must be paid to the incoming system air quality. This can be specific to the area in which the facility has been constructed such as an agrarian or industrial area. An industrial area may have a more corrosive or chemical laden air quality and an agrarian area may have a higher level of seasonal air borne particulate and bio-burden. These issues must be carefully considered when selecting filtration systems so as to minimize the possibility of product contamination.

Most often, however, building intake re-entrainment or its own effluent is the greater problem. Careful consideration must be made as to the impacts of building exhaust and relief systems, loading docks and other incidences of vehicle exhaust and electrical generator exhaust. Analysis must be made of the subject building's impact on itself and other surrounding buildings, and their impact on the subject building. Potential future building activities should also be considered.

Rooftop activity safety should also be analyzed and a safety rooftop environment should be provided for routine maintenance activities.

Noise Considerations

Given the overriding concerns for durability and cleanability in process spaces, little can be done to dampen the finished surface acoustic qualities. By definition a cleanable space has smooth, hard finishes with simple geometries that reflect rather than absorb sound. This makes the control of noise contributed by utility systems critical in these spaces. Sound attenuation can be added to supply and exhaust air systems. Dust collection inlets, however, tend to be the greatest contributor to space noise and absolute attention to design parameters can minimize the sound radiated from these inlets.

Manufacturing facilities also tend to utilize large process and utility equipment that can radiate noise to the outdoor environment. Local ordinances and community goodwill may require that noise generated by this equipment be minimized. Methods of enclosure and the specification of sound attenuation devices can significantly reduce noise transmitted outside of the facility.

Cost Considerations

Pharmaceutical manufacturing facilities and processes are extremely costly facilities to design, construct, and operate. When designing a facility and process, careful consideration must be made of the initial construction cost, balanced against life cycle operating costs. Careful analysis must be made of all of the components that comprise a facility or process design. A cost cutting measure taken during the initial capital expenditure can multiply into huge operating costs by years of inefficient operation. Conversely, a complex, cost intensive project can take too long to build and commission, which may affect speed to market and ultimately production and sales.

Heating Systems

Heating of facility and process systems is generally accomplished utilizing steam or hot water as the heat source. There may also be intermediate methods of heat transfer utilizing a secondary steam or heating hot water system. Heating can also be provided by electric means that is easily controlled but is expensive to operate and therefore not in widespread use.

Primary steam is usually generated by a central boiler system. Steam is generally distributed throughout the facility at higher pressures (100 psig or more) because of the smaller piping required in the distribution network.

Primary steam is reduced in pressure near concentrated points of use. Points of use include steam heating coils, steam-to-steam heat exchangers, steam-to-water heat exchangers, jacketed heat exchange process, or direct injection for some methods of humidification. The pressure is reduced because lower pressure steam is easier to control and has a greater latent heat, the heat that is actually available through steam condensation. Generally, points of use are grouped together on central pressure reducing stations. Piping for the plant steam systems is generally welded, flanged, or screwed black steel.

Steam used for sterilization of containers or equipment or that comes in direct contact with the product through a process or though humidified room air in an open product space must be "clean steam." This steam is produced in a dedicated heat exchanger or boiler supplied with purified feed water that is also free of chemical additives. Piping for clean steam is preferably welded stainless steel.

Heating can also be provided by a heating hot water system that uses plant steam or a hot water boiler as the heat source. Heating hot water is generally used for space heating utilized in room radiation or convection units or hot water coils in the supply air distribution system. Electric resistance heating is also an option but is an expensive energy source.

Heating of primary air at the central air handling unit is generally accomplished using hot water or low pressure steam. Incoming ventilation air on high outside air volume systems in colder climates is generally heated utilizing low pressure steam or a separate hot water system with a concentration of propylene glycol sufficient to prevent water system freezing.

It is preferred that heat required in a jacketed heat exchange process such as a kettle that has one level of product containment (the kettle wall) be a non-plant process. This process should utilize a secondary heat source that could be an independent water or steam system utilizing plant steam as the primary heat source. This prevents plant system contamination in case of a boundary wall failure.

Cooling Systems

Cooling of facility and process systems is generally accomplished utilizing chilled water, condenser water, or direct refrigerant expansion (DX) as the heat sink. In isolated cases, a water/anti-freeze solution or other heat exchange fluid may be utilized, generally without a phase change. There may also be an intermediate method of heat transfer utilizing a secondary chilled water system in concert with the plant systems outlined above.

Primary chilled and condenser water is usually generated by a central cooling system. It is then distributed throughout the facility to points of use that include cooling coils, heat exchangers, and jacketed heat exchange processes. Piping for

Typical Heating System: Major Component Configuration

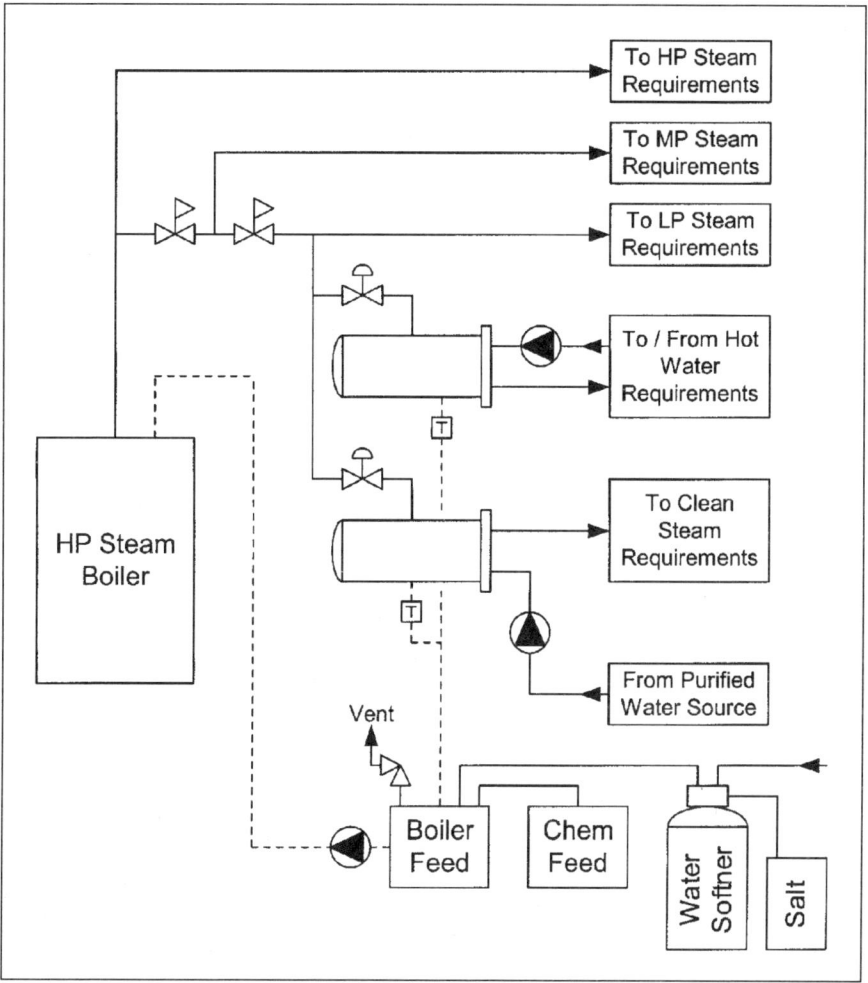

Note: All components may not be required.

these plant water systems is generally welded or screwed black steel. Mechanical coupling systems are also utilized.

Plant chilled water is generally produced utilizing water-cooled or air-cooled chillers. Chilled water supply temperatures are usually in the range of 40°– 45°F and are determined by the requirements of the cooled medium, generally air.

Condenser water cools the condenser side of the chiller and is of a higher temperature. Condenser water supply temperatures are usually in the range of 85°– 95°F, in the summer. Non-summer condenser water supply temperatures can generally be maintained at lower temperatures. Water is generally cooled by open cooling towers or closed circuit coolers. Open towers utilize outside air to cool the water directly.

Closed circuit coolers circulate the water through tubing in the tower that is air cooled and sprinkled with water.

Condenser water can also be used to cool processes besides chiller condensers. These include cooling of purified water processes, refrigerated processes, and jacketed processes. If the process does not require the lower temperatures of chilled water, condenser water can be a cost effective solution, as it does not require the additional energy of the mechanical refrigeration process.

It is preferable that cooling required in a jacketed heat exchange process such as a kettle that has one level of product containment (the kettle wall) be a non-plant process. This process should utilize a secondary cooling source that can be an independent cooling water system utilizing plant chilled or condenser water as the primary heat sink, or a direct refrigerant expansion system. This prevents plant system contamination in case of a boundary wall failure.

Cooling of space or process supply air is generally accomplished at the central air handling unit. Incoming ventilation air on high outside air volume systems may require additional dehumidification that the chilled water system cannot achieve (see the discussion of Dehumidification Systems below). Terminal cooling is often required when an area with lower environmental temperature or humidity levels is served by a central system without these requirements.

Typical Cooling System: Major Component Configuration

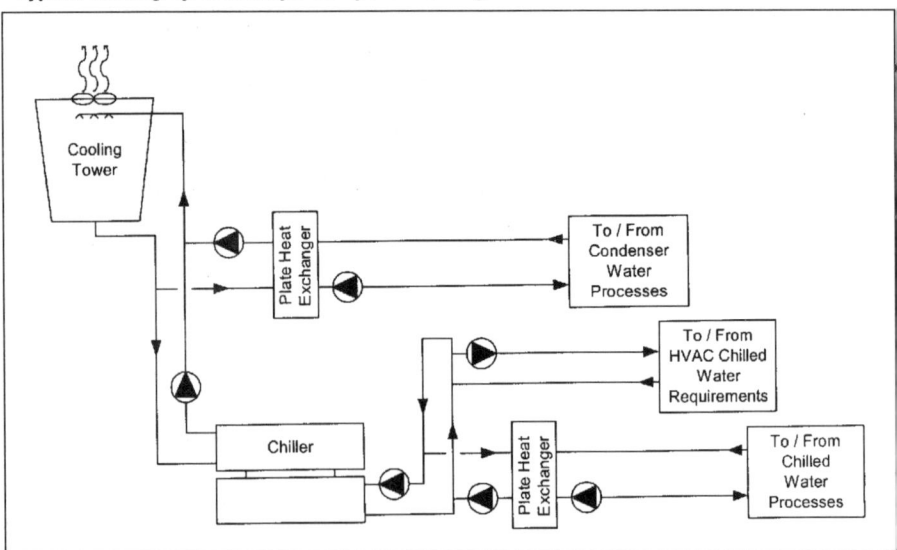

Note: All components may not be required.

Humidification Systems

In most cases, air supplied to the space or process will require the addition of moisture to maintain relative humidity conditions. Moisture is generally provided utilizing steam injection and in some cases atomized water utilizing compressed air. In the cGMP environment, the added moisture cannot be a source of contamination. Its source is therefore generally purified water that is then atomized or converted to clean steam. These humidifiers are typically constructed of stainless steel.

Dehumidification Systems

In cases of high latent loads from processes or high quantities of outside ventilation air, the building cooling system may not be capable of the higher dehumidification requirements. Several moisture removal methods are available. These include low temperature latent cooling used in concert with reheating, solid and liquid desiccant drying systems, and the injection of sterile, dry compressed air into the air stream. In all cases, room or process air can be treated centrally or locally. All methods must consider minimization of product contamination.

Supply Air Handling Systems

Air systems have the greatest influence over the environment within the space or process that it serves. It assists in determining the temperature, moisture level, and cleanliness of that environment. It also assists in the relative pressurization of the space or process.

Space Supply Air Handling Systems

Supply air systems are divided into four specific components: prime movers, distribution, terminal control equipment and terminal distribution equipment.

Primer Movers. Prime movers on the supply air system are generally enclosed in an air handling unit comprised of several components. The device that drives the air is a fan. The largest consideration for supply air fans in this industry is generally capacity control and turndown capability to accurately match the requirements of the supply air system.

Coils are used to transfer heat into or out of the air stream. As described in the heating and cooling discussions above, many heat transfer fluids may be used for heating and cooling.

Humidification devices are often placed inside of the air handling unit but can also be installed within the ductwork outside of the unit, saving unit casing cost. Primary concerns in their specification are the moisture source and carryover, which are both potential contributors of biological and or chemical contamination.

Air systems tend to be noisy. Contributors are primarily fans, dampers and terminal air control boxes. Sound attenuation is often place in or near the air handling unit to decrease the radiated noise of the fan. Concerns here are the type of attenuator, which could also be a source of particulate and microbial growth.

Filters are generally the first and last devices in the pharmaceutical manufacturing air handling unit. Intake pre-filters protect the unit components from dirt and contamination. Final filters at the unit discharge protect the system and ultimately the space and process. Terminal filter are also often specified.(See discussion under Terminal Distribution Equipment below.)

Typical Air Handling Unit Configuration

Note: All components may not be required.

Distribution: Distribution is generally sheet metal ductwork, although it can be piping or other materials. The greatest consideration is often the material. Galvanized sheet steel is most often used, but is difficult to sanitize. If the material is open to product or product space or must be frequently decontaminated, it is often specified as stainless steel. Another important consideration is accessibility, both inside and out for cleaning testing. Other considerations for the greater design, although not specific to the pharmaceutical industry, are the size of the ductwork and leakage rate.

Terminal Control Equipment: This includes air volume control boxes, terminal heating and cooling coils, terminal humidification and sound attenuation. Air volume control boxes control the air quantity delivered to the space and control space relative pressurization in concert with other supply, return and exhaust boxes within the space and adjacent spaces. Terminal cooling coils provide for space sub-cooling and or dehumidification. Terminal heating coils provided for reheat of space air to support dehumidification and room temperature control. Accessibility for maintenance is the primary concern for these devices. Terminal humidifiers provide additional moisture to the space greater than the system can. As with central humid-ifiers, the primary concern is potential contamination from the moisture source or carryover. Terminal sound attenuation masks the noise from terminal boxes and, as with central attenuators, proper selection of the attenuator type is important to limit potential contamination from particulate and microbial growth.

Terminal Distribution Equipment: These includes diffusers, registers and grilles, and terminal filtration. Diffusers, and registers and grilles introduce air into the space. Proper application of the different types of devices is critical to maintain effective distribution. The airflow direction into the space is important. Unidirectional diffusers are often specified instead of the aspirating type to provide, in concert with the exhaust terminal device, a "sweeping" effect in the room to more effectively remove particulate from the space. Another important consideration is device cleanability within the space. The device cannot be a source of contamination. Terminal filtration is applied most often where space cleanliness is paramount. While this application of filtration can protect the space and product from contaminant within the air system, it can also protect the air system from product or contaminant within the space in case of system failure. Important considerations for the selection and placement of terminal filtration are its location, change out requirements, and accessibility for testing.

Other Design Concepts: There are many other important design concepts; discussion of some of them follow.

The *supply air system*, more than any other system, controls the space temperature and relative humidity. Utilizing cooling and heating coils and methods of humidification and dehumidification, all within the supply air stream, each space is controlled to maintain the required criteria.

Space relative pressurization is determined primarily by requirements of the product, but also by characteristics of the product that may adversely effect personnel. Space containment and isolation techniques, in general, can protect the product, the operator, or both. Where product contamination control is required, the space relative pressurization must be designed to ensure that the movement of exfiltrated air is from the clean to the less clean areas. In some cases, especially when dealing with hazardous products (e.g., high potency compounds), this relative pressurization and resultant air movement is sometimes reversed to contain the hazard and protect personnel. In these cases, product contamination can be controlled by the use of special laminar flow hoods or personal isolation suits, and or positive and negative pressurization utilizing airlocks. Some operations may require flexibility for either positive or negative pressurization, depending on the application. A pressure differential of at least 0.05 inches water gage with all doors closed is preferable between spaces with a pressure differential requirement. Space relative pressurization is generally maintained by utilizing air control devices that serve each space. See the Isolation and Containment section for more discussion on this topic.

In order to achieve specific cleanliness classifications, clean, HEPA (high-efficiency particulate air) filtered air is provided to the space. HEPA filtration is generally 99.97% or 99.997% effective on particles 0.3 microns or larger as measured by the DOP method. DOP, or dioctylphthalate, is a particulate matter that measures 0.3 microns in diameter or larger, and is used in the testing of HEPA filter material.

Air is often terminally filtered to avoid contamination through ductwork. If the room is clean, and the air is clean, and the space is positively pressurized, the only source of contamination to the product and process is from personnel or materials brought into the environment. By increasing the amount of clean air provided to the space, the density of contaminants is reduced by dilution. Many articles and papers have been published discussing the association between cleanliness class and the amount of clean air that must be delivered to the space.

The density of contaminants is also affected by the physical relationship of the source to the product as well as the airflow patterns around them. A unidirectional or laminar flow of air should be provided with a minimum velocity of 90 feet per minute at the aseptic critical zone. Also, placing a source of contamination upstream of the product area must be avoided.

A means of avoiding local contamination and providing for a higher level of cleanliness at the critical area is to supply air at the point of use (directly over a filling line, for example) in an enclosed or semi-enclosed environment. Semi-enclosed environments include laminar flow hoods or curtained laminar flow modules. Totally enclosed environments are completely enclosed stationary or portable equipment that house the critical procedure and sometimes the entire process in a controlled micro-environment. The popularity of these technologies is growing in the sterile process environment.

FDA cGMP regulations for finished pharmaceuticals concerning HVAC systems are somewhat general. The proposed regulations dealing with large volume parenterals, however, are more rigorous.

Process Supply Air Handling Systems

Air can be utilized in the manufacturing process in various ways. It can be used to draw off dust and solvent fumes; it can be used to dry a granulation as in a fluid bed dryer and tray dryer; it can also be used to dry a tablet coating as it is applied as in a film or sugar coating pan. (Process exhausted air and its treatment is discussed later in the exhaust air systems section.)

The process supply air stream characteristics determine the environment within the process. These include temperature, relative humidity, and cleanliness. The process supply air temperature and relative humidity are solely determined by the product and process requirements. Air can be dehumidified, cooled, heated, and humidified, as required. The process supply air cleanliness is also determined by the product and process requirements. Because the air comes in contact with open product, it is often filtered through a high efficiency particulate air (HEPA) filtration system.

Process air is generally provided to each process by an individual air handling unit which may include a supply air fan, dehumidification, cooling coils, heating coils, clean steam humidifier, and final filtration, as required. Some processes utilize a powerful exhaust fan that precludes the need for a supply fan. Dehumidification, humidification, heating, and cooling can be applied, although heating is most often required. Final filtration of the supply air is usually mandatory.

Cross contamination prevention is a regulatory requirement. Process air handling systems should not be common to each other without positive separations systems (reliable fan operation, back draft dampers, air control dampers, etc.). As always, it is better to avoid the possibility of a problem by utilizing completely individual systems.

The distance between the air handling unit components and the process is generally critical. Equipment and control reaction times and maintainability and accessibility will govern the location of support equipment relative to the process.

The air handling equipment is designed for the process that it serves. Air quantities and pressures, heating, cooling, moisture addition, and filtration are all potential requirements of the process. Some processes do not require supply air fans as the exhaust blower maintains all airflow. All air supplied to a process with open product requires high efficiency filtration to prevent product contamination.

See the Exhaust System Safety discussion in the following section.

Exhaust and Return Air Systems

Exhaust systems can have a great influence over the environment within the space or process that they serve. They evacuate contaminant or contaminated air to be filtered or processed in some other manner and returned to the supply air unit or to the atmosphere. They also assist in the relative pressurization of the space or process and can aid in the removal of unwanted heat and moisture from within a space or process.

Space Exhaust Air Systems

Several different types of exhaust air systems can serve each space. The general room air exhaust or return air system normally aids in maintaining the pressurization, temperature, and relative humidity environment of the space, as well as the dilution of airborne contaminants to maintain cleanliness or a non-hazardous environment. Other exhaust systems including dust collection and local scavenging systems for solvents, etc., generally remove air with more concentrated contaminants at the source. This can include vapor, fume, or particulate contamination, or even excess heat. Terminal capture device design is extremely important as the more effective a collection device is, the more contaminant it removes from the source and the less air it uses.

Generally, room air that is difficult to treat for contaminants or from which it is impractical to remove excess heat before reuse in the space is exhausted to the outdoors. Regulations may require, however, that the air be treated before being released to the environment. If there is manageable contaminant and heat content, the air is generally returned to the space after processing (filtering) and cooling and dehumidification.

The air in exhaust systems with more concentrated contaminants is generally treated and released to the environment. This treatment may take the form of filtration or vapor/fume removal.

Consideration should be made that manifolded systems tend to have concentrations lowered due to system dilution from unused points. Diluted air streams are safer but tend to make contaminant removal more difficult and expensive.

A major consideration in particulate transport systems is the transport velocity. Low velocity will cause particulate to drop out of the air stream. High velocity causes high distribution pressures and requires more energy for transport. This concept is especially important in dynamic operation of manifolded systems.

The potential for static electricity generated by the particulate movement must also be carefully considered, primarily from a safety standpoint. Distribution systems must be properly grounded to prevent discharge.

Cleanability is also an important consideration, primarily in material selection and provision of access into the distribution system.

See Exhaust Air Filtration, Dust Collection, and Vapor and Fume Handling and Treatment sections (following) for discussion of exhaust processing methods.

Process Exhaust Air Systems

Air supplied to an open product process cannot be returned and must be exhausted. Inherently, process exhaust may have particulate, solvents, or other vapors or fumes. These, of course, may require treatment before release to the environment. (See Exhaust Air Filtration, Dust Collection, and Vapor and Fume Handling and Treatment sections below for discussion of exhaust processing methods; see the Exhaust System Safety section for discussion of explosion isolation, venting, and containment.

Contaminant Characterization and Handling

Space and process contaminants can include unwanted particulate, vapor, fume, or biological. These can be a nuisance or a hazard to product quality and personnel health and safety from a chemical or biological standpoint.

The handling of the contaminant must be carefully considered, including the removal from the space or process and the support of dilution within the space or process, the collection and handling of the contaminant or contaminated air, and the

Technology / Contaminant	Particulate	Organic Vapor	Inorganic Vapor	Biological
Particulate filtration	X			X
Carbon bed filtration		X		
Wet scrubbing	X		X	X
Incineration		X		X
Adsorption		X		
Absorption		X		
Condensation		X		

treatment of this effluent. The following table generalizes primary treatment techniques and their application.

Exhaust Air Filtration

Particulate laden air is treated with filtration to remove the contaminant to an acceptable level. Efficiency of the filtration system is measured by the percentage of particulate above a given size that is removed from the air stream that it is serving. Filter efficiencies generally range from 30% to 99.999% (these are called high efficiency particulate air or HEPA filters). Filtration can be done in stages of efficiency to provide the appropriate overall effectiveness. For example, suppose that a high degree of filtration efficiency is required, say 95%, for a reasonably dusty environment such as a coating process. 95% efficient filters alone would continually overload in a short period of time and would require extremely frequent and costly replacement. A staged filter system, utilizing 30% and 60% pre-filters and 95% final filters would provide a much more effective system and require less expensive filter replacements. Where the level of particulate in the air stream is extremely high or when unacceptable levels of fumes or toxic chemicals are present, alternate methods of removal must be employed. Careful consideration to filter change out and potential exposure to filtered contents must be made when selecting filtration systems. Methods for removal of filter media are available to minimize or eliminate open handling of contaminated filters.

Dust Collection

Extremely high levels of particulate require larger filter surface areas and a means of collecting the particulate build-up from the filtration material. A dust collector is essentially a plenum. Particulate, which has been conveyed to the collector at high duct transport velocities, settles in the comparably lower velocity of the plenum. The particulate is then collected outside of the plenum, either via gravity to a container below or, in the case of larger installations, by a method of material conveyance such as belt or screw conveyor.

Filters are generally located within the dust collector to capture the finer, more buoyant material. These filters are usually bags or cartridges. The downstream side of the filters are pulsated either mechanically or via a blast of compressed air to shake loose material collecting on the filter media. High efficiency final filters may also be included, depending on overall system filtration efficiency requirements. As with exhaust system filtration described above, careful consideration to duct collector media change out and potential exposure to collected contents must be made when selecting dust collectors. Methods for removal of filter media are available to minimize or eliminate open handling of contaminated filters.

Filtration is not always required, however. In the case of the cyclone separator, a high efficiency of particulate removal can be attained with a correct configuration, without the requirement for downstream filtration.

Small separators or collectors are sometimes required at the process point of use for product accounting purposes or potent material containment requirements.

Vapor and Fume Handling and Treatment

If the air exhausted from a process contains airborne toxic or otherwise harmful chemicals, it is probable that the Clean Air Act will require these materials be removed from the air before release into the environment. These chemicals include organic and inorganic vapors and particulate. Organic vapors and particulate are most often found in the pharmaceutical manufacturing environment. (Particulate filtering is discussed in the Dust Collection section above.) Organic vapors can be dealt with in several ways. These include incineration, adsorption, condensation, and absorption.

Incineration converts organic vapors to carbon dioxide, water, and other elements using combustion. When these vapors are present in low concentration, a supporting fuel such as natural gas may be required to assist in burning the vapors.

Adsorption is the process by which organic substances are retained on a granulated surface. Some of these include activated carbon, silica gel, and alumina. Activated carbon is most effective and efficient.

Absorption is the process by which contaminants are transferred from a gas stream to a liquid stream. Some of these include water, caustic soda, and low volatility hydrocarbons.

Condensation is the process by which the air stream is cooled or pressurized to the point of condensation of the organic compound to be removed. The condensate can either be recovered and purified for further use or disposed of in an approved manner.

Process effluent that requires particulate and vapor or fume treatment can be staged such that particulate is removed utilizing filtration, and then fumes or vapors are treated utilizing one of the methods outlined above.

Exhaust System Safety

In many processes, volatile materials are used. These materials may be a flammable solvent, a dust or powder, or a combination of the two. In order for an explosion hazard to exist, a heat source, a fuel source, and an oxidizer are needed in sufficient quantities.

Explosions are classified as deflagration or detonation. A deflagration is an ignition and burning with a flame front. A detonation, which can be extremely violent, is a deflagration whose flame front velocity has exceeded the speed of sound. It is critical that a deflagration be contained and controlled and not allowed to become a detonation.

There are several control methods including containment, isolation, venting, and arresting. These can be used separately or in combination with one another, depending on the size and volatility of the process. In smaller, less volatile processes, the equipment or distribution may be able to withstand an explosion. Generally, upon ignition sensing, the process must be isolated from other systems utilizing high-speed explosion dampers so that the equipment will contain the explosion. In larger and more volatile processes, the equipment cannot withstand the full force of the explosion and the process must be vented. In these systems, upon ignition sensing, the process will be isolated from other systems and, as the resulting pressure rises in the process, a vent will release to the outdoors and the explosion will be released. In all cases, the reaction times of these systems are measured in fractions of a second and their selection is extremely critical.

Arresting is a process of removing the heat from the flame front. Arresting devices, placed in the air stream, are extremely efficient heat dissipaters. When a flame front passes through an arrestor, the heat is removed, even as the fuel and oxidizer is present.

To help avoid explosions, the system must be completely grounded to prevent build-up of static electricity, and devices and equipment should be spark proof and/or purged with an inert gas.

Mechanical Systems Instrumentation and Control

Similar to other pharmaceutical facilities, manufacturing facilities rely on Building Automation Systems (BAS) for coordinated control of the building mechanical and electrical systems. These may also be referred to as Building Management Systems (BMS) or Facility Management Systems (FMS). The BAS is separate from process control systems associated with manufacturing process equipment. The modern BAS consists of a network of Direct Digital Control (DDC) controllers and/or control panels. These DDC panels are distributed controllers interfaced to their associated building systems through inputs and outputs. Examples of inputs are space temperature and relative humidity, airflow, room differential pressure, and valve and damper position indication. Examples of outputs are a fan start command, variable frequency drive (VFD) speed control, and valve or damper modulation. Inputs come from instrumentation such as temperature sensors and valve limit switches. Outputs go to control devices such as starters, variable speed drives and automatic control valves.

The BAS is programmed to execute a sequence of operations for each building system to maintain building conditions within design parameters and to operate the equipment efficiently and reliably. In order to achieve the required reliability, sequences of operation must include different operating scenarios as well as planned failure modes. These include system operation upon the loss of building electric power and failure of a major components or equipment devices. While each DDC controller operates in a stand-alone fashion, the controllers are networked together for coordinated operation and response to changes in conditions.

In addition to direct inputs and outputs through instrumentation and controls, other building systems and equipment are often integrated with the BAS through network communication interfaces. Chillers, variable speed drives and lighting control panel boards are examples of intelligent building equipment with self-contained microprocessor controls that commonly interface with the BAS. There are many available methods for interface. These include "open protocols" established by standards organizations or manufacturers' associations; older standard serial communication schemes; and proprietary interfaces developed by individual BAS manufacturers and third-party software vendors. The specifications for the intelligent building equipment and the specifications for the BAS must both indicate requirements for the network interface, and should require coordination of the communication interface between the equipment supplier and the BAS supplier.

The BAS may also monitor critical equipment such as freezers, refrigerators, and controlled environment rooms that supports the manufacturing process. These monitoring functions may also be provided through a separate independent system. These functions need to be established early in the design process so that BAS panels are located where required and with adequate capacity to accommodate the full range of requirements.

The BAS can also aid in preventive maintenance by automatically generating maintenance work orders on a scheduled or run-time basis. They can be interfaced with fire and security alarm systems to provide comprehensive monitoring and reporting capabilities. All of these capabilities can be provided on a single-building basis or for an entire building complex or campus.

Control of space conditions within established parameters is important to product quality, so these conditions must be monitored and archived as part of manufacturing records. Many BAS suppliers have developed reliable and secure data archiving software designed and qualified to meet industry guidelines for electronic record keeping. The need for this level of qualification must be determined during design and included in the system specifications. Often this application will require a more stringent level of quality control and documentation, including validation of the BAS or a portion of the BAS. Validation requirements for the BAS must be considered during design and addressed in the facility validation plan. Because validation increases the cost of BAS, it is sometimes appropriate to segregate the BAS into discrete segments for building system control and general monitoring and for monitoring and archiving of critical space conditions. With this approach, the more stringent quality control and documentation requirements associated with validation may be applied only to the segment of the system monitoring critical conditions.

Important design considerations include the implementation of well thought out sequences and consideration of dynamic turndown and system diversity. Accuracy must be carefully considered in component types and repeatability. Accuracy costs money and selection can easy reach a point of diminishing returns. Carefully written failure sequences can lead to the capital savings by avoiding purchasing redundancy and backup generation while minimizing productivity losses. Maintenance is an especially important consideration when it comes to instrumentation. Devices must be periodically calibrated according to an established plan.

PROCESS AND PIPING SYSTEMS

Introduction

The process and piping systems disciplines, including plumbing, gases, true process systems, and fire protection, provide a critical role in the manufacture of pharmaceutical products. The FDA through the current Good Manufacturing Practices and guidelines, has set strict facility requirements for the process and piping systems environment.

Water Systems

Domestic Cold Water

Water supplied by the local authority to the building or site is generally referred to as domestic cold water. The facility domestic cold water is the base for all other water qualities required by the processes. The water quality may be adjusted before any use in the facility by filtering, softening, or chlorinating. The potable water must be supplied under continuous positive pressure in a plumbing system free of defects that could contribute contamination to any drug product. The base water quality must be potable as defined by the Environmental Protection Agency's Primary Drinking Water Regulations set forth in 40 CFR Part 141.

Domestic cold water is generally used for the following purposes:

- General non-purified water usage including toilet rooms, equipment wash (not including final rinse), water fountains, etc.
- Source water for the domestic hot water system
- Source water for further purified water systems
- Makeup water for HVAC water systems

It is permissible for potable domestic cold water to be used for cleaning and initial rinse of drug product contact surfaces, such as containers, closures, and equipment if, as stated above, it is considered to be potable water, meets the Public Health Service drinking water standards, has been subjected to a process such as chlorination for microbial control, and contains no more than 50 microorganisms per hundred milliliters.

To prevent cross contamination from systems or processes, an air gap (in the case of an open fill) or a backflow preventer must be employed. This prevents contaminants (including product) from infiltrating supply water systems. Often, the prevention device is placed centrally in the system, providing separate potable and non-potable water systems, thus avoiding the requirement for multiple devices that require frequent inspection and maintenance.

Domestic Hot Water

The domestic hot water system utilizes domestic cold water as a source. Water is heated generally by steam or electric resistance and stored for use. Domestic hot water is generally circulated throughout the facility so that hot water is readily available without waiting for "warm-up." Domestic hot water is used for ordinary facility usages such as toilet rooms, equipment wash (not including final rinse), etc. Other hot water requirements are satisfied by heating the purified water. As with the domestic cold water system, often a cross contamination prevention device is placed centrally in the hot water system, providing separate potable and non-potable hot water distribution systems, thus avoiding the requirement for multiple devices that require frequent inspection and maintenance.

Purified and Process Water Systems

Water requiring a higher quality for processes or products is purified utilizing domestic cold water as a source. There are many grades of purified water and these are generally determined by the product or process.

Drainage Systems

Drainage systems remove effluent from spaces, systems, or process. Generally, the drainage system type, construction materials, and segregation and treatment requirements are dictated by the effluent involved, whether it be product-laden water, final rinse water, toilet room effluent, mechanical system drainage, solvent, acid or caustic, etc. In all cases, backflow considerations are critical. Different drainage system types are discussed in the following sections.

Sanitary Waste System

A separate sanitary waste drainage and vent system is provided to convey waste from toilets, lavatories, non-process service sinks and floor drains. Sanitary drainage is connected to the site sanitary sewer system generally without treatment. Any other materials or product that may present a hazard or environmental problem in the sewer system must be conveyed by a separate waste and vent system.

Laboratory Waste System

A separate laboratory waste drainage and vent system is often provided in cases where acids or caustics used in laboratory processes must be sampled and potentially neutralized before disposal into the sanitary waste system. A batch or continuous neutralization system may be utilized.

Process Waste System

A separate process waste drainage and vent system is often provided in cases where products used in the manufacturing process must either be contained separately or treated before disposal into the sanitary waste system. If they are contained, they are usually removed by tanker truck and disposed of offsite.

Because the drainage may be potentially hazardous and certainly poses a potential contamination and environmental threat, the piping distribution system must either be protected (double wall piping system) or provided in a location that is easily monitored (i.e., exposed service corridors).

Hazardous Material Waste and Retention

Separate hazardous waste drainage and vent systems are provided in cases where hazardous materials such as solvents, toxins, radioactives, high concentrations, etc. must be contained. Generally these systems are limited in distribution and highly contained. They can either be local such as "in-lab" safety containers or larger as in the case of a solvent spill retention system in a dispensing area. These systems must maintain isolation of the hazardous material for other drainage systems.

Storm Drainage System

A separate storm drainage system is provided to drain rainwater from all roof and area drains. This system is generally not combined with any other drainage system.

All precautions must be taken to ensure that contaminated fluids cannot flow into the storm drainage system.

General loading dock apron area drains can connect to the site storm drainage system and are generally provided with in-line sand and oil interceptors. In case of potentially hazardous material spills, valving is generally provided in the drainage system to isolate the drainage area.

Plumbing Fixtures and Specialties

The FDA requires that adequate personnel washing facilities be provided, including hot and cold water, soap or detergent, air dryers or single-service towels, and clean toilet facilities easily accessible to working areas. Gowning areas are also required and must be equipped with surgical-type hand-washing facilities and warm-air hand-drying equipment. Other fixtures must be provided to meet specific facility requirements and those of the local building codes and standards.

Gas Systems

Many types of gases are utilized in the manufacturing process. The most prevalent of these include compressed air use in process and controls, breathing air for hazardous environments, nitrogen, vacuum, vacuum cleaning, natural gas, propane, and other process systems.

All gases used in manufacturing and processing operations, including the sterilization process, should be sterile filtered at points of use to meet the requirements of the specific area. Gases to be used in sterilizers after the sterilization process must be sterile filtered. Any gases to be used at the filling line or microbiological testing area must also be sterile filtered.

The integrity of all air filters must be verified upon installation and maintained throughout use. A written testing program adequate to monitor integrity of filters must be established and followed. Results are recorded and maintained.

Compressed Air

In general compressed air should be supplied by an "oil-free" type compressor and must be free of oil and oil vapor unless vented directly to a non-controlled environment area. It should also be dehumidified to prevent condensation of water vapor (generally to around -40(F dewpoint). Centrally distributed compressed air is generally provided at 100 to 125 psig and reduced as required.

Breathing Air

Breathing air is generally provided for use to personnel working in hazardous environments. It can be provided centrally through a breathing air distribution system or at the local level with "backpack" type breathing air units worn by each person. Personal units are more cumbersome but less expensive than central units. In either case, the system must be designed in accordance with the delivery device employed by the user. Air must be purified to meet OSHA Grade D breathing air requirements.

System reliability must be provided in the design with redundancy or storage to provide for "escape time" in case of equipment failure.

Nitrogen

Nitrogen is an inert gas generally utilized in the pharmaceutical laboratory and manufacturing environments primarily for the purging of electrical equipment in volatile or explosive environments. Cryogenic uses are limited in the pharmaceutical manufacturing industry. If it is utilized extensively throughout the facility, a central distribution system will generally be provided. Nitrogen, however, can be provided locally utilizing small individual bottles or generators. In the central system, nitrogen may be distributed at 100 to 125 psig with pressure regulation as required. Laboratory nitrogen is generally provided at lower pressures (40 to 90 psig).

Vacuum

Vacuum is utilized throughout pharmaceutical laboratory and manufacturing facilities. A great deal of vacuum is utilized in the encapsulation and tablet compression areas. Vacuum is generally generated at between 20 and 25 inches Hg and provided at between 15 and 20 inches Hg at the inlet. Once again, process and equipment requirements will dictate pressures and quantities.

Vacuum Cleaning

Vacuum cleaning is utilized throughout the pharmaceutical manufacturing environment for dry particulate and powder pickup. It can be provided centrally through a vacuum cleaning distribution system or at the local level with individual vacuum cleaning units. Individual units are more cumbersome, require stricter cleaning regimens between uses, can be a source of cross contamination, but are less expensive than central units. Vacuum cleaning is generally generated at between 5 and 10 inches Hg and provided at about 2 inches Hg at the inlet. This reduced pressure range compared to the vacuum system described above may be more conducive to some processes.. Once again, specific space and process and equipment requirements will dictate pressures and quantities.

Natural Gas and Propane

Natural gas and propane are sometimes required in the pharmaceutical laboratory environment for such processes as maintaining solvent oxidization and heating hot water and steam. Gas is generally distributed to laboratory outlets at 5 to 10 inches wg.

Process Piping Systems

Process piping systems, those that deal directly with the product or process equipment, include tanks, vessels, pumps, heat exchangers, piping, clean- and sterilize-in-place systems, vacuum material transfer systems, etc. These are discussed in other sections of this text.

FIRE PROTECTION SYSTEMS

Overview

This section describes, in general terms, the various automatic fire suppression and protection systems and their application in a pharmaceutical manufacturing facility.

Pharmaceutical manufacturing facilities are typically provided with automatic fire suppression and protection system throughout. The provision of specific suppression and protection throughout the facility might be the consequence of a strict code requirement, a trade-off for increased allowable building area or height, or simply good life and fire safety design practice.

Design Codes and Standards

Fire protection systems are designed and installed in accordance with locally adopted building codes and NFPA Standards. Underwriter's requirements and guidelines (FM, IRI, Kemper, CIGNA, etc.) may also be incorporated as applicable.

Definitions

Sprinkler Systems

Wet Sprinkler System: A sprinkler system with automatic sprinkler heads attached to a piping system containing water and connected to a water supply, so that water discharges immediately from sprinkler heads that are opened directly by heat from a fire.

Dry Pipe Sprinkler System: A sprinkler system using automatic sprinklers attached to a piping system containing air or nitrogen under pressure which, when released during the opening of the sprinkler heads, permits the water pressure to open a "dry pipe valve." The water then flows into the piping system and out of the opened sprinkler heads.

Preaction Sprinkler System: A sprinkler system using automatic sprinklers attached to a piping system containing air that may or may not be under pressure, with a supplemental detection system (smoke, heat, or flame detectors) installed in the same areas as the sprinklers. Actuation of the detection system opens a valve that permits water to flow into the sprinkler piping system and to be discharged from any sprinkler heads that may be open. Preaction systems can operate by one of the following three basic means:

- Systems that admit water to the sprinkler piping upon operation of detection devices (single interlock).
- Systems that admit water to the sprinkler piping upon operation of detection devices or automatic sprinklers (non-interlock).
- Systems that admit water to sprinkler piping upon operation of both detection devices and automatic sprinklers (double interlock).

Deluge Sprinkler System: A sprinkler system using open sprinkler heads attached to a piping system connected to a water supply through a valve that is opened by the operation of a detection system (smoke, heat, flame detectors, etc.) installed in the same areas as the sprinklers. When the valve opens, water flows into the piping system and discharges from all attached sprinkler heads.

Antifreeze Sprinkler System: A wet pipe sprinkler system using automatic sprinkler heads attached to a piping system containing an antifreeze solution and connected to a water supply. The antifreeze solution is discharged, followed by water, immediately upon operation of sprinkler heads opened directly by heat from a fire.

Deluge Foam-Water Sprinkler and Foam-Water Spray Systems

Foam-Water Sprinkler System: A special system of piping connected to a source of foam concentrate and a water supply, and equipped with appropriate discharge devices for extinguishing agent discharge and for distribution over the area to be protected. The piping system is connected to the water supply through a control valve that is usually actuated by operation of automatic detection equipment (smoke, heat, flame detectors, etc.) installed in the same areas as the sprinklers. When this valve opens, water flows into the piping system and foam concentrate is injected into the water; the resulting foam solution discharging through the discharge devices generates and distributes foam. Upon exhaustion of the foam concentrate supply, water discharge will follow the foam and continue until the system is shut off manually.

Foam-Water Spray System: A special system of piping connected to a source of foam concentrate and to a water supply and equipped with foam-water spray nozzles for extinguishing agent discharge (foam or water sequentially in that order or in reverse order) and for distribution over the area to be protected. System operation arrangements parallel those for foam-water sprinkler systems as described previously.

Closed-Head Foam-Water Sprinkler System: A sprinkler system with standard automatic sprinklers attached to a piping system containing air, water, or foam solution up to the closed-head sprinklers, that discharges foam or water directly onto the fire after the operation of a sprinkler(s). This system can also be a dry-pipe or preaction type system.

Standpipes

Standpipes are designed and installed in accordance with locally adopted building code and NFPA Standards. Typically, standpipes are required if the floor level of the highest story is more than 30 feet above the lowest level of fire department vehicle access, or if the floor level of the lowest story is located more than 30 feet below the highest level of fire department vehicle access. Standpipes are also typically required if any portion of the building floor area is more than 400 feet of travel from the nearest point of fire department vehicle access.

The installation of standpipes and hose stations may be desired independent of code requirements, especially if there is an on-site emergency response organization trained to respond to fire emergencies.

Fire Water Source and Conveyance

The water supply for automatic fire suppression and protection is provided in accordance with the locally adopted building code and NFPA Standards. If an adequate supply of water is not available from a public source, an on-site source of water will need to be provided. If the source of water has inadequate pressure to provide the required sprinkler protection, a fire pump (electric or diesel) must also be provided. The decision whether the pump is electric or diesel should be made based on the availability of electricity, reliability issues, underwriter requirements, maintenance issues, and cost.

General Design Requirements

The building will typically be provided with one or a combination of systems to provide automatic fire suppression and protection throughout the building. Suppressing agents other than those mentioned above (such as CO_2, Dry Chemical, Foam and Halon alternatives) can be used to address specific hazards, and would not be used as a suppression agent throughout.

In general the first choice for automatic fire suppression is a wet-pipe sprinkler system. This most common type of system provides the quickest actuating, most reliable, and least expensive type of suppression for most applications. Wet type sprinkler systems are generally used throughout most of the facility and designed in accordance with local building code and NFPA Standards.

Protection of spaces for storage, handling, and dispensing of flammable and combustible liquids are designed in accordance with local building code and NFPA Standards. Due to containment requirements in the event of fire and subsequent sprinkler discharge as well as flammable/combustible liquid discharge, these spaces are prime candidates for low expansion foam-water sprinkler systems such as a closed-head foam-water sprinkler system. High expansion foam and dry chemical systems are also applicable to these spaces.

In areas which are susceptible to water damage or where contamination is a concern, the use of preaction sprinkler systems are appropriate. These space may include, computer rooms, high voltage electric rooms, telecommunications rooms, sterile areas, containment areas, and other GMP spaces. At a minimum, a single-interlock preaction system can be provided. Where the accidental or unnecessary discharge of water is a concern, a double-interlock preaction system can be provided.

Dry-pipe valve systems are appropriate for use in unheated spaces such as remote detached buildings, warehouses, outside loading docks, combustible concealed spaces, parking garages, etc.

Antifreeze sprinkler systems are also appropriate for unheated spaces but are typically limited for applications requiring twenty sprinkler heads or less, such as small loading dock areas or a vestibule. Caution must be taken with the application of these systems to support local water company requirements regarding to cross-connection control (backflow prevention) due to the addition of the antifreeze to the sprinkler system.

Control and Monitoring

Water flow detection and alarms are typically provided for each floor, zone, or specific hazard space and are monitored by the building fire alarm system. Each floor or zone is equipped with electrically supervised water supply control valves that are also monitored by the building fire alarm system. Other items such as fire detection and loss of air pressure are monitored for preaction, dry and deluge type systems.

Portable Fire Extinguishers

Portable fire extinguishers are provided to suit the type of hazard and are provided in accordance with locally adopted building codes and NFPA 10 "Portable Fire Extinguishers." Extinguishers are typically the dry chemical multi-purpose ABC type, but can be water, CO_2 or other substance depending on the occupancy and hazard involved.

BIBLIOGRAPHY

ACGIH Industrial Ventilation Manual
AGS Guideline for Gloveboxes
ANSI Z 9.2: Local Exhaust Ventilation Systems
ANSI / AIHA Z9.5: American National Standard for Laboratory Ventilation
ANSI / ASHRAE 110: Method of Testing Performance of Laboratory Fume Hoods
ASHRAE Fundamentals and Applications Handbooks
ASHRAE 1: HVAC Commissioning Process
ASHRAE 55: Thermal Environmental Conditions for Human Occupancy
ASHRAE 62: Ventilation for Acceptable Indoor Air Quality
ASHRAE 90.1: Energy Standard for Buildings Except Low Rise Residential Buildings
Code of Federal Regulations, Title 21: Food and Drugs, Chapter 1: Food and Drug Administration, Department of Health and Human Services
Subchapter A—General
Subchapter C—Drugs: General
Subchapter D—Drugs for Human Use
Subchapter F—Biologics
Subchapter H—Medical Devices
Chapter 2: Drug Enforcement Administration, Department of Justice Discussions of Controlled Substances
Federal Standard 209E, Clean Room and Work Station Requirements, Controlled Environment
ICC/IMC 510: Hazardous Exhaust Systems
ISO 14644: Cleanrooms and Controlled Environments
ISPE Baseline Guides
NFPA 30: Flammable and Combustible Liquids Code
NFPA 68: Venting of Deflagrations
NFPA 69: Explosion Prevention Systems
NFPA 45: Standard on Fire Protection for Laboratories Using Chemicals

NSF 49: Class II (Laminar Flow) Biosafety Cabinetry

OSHA 29 CFR 1910.1450: Occupational Exposure to Hazardous Chemicals in Laboratories (with Appendices)

Prudent Practices for Handling Hazardous Chemicals in Laboratories

Remington's *Pharmaceutical Sciences*, Mack Publishing Company

Scientific Equipment and Furniture Association: SEFA 1.3–Laboratory Fume Hoods: Recommended Practices

SMACNA Technical Manuals

U.S. Dept. of Health and Human Services, Centers for Disease Control and Prevention: *Biosafety in Microbiological and Biomedical Laboratories, United States Pharmacopoeia (USP)*

World Health Organization: Good Practices for the Manufacture and Quality Control of Drugs

6
High Purity Water

Author: Gary V. Zoccolante

Advisor: Teri C. Soli

INTRODUCTION

The importance of process water to a pharmaceutical manufacturing facility cannot be overstated. Production of water used for drug manufacturing is a great challenge in every aspect of design, implementation, and maintenance. Water is the most widely used material in pharmaceutical manufacturing and is often the most costly. The percentage of water in finished products varies from 0 to greater than 90%. A greater volume of water is used in cleaning and rinsing processes than in formulation in most facilities. Regardless of the water volume used in actual drug formulation, all pharmaceutical water is subject to current Good Manufacturing Practices (cGMPs) even when the water does not remain in the finished product.

Water treatment systems are often investigated in great depth by the U.S. Department of Health and Human Services Food and Drug Administration (FDA) inspectors. Poor design and inadequate maintenance of water systems has led to countless FDA 483s, warning letters, and, in some cases, recall of pharmaceutical products.

Optimization of pharmaceutical water systems is a risk management exercise that requires extensive utilization of Good Engineering Practices (GEPs). The decisions regarding water quality, method of generation and distribution, sanitization method, instrumentation and control, data acquisition, and countless other construction and maintenance specifications are all based upon the impact of the consequences of water system success or failure. Optimization is a delicate balance of acceptable risk and available financial resources.

Good Manufacturing Practices (GMPs)

One of the most significant issues in water system design and operation is that although the GMP requirements are well documented in writing, they are very general and subject to continually tightening interpretation as current Good Manufacturing Practices or cGMPs. FDA establishes cGMP requirements beyond those that are documented in legal compendia, but rarely publishes written guidelines with any level of detailed engineering guidance.

Most of the GMP requirements for water are derived from broad statements in 21 CFR Part 211: Current Good Manufacturing Practices for Finished Pharmaceuticals. These general statements relate to the requirement for water used in production or cleaning processes to not "alter the safety, identity, strength, quality or purity of the drug product." These statements directly open all water system unit operations, contact surfaces of equipment and piping, installation, and maintenance to FDA scrutiny. All materials must be proven to be compatible with the product and process, and must not contribute objectionable contaminants.

Additional 21 CFR Part 211 GMP requirements for verification of proper cleaning and sanitization procedures mandate written records and procedures for these steps. All rinse and cleaning water qualities must be proven to be appropriate.

Most of the engineering details that are considered to be "cGMP requirements" have evolved over decades of system development since the birth of the concept of GMP manufacturing. Several key concepts of cGMP production of water have been adopted from the long considered but never adopted "Good Manufacturing Practices for Large Volume Parenterals," (21 CFR Part 212). This legislation was proposed in 1976 and finally removed from consideration in 1994. Although this document was never approved, many concepts it proposed have become commonplace in pharmaceutical systems. Some of these concepts include storage tank vent filters, minimal piping dead legs, sloped and fully drainable distribution systems, flushed pump seals, double tube sheet heat exchangers, and elimination of use point filters. These concepts and others will be discussed in more detail in the system design sections of this chapter.

Due to the perceived ambiguity of cGMP regulations, great disparity exists in both individual and corporate views regarding what constitutes a cGMP-compliant water system. System costs may vary by more than an order of magnitude from company to company with all groups believing that each system is optimized for cGMP construction and good design practice. The proper materials of construction, surface finishes, level and accuracy of instrumentation, automation level, data acquisition and trending, sanitization methods, system and component draining, use of microbially retentive filters, and many other factors are open to interpretation. The most difficult part of water system design is the development of what are the actual cGMP requirements when little written documentation of design details exists. Significant capital and operating cost savings are available to those who properly interpret the cGMP requirements and do not over-design the system.

KEY CONCEPTS AND PRINCIPLES

Pharmacopoeia

It is important to understand the roles of the FDA and the United States Pharmacopoeia Convention (USPC). USPC is a private not-for-profit organization established to promote public health. USPC works closely with the FDA and the pharmaceutical industry to establish authoritative drug standards. These standards are enforceable by the FDA. More than 3800 standards monographs are published in the *United States Pharmacopoeia* (USP) and *National Formulary* (NF). The monographs for water used in pharmaceutical manufacturing for products used in the United States are published in the USP.

Other pharmacopoeial regulations such as the requirements of the *European Pharmacopoeia* (PhEur) and *The Society of Japanese Pharmacopoeia* (JP) may need to be considered in the water system design and water quality testing for products that are exported from the United States. The ultimate destination of drug products or drug substances determines the regulatory requirements that must be satisfied.

Water Quality Requirement

The types of water defined in the pharmacopoeial monographs such as Purified Water and Water for Injection (WFI) are known as compendial waters. Other quality waters used in manufacturing, not defined by USP or other recognized compendia, are known as non-compendial waters. Non-compendial waters can be used in many applications such as production of many Active Pharmaceutical Ingredients (APIs) and in many cleaning and rinsing steps.

Non-compendial waters are not necessarily lower quality than compendial waters. Non-compendial waters range from water that is required only to meet the U.S. Environmental Protection Agency (EPA) National Primary Drinking Water Requirements (NPDWR), to water that is specified to exceed the requirements for Water for Injection. Non-compendial water systems are not necessarily less tested, maintained or validated than compendial waters, and they are subject to the same cGMP requirements

The water quality specification required for manufacturing is a function of several factors such as where the product will be shipped. If production is for the United States only, the water specification will be principally based on USP requirements. Shipment to Europe will require compliance with PhEur requirements, and, similarly, shipment to Japan will require compliance with JP requirements. Many other countries utilize USP, PhEur, or JP regulations or have their own requirements. In addition to pharmacopoeial requirements, water specifications reflect product and process requirements and corporate views towards FDA and cGMP regulations.

Microbial control methods for water systems frequently impact the total cost of water production more than attainment of the chemical attributes of water outlined in the USP and other appropriate compendia. The chemical attributes of compendial water listed in the monographs of the governing pharmacopeial groups are generally easily met with a properly designed and maintained system.

The microbial requirements are not stated in the USP monographs as of this writing, but the maximum action levels are documented in the USP 28 General Information Chapter <1231> and have been defined by the FDA in the 1993 FDA "Guide for Inspections of High Purity Water Systems." Although the chemical quality of water must be met consistently at points of use, proper microbial control is the focus of many FDA inspections.

Design and Cost Factors

The capital and operating costs for pharmaceutical water systems can vary significantly as a function of the selected processes and materials of construction. Water for injection (WFI) systems have fewer acceptable options for generation, storage, and distribution. The microbiological requirements are much tighter for WFI than for purified water, and WFI is generally utilized for the most critical pharmaceutical applications. Most WFI systems utilize distillation, are similar in construction, and tend to favor conservative approaches to system design, as will be detailed later in the chapter. Recent USP changes have expanded those approaches if they can be proven to be equal or superior to distillation.

Purified Water can be generated by an almost unlimited combination of processes, and can be stored and distributed utilizing a wide variety of methods and materials. The uses for Purified Water vary greatly in microbiological specifications and criticality. There is generally a greater disparity in process, cost, and risk in purified water systems than in WFI systems.

The selection of an appropriate sanitization method for generation, storage and distribution equipment can impact capital and operating costs significantly. Thermally sanitizable systems generally have higher capital costs due to a greater content of stainless steel components, but usually require considerably less labor for sanitization and have less downtime. Thermal sanitization is easier to automate and validate and typically allows attainment of lower microbial levels.

Chemically sanitized equipment has been proven to be acceptable in many applications and may have a lower capital cost, but generally requires more labor to prepare chemicals, verify attainment of proper chemical level during sanitization, and prove proper removal of residual chemical in rinse steps

Future needs and system expansion should be considered at the time of system design. Some unit processes may be practically expanded with a reasonable capital investment while others are extremely difficult to expand without additional space, equipment, and controls. Reverse osmosis units that are designed for expansion may have increased capacity within the original dimensions through addition of pressure vessels and membranes. Column based processes such as softeners and activated carbon units are generally impractical to expand without additional unit implementation. Low cost processes such as softeners are often best oversized initially to allow for anticipated expanded flows in the future.

Sampling

A sampling and testing plan must be developed for every pharmaceutical water system. This is a cGMP requirement, is certainly a Good Engineering Practice, and is necessary for monitoring system operation and control. It is important to design sampling points into the unit processes to be able to monitor each process for validation, normal operation, and troubleshooting. Test protocols and frequency must be established for each unit process as well as every use point.

Samples for quality control purposes, as opposed to process control purposes, must be collected in an appropriate manner. As an example, use-point samples for hose connections must be collected from actual production hoses using the same flush cycle used in production to prove proper water quality.

Unit process tests should be based on the expected unit performance (e.g., effluent chlorine level for an activated carbon unit employed for dechlorination). Use-point testing must be sufficient to prove compliance with both chemical and microbial requirements. Most of the chemical requirements may be proven with online or laboratory conductivity and Total Organic Carbon monitoring from a single distribution system sample location. Periodic use-point testing is required to verify the single loop sample location.

A single distribution loop sample for microbial performance is not acceptable. Each use point must be tested at a sufficient frequency to prove that the system is in microbial control. The 1993 FDA Guide to Inspections of High Purity Water Systems suggests microbial testing at a minimum of at least one use point per day and that all use points are tested at least once weekly.

Validation

It is accepted that all pharmaceutical water systems will be validated. The validation plan must be completed to some degree prior to specification of the water system. All equipment suppliers, contractors, commissioning agents, and other implementation parties must be aware of the requirements for documentation, automation lifecycle, commissioning/validation overlap, and many other factors to ensure a successful validation. Critical information such as proper lifecycle methodology, instrument certifications, material certifications, weld documentation, etc. often cannot be created after the fact if the requirements are not known prior to the manufacturing and installation. The most successful validations generally occur when the validation group has been involved throughout the project design phase. The ISPE Baseline Pharmaceutical Engineering Guide, Volume 5: Commissioning and Qualification provides a practical approach to system qualification.

Additional Information Sources

The ISPE Baseline Guide, Volume 4: Water and Steam Systems provides an excellent overview of all aspects of pharmaceutical water. The 1993 FDA Guide to Inspections of High Purity Water Systems provides insight into areas that inspectors may pursue.

Books providing excellent information regarding pharmaceutical water system design, operation, and validation are *Pharmaceutical Water: System Design, Operation, and Validation* by William V. Collentro, and *Pharmaceutical Water Systems* by Theodore A. Meltzer.

Monograph Requirements

USP 28 (as of this writing) includes monographs for eight types of pharmaceutical water. Three types of bulk water are defined as well as five types of packaged waters. The three bulk waters are USP Purified Water (PW), USP Water for Injection (WFI), and USP Water for Hemodialysis. The packaged waters are Bacteriostatic Water for Injection, Sterile Water for Inhalation, Sterile Water for Injection, Sterile Water for Irrigation, and Sterile Purified Water.

Most pharmaceutical products are manufactured with either PW or WFI. PW and WFI have the same chemical purity requirements. The monographs require that the water purity is proven by conductivity and total organic carbon (TOC).

The conductivity requirement using USP <645> can be met with online testing (Stage 1) or in laboratory testing (Stages 1, 2, or 3). The Stage 1 conductivity test requires measurement of conductivity and water temperature. The conductivity limit varies from 0.6 microsiemens/centimeter (µS/cm) at 0°C to 3.1 µS/cm at 100°C. Intermediate values include 1.3 µS/cm at 25°C and 2.7 µS/cm at 80°C.

Stage 1 conductivity requirements can be reliably attained with a variety of system configurations using common water purification processes. Most pharmaceutical water systems are designed to meet Stage 1 conductivity to take advantage of online testing to provide significant data for trending and to minimize laboratory testing. Point-of-use testing generally requires laboratory analysis. Pharmaceutical water that does not meet the Stage 1 conductivity limit can be laboratory tested to meet the Stage 2 or 3 limit.

The TOC test is a limit response test with a theoretical limit of 500 parts per billion (ppb). The test is designed to accommodate virtually any TOC analyzer that meets the USP suitability requirements

The microbial limits for USP Purified Water (PW) are not defined in the legally binding monograph. The General Information Chapter <1231> Water for Pharmaceutical Purposes states that a maximum of 100 colony forming units per milliliter (mL) may be used as an action level and this is also stated in the 1993 FDA Guide to Inspections of High Purity Water Systems. The requirements of this General Information section are not legally binding, but FDA has stated publicly on many occasions that this is the maximum microbial level acceptable for USP PW.

The actual action level may be much lower than the maximum action level of 100 mL and is determined by the manufacturer (subject to FDA approval) as a function of product, process, and system performance. Some products and processes require an absence of certain objectionable species such as *Pseudomonas aeruginosa* as well as a low total viable plate count.

Water for Injection (WFI) has the same chemical requirements as PW and has a limit of 0.25 endotoxin units per milliliter (EU/mL). The microbial level for WFI also is absent from the monograph but is stated to be a maximum action level of 10 cfu/100 mL in USP Chapter <1231> and this is in agreement with FDA views.

The USP 28 PW monograph states "Purified Water is water obtained by a suitable process." This essentially leaves the process selection open to all technologies.

The USP 28 WFI monograph states "Water for Injection is water purified by distillation or a purification process that is equivalent or superior to distillation in the removal of chemicals and microorganisms." Several prior volumes of USP limited WFI production to distillation or reverse osmosis.

Distillation currently produces over 99% of USP WFI. Other processes such as a combination of reverse osmosis, deionization, and ultrafiltration have a significant history of production of WFI quality water for rinsing, API production, and other uses. Distillation was the only allowable process for WFI production for decades and became the standard method of production. The revised USP 28 WFI monograph may stimulate an increase in alternative system designs if the alternative designs are evaluated to be as reliable as distillation and more cost effective.

WATER QUALITY SELECTION

The water quality or qualities selected for the pharmaceutical process must be consistent with the final product requirements. The final rinse water must be the same quality as the water used in manufacturing. Oral products must use a minimum of USP PW for manufacturing and PW is normally used as final rinse water. Since the

Water Quality Decision Tree

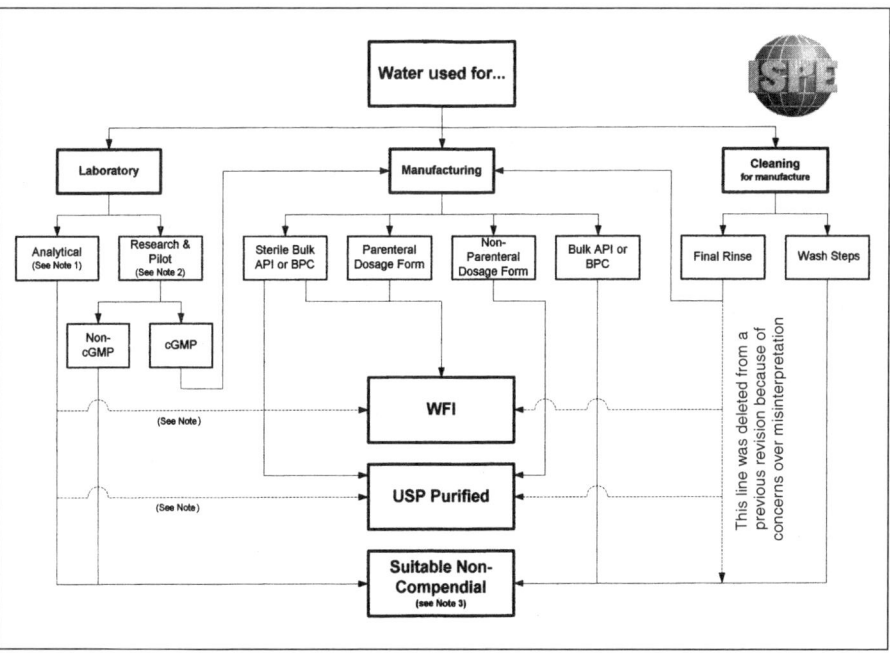

Note: Commitments made in drug applications override suggestions of this decision tree.
Source: Reprinted with permission of ISPE Baseline Pharmaceutical Engineering Guide, Vol. 4, Water and Steam Systems, 2001.

Laboratory Water

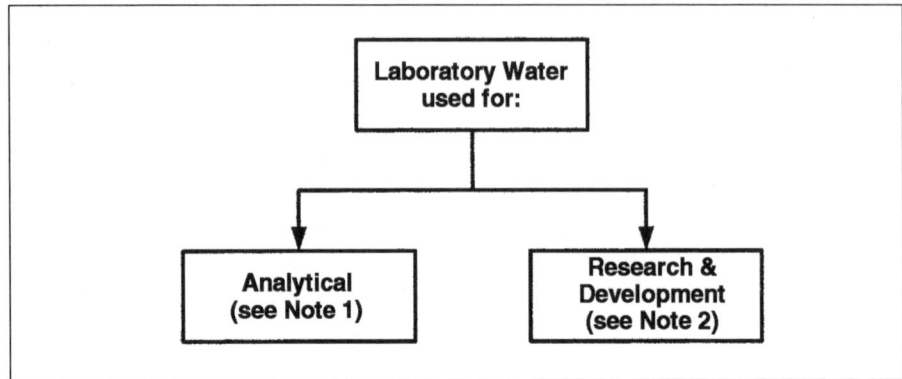

Note 1: Some analytical methods require USP Compendial Waters.
Note 2: If both cGMP and non-cGMP operations occur in the same facility, follow the cGMP path

method of manufacture for PW is not stated by USP, there is little advantage to use of non-compendial water for final rinse water where PW is acceptable.

Parenteral products must use a minimum water quality of USP WFI for manufacturing and WFI is used in most plants for final rinse water. It is acceptable to use "WFI quality" non-compendial water for final rinse in parenteral processes if practical. Production of non-compendial "WFI quality" water may or may not be less expensive than WFI.

The ISPE Baseline Guide Volume 4: Water and Steam Systems recommendations, and expanded views for laboratory, manufacturing and cleaning are shown in the following.

Water for Manufacture

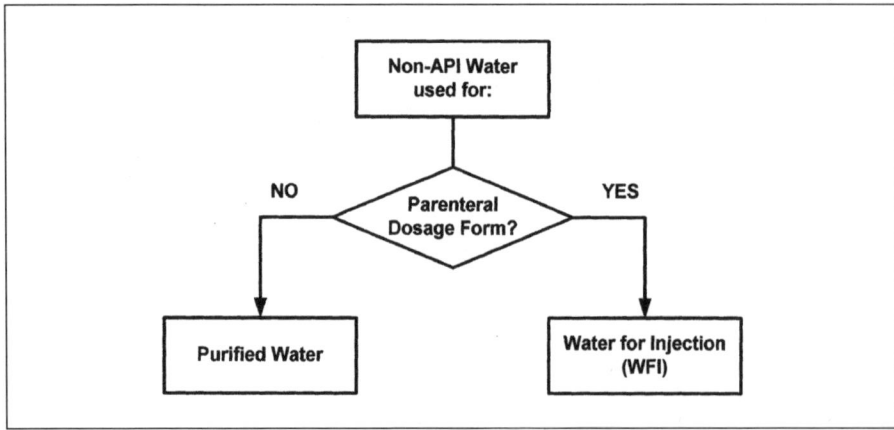

Cleaning Water for Manufacture

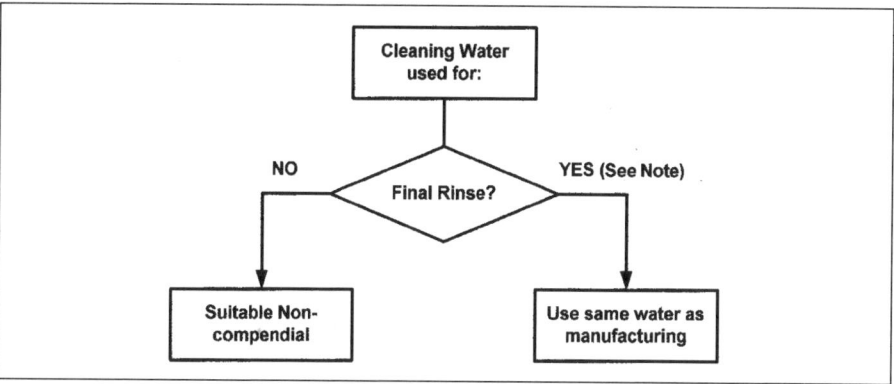

Note: A suitable non-compendial water may be used where the product contact surface is subsequently sanitized.

The water quality requirements for Active Pharmaceutical Ingredients (API) and Bulk Pharmaceutical Chemicals (BPC) are complex. The minimum water quality permitted in API or BPC manufacturing is water meeting the U.S. Environmental Protection Agency (EPA) National Primary Drinking Water Requirements (NPDWR) or equivalent. APIs use a wide range of waters for manufacturing, initial rinses and final rinses, up to and including WFI.

API Process Water Decision Tree Minimum Water Quality

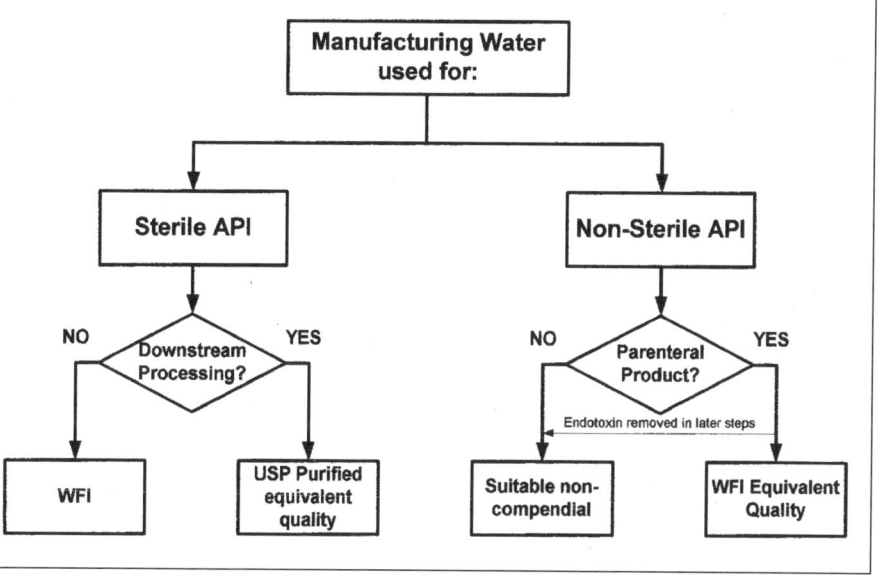

API Cleaning Water Decision Tree

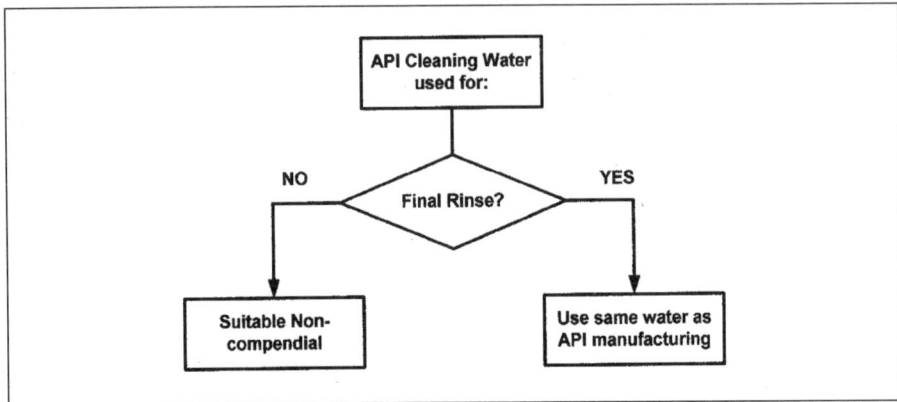

The ISPE Baseline Guide, Volume 4: Water and Steam Systems water quality recommendations for API manufacturing are shown below.

FDA may expect WFI to be used in certain inhalation products depending upon use. Water quality exceeding USP, PW, or WFI requirements may be required for some products such as intrathecals. A large volume parenteral product may have to be produced with water with endotoxin limits well below WFI limits dependent upon the expected patient weight and the dosage volume. The manufacturer is required to determine the appropriate water quality.

Foreign Pharmacopoeial Requirements

The *European Pharmacopoeia* 5 has monographs for PW and WFI as well as a third bulk water, Highly Purified Water. The EP 5 PW requirements are similar in many respects to the USP 28 PW as of this writing. The chemical purity is defined by TOC and conductivity, but also by traditional pass/fail tests for nitrates and heavy metals. The allowable PW conductivity is higher than USP limits.

EP 5 requires WFI to be produced by distillation without exception. The chemical requirements are the same as EP 5 PW with the exception that the conductivity limit is equivalent to USP limits. The microbial requirements are the same as USP WFI. The EP 5 endotoxin requirements are the same as USP although the units are expressed as IU/mL rather than EU/ml.

Determine System Capacity Requirements

One of the most critical and difficult steps in the programming of a water system is determination of the optimum generation and storage/distribution system sizing. Optimization requires accurate information regarding individual use-point demand and the total manufacturing cycle. Users must provide data regarding flow, pressure, and temperature for each use point over a daily and weekly schedule. At times this information is estimated prior to confirmation of the production cycle.

All parties involved must resist the tendency to overestimate consumption or the system may be significantly oversized. Significant system over-sizing wastes capital, can lead to microbial issues during operation, and can needlessly increase wastewater generation.

Future needs should be considered during system design. Systems can often be designed to run at low flows initially and to be operated at higher flows later as production needs increase. Good engineering practice minimizes capital expenditure without incurring unacceptable risk.

A *usage chart* can help to organize the usage data. Each point can be plotted over a 24-hour period and total consumption can be calculated. These data can be compared with makeup rates and tank level to ensure proper operation. A sample usage chart is shown below.

Water Options Planning
Typical total usage chart.

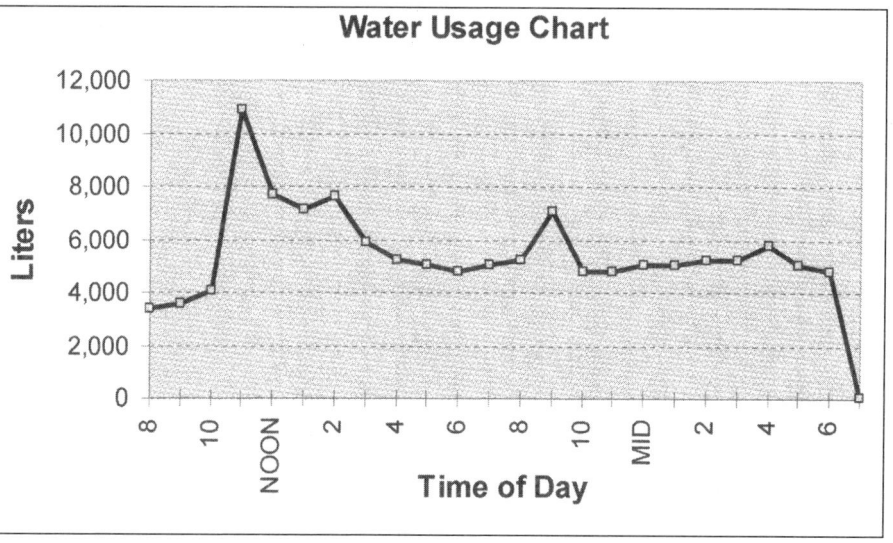

Source: Reprinted with permission from ISPE Baseline Pharmaceutical Engineering Guide, Vol. 4, Water and Steam Systems, 2001.

The information in the usage chart can be plotted to show storage tank level under estimated usage conditions. A sample plot is shown below. The tank level cannot be allowed to go below the tank low level value or the system distribution pumps will be shut off for pump protection. This would stop production water flow, halt water-related production activities, and require system sanitization if the shutdown is prolonged. No single configuration of makeup flow rate and storage volume is necessarily perfect for any given set of conditions. Users have different degrees of conservatism, tolerable risk, and budget constraints. System designers should consider the impact of abnormal situations such as a process failure or cleaning cycle that may require more makeup water than normal.

Water Options/Planning
Typical storage tank level chart.

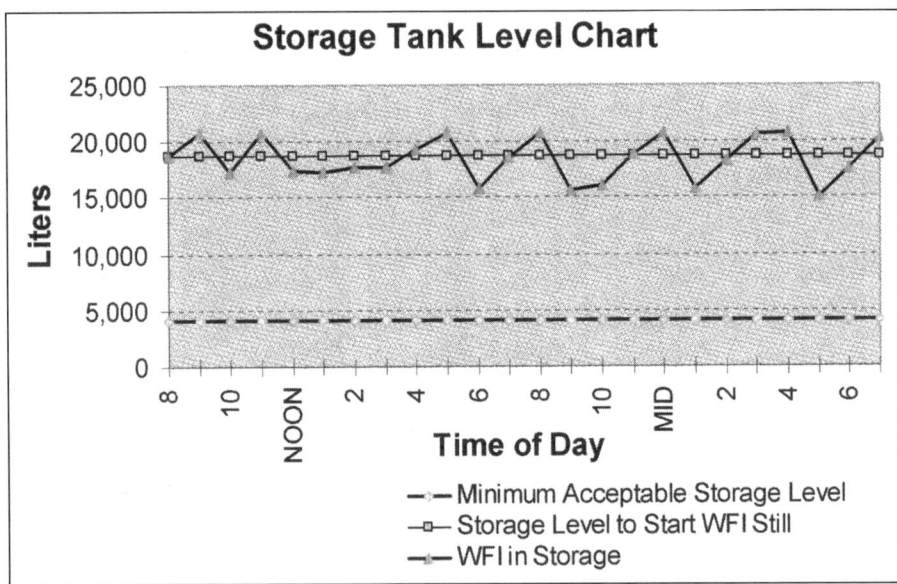

Source: Reprinted with permission from ISPE Baseline Pharmaceutical Engineering Guide, Vol. 4, Water and Steam Systems, 2001.

Determine the Optimum Generation System

Good design practice can be applied in selection of the pharmaceutical water generation system process and equipment specification. Generation system selection should be based upon accurate source water information, proper water quality specifications, lifecycle cost analysis, sanitization methods, reliability, maintenance requirements, and several other possible factors.

Pretreatment

Most pharmaceutical water systems include pre-treatment equipment, primary (or final) treatment equipment, and sometimes polishing equipment. The primary treatment processes most commonly implemented in pharmaceutical water systems includes reverse osmosis (RO), ion exchange (IX), and distillation separately or in various combinations. Typically polishing technologies are not used downstream of distillation.

Pretreatment equipment selection must be made after selection of the primary treatment equipment. Pretreatment equipment must be properly selected to protect the final treatment equipment and, in some cases, to meet the final water quality requirements.

Pretreatment equipment typically is implemented to control scale, fouling, and oxidation of final treatment equipment. Scale or precipitation occurs when the solubility of sparingly soluble salts is exceeded in the concentrate streams of RO and distillation units. Scale is commonly controlled with several process options. The options are briefly discussed below. More information is available in the ISPE Baseline Guide, Volume 4: Water and Steam Systems and other pharmaceutical water system design books.

Scale Control

The most common form of scale control is the use of water softeners upstream of stills and RO units. Water softeners utilize cation exchange resin in the sodium form to remove divalent cations such as calcium, magnesium, barium, and strontium. The most common forms of scale in reverse osmosis units and stills are calcium carbonate, calcium sulfate, calcium fluoride, barium sulfate, strontium sulfate, and silica. Softeners cannot control silica scale but can prevent formation of the other forms of scale through the removal of calcium, magnesium, barium, and stronium from the feed water in exchange for sodium. Sodium salts are highly soluble.

Softeners operate on a batch basis and are regenerated with a sodium chloride brine solution. The method of brine introduction and brine volume can be optimized to reduce operating cost.

Softener construction varies broadly. Vessel construction is typically plastic-lined, reinforced fiberglass (FRP), lined carbon steel, or stainless steel. Piping materials are typically PVC, copper, or stainless steel. Multi-port valve units are used as well as individual valves. All of these designs are proven in thousands of applications.

Instrumentation commonly includes a flow monitor to measure service and backwash flows and inlet and outlet pressure gauges. Hardness monitors can be used on the effluent to detect the breakthrough of hardness and can be used to initiate regeneration of the softeners.

Anti-scalant/anti-foulant chemicals can also be used to control scale and fouling in RO units. Several anti-scalant chemicals are very effective in inorganic scale control including all of the calcium salts previously mentioned and various silica compounds. These chemicals also have anti-foulant properties and can be very useful in minimizing particulate fouling. The anti-foulant properties limit deposition of inorganic and organic particulates and colloids. The capital cost of anti-scalant systems is generally significantly less than the capital cost of water softeners. The operating cost may be higher or lower dependent upon feed water quality.

Anti-scalant chemicals have been successfully utilized in RO feed water applications for decades but some issues must be addressed. The application rate of the anti-scalant chemical must be correctly projected and adjusted to be the correct rate. Under application of the chemical may result in significant scaling of the RO or distillation equipment, and over application may lead to significant membrane fouling requiring frequent cleaning.

Adjustment of feed water pH can also be utilized to minimize scale in RO systems. Lowering of the pH increases the solubility of most sparingly soluble salts. Lowering of pH converts some bicarbonate to carbon dioxide that is not removed by RO. The system design must address this carbon dioxide or an alternate scale control method must be implemented.

Fouling Control

Pretreatment equipment is often included to minimize fouling in RO primary treatment systems. Fouling is a mechanical coating of membranes rather than a chemical precipitation such as scale. Fouling occurs from common feed water contaminants such as silt, dissolved organics, colloids, heavy metals, and microorganisms. Different pretreatment processes are utilized for the different foulants.

Silt, colloids, and other types of particulate are generally controlled through different methods of filtration. Large particulate or suspended solids are typically minimized through pretreatment steps such as multi-media filtration, disposable cartridge filtration, nanofiltration, and ultrafiltration, or through a clarification or flocculation process.

The most common particulate fouling control is use of a multi-media filter as the first component of the pharmaceutical water system. Multi-media filters are pressure filters generally employing three active layers of media filtration in a pressure vessel utilized in a downward service flow. The active layers vary but are most commonly anthracite followed by a layer of sand with a final filtration layer of fine garnet. Multi-media filters can generally filter down to the 7–10 micron range, although not on an absolute basis.

Multi-media filters are sized as a function of the pretreatment requirement and the feed water quality. Multi-media filters are generally sized larger to provide better filtration ahead of reverse osmosis systems than ahead of either distillation units or demineralizers. The flow rate of multi-media filters upstream of reverse osmosis units is generally in the range of 5–8 gpm per square foot of filter surface area, with a maximum of 10 gpm per square foot for continuous duty. When multiple filters are used, the instantaneous velocity through the filter will obviously increase when one of the filters is out of service in a backwash or maintenance mode. It is not an issue to increase the velocity through the remaining filters in service for the brief period of filter backwash and rinse.

The most common alternative to multi-media filtration is an inexpensive disposable cartridge filter or bag filter. These filters reduce the capital cost and reduce the generation of wastewater, but generally increase operating cost. Manual labor is required to change the cartridges or bags and the media replacement cost can be significant in some applications. Disposable cartridge filters and bag filters are available in a very wide range of materials, filtration ratings, and costs. Disposable cartridge filters and bag filters can filter just as effectively as

Multimedia Depth Filtration

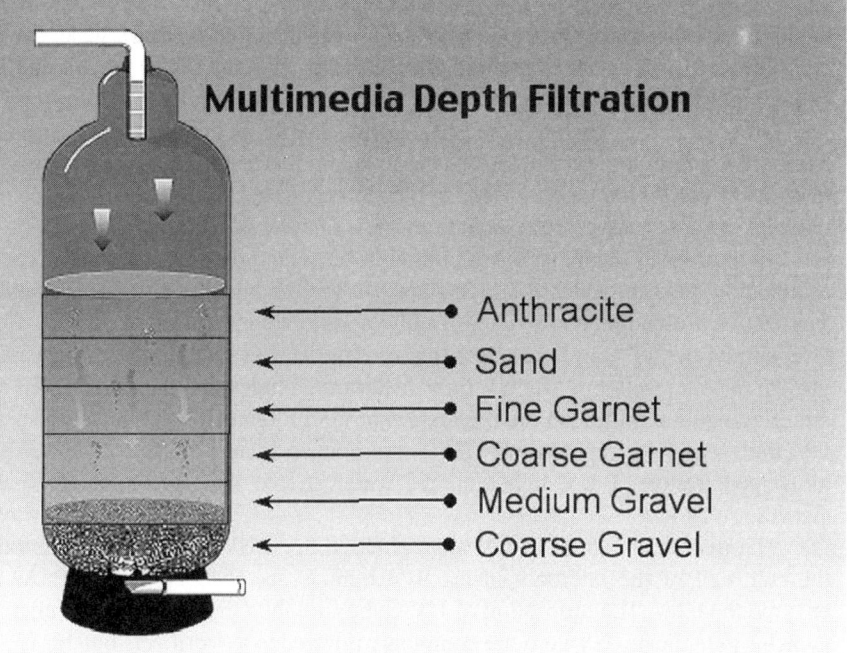

multi-media filters or better as a function of the disposable filter micron rating. In cases of high flow and high suspended solids, multi-media filters are generally the better choice since they are typically automatically backwashed and necessitate very little labor.

Organic fouling reduction is not always included in RO pretreatment. When organic fouling reduction is included, it is generally an organic scavenger, activated carbon filtration, or ultrafiltration.

Organic scavengers utilize specially selected anion resins in a pressure vessel configuration very similar to water softeners. The anion resin selected has the ability to remove a wide variety of dissolved organics from feed water and have the ability to have the organics eluted from the resin during a regeneration process.

Activated carbon has been used in several applications for organic reduction as well as dechlorination. The reduction of organics varies greatly with time in service, carbon type, application, and feed water properties. The reduction of organics through use of activated carbon may range from only a few percent to as high as perhaps 80%. It is difficult to predict the effectiveness of organic reduction with activated carbon without pilot testing.

Pretreatment systems must also address the issue of microbial fouling of final treatment equipment. Microbial fouling is an issue in membrane systems such as reverse osmosis and ultrafiltration and also media processes such as multi-media filters, disposable cartridge filters, softeners, and activated carbon units.

Microbial fouling can be effectively controlled through the presence of residual chlorine in the feed water to many processes. Some of the processes such as multimedia filters, disposable cartridge filters, and softeners, for example, generally tolerate levels of chlorine that are high enough to control microbial growth and low enough to avoid significant media oxidation.

Other processes such as some RO, ultrafiltration, or microfiltration processes frequently incorporate membranes or media that are not chlorine tolerant. Residual feed water chlorine is not a viable option in this case. Microbial fouling control methods in these cases often include the use of ultraviolet light upstream of the process in order to moderate the microbial level in the process feed water, frequent sanitization with hot water at temperatures of 80⁰C or higher, or frequent chemical sanitization with a range of oxidizing and non-oxidizing biocides.

Ultraviolet (UV) light has been utilized for decades to control microorganism growth in water systems. The UV light spectrum includes several wavelengths that are effective in minimizing the replication of microorganisms in the water stream. UV units typically incorporate UV lamps housed inside of quartz sleeves that allow penetration of UV light into the water stream that surrounds the quartz sleeves.

The microbial control of UV units is based upon UV radiation penetration of the cell wall of the microorganisms. UV light is absorbed by DNA, RNA, and enzyme modules. The absorption of UV energy inhibits the ability of the microorganisms to replicate. UV units are commonly referred to as sterilizers but this is generally inaccurate since UV units typically only provide a significant reduction in microbial counts from the influent stream to the effluent stream, and are not expected to sterilize the process stream.

Oxidation Control

Another critical part of pretreatment systems is the implementation of a process to remove feed water disinfectants from the process stream. Most municipal feed waters utilize chlorine or chloramines for bacterial control. Many private supply systems utilize injection of chlorine for the same microbial control purpose. The chlorine or chloramines are damaging to many pretreatment and final treatment components. Ammonia can be a byproduct of dechloramination and the system must be designed to remove the ammonia or USP conductivity limits may not be met.

Distillation units and RO units that include the widely used thin film composite membranes are subject to extreme damage from chlorine compounds. Most distillation units are only rated up to 0.02 ppm free chlorine and most manufacturers recommend that non-detectable levels should be present. Manufacturers of thin film composite RO membranes have various rating systems for chlorine tolerance. Most are rated in chlorine ppm/hours of contact, but none of the manufacturers provide any membrane warranty if oxidation of the membrane is present. The reality is that chlorine should be at non-detectable levels ahead of all distillation and thin film composite RO systems for the most reliable operation.

Dechlorination or dechloramination is accomplished in most pharmaceutical systems through implementation of activated carbon, injection of sodium sulfite compounds, or through the use of UV light. All of these processes have significant advantages and disadvantages.

Activated Carbon: Activated carbon had been by far the most widely used dechlorination process until recent years. Activated carbon is still used in approximately 50% of new systems that are implemented in the pharmaceutical industry. It is capable of removing chlorine or chloramine to virtually non-detectable levels, preparing the effluent water for further purification in final treatment processes. The activated carbon process is relatively passive and typically does not require significant operator attention other than the sanitization process.

The principal issue with activated carbon use is the potential effluent microbial level. Activated carbon units can provide an ideal environment for microbial growth. This issue is well managed with regular sanitization with clean steam or hot water at 80°C or higher. Steam is very effective, but the carbon unit must be well designed to avoid channeling of steam through the carbon bed. The channeling could leave unsanitized cold areas.

Hot water is more easily distributed to provide complete heating of the carbon unit and plant steam can be utilized as the heating source. Both hot water and steam can effectively control microbial levels in carbon units.

Activated carbon is generally provided on either a deep bed column basis where the carbon remains in service from generally a minimum of 6 months to a maximum

Multimedia Depth Filter

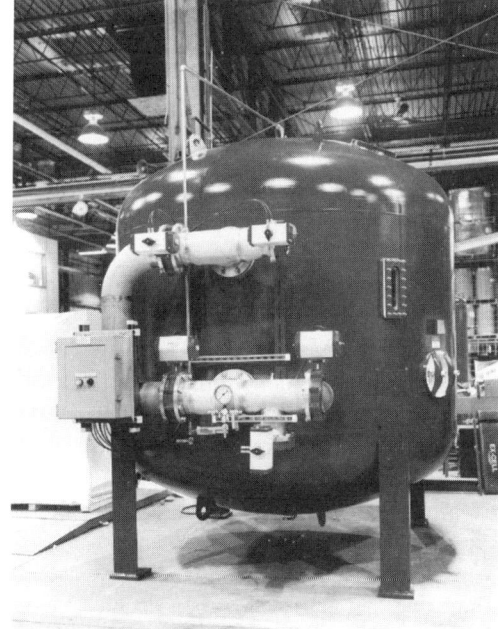

Source: Courtesy of USFilter, a Siemens company.

of approximately 2 years or on an easily disposable basis where the carbon may be changed as frequently as every 2 weeks. Both methods of carbon implementation have been widely used with success in pharmaceutical systems.

Activated carbon units are normally provided with inlet and outlet pressure gauges and flow instrumentation to ensure appropriate backwash flow rates. Thermally sanitized activated carbon units are typically provided with temperature indication to ensure that appropriate temperatures are reached for the thermal sanitization procedure. Dual thermally sanitizable carbon units are shown below.

Sodium Sulfite: The use of sodium sulfite compounds (sodium sulfite, sodium bisulfite, or sodium metabisulfite) has increased significantly in recent years. Injection of sodium sulfite compounds for dechlorination or dechloramination is almost always the lowest capital cost alternative for this process.

Sodium sulfite injection can be very effective for removal of chlorine or chloramines (combined chlorine). The application rate varies with the compound utilized. Applying sodium sulfite at the correct rate is one of the issues in use of this technology for dechlorination. Sodium sulfite systems must address feed water chlorine/chloramines spikes as complete removal is required without excessive over-application of sulfite

Under application of sodium sulfite can lead to residual chlorine or chloramines and, therefore, may result in oxidation of downstream equipment. Over application of sodium sulfite can lead to rapid fouling of reverse osmosis units.

Instrumentation of sodium sulfite injection systems varies. Instrumentation to measure free chlorine or combined chlorine should be incorporated to ensure proper performance of the system. Oxidation/reduction potential (ORP) monitors are commonly used for this purpose. Monitors to directly measure free chlorine or combined chlorine have also been used.

UV Light: The newest alternative method for dechlorination in pharmaceutical water systems is use of UV light. Low pressure and medium pressure units can be effectively utilized, as is the case in microbial control. Extremely high intensity levels are required for quantitative reduction of free or combined chlorine. The range of UV light energy can vary from 10 times the energy required for microbial control to as high as 150 times the energy required for germicidal control.

Many factors are considered when sizing UV units for dechlorination or dechloramination. These factors include the disinfectant utilized, the range of concentration of disinfectant in the feed water, water temperature, feed water total organic carbon level, and the UV unit that is to be utilized. Ultraviolet light is very effective in reduction of free or combined chlorine levels, but significant energy must be applied to reduce typical feed water levels to non-detectable levels.

The greatest advantage of UV dechlorination is that no microbial risk exists, as is the case with both sodium sulfite injection and activated carbon dechlorination. The massive doses of UV light applied are lethal to feed water microbes. The capital cost is generally higher than sodium sulfite injection but lower than or equal to thermally sanitized activated carbon units.

The principal disadvantage of UV light dechlorination is that attainment of chlorine levels below the limit of detection is quite difficult without using significant UV light energy levels. The effectiveness of UV dechlorination is a direct function of the feed water disinfectant level and the UV energy level applied. Significant increases in feed water disinfectant level such as those encountered when coliform microorganisms are detected in municipal feed water may present a challenge to UV light dechlorination. Sodium sulfite injection can be used as a supplemental dechlorination method when peak chlorine levels are encountered.

It is obvious that significant advantages and disadvantages exist with all of the common methods of pharmaceutical water system dechlorination. Great debate exists regarding the most effective method of dechlorination but all of the technologies have been employed successfully.

Primary (Final) Treatment

Water systems may incorporate one or more final treatment processes. The most commonly implemented primary treatment processes for USP PW and WFI production are reverse osmosis (RO), ion exchange (IX), and distillation. These processes may be used individually or in various combinations.

Reverse Osmosis

Reverse osmosis (RO) is a process utilizing a semi-permeable membrane capable of removing dissolved organic and inorganic contaminants from water. Water can permeate through the membrane while other substances such as salts, acids, bases, colloids, bacteria, and bacterial endotoxins are quantitatively rejected and concentrated in a waste stream. RO can reject up to 99.5 % of the inorganic salts that comprise the largest contaminant group of raw feed water. Rejection of organics, microorganisms and endotoxins can also be multiple logs. The only feed water contaminant group that is not effectively rejected by RO is dissolved gases.

Many water purification processes are operated on a batch basis. Contaminants are removed in a process and collected on the process media. The contaminants are then removed in a regeneration or backwash procedure and the removal/regeneration is repeated. RO is a continuous pressure driven process that depends on cross-flow contaminant removal into the waste or concentrate stream for effective operation.

The recovery (i.e., percent of feed water that becomes purified product water) of RO systems is typically about 75%. The recovery can range from as low as 25% to levels approaching 90%. The significant wastewater generated from the RO process is a significant concern in many facilities. Higher recovery rates reduce wastewater, but can lead to more frequent RO cleaning requirements and lower product water quality. Lower recovery rates improve product water quality and process reliability, but can increase water consumption unless the RO wastewater is utilized elsewhere. RO wastewater can often be utilized in cooling tower makeup or other applications and then RO can be a very efficient process from a standpoint of water conservation.

The output of an RO array of membrane modules is a function of the applied trans-membrane pressure (feed pressure minus product pressure) and the feed temperature. The product water output of a fixed membrane area increases with an increase of pressure or temperature. If low cost heat is available, it may be wise to heat the feed water in cold water applications to somewhere in the range of 50°F to 70°F. This reduces the feed pump pressure and energy requirement. Low cost heat is generally not available and, in most cases, the lowest energy cost application of RO is to use low temperature feed water from the source with higher applied membrane driving pressures. System optimization requires an analysis of the best temperature/pressure combination.

Most pharmaceutical RO units incorporate membranes utilizing thin film composite membrane construction. Thin film composite membranes are degraded rapidly in the presence of chlorine at municipal drinking water levels. The dechlorination of the feed water does allow the opportunity for some bacterial growth to occur and sanitization methods must be taken into account. All RO units can be configured to be compatible with a range of chemical sanitization agents. Many units are supplied with RO membrane modules that allow hundreds of sanitization cycles with water at 80°C. The hot water sanitization is extremely effective in microbial control, but does not generally eliminate the need for periodic membrane chemical cleaning. Hot water sanitization is typically significantly more effective than chemical sanitization.

RO can be successfully implemented in pharmaceutical systems in several ways. The most common application of RO in pharmaceutical water systems is utilization of RO upstream of an ion exchange process to produce USP Purified Water. The combination of RO and ion exchange easily exceeds the requirements for conductivity, total organic carbon, and microbiology when properly applied. RO units can be implemented upstream of off-site regenerated ion exchange units to reduce the cost of resin replacement and are frequently utilized upstream of continuous electrodeionization (CEDI) units to provide appropriate feed water quality. RO units are utilized upstream of regenerable deionizers to reduce regenerant acid and caustic consumption. All of these combinations of reverse osmosis and ion exchange technologies reliably produce USP Purified Water and can be designed to meet even higher non-compendial standards.

RO is also used to pretreat the feed water to a polishing RO unit. These systems are known as product staged or two-pass RO and are generally capable of producing water that meets the requirements of the USP Purified Water for TOC and conductivity. Some installations produce water that meets the USP Stage 1 conductivity level allowing on-line measurement, while others produce water that passes the Stage 2 or 3 laboratory tests.

RO is commonly implemented as part of a pretreatment system for still feed. RO units alone, or with ion exchange, produce feed water meeting the still requirements for chloride, silica, and other contaminants. The reduction of endotoxin in the still feed stream ensures extremely low endotoxin levels in the distillate. A RO unit is shown below.

Dual Activated Carbon Filters

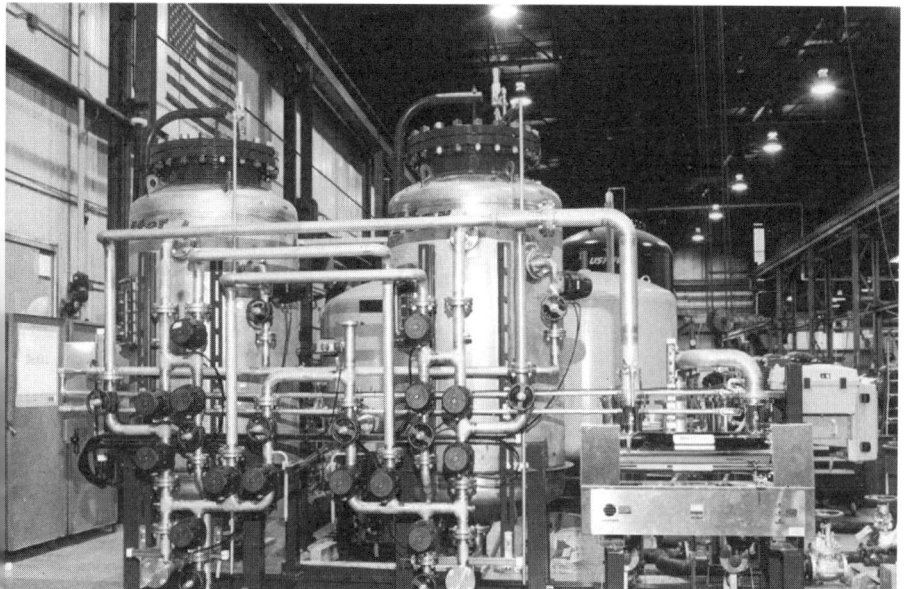

Source: Courtesy of USFilters, a Siemens company.

Microbial levels in the RO product water can also be an issue. RO can control product water microbial levels to meet WFI requirements (less than 10 cfu/100 ml) when properly designed and maintained. Most RO applications do not require micro-

Reverse Osmosis/Continuous Deionization (RO/CEDI) Process

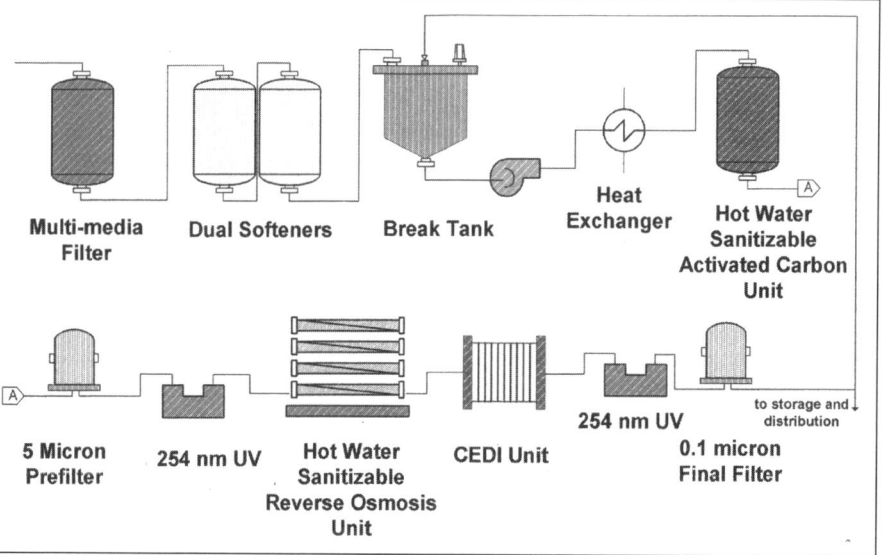

bial levels even approaching WFI requirements. The product water microbial levels from most RO units meet USP Purified Water specifications. High RO product water microbial levels generally occur as a result of poor sanitization procedures, infrequent sanitization, or poor preteatment design and maintenance. RO membranes are now available for continuous operation at 80°C. This operation is self-sanitizing and allows RO to consistently meet the WFI microbial requirement of less than 10 cfu/mL.

The common RO pretreatment processes and complete RO systems have been reviewed earlier in this chapter.

RO is widely used for final treatment in pharmaceutical water because the process removes a wide variety of contaminants with minimal chemical consumption and reasonable energy costs. The process is reliable when the pretreatment and RO systems are properly designed and maintained. The membrane barrier protects the finished water from contamination under normal and most peak feed water contamination conditions.

Ion Exchange

Ion exchange is incorporated in many USP Purified Water systems, WFI systems, and non-compendial systems. The common ion exchange processes are off-site regenerated ion exchange, in place regenerated ion exchange, and continuous electrodeionization. All of the processes incorporate cation exchange resin for cation removal and anion exchange resin for anion removal. The processes have similarities in performance, but can differ significantly in capital cost, operating cost, chemical consumption, wastewater generation, maintenance requirements, microbial control, and outside service requirements.

All ion exchange technologies can support microbial growth, and sanitization methods must be incorporated. Hot water sanitization, chemical sanitization, and frequent chemical regeneration have all been successfully implemented in pharmaceutical water systems.

Off-site and in place ion exchange resins are the same materials. The difference is simply that off site regeneration transfers the regeneration process to outside service companies. In place regeneration requires pharmaceutical companies to implement chemical storage, chemical handling, and neutralization equipment to perform resin regeneration. The ion exchange capability of ionized solids removal is the same regardless of off-site or in place regeneration. The decision for off-site versus in place regeneration is based upon consideration of capital cost, operating cost, chemical handling, process control, and other factors.

Off-site regenerated resin systems are generally much lower in capital cost than in place regenerated systems because significant chemical handling equipment and piping is eliminated. The outside services of a resin regenerator are required unless new resin is purchased for each exchange. Most systems use regenerated resin, but some pharmaceutical companies do purchase new resin for each exchange because it is felt that quality control is improved. Many quality resin regeneration companies exist, but all should be periodically audited to ensure that the resin regeneration process is accomplished in a GMP manner.

Off-site regenerated ion exchange resin systems can be the only final treatment utilized to produce USP Purified Water or may follow reverse osmosis to remove the ionic contaminants that have passed through the RO process. Ion exchange, whether regenerated off-site or in place, can remove ionized contaminants to virtually immeasurable levels. The decision to utilize ion exchange alone or to use RO upstream of ion exchange is generally based on cost and technical considerations.

Ion exchange units can reduce feed water total organic carbon, but not necessarily to USP levels on all water supplies. RO may be implemented upstream of ion exchange units to ensure consistent USP TOC attainment. Ion exchange systems without RO pretreatment reliably produce USP Purified Water in many installations where the feed water TOC levels are not too high.

Since RO typically removes greater than 98% of feed water ionized solids, the throughput of downstream ion exchange units is increased substantially. When RO is implemented upstream of off-site regenerated ion exchange units, the payback is fast in most cases. If TOC attainment is not an issue the decision to utilize RO pretreatment is usually based on whether or not the additional capital cost of RO equipment is offset within reasonable time by reduced resin regeneration costs.

All ion exchange systems (no ROs) are generally limited to relatively low daily makeup volume on relatively low total dissolved solids feed waters. Polishing components such as UV light microbial reduction units, disposable cartridge filters, and even ultrafilters are commonly placed downstream of the ion exchange units. The disposable cartridge filters may be rated in the range of 5 micron removal for resin fines or may be as tight as 0.1 micron absolute for microbial retention.

High makeup volume systems more commonly use continuous electrodeionization or in place regenerated ion exchange units for the ion exchange polishing process. Systems implementing pretreatment and in place regenerated ion exchange (but no RO) were the dominant USP Purified Water generation system design for decades until about 1990. At that time RO based systems began to claim a majority of new large volume systems. Large volume regenerable ion exchange systems are rare in new applications as most companies wish to reduce chemical consumption and utilize membrane technology or distillation.

In place regenerated ion exchange systems are still utilized downstream of RO in some new systems. In place regeneration can offer lower operating costs than off site regeneration. The regeneration of resin with acid and caustic can provide excellent microbial control of the demineralizers if the regeneration is frequent enough. Some ion exchange units that are regenerated every one or two days have effluent microbial levels that are equal to or better than membrane systems. When regeneration frequency becomes less frequent than once per week microbial issues may occur. An in place regenerated separate bed ion exchange unit is shown below.

Most systems that use in place regenerated ion exchange units also utilize ultraviolet and filtration devices downstream for control of microbial levels and resin fines (particulates). The cost of microbially retentive filters downstream of ion exchange units can be excessive on high colloidal level feed waters when RO is not employed upstream.

Pharmaceutical Reverse Osmosis Unit

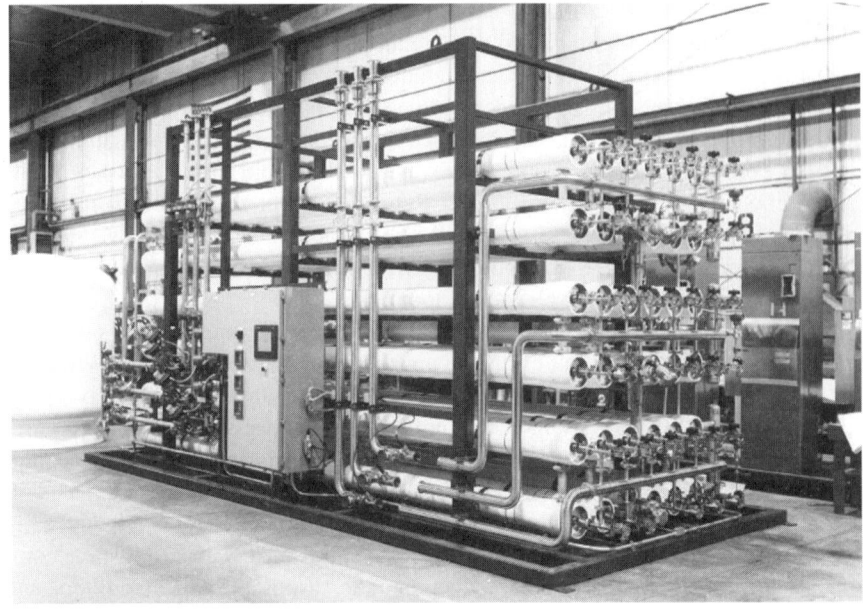

Source: Courtesy of USFilter, a Siemens company.

The final ion exchange process that is commonly used in pharmaceutical water production is continuous electrodeionization (CEDI). CEDI devices are able to remove ionizable contaminants from water without the requirement for chemical regeneration. CEDI units use ion exchange membranes, ion exchange resin, and DC electrical potential to transport ionized species from a feed stream into a concentrate stream. Some of the ion exchange resin in the unit is continuously regenerated with H^+ and OH^- that are created from splitting of a minor portion of the feed water stream.

Almost all CEDI units are placed downstream of RO. The RO unit upstream improves the feed water quality to a level suitable for feed to CEDI. The RO unit also minimizes the conductivity level of the RO product stream making the removal of the remaining ionized contaminants by CEDI practical. For reliable operation, CEDI feed water must be relatively low in hardness, organics, silica, suspended solids, total dissolved solids, and free of oxidizing agents.

CEDI units typically exhibit bacteriostatic or bactericidal effects within the electric field. This can significantly retard microbial growth within the resin membrane matrix. This effect does not extend into piping areas outside of the electric field so periodic sanitization is still required. Some units can be chemically sanitized or sanitized with hot water up to 80°C while others can only be chemically sanitized. Field data show that chemical sanitization can be effective, but hot water sanitization is generally more effective.

The post-treatment considerations for CEDI are similar to other ion exchange processes. Many systems use UV light downstream for additional microbial control. Some systems also use post-filtration for particle control or additional microbial control. Other systems rely on the hot water sanitization microbial control and use no post-treatment.

The selection of the best ion exchange process for each application is generally made on an analysis of capital cost, operating cost, user history, chemical handling requirements, outside service considerations, microbial control, maintenance requirements and sanitization methods.

All of the ion exchange processes are well proven in thousands of applications and are frequently combined with RO to easily exceed all USP Purified Water attributes. All of the processes have been utilized successfully in production of USP WFI and many grades of non-compendial water. The advantages and disadvantages are further discussed in the USP Purified Water system discussion.

Distillation

Distillation is one of the oldest water purification processes and has an extensive history in the production of pharmaceutical water. Distillation is the predominant process used worldwide for production of WFI, and is also used to produce Purified Water and non-compendial waters. As stated earlier, distillation is the only process allowed by EuPhr for production of WFI. Distillation utilizes phase change from liquid to vapor and removal of entrained liquid droplets to purify water. This process can, with appropriate pretreatment, reduce feed levels of ionized solids, suspended solids, organics, certain gases, microorganisms, and endotoxins to USP WFI and PW requirements.

The basic process requires energy in the form of steam and/or electricity to evaporate feed water, disengage entrained water droplets, and condense the vapor to pure water. The evaporator and droplet disengagement features differ among manufacturers and basic still types. The dominant still types are Multiple Effect (ME) and Vapor Compression (VC). Both are capable of cGMP production of WFI and PW. These types do differ in energy consumption, pretreatment requirements, cooling water requirements, and maintenance needs, however.

Multiple effect stills incorporate more than one evaporator in order to recover the latent and sensible heat from pure vapor for reuse and an increase in operating efficiency. The number of evaporators, or effects, may be as few as two or as many as ten; standard units generally incorporate from three to eight effects. The feed water is evaporated in the first evaporator or effect. The vapor produced in the first effect becomes the heating medium in the second effect. The first effect pure vapor is condensed in the second effect heating section, and eventually travels to the condenser for final cooling and recovery as pure distillate. The pure vapor generated in each effect is utilized as the heating medium in the next effect throughout the multiple effect still. The pure vapor from the last effect goes directly to the condenser. Multiple effect stills also use multiple heat exchangers to recover energy from condensate, blow down and inter-stage condensate to improve efficiency.

The multiple effects are utilized for efficiency and the water is only evaporated once, not multiple times. The distillate quality is the same as from a single effect still. A common myth is that distillate from, for example, a three effect still is triple distilled.

An increase in the number of effects increases the capital cost of the still for a fixed output and reduces the operating cost through reduction of heating steam and cooling water. Economic optimization requires a balance of the capital cost increase against a reasonable payback period.

Since a temperature differential between heating medium and feed water must exist in each effect, an increase in number of effects is usually accompanied by an increase in the first effect heating steam temperature. Multiple effect stills operate at higher temperatures than vapor compression stills. The feed water quality requirements are generally higher for multiple effect than vapor compression stills to minimize evaporator scale. The specifications vary with manufacturer and blow down rates, but most multiple effect pretreatment systems significantly reduce silica, chloride, hardness, total dissolved solids, and oxidizing disinfectants to low levels. Many multiple effect pretreatment systems incorporate either product staged RO or reverse osmosis and ion exchange to provide extremely reliable multiple effect still operation.

Multiple effect stills share the vast majority of the still marketplace with vapor compression. Some prefer multiple effect distillation because they believe that the minimum number of moving parts in multiple effect stills is a maintenance advantage. As stated previously, the water quality produced by the various still types is usually not a significant consideration. The final distillate quality from any well-designed still meets WFI or PW requirements with proper feed water. The distillate conductivity is often more a function of feed water quality than still design.

Vapor compression stills also recover latent heat from previously evaporated pure vapor for efficiency purposes. Feed water is evaporated on a surface of a tubular heat exchanger in an evaporator section. The heat source is most commonly steam, but can be electric in smaller units. The pure vapor is drawn into a compressor and in the compression cycle the pressure and temperature of the pure vapor is increased. The higher temperature pure vapor exits the compressor and enters a heat exchange unit in the evaporator where the latent heat is transferred to feed water and more pure vapor is produced. The condensed pure vapor loses sensible heat in an additional exchanger or exchangers, and a classical condenser with cooling water is not required.

Vapor compression stills are generally regarded as the most efficient still option. These stills are used in most very high volume applications and can be found in multiple units in some facilities producing several hundred gallons per minute of distillate. Vapor compression stills can also produce very small distillate volumes and compete with multiple effect stills across a broad spectrum of flows.

The pretreatment systems upstream of vapor compression stills vary greatly with feed water quality, corporate standard designs, and personal preferences. Vapor compression stills have an upper limit on silica in the evaporator. Feed water silica level may necessitate ion exchange or RO as pretreatment for reliable operation and minimum blow down. When silica is not a factor, many vapor compression installations use simple pretreatment systems that may include particle filtration, softening and dechlorination. Some facilities prefer this simple pretreatment scheme while others believe that still reliability is increased and maintenance decreased through implementation of RO or ion exchange as vapor compression pretreatment. The FDA Guide to Inspections of High Purity Water Systems notes that WFI endotoxin

Pharmaceutical Separate Bed Deionizer

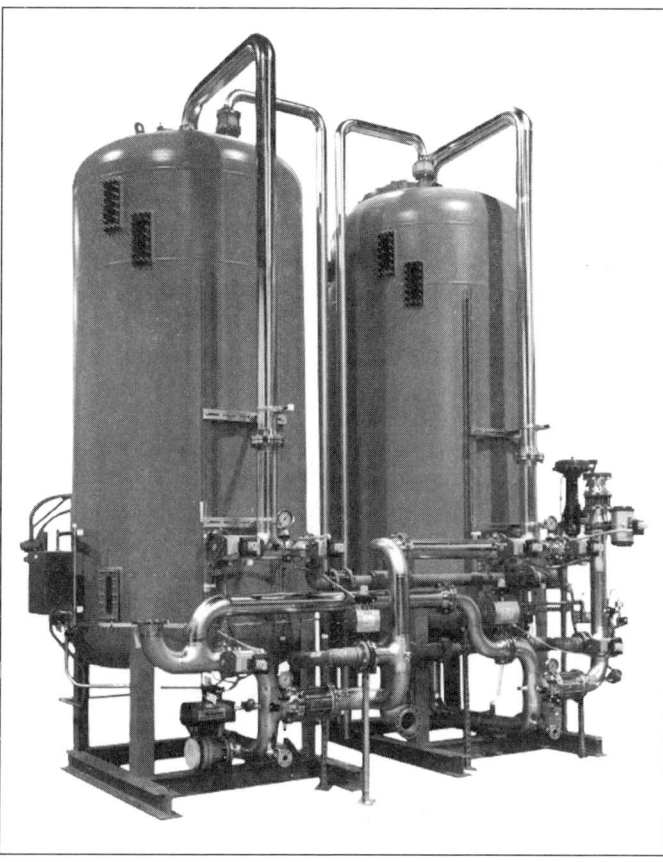

Source: Courtesy of USFilter, a Siemens company.

failures have occurred when no membrane pre-treatment was utilized upstream of stills. The Guide states that system design and performance should be evaluated to ensure that the system is in a state of control.

The presence of chloramines in still feed water can cause pretreatment changes for multiple effect or vapor compression stills. Stills cannot remove ammonia; and ammonium is converted to ammonia in a hot distillation process. The presence of even a small amount of ammonium in the distillate can cause a significant increase in distillate conductivity. The still pretreatment system must be capable of ammonia removal when ammonia is present in the feed water or ammonia is generated in other process steps.

PHARMACEUTICAL WATER SYSTEM DESIGN

Pharmaceutical facilities may utilize a single grade or multiple grades of water. The water requirements may include the compendial grades of USP WFI or PW or various non-compendial grades. The first decision is whether a single grade of water is the best regulatory and economic choice or if multiple grades provide more logical operation. A higher grade of water such as USP WFI can also serve as a lower grade such as USP PW. USP PW, of course, cannot be used as USP WFI. The cost to produce USP WFI may be higher than the cost to produce USP PW, therefore significant analysis is usually required to optimize system design.

Consider a facility that requires both USP Water for Injection and USP Purified Water. The facility could be best served by production of only WFI to serve both WFI and PW if several factors exist. If the WFI quantity required significantly exceeds the PW requirement, if all or most of the water is used hot (>65°C), and if the WFI and PW use are reasonably congruent, a single WFI system with hot storage is probably the best choice.

If the PW requirement is greater than the WFI requirement, the PW is used at ambient temperature, the WFI and PW use points are reasonably divergent, or heating and cooling resources are limited or expensive, separate systems to produce and distribute WFI and PW are probably more logical. When several factors favor each choice of either a single system or multiple systems, the choice can be difficult.

The change in allowable method of production of WFI in USP 28 may open more system configurations to acceptablility to produce WFI and PW in a single generation system. Historically single systems to produce both WFI and PW have been distillation based, but USP 28 allows consideration of alternate technologies.

After the choice of single or multiple water systems is made, the systems must be optimized for generation method and storage/distribution method. Generation systems will generally comprise several of the pretreatment, final treatment, and polishing components previously discussed.

USP Purified Water (PW) and Water for Injection (WFI) Generation Systems

Proper design of USP water systems requires consideration of many factors. Major factors include USP specifications, cGMP requirements, feed water quality, required system availability, raw water cost, plant wastewater discharge limits and costs, labor availability, outside service availability and competence, chemical handling, utility availability, and cost and designs with prior successful history. Previously successful system designs should always be weighed against other viable options unless the prior system design is obsolete or not cGMP.

The ISPE Baseline Water and Steam Guide Committee, after meetings with FDA personnel, recommended that the specified water quality for pharmaceutical use must be met at the outlet of the generation system as well as at the use points. Although some water quality parameters (particularly microbial levels in hot or ozonated storage systems) may improve in storage, the water quality should not fail as generated and should not depend upon improvement in storage to comply with the quality specifications. Some laboratory systems or production systems with extremely low conductivity requirements do successfully implement polishing techniques such as ion exchange, ultraviolet light, and submicron filtration in distribution to maintain quality standard.

System configurations based upon RO, ion exchange, and distillation will be reviewed. Distillation-based systems have an extensive history of production of both USP WFI and PW. The alternate designs have been primarily utilized for PW production with a few WFI applications when a final RO unit was implemented. All designs will be assessed for the capacity to produce both compendial waters.

Most high volume USP Purified Water systems utilize RO as the primary purification process with varying additional polishing processes. A technology map (below) shows the most common options for the basic reverse osmosis based USP PW systems. The number of process steps implemented is usually a function of feed water quality, finished water quality specification and risk assessment. The addition of an appropriate final endotoxin and microbial reduction process would allow production of WFI quality water if the process is proven to be equal or superior to distillation. The first pretreatment purification step is primary filtration for reduction of coarse suspended solids.

RO System Technology Map

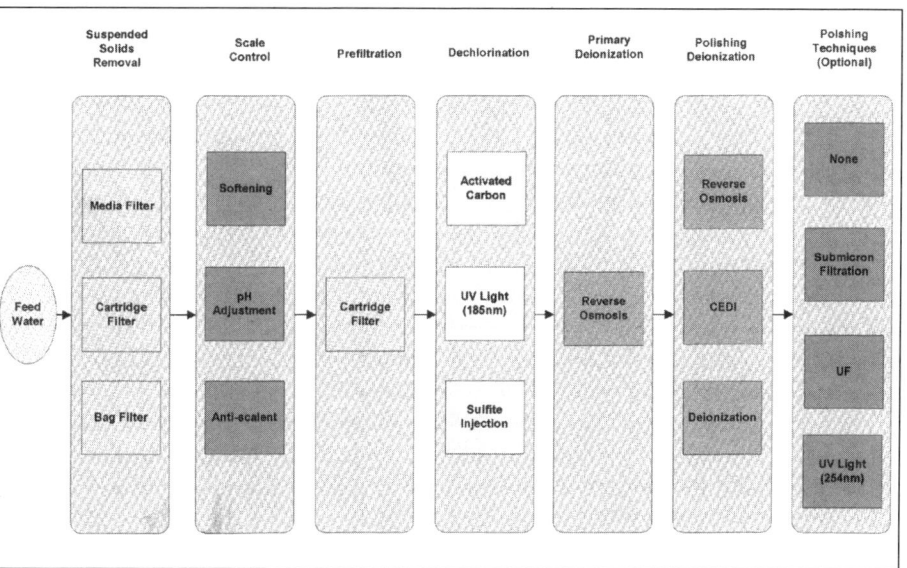

Source: From ISPE Pharmaceutical Water Basic Systems, 2004.

Multimedia filtration is selected when labor is minimized or the expected suspended solids level is low. Disposable cartridge or bag filters minimize capital cost and are a good choice for low suspended solids or low flow applications.

Scale control is the next pretreatment step. Softening for hardness removal is by far the most popular choice. Addition of antiscalant chemicals is a lower capital cost option. Although not used in nearly as many applications as softening, it is popular where discharge of softener regeneration brine is an issue. Reduction of pH is also used in a small number of systems. The scale control through reduction of pH is very effective, but the negative consequences of carbon dioxide generation limit use of this low capital cost option.

Disinfectant removal is accomplished through implementation of activated carbon, sodium sulfite injection, or UV light. Activated carbon may be the highest capital cost option when thermal carbon sanitization is included. Activated carbon is used in a majority of systems when all flow rates are considered, because the activated carbon requires little operator attention and can remove any municipal level of chlorine or chloramines. Sodium sulfite injection is the lowest cost option. Dechlorination is effective, but the application rate must be carefully controlled to avoid RO fouling or membrane oxidation.

UV light can be very effective. The sizing of UV must take peak chlorine or chloramines levels into account.

Final particulate removal prior to RO is accomplished with disposable cartridge filtration. The optimum filter rating is often determined in service. The filter particulate retention and cost must be balanced against RO cleaning frequency and down time for the application.

The final pretreatment option is microbial reduction though application of UV light. Many companies prefer to place UV light units downstream of activated carbon units to reduce the effluent microorganisms.

The primary treatment process of RO reduces the inorganic, organic and microbial contaminants to or near USP PW requirements. USP PW TOC and microbial levels are very likely to be met in the RO product water. The conductivity requirement is generally not met after a single pass through RO and further polishing is typically implemented.

A second pass of RO is a popular option at this point in the system for feed to multiple effect stills, USP PW production, and in some cases, USP WFI. The still feed option is popular as chloride, silica, and conductivity requirements are often met. Some systems also meet the USP PW conductivity limits out of the second RO pass. The product water meets Stage 1 conductivity requirements in some applications and Stage 2 or 3 in others. This design is excellent for low TOC and microbial levels.

Most USP PW systems utilizing RO as the primary process implement an ion exchange (IX) process to ensure consistent attainment of USP conductivity with variation in feed water and RO performance. All of the ion exchange, also known as deionization (DI), combinations with RO allow consistent production of USP PW water.

Automatic in place regenerated mixed bed DIs provide process control, but require chemical handling. Off site regenerated IX units allow conductivity attainment at minimal capital cost. Some internal process control is lost as outside service is required. The final option is continuous electrodeionization or CEDI. This option is popular when chemical handling is undesirable and off site regenerated resin is not cost effective or does not meet quality assurance requirements.

Many RO/DI-based systems incorporate one or both of the optional post IX polishing options shown in the preceding figure. UV. Ultraviolet light bacteria reduction follows a majority of IX units in systems where microbial control is desired. This process is not implemented when resin regeneration or hot water sanitization provides sufficient microbial control.

Microbially retentive filters with ratings of 0.02 μm to 0.45 μm are often implemented to produce extremely low bacteria levels in RO/DI water. These filters allow consistent attainment of low total plate count levels and are very useful where indicator organisms limits such as *Pseudomonas aeruginosa, Burkholderia cepacia*, or an absence of gram negatives exist.

The final option shown in the figure is ultrafiltration. This option can provide the endotoxin and microbial control necessary to produce WFI quality or WFI water. Ultrafiltration modules are available in polymeric and ceramic construction. Both membrane types have extensive history in production of WFI quality water. Some ultrafiltration membranes can be run continuously hot at 80°C or higher for self-sanitizing operation.

Systems using the many RO and IX options shown in the figure are popular because they provide consistent USP PW or now WFI water with minimal chemical consumption and are often the lowest evaluated life cycle cost.

Distillation is the primary treatment process in some USP PW applications. This can occur when distillation is used to produce both PW and WFI or just PW. The next two figures show the pretreatment and distillation options.

Primary filtration may or may not be required to protect other pretreatment components such as softeners and activated carbon units. The choice of no filtration, multi media filter or disposable filter is based on the same logic as the RO based systems previously discussed.

Multiple Effect Distribution Technology Map

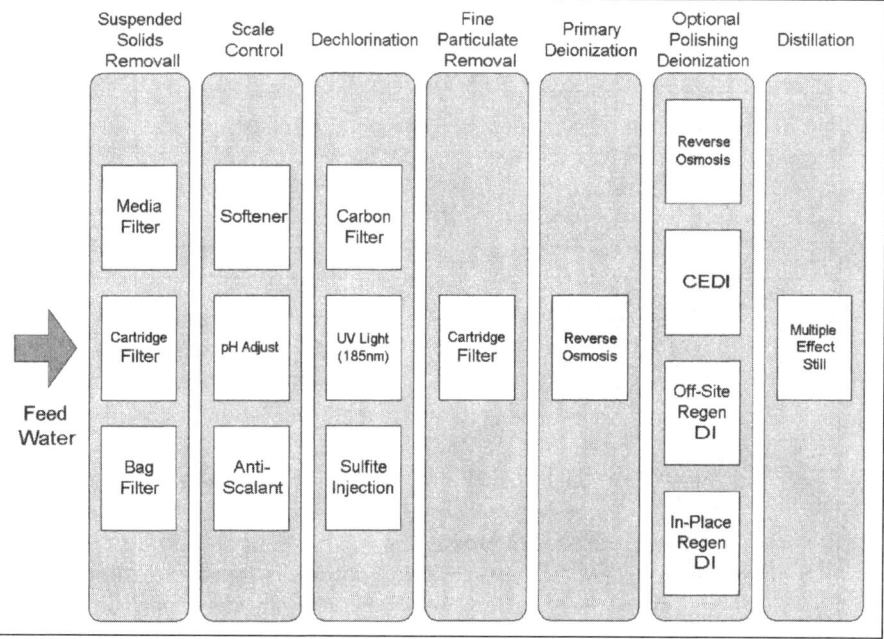

Source: From ISPE Pharmaceutical Water Basic Systems, 2004.

Vapor Compression Distribution Technology Map

Source: From ISPE Pharmaceutical Water Basic Systems, 2004.

Almost all distillation pretreatment systems utilize softening for scale control of the still directly, or to protect a pretreatment RO unit, if implemented, from scale. The use of just softeners as the only scale control is more common for vapor compression stills than for multiple effect stills. Softening of still feed water can provide adequate protection against hardness-based salt scale, but does not eliminate silica scale if sufficient feed water silica is present to make silica scale an issue. The softening can also be accomplished with nanofiltration rather than regenerable softeners.

All stills need protection from chlorine corrosion if feed water disinfectants are present. Activated carbon is currently the most popular choice. Sodium sulfite injection and UV light are used in a relatively small population of distillation feed water systems. The tolerance for feed water free chlorine is generally even lower for stills than most RO units. Either process can require extremely expensive repair when feed chlorine is not reduced to extremely low levels in accordance with the manufacturers recommendations.

A disposable cartridge filter typically follows media based pretreatment processes such as activated carbon and softening units. The cartridge removal rating can be relatively coarse and is usually in the 5 to 10 micron range.

The most critical choice in still pretreatment system design is the decision to implement inorganic solids reduction or not. This decision has significant capital cost, operating cost, maintenance, and reliability consequences. The still selection (multiple effect or vapor compression) must be made simultaneously to optimize the system. The still feed water requirements for conductivity, silica, hardness, chloride, and other factors must be known.

Some vapor compression still installations operate successfully without RO or IX processes upstream. Still blow down is generally significantly higher than the rate for RO or DI feed. Others implement RO, IX or RO/IX upstream to either meet requirements for silica, product water conductivity guarantees, guarantee low endotofin performance, or simply to minimize maintenance and maximize reliability.

Most multiple effect installations incorporate a minimum of RO as feed water inorganic level control. Multiple effect stills typically limit chloride, silica, and feed conductivity as a minimum. Single pass ROs can meet these requirements on relatively low total dissolved (TDS) solids waters. Product staged, or two pass, RO is very popular on higher TDS waters to meet the feed requirements. RO and any one of the IX processes are often combined to produce multiple effect feed water with minimal inorganic, organic, microbial, or endotoxin contaminants. A final filter for retention of resin fines may be used after the final IX process.

Another group of USP PW systems utilizes ion exchange processes without RO pretreatment or distillation post-treatment. The figure shows options for ion exchange based PW systems.

IX system process selection may be based upon in-place regenerated or off-site regenerated resin. The first process step is coarse suspended solids reduction and the selection of either multimedia filtration or a disposable filter, as in the cases of RO or distillation based systems.

Dechlorination typically follows filtration and the complete removal of chlorine or chloramines is not as critical as pretreatment to RO or stills. The IX resins used in most pharmaceutical systems are tolerant of low levels of chlorine. Activated carbon is the most common selection as the carbon media can also provide some protection against anion resin organic fouling if the carbon is sized and maintained correctly. UV light is an excellent choice since total dechlorination is not critical and the UV light can provide microbial control.

Some IX based systems employ anion resin organic scavenging units on high feed TOC feed waters. These units can provide more consistent and greater TOC reduction than activated carbon on many feed water supplies. This unit process can help to meet the final USP TOC requirement as well as to protect the IX anion resin from organic fouling.

Coarse cartridge filtration is frequently employed before IX units if multimedia, carbon, or organic scavenging units are upstream. These filters would serve little purpose if no media beds are implemented upstream.

The primary IX process for conductivity attainment may be mixed bed DI, separate bed DI, or both. Mixed bed DI can meet the USP conductivity requirement on

Ion Exchange Technology Map

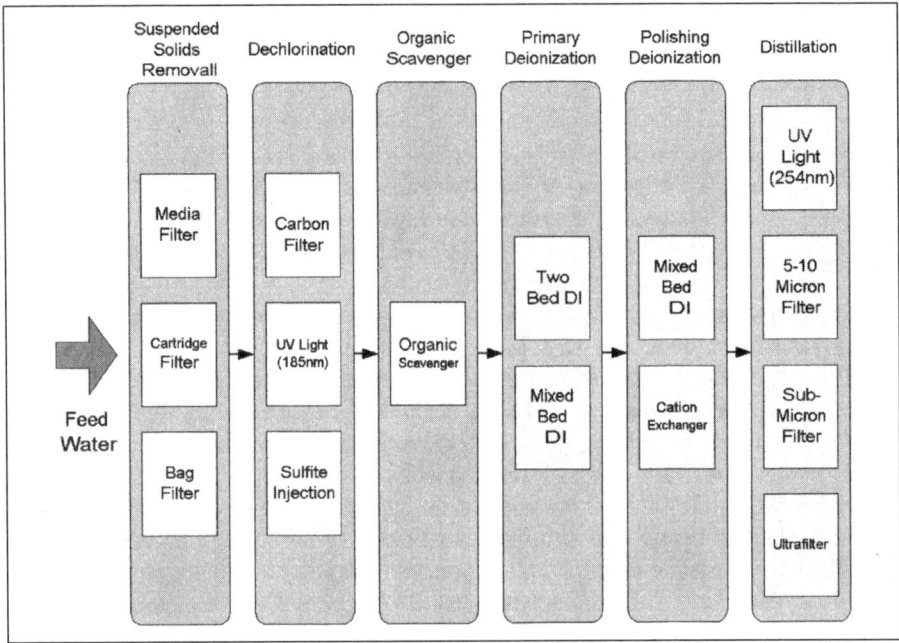

Source: From ISPE Pharmaceutical Water Basic Systems, 2004.

almost any EPA qualified feed source. Separate bed DI units may be implemented upstream for in place regenerated systems to take advantage of the simpler separate bed regeneration procedure for the bulk of regenerations. Separate bed units may be employed in off-site regenerated systems if the economics are favorable.

Counter-current regenerated separate bed DI units can meet the USP conductivity limits without mixed bed polishing on many feed waters. The final reason to consider separate bed DI units is the superior microbial control impact of the pH shifts through the resin beds.

Most systems utilizing ion exchange resin use filtration downstream of resin beds. Filtration rating from coarse (5 to 10 µm) for resin fine retention to as 0.2 µm or tighter for microbial retention. The operating cost of microbial retentive filters may be high on high colloidal content feed waters.

UV light units are also common downstream of DI units for microbial control. The necessity is based on microbial limits and other microbial control methods as in RO/DI system design.

All of the DI options discussed have been utilized successfully in thousands of applications. The greatest risk in DI systems that do not utilize RO upstream is failure to meet the USP TOC requirement if the feed water is high in TOC. Several DI systems have successfully utilized ultrafiltration and/or organic scavenging units to compensate for no RO membrane on difficult water supplies.

All IX resins can contribute high TOC levels when first placed in service. This TOC contribution can cause failure of the USP TOC requirement. Special resins that have been through a TOC extraction process can be implemented to eliminate the problem. These resins should be used when new resin is used in off-site regenerated units. New regenerable units can use these resins or go through several exhaustion and regeneration cycles of standard resins to provide low TOC levels.

The most significant advantages of DI based systems are: (1) potential low capital cost if no chemicals are used or if chemical handling and neutralization equipment exist; (2) higher water recovery than RO based systems if RO wastewater is not reused; and (3) excellent flow rate flexibility.

The principal disadvantages are chemical handling for in-place regenerated systems and process control issues for off site regenerated systems. Operating costs can be high or low as a function of feed water source, resin regeneration cost and water consumption.

Storage and Distribution Systems

Process Considerations

The design requirements for storage and distribution systems vary with the water quality specifications, generation system quality, and risk assessment. The storage and distribution system must maintain the water quality within the specified quality limits. Deterioration of quality is acceptable as long as the quality attributes do not fall out of specification.

The USP WFI mongraph requires the system be designed to "protect [WFI] from microbial contamination." The FDA expectation for maximum WFI microbial level is 10 cfu per 100 mL. This requires a conservative storage and distribution system design. The FDA expectation for PW is a maximum of 100 cfu per mL. This is three logs higher than the WFI specification and allows consideration of some designs that are not practical for WFI.

Almost all WFI distribution loops are constructed of sanitary 316L or 316 stainless steel tubing, fittings, and valves. The 316L or "low carbon" material is required for proper welding of welded assemblies. These systems use orbitally welded joints where possible and use sanitary "tri-clamp" joints for mechanical connections. Most piping is pitched to allow for complete drainage for steam sanitization (if utilized) or maintenance.

This construction is considered by most to be cGMP and is one of the cGMP common practices to come from the previously discussed GMPs for LVPs. Most companies utilize this construction unless technical considerations favor alternate construction.

A few WFI distribution systems are constructed with PVDF plastic piping because the products cannot be made with the metal levels in WFI that arise from contact with stainless steel. Some companies favor PVDF because passivation initially and periodically is not required as with stainless steel systems.

PVDF piping can be operated continuously at 80°C with continuous piping support and expansion loops. PVDF can be intermittently sanitized with low pressure steam or hot water. Hot water is sufficient and presents less of a risk of exceeding the rated temperature than steam. The PVDF piping costs are often similar to 316L stainless steel piping when the stainless steel is properly specified.

Almost all WFI systems are operated at continuous high temperature (>65°C) or intermittently high temperature. Few variations exist and, since almost all WFI systems are sanitary 316L SS construction, most WFI systems are quite similar in design. The differences exist in instrumentation, surface finish, and other details.

Most PW storage and distribution systems are variations of a few basic designs. Water can be stored at continuous high temperature (>65°C), ambient with intermittent hot water sanitization, ambient with continuous or intermittent ozone, ambient with periodic chemical sanitization, or cold (generally <10°C) with periodic sanitization. When water is stored at continuous high temperature, the water may be distributed at high temperature or ambient temperature.

All of these designs have been employed successfully, but the risk of microbial contamination can vary significantly. The materials of construction and cost can also vary significantly.

Continuous Hot Storage

A typical continuous hot storage and hot distribution system is shown in below. The water may be used hot or may need some method of heat exchange if colder temperatures are required. The continuous hot system is self-sanitizing and microbial problems are virtually always external to the sanitary system. Poor hose practices, airborne contamination, poor sampling practices, or other factors may contribute to unacceptable use point microbial counts, but poor counts from the sanitary system are unlikely.

Hot Storage and Hot Distribution System

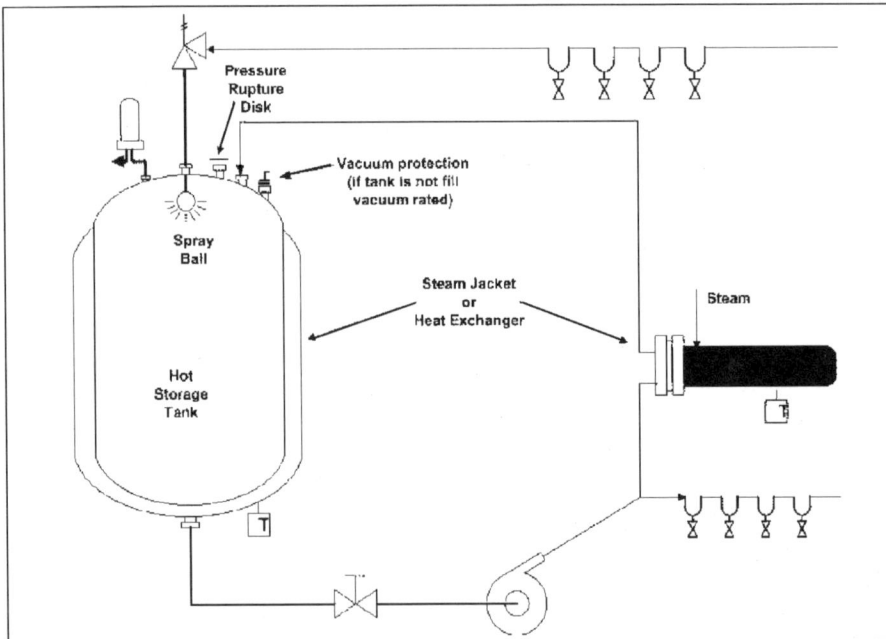

Source: Courtesy of USFilter, a Siemens company.

A continuous hot system is generally considered to be the most conservative and lowest risk storage system design. The capital cost is relatively high as almost all hot systems are constructed from 316L stainless steel sanitary components and require insulation.

Continuous hot system operating cost may not be high if all of the water is used hot for manufacturing. This situation would be ideal for continuous hot operation.

Most facilities require cooled water for manufacturing and the energy costs for heating and cooling may be significant. A very significant percentage of the pharmaceutical industry incurs these high energy costs to ensure a low risk system operation.

Use point heat exchangers for cooling or cooled sub-loops are commonly employed where hot water is not suitable for manufacturing. The ISPE Baseline Guide Volume 4: Water and Steam Systems provides guidance regarding use point heat exchanger implementation options. The Guide also illustrates the energy efficient implementation of self-contained cooled sub-loops off hot storage tanks. The key point is to recirculate all or most of the cooled water back to the sub-loop rather than constantly reheating all of the unused cooled water for return to the hot tank.

Ozonated Storage

An excellent alternative to continuous hot storage with cooled water for usage is continuously ozonated storage as shown below. The continuous application of ozone

Ozonated Storage and Distribution System

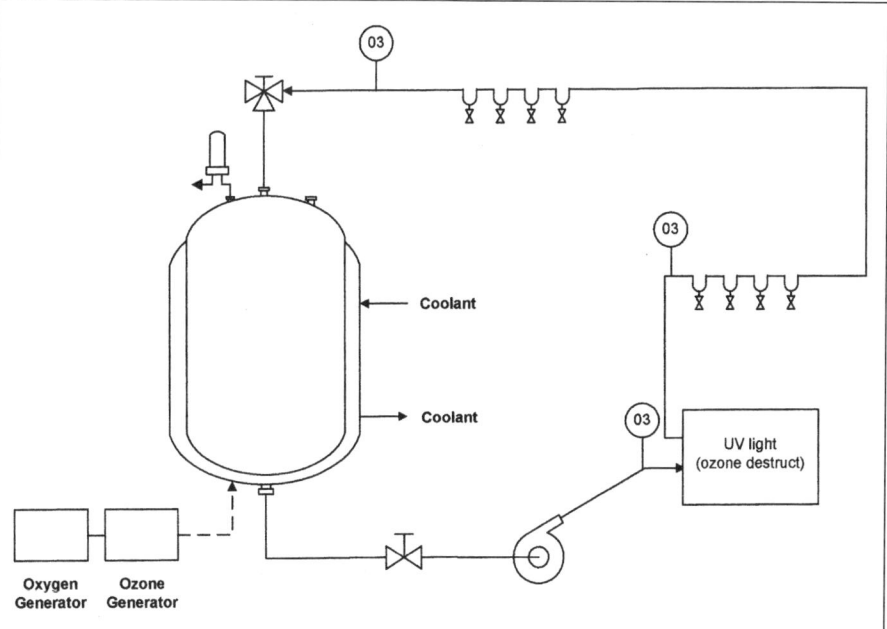

Source: Courtesy of USFilter, a Siemens company.

ensures low microbial counts in storage and the stored ozonated water can be used to periodically sanitize the distribution system. Ozone can destroy most (i.e., those not embedded in biofilm) microorganisms in seconds of contact time, is easily removed from manufacturing water with UV light, and has been successfully documented in many installations. Microorganisms embedded in biofilm necessitate significantly longer ozone contact time for destruction.

Pharmaceutical companies must demonstrate that ozone has been completely removed from water for manufacturing. Residual ozone in USP Purified Water or Water for Injection utilized in manufacturing would violate the monograph prohibition of "added substances." Online monitors are typically utilized to prove the absence of ozone in distributed water.

The residual ozone in water from storage is removed with inline UV units downstream of the distribution pump. These UV units use approximately three times the energy, per gallon processed, as UV units sized for microbial control. Distribution system sanitization is easily automated and accomplished by shutting off the UV units when system sanitization is desired. The ozonated water from storage is allowed to enter the distribution system and sanitization is accomplished.

Continuous addition of ozone to stored water will cause an increase in conductivity. The increase may cause the conductivity to rise above the USP conductivity limit during lengthy periods of low or no water usage. This issue is eliminated or minimized through repurification of some of the stored water, use of appropriately low applied ozone levels, or purging of some stored water resulting in addition of low conductivity makeup water to storage.

Since ozone is an extremely strong oxidizing agent, material compatibility must be addressed in system design. Most ozonated systems use components constructed of 316L or 316 stainless steel. PVDF piping, fittings, and valves are also very compatible with ozone. Gaskets and other elastomers must be carefully selected.

The capital cost of most ozonated systems is similar to continuous hot systems. The operating cost of ozonated systems may be much lower than continuous hot systems if the makeup water is generated at ambient temperature and the water is used at ambient temperature.

Ambient Storage

Many systems utilize ambient temperature water storage without continuous or intermittent ozone. These systems rely on periodic hot water sanitization (80 to 121°C) or chemical sanitization. Properly designed sanitary 316 stainless steel systems with daily hot sanitization are commonly used with great success in both WFI and PW applications. Many systems operate successfully with hot sanitization less frequently than daily, but the microbial risk increases.

Chemical sanitization is the least desirable of all sanitization options. Chemical sanitization is usually implemented as a result of budget limitations rather than technical superiority. Chemical sanitization is limited to PW applications and is typically used with plastic piping (polypropylene or PVC) to minimize capital costs.

Chemical sanitization is usually considerably more time consuming than thermal or ozone sanitization and less effective. The required contact time with organisms is greater and other time factors apply. Each use point must be drained and tested to prove the presence of chemical during sanitization and the absence of chemical after rinsing. Higher microbial counts after sanitization may occur for a short period if the biofilm is disturbed, but not completely inactivated.

Plastic piping systems with chemical sanitization can be successfully implemented. This design is best utilized when the acceptable microbial counts at use points are relatively high. Frequent sanitization helps. A properly designed and maintained makeup system with tight microbial control also helps significantly

Distribution Storage Tank Design Considerations

Distribution tank capacity optimization was reviewed earlier. Other design specification considerations include material, surface finish, pressure rating, vacuum rating, temperature rating, access, fitting number and type, instrumentation, spray balls, vent filters, rupture disks, nitrogen blanketing, support, steam jacketing, and insulation.

Tank Atmospheric Isolation

Proper isolation of WFI or PW in storage is an absolute cGMP requirement. An appropriate hydrophobic, integrity testable, microbial retentive vent filter or nitrogen blanketing is acceptable. The filter, normally rated at 0.2 μm absolute or tighter, should be heat traced in hot applications to prevent filter plugging due to condensation. Proper integrity tests for vent filters prior to and after use must be implemented.

Proper pressure and vacuum protection should be provided. A pressure rupture disk is often implemented. A vacuum rupture disk is usually implemented if the tank is not rated for full vacuum. Rupture disks can be equipped with an alarm function to notify operators of rupture and tank atmospheric exposure. Relief valves are utilized in lieu of rupture disks in some instances.

Distribution Piping Design Considerations

The optimization of the distribution system configuration, tubing or pipe size, and flow rate or rates requires significant thought. The distribution system must be able to deliver the proper flow and pressure to all users under varying demand. The flow rate in each individual loop is generally at least 50 % greater than the maximum instantaneous demand to allow proper pressure control and to avoid water hammer incidents. The system must be maintained at a positive pressure or system sanitization would be required if air is presumed to have entered the system.

The number of parallel loops is normally minimized for cost and control purposes. One serpentine loop is ideal for control, instrumentation, ease of balancing, and sometimes capital cost. Each individual loop length is ultimately constrained by pressure drop. Multiple loops are generally used in large systems to limit the pressure drop in each loop to ensure that water can be delivered to all users at the required pressure and flow. Each loop is normally individually instrumented to monitor proper flow, pressure, and temperature.

Continuous Recirculating or Non-recirculating Configuration

Although many consider continuous recirculation of water a cGMP requirement, this is not true. Most systems do continuously recirculate at reasonable velocity in an attempt to minimize microbial attachment to piping surfaces. This is logical and somewhat effective, but not a regulatory requirement.

Non-recirculating or "dead-end" systems can be validated and pass audit if continuous flow or proper flushing and sanitization procedures are implemented and documented. Some non-recirculating systems have continuous usage and are dynamic at all points without having to bear the cost of return piping back to the tank. Other systems utilize timed flushes for drainage and/or effective sanitization to demonstrate proper microbial control.

Dead Legs

Extreme attention is paid to piping layout to minimize dead legs in order to minimize microbial growth opportunity and to meet cGMP expectations. The older interpretation of an acceptable dead leg meeting GMP guidelines was a maximum of six pipe diameters (using the branch diameter) measured from the centerline of the main run to the center of the branch isolation valve. The six pipe diameter dead leg "rule" was based upon hot (nominal 80°C operating temperature) sanitary stainless steel tubing distribution systems. The current view is to limit the dead leg to three pipe diameters (branch diameter) or less measuring from the pipe wall of the main run to the center of the branch isolation valve in similar systems. When plastic piping materials or ambient operating temperatures are utilized the dead legs should be as close to zero as possible.

Distribution Piping Velocity

A long standing rule-of-thumb in pure water system design has been a goal of 5 feet per second water velocity in distribution system. The theory is that the turbulence produced by the high velocity will inhibit microbial attachment to piping surfaces and minimize biofilm formation. This rule-of-thumb is not a cGMP requirement and is not completely effective in practice. No evidence exists to indicate that FDA inspectors seek a particular minimum water velocity.

Data indicate that microbial attachment can eventually occur at almost any velocity or Reynolds number (a common measure of turbulence). Biofilm control is best achieved through effective sanitization methods and continuous measures such as high or low temperature, residual ozone, UV light, and filtration.

Water velocities as low as 2 feet per second have proven to be sufficient. From a practical point extremely low continuous velocities are unlikely because this would require large pipe diameters at increased capital cost. Most systems utilize water velocities in the range of 3 to 10 feet per second to minimize pipe diameter and cost. Higher velocities would produce unacceptably high pressure drops in long piping runs.

The most important consideration is to avoid designing for a high absolute minimum velocity under all possible operating conditions. This difficult constraint may result in small return lines, high pressure drop, and validation difficulties.

Distribution Piping Material

Although the term distribution piping is used in this chapter and is the common term for a water distribution network, tubing is more common than pipe in distribution systems. Stainless steel tubing (316L) is used in almost 100% of WFI systems, as discussed earlier. Sanitary stainless steel tubing for WFI distribution is a regulatory expectation and alternative designs should be based upon technical considerations rather than economic considerations. Almost all new PW systems in large manufacturing facilities also use 316L stainless steel tubing construction.

Pipe, rather than tubing, is utilized in some manufacturing and laboratory applications. The pipe is almost always plastic material and may be utilized for economic or technical considerations. The economic considerations may be considerable if PVC or polypropylene piping is utilized rather than 316L stainless steel tubing and fittings. A sanitary stainless steel tubing system is typically five to eight times the cost of a PVC system and two to four times the cost of a polypropylene piping system.

The piping or tubing material selection must be compatible with the continuous or intermittent sanitization method. Continuous hot or ozonated systems are restricted to stainless steel or PVDF. Polypropylene and PVC systems are typically chemically sanitized although a small percentage use intermittent ozone sanitization. Polypropylene is not ozone compatible. Chemical, heat, or ozone compatibility should always be confirmed by the piping manufacturer.

The choice of distribution material and joining method is a critical choice relative to the microbial limit specification. Almost any configuration can be properly maintained to meet the PW maximum allowable microbial action level of 100 cfu/mL. Lower levels and the absence of indicator organisms such as *Pseudomonas aeruginosa* or *Burkholderia cepacia* are more consistently achieved with sanitary stainless systems. Extremely low microbial levels can be achieved with piping, but continuous heat or ozone is recommended.

Plastic piping can contribute excessive organic extractible contaminants when usage is low and the piping is new. Some low usage plastic systems require periodic purging of water from storage or use of TOC reduction UV units to control TOC levels.

Joint Method

Stainless steel sanitary tubing systems joints are automatically orbitally welded where possible, hand welded where necessary, and manually clamped in a sanitary manner for instrumentation and access. PVDF and polypropylene are joined with welded joints where possible and joined mechanically where necessary. Different weld methods are available and produce varying degrees of weld surface smoothness. Smooth surfaces are desirable for the lowest microbial requirements. Smooth surfaces cannot completely inhibit microbial attachment, but the initial attachment can be delayed. A smooth surface is particularly important with intermittent chemical sanitization.

PVC systems use solvent welded joints for most joints and incorporate flanged and threaded mechanical joints. These joints are more likely to contribute to microbial issues than welded joints. PVC systems are generally used where low microbial levels are not required.

Surface Finish

Stainless steel tubing systems are normally specified for surface finish. WFI surfaces are normally in the range of 15 to 20 Ra in micro-inches, and PW system stainless surfaces are normally range 25 to 40 Ra in micro-inches. Surface finish is generally less critical where continuous sanitization with heat or ozone is implemented than in ambient non-ozonated systems. Most self-sanitizing systems still use highly polished tubing regardless of the technical justification.

Plastic systems are not specified for surface finish. PVDF surfaces are typically smoother than the highest mechanical polish stainless steel surfaces. Polypropylene piping surfaces are also extremely smooth. PVC surfaces provide the most surface crevices in the common plastic piping materials.

Total System Draining

Systems incorporating steam sterilization or sanitization should be designed to facilitate complete draining prior to steaming. These systems must also be designed to allow complete venting of air. Systems that use hot water, ozone, or chemical sanitization are frequently designed for complete draining but it is not absolutely necessary. Flushing residual chemicals out of systems can be validated.

Distribution System Polishing Components

Ideally the water quality specifications are met out of the generation system and no polish processes are required in distribution. Continuous hot systems typically incorporate no additional purification processes in distribution. Ozonated systems implement UV light units for ozone removal, but typically use no other distribution processes.

Ambient non-ozonated systems are the most likely to incorporate distribution polishing technologies. These processes may be used to improve or maintain conductivity, TOC, or microbial levels. IX processes may be incorporated where extremely low conductivity values are required. These conductivity values are generally well below USP allowable values. These extremely low conductivity requirements should be questioned and justified.

Implementation of an IX process generally involves UV light units and/or filters for microbial and particulate control. UV light units, similar to those reviewed earlier can provide adequate microbial control downstream of IX and are not a regulatory issue. Filters implemented for particle control downstream of IX are also not a regulatory issue.

Microbial retentive filters in distribution or at use points can be very effective, but generate significant cGMP debate. The only written prohibition of filters in distribution was in the previously discussed GMPs for LVPs. Since these requirements were never adopted, the use of microbial retentive filters is subject to interpretation.

Almost if not all pharmaceutical companies ban the use of microbial retentive filters in WFI distribution because they believe that FDA acceptance is unlikely. The FDA does not disallow inline or use point filters if they are properly validated and maintained, but many firms do not do this properly. Use point filters can mask system microbial control problems. Proper microbial sampling should be done upstream and downstream of filters to ensure that the entire system is in proper microbial control.

Many companies also shun filter use in PW distribution for similar logic. Some companies use a single bulk filter after distribution ion exchange units in PW applications. The effectiveness of microbial retentive filters has been proven for decades in pharmaceutical, microelectronics, chemical process, and other applications. The issue has nothing to do with effectiveness, and is strictly a perceived regulatory issue.

Many people believe that a single bulk filter, used as part of a total microbial control plan and properly maintained, is perfectly appropriate for pharmaceutical use in PW applications. Multiple use point filters are rarely necessary and are used extremely infrequently.

Some low endotoxin non-compendial or PW systems utilize an ultrafiltration unit in distribution to ensure extremely low endotoxin levels. These units are similar to the units described earlier, but are generally sanitary in construction. These systems typically produce water with endotoxin levels well below USP WFI requirements.

SUMMARY

Water is often the most expensive utility in pharmaceutical plants. Considerable capital and operating cost reductions can be realized through optimization of water quality specification, generation system design, storage and distribution system design and proper maintenance. The FDA is not an engineering agency and does not publish strict engineering guidelines. Many individuals have expressed a desire for greater FDA detailed engineering requirements. This is not likely to occur and this provides an opportunity for companies to optimize water generation and distribution and prove that the system is appropriate for the application through proper validation.

7
Automation and Process Controls

Author: David Lonza

INTRODUCTION

Pharmaceutical manufacturing and laboratory operations are based on FDA Quality System Regulations, namely Current Good Manufacturing/Laboratory Practices, and Organizational Goals. The common objective of these regulations and industry practices is to *consistently* meet the desired end product quality by continuously monitoring and controlling process variance within acceptable limits. In order to achieve this, the FDA requires the industry to achieve and maintain what is known as a "validated" state on all critical processes, equipment, utility systems and facilities used for pharmaceutical operations. The application of automation and control system technology to pharmaceutical facility and process control is arguably the single most important enabler in recent times. Achieving uniform end product quality, ensuring regulatory compliance, and gaining higher cost efficiencies is the ideal balance that all pharma and bio companies strive to achieve. Automation technology also helps manufacturers to gain competitive advantage by allowing effortless scaling of unique and sophisticated biochemical processes in commercial manufacturing. This chapter discusses the trends and typical applications of automation and control system technologies in the bio-pharmaceutical industry.

*Editor's Note:*_____

> The use of computer assisted technicians continues to be a subject of much debate and regulatory development. The FDA guidance for industry (21 CFR, Part II, Electronic Record; Electronic Signatures—Scope and Application) was released in February 2003. (The previous guidance was rescinded in January 2003.) The new guidance is still much discussed within the industry and its regulators. The FDA's guidance recommends that regulated organizations "base your approach on justified and documented risk assessment."

AUTOMATION AND CONTROL SYSTEMS EXPLAINED

A *control system* is a set of hardware and software components used to monitor and control one or more devices. When multiple devices are being controlled in a co-ordinated fashion, it is referred to as *process automation*. A control system may be passive; that is to say, it provides information on the status of the process to an operator who then decides whether control actions are required and, if so, submits the necessary commands to the system. The control system then passes these commands to the appropriate device(s) in the form understood by that device. In the case of simple devices this may be an electrical signal with well-defined characteristics, whereas in the case of a more complex device this may be a complex formatted message. Control systems are often not purely passive and in many cases may be programmed to perform actions in an automated fashion. In such cases these systems are referred to as *automation and control systems.*

Typical components of an automation and control system include the following:

- *Controllers:* The intelligence to collect, store, communicate data and signals, and trigger actions according to a predetermined sequence and control logic is built (programmed) into controllers such as programmable logic controllers or programmable computers.
- *Instruments:* The collection of information about process parameters such as temperature, pressure, humidity, etc. is achieved through the use of instruments, sensors, and transmitters.
- *Field devices:* Physical action is achieved through the use of components such as actuators and valves.
- *Networks:* Communication of data and signals is achieved through field wiring and data transmission network components.
- *Human machine interface:* The capability to allow human intervention, for example in passive control systems, is achieved through the use of human machine interface such as an industrial computers or control panels.

Typical Automation System Components

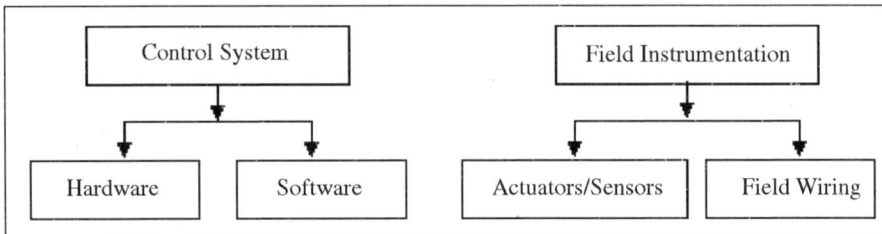

Control Strategies

Automation systems employ multiple strategies to accomplish the control functionality using various available hardware and software technologies depending on the need and other economic considerations. The end result is achieved by a set of hardware components made functional by programming software. The two main control system strategies or technology frameworks and their components are:

- Programmable Logic Controllers (PLC)-based control systems
- Distributed Control Systems (DCS) (e.g., Supervisory Control and Data Acquisition or (CADA)

Programmable Logic Controllers (PLCs). Earliest automation and control technology was based on relay control circuits. PLCs were found as a replacement for relay control circuits by providing flexible capabilities such as reprogrammable units. A typical PLC consists of a microprocessor, memory, input/output circuits and terminals, and a programming interface. Memory is usually battery-backed in order to avoid losing a program during power loss. PLCs are still preferred over other options for many types of process control applications due to their high reliability even in extreme industrial conditions.

Typical PLC

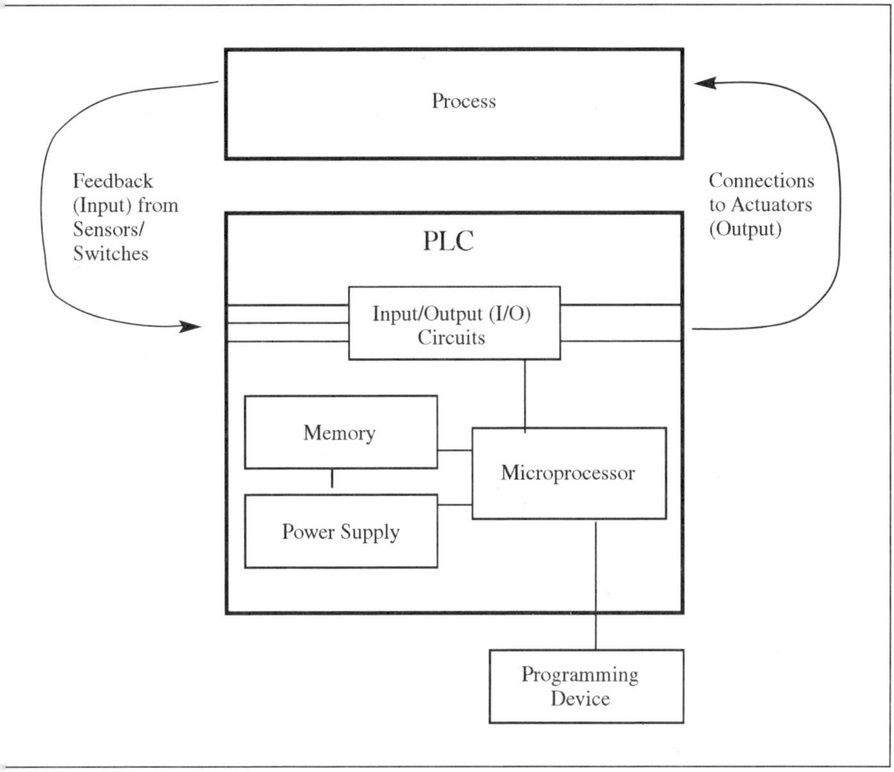

Process

Feedback
(Input) from
Sensors/
Switches

Connections
to Actuators
(Output)

PLC

Input/Output (I/O)
Circuits

Memory

Microprocessor

Power Supply

Programming
Device

Components of a Typical PLC

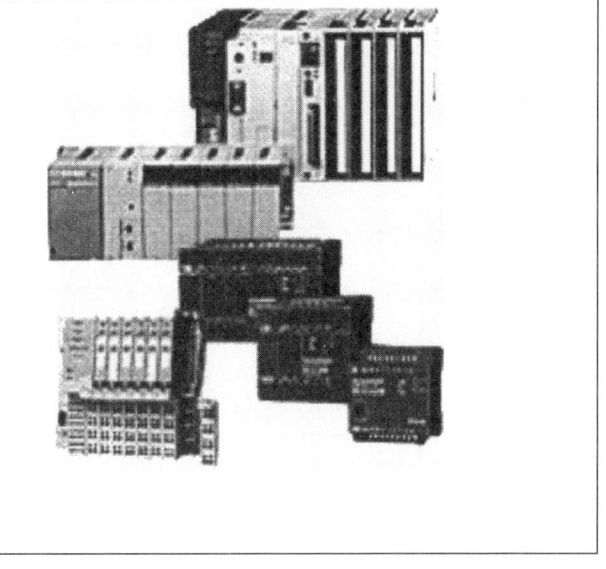

Evolution of Control Mechanisms

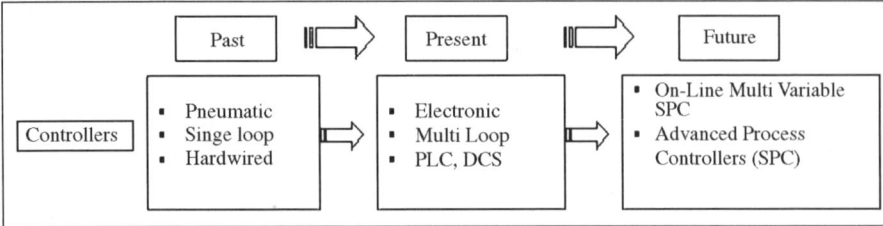

Distributed Control System DCSs. Distributed control systems (DCSs) is a method where control of a process is distributed among different unit processes while retaining central monitoring and supervisory capabilities. These unit processes may be related or unrelated. A typical DCS is a hard-wired system that exists within finite boundaries, such as a process plant or within a factory. True distributed control systems use localized control that in turn, for example, is controlled by the operator located at a central location. Distributed control Systems consist of the following components:

- Main and remote control panels
- Data communication infrastructure
- Human machine interface and database software

Control System File

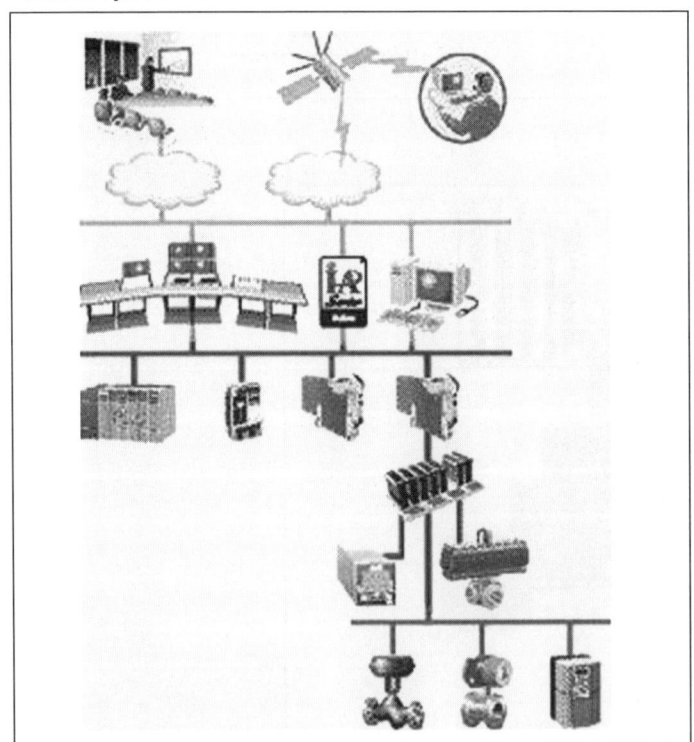

A DCS may be as simple as one PLC remotely connected to a computer located in a field office or a number of remote control panel mounted control systems networked to each other and a main or central control panel mounted control unit. These remote or main control panels may be PLC- or PC-based, but will most likely consist of specially designed cabinets containing all of the equipment necessary to provide input/output (I/O) and communication. DCSs typically allow most remote nodes to operate independently of the central control unit should the facility go off line or lose communication capability. Each remote node will also be able to store the minimum process data required to operate in the event of such a failure. In years past, DCSs were the choice for complex batch operations. Today, DCSs are finding their way into Building Automation Systems (BAS) as well as simple non-batch processes.

Evolution of Field Instrumentation

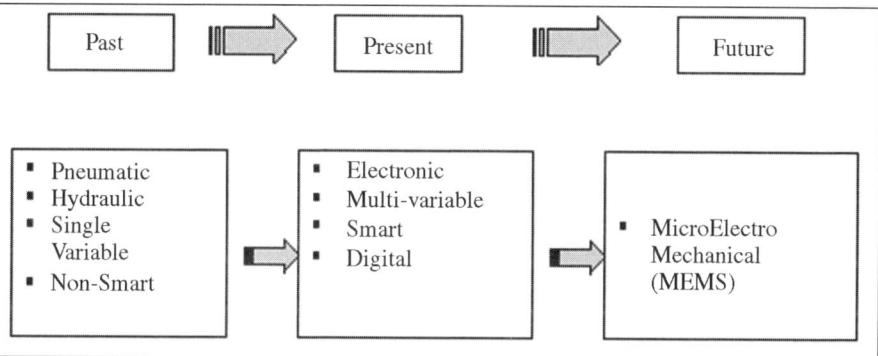

Field Instrumentation and Devices

Field instrumentation consists of measuring units such as sensors that measure and send absolute or relative information about one or more of process parameters such as:

• Temperature
• Pressure
• Humidity
• Flow
• Conductivity
• Level
• State of a process

Field instrumentation is broken down into two categories: analog and discreet. Analog instrumentation can be described as sensors that have a range, such as temperature or humidity. Typical analog field instruments include temperature sensors, pressure sensors, humidity sensors, and torque sensors. An example of an analog input could be a signal from a temperature sensor, ranging from 0°C to 100°C, or anywhere in between. The temperature will correspond to the output of the sensor to the control system. A typical analog output could be to an analog valve. These valves have the ability to open with a 0–100% range control or any value in between. For instance, process temperature setpoint can be 75°C. Discreet sensors, on the other hand, have no range. They have two distinct states, open/on or closed/off. Discreet devices are found in many applications; an example is a valve limit switch that sends an indication back to the controller that it is open. A discreet output could be a signal to close the valve.

For biopharmaceutical applications, the choice of instrument specification is driven by the nature of application (product contact and non-product contact), and criticality of the sensing parameter to end product quality. For product contact applications, care must be taken to specify sensors or sensor housings made of materials that do not have any harmful effects on the product characteristics upon contact. Also instruments related to critical process parameters are required to be calibrated more frequently in the field, and the records generated by them must be archived for regulatory reasons.

Process controllers use information generated by these instruments and transmitters to control the state of field devices such as valves and actuators to maintain the process parameters within preprogrammed limits. Process sensors measure a single variable and use analog circuits to convert the process variable into an electrical signal to feed a controller or a display unit. The current trend is shifting to using one sensing element to make multiple measurements. For example, a Coriollis mass flow meter can measure mass flow rate, temperature, and density of the fluid using a single element. The advancement in digital technology has also considerably reduced the time to calibrate a typical transmitter. Innovations such as the Field bus technology has made it possible to communicate more data, such as calibration records, vendor model and problem diagnostics from the field devices to the control system.

Another trend is the use of *MicroElectroMechanical* sensors (MEMS) which will be embedded in physical and analytical measuring devices. Performance requirements drive most of this shift. Higher data rates will be necessary because of increased sampling frequency, number of parameters being monitored, and resolution requirements. Such improvements in technology have also resulted in ease of installation and use and cost effectiveness.

Human-Machine Interface (HMI)

Every plant or a major process suite will have a control room from which the plant manager, supervisor, or operator can monitor and control a process. When using a DCS, the control room is the center of activity and provides the means for effectively monitoring and controlling the process or facility. The control room contains the HMI or Human-machine Interface, a computer that runs specialized software designed for providing the interface to process through graphic media. There may be multiple consoles, with varying degrees of access to data. In most cases, each operator or manager is given access rights to allow an appropriate level of access and control of the system. The plant manager, for instance, may have complete control over the facility, while a technician may only have access to monitoring and/or changing certain process parameters data (set points) on a particular process. This is done to avoid process upsets and will be designed, specified, and built into a control system used for biopharmaceutical applications as a regulatory compliance requirement. This also offers a degree of security, ensuring that only properly trained and authorized personnel can operate the various parts of the process or facility.

The features of an HMI vary by vendor. Each presents the operator with a graphical version of the local or remote process. Depending upon the skill of the operator and the level of sophistication of the interface, the process may be represented by anything from simple static graphics and displays to animation and voice alerts. Most packages offer the operator wide latitude on the design of the interface.

An HMI Screen

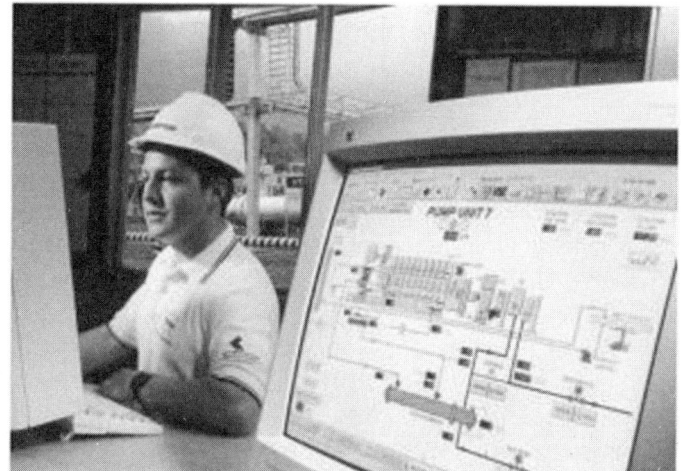

Source: Courtesy of Emerson Process Management.

A Simple HMI Screen

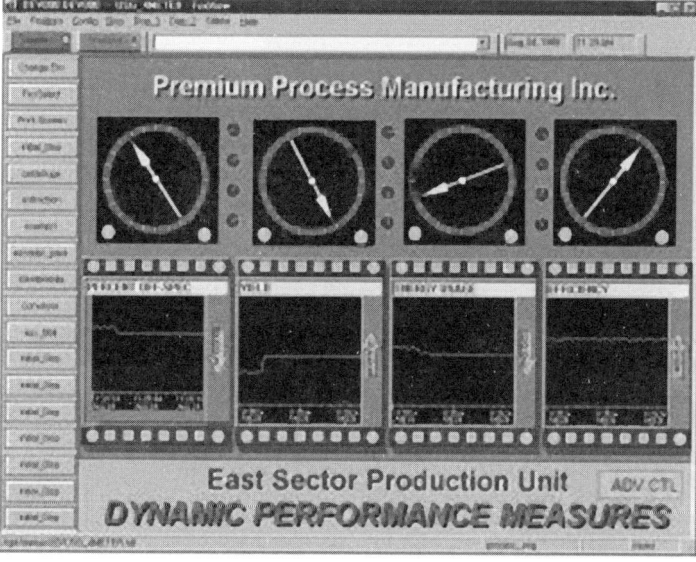

Source: Integrated Controls Group.

Evolution of HMI Technology

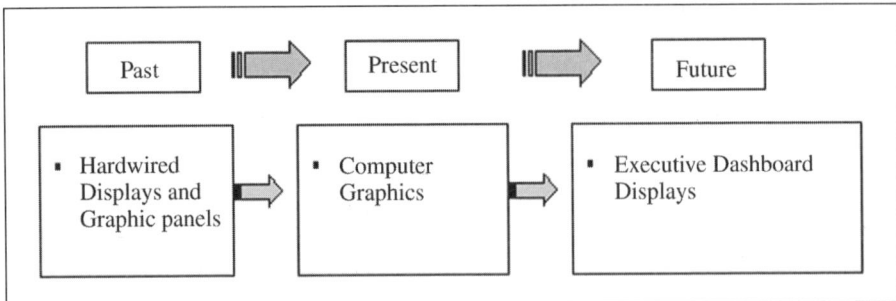

A recent trend in HMI technology is the use of process dashboards that not only gives a snapshot of the process's scientific parameters, but also gives a real-time view of the shop floor economics for management reporting and decision making.

Process Dashboard Example

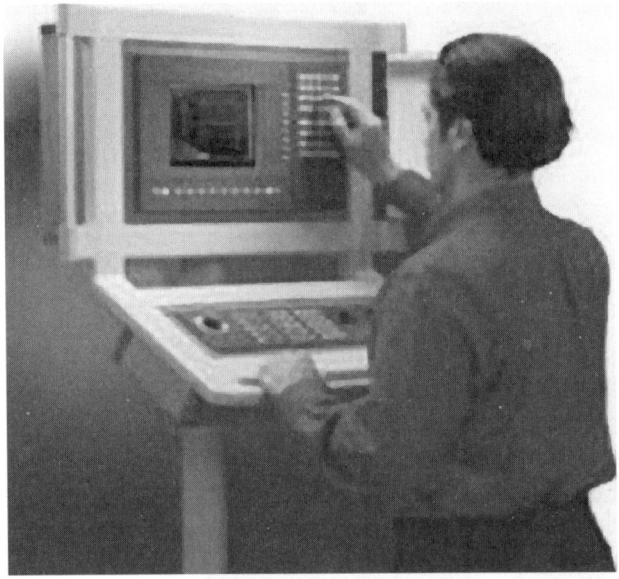

AUTOMATION AND CONTROL SYSTEMS SOFTWARE

Automation and control system hardware, instrumentation, and field device components already discussed are brought together to perform monitoring and control functions by building the intelligence into the system. This is accomplished through the use of application software that includes the following components in a control system:

HMI User View

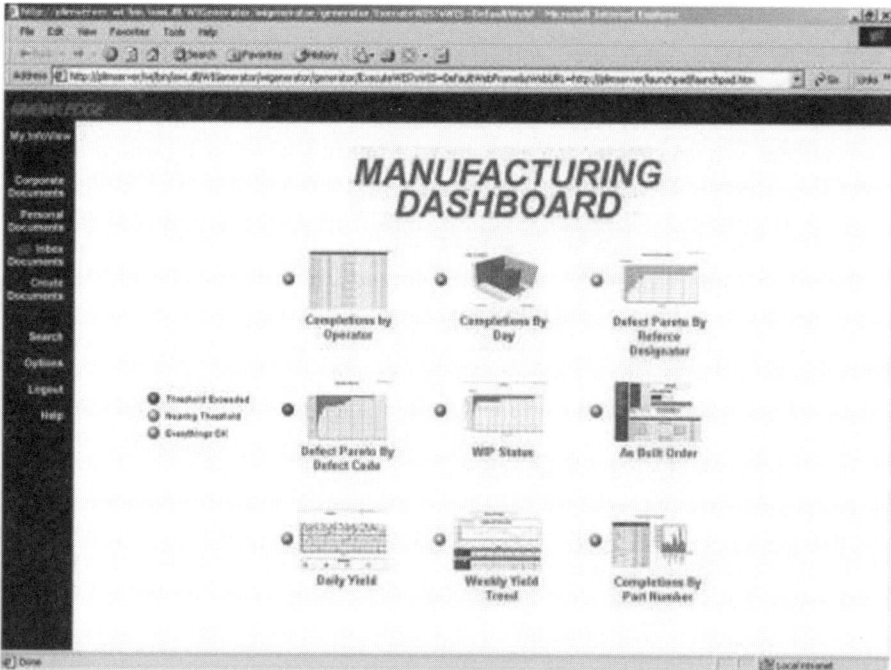

HMI Screen

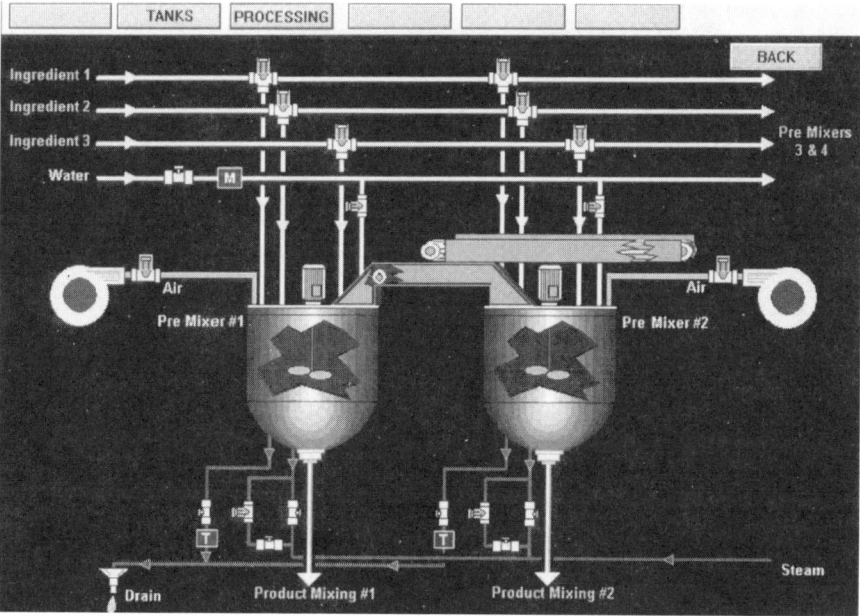

- PLC/SCADA software program and I/O database
- HMI software program

PLC/SCADA application software packages provide an easy programming interface to add/modify functionality of the controllers. These packages range from simple user interfaces for ladder logic programming to applications that provide documentation, version control, and change management features along with programming capabilities for regulatory compliance requirements.

HMI software programs are used to configure/program the User Interface (UI) application of the control system. These programs help build features such as graphic reporting, trending, visual alarm generation, screen customization, security features, access rights, and electronic signatures.

The common thread to the control system and HMI software application is the I/O database. The database contains all of I/O points defined for that DCS. This does not mean that all process data will be monitored and controlled; it means that only the data defined by the designers to be monitored and controlled will be available to the DCS. This database is usually a result of detailed evaluation of the process by the designer who typically has the responsibility, with operator input, to design the most effective control schemes for a particular process or facility. The control software uses the database as a reference to address each remote I/O point accurately. Each database entry corresponds to an entity on the system, whether it is a physical point, an internal point, or a "soft" point such as an alarm, timer, or screen entity.

Control System Software

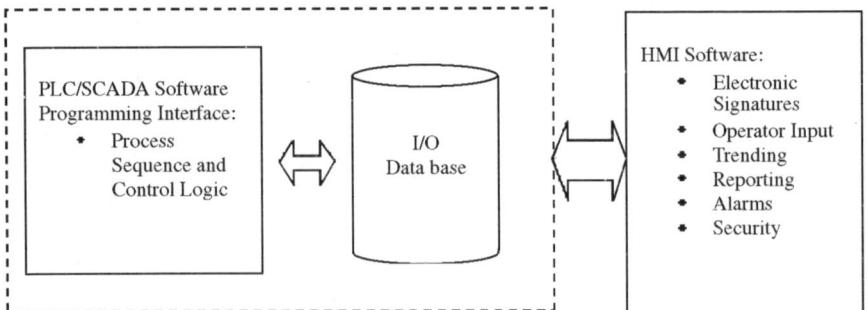

There are a wide variety of control systems and HMI software applications. Choices are normally driven by considerations such as features, hardware selection, and compatibility with existing systems, ability to meet regulatory requirements in a pharmaceutical environment, and ease of use or minimal training requirements for the engineers.

Typical Automation and Control Applications in the Bio-Pharmaceutical Industry

Drug products are required to be manufactured in controlled environments, as they are highly sensitive to environmental factors such as air quality, temperature, and humidity. The Food and Drug Administration (FDA) defines general conditions in various regulatory guidelines including current Good Manufacturing Practices (cGMP). Automation and Control Systems can help achieve cGMP and quality standards by ensuring that environmental and product contact air quality, temperature, humidity and differential pressure are constantly monitored and controlled within acceptable limits. Predictability in these environments and processes is necessary to ensure that end products meet quality requirements. Control of these environments is also necessary to avoid change environments and processes as required by different products manufactured in the facility. Also, the risk of cross contamination or contaminants is high in facilities that are engaged in making multiple products. This require maintaining strict control of the differential pressure between processing suites and passageways.

Building Automation Systems (BAS)

Design

Over the past 10 to 15 years building automation systems (BAS) have become increasingly more and more an integral part of facility designs. Up until the early 1980s automatic temperature control systems consisted of mostly pneumatic and electrical control systems. The closest thing to a front-end system was a control panel that had a variety of gauges and pilot lights to tell building operators the status of their mechanical systems. In the mid to late 1980s building designs began to be inclusive of BAS and this has steadily increased over the years.

BAS have proven to be vital to the functionality of a building. The first approach in a BAS design is to generate a Statement of Criteria and a Basis of Design (SOC and BOD) document. In general terms the document outlines what the BAS will contain and how it will control and monitor the building mechanical, electrical, and life safety systems. The document is inclusive of the following type of system proposed, graphical user interfaces (GUI), network type, the interface to existing systems, control and monitoring of applicable systems, hours of operation of the various systems, etc. When the BAS is to be integrated with other vendors systems, OPC and OLE (OLE for Process Control) must be utilized to be a gateway between the various systems keeping an open system.

Normally before the SOC and BOD are done you have met with the client and discussed the project. For the renovation of an existing building the project team will have done a thorough survey of the existing building. Normally clients will give input on the BAS; sometimes, however, the client does not have any personnel with instrumentation and control experience and so they rely on your expertise to guide the BAS design. Almost always there is a total construction budget the design must follow, so a rough estimate is done once SOC and BOD are completed. Typically the engineering firm does the initial BAS estimate by trying to generate a total controls I/O points list and calculating a cost per point.

Once the client approves the BOD, the detailed design and construction documents are started. At this point in the design the BOD is expanded and detailed to the point where the BAS can be built. Instrumentation and control drawings are generated detailing all of the mechanical and electrical systems that will be either controlled and/or monitored. All the I/O points will be documented for each system. The instrumentation and control drawings will consist of airflow diagrams and hydronic systems diagrams. A system architecture riser diagram is done showing the layout of the various controllers, the location of operator workstations, gateways to other systems, etc. In addition a symbols and abbreviations drawing is generated.

Specifications are written to detail the requirements of the BAS controllers, operator workstations, instrumentation and control devices, control valves and damper, etc. The specific details are generated stating the requirements of each control device, valves, dampers, and air measuring devices. Sequences of operations are generated detailing the operation of each mechanical system. Each system has a sequence of operation explaining in detail how each component of the system operates. Safety operation is included to explain what happens in the event of an emergency (smoke, freeze condition, etc.). Also a sequence is written for loss of normal power, and what happens to the various systems. An event sequence must be written to detail what system will be shutdown by the BAS and in what order in the event of loss of power and what systems will run on emergency power. When power is restored, the event sequence will specify how the BAS will energize the various systems and in what order.

Last but not least the specifications include the various BAS requirements along with performance requirements. The responsibilities of the BAS vendor are mentioned regarding codes, installation procedures, training, warranty, etc. Once all of these documents are prepared including the instrumentation and control drawings, they are all combined and referred to as the Functional Requirement Specification (FRS). These will be the documents the BAS vendor will use to construct the system.

BAS Build

The FRS is issued to the BAS vendor who has been awarded the project; these documents are then utilized to generate detailed shop drawings to be submitted for approval. Once the shop drawing process is completed and shop drawings are approved, the installation can begin. One of the most important aspects of a BAS installation is to closely coordinate construction schedules with other suppliers and vendors to ensure that the BAS vendor is following along the appropriate timeline. The first task in installing a BAS is to order approved valves and release them to the mechanical contractor for installation. Industrial type valves can require long lead times, taking 6–10 weeks before they are available.

In addition any flow meters and temperature sensor thermowells must be sent to the mechanical contractor for installation. The same goes for automatic dampers and air measuring devices (AMD) to be mounted by the sheet metal contractor. It is important to coordinate damper and AMD sizes with the sheet metal contractor because duct sizes may have changed slightly since the latest construction documents were released. It is common in the shop drawing process for duct sizes to change slightly. These are typically items that the BAS vendor furnishes but are installed by the mechanical contractor. Once these tasks are resolved the installation can begin.

The next task is to study the floor plans and strategically plan conduit sizes and layouts to be as efficient as possible. It is crucial to follow all applicable codes and specifications. One code to bear in mind for BAS is to make certain the class 1 and class 2 wiring circuits are kept in separate raceways (covered in NEC article 725). Briefly, a class 2 circuit is one that is 24 volts AC or lower, and a class 1 circuit is one that is above 24 volts AC. Most times these two types of circuits are present on the same control panel. This is acceptable as long as there is an appropriate barrier between them.

Even if the code permitted these two types of circuits to be together, it would not be recommended. The reason for the separation is that the noise from the class 1 circuit(s) would probably cause noise and disrupt the control signals. It is important to spend the extra time ensuring that high and low voltage circuits are kept completely separate. Once the conduit layouts are completed, submit the marked up floor plans to the project Engineering firm for approval. This will ensure that the BAS condiut runs will not conflict with other conduits, piping, support beams, etc. Upon completion of the conduit layouts, wiring may begin.

Once the wiring process has begun, the control panels should be built in the panel shop. Often it is a good idea for the control panel enclosure to be sent to the job site to be hung. This way the electrical contractor can complete the conduit runs before the control panels are completely assembled between the control devices and the control panels. Also wiring can be pulled from the control devices to the control panels. Meanwhile the control panel can be assembled on the back plane of the control panel and inserted into the enclosure. For this reason it is always a good idea to utilize control panels that contain a back plane.

At this point things should be making very good progress as many things are being done simultaneously, closing in on a successful installation. Once all control devices are completely installed and wired, it is time to terminate everything within the control panels. It is important that the control panels are not powered until all control points have been successfully terminated keeping the correct control signals in order. It is critical to make certain that all the correct control devices have been terminated at the appropriate control panel terminals. Once all of the above has been completed, point-to-point wiring check out can begin.

Point-to-point wiring check out consists of checking for wiring continuity from the control device back to the appropriate terminals. This is done for each and every control point. A procedural checklist is recommended for this task to keep order and efficiency. If continuity is not found for a control device, then the wires must be traced until the problem is resolved. In addition all of the network wiring must be checked out to ensure completion as well. Once all of the above has been accomplished successfully, then a site acceptance test must be scheduled with the owner, validation, construction manager, and possibly the engineering firm.

BAS Validation

First order of business is to determine what are the validated GMP (Good Manufacturing Practices) systems and what are non-validated (non-GMP) systems. The difference between the two is additional procedures and requirements for approval, testing, and qualification—you do not want to invest the resources to validate a system unless it is absolutely required. This process is normally done upfront because different quality control devices might be required for GMP vs. non-GMP systems.

It is important that a binder be created containing all of the factory calibration certificates for each and every control device. This makes it easier for the validation team to follow through for all of the control devices and approve them if they all have the appropriate NIST tracability and factory calibration. Documentation is half the battle in validation.

Site acceptance will entail going through each system in detail and performing a system operational test for each control loop, etc. Each control loop will be fully tested to verify that it does what it is supposed to do. In short, you run through each P&ID loop, and check the sequence of operation, and walk the system through the checks and balances. Basically, try and simulate the system operation to see how everything responds and make the necessary changes to your programming as you go—It's next to impossible to fully simulate a real life system operation.

The validated portion of the BMS must have full capabilities to trend system data for a period of time and be able to store that data for batch record purposes. Typically, you also want to print these data for several reasons but mostly for batch records. Also you must ensure that complete change control is in place, with only authorized personnel having access to the validated system through the graphical user interface (GUI) or the human machine interface (HMI) screens.

In addition, Standard Operating Procedures (SOP) should be in place for what do to in all scenarios with the BAS from changing setpoint for various control loops to overriding system operation. All personnel that will be involved in this operation must be documented and trained. You will need a administrator type person in place as well, with full rights through the front-end system and who can add and delete users as well. For security purposes you should only have one or two people with these capabilities. All changes to the system must be fully documented. The system must have the ability to record every single activity on the system.

Client preference determines the setup of the BAS networks for the GMP vs. non-GMP systems. Some clients do not mind having their GMP and non-GMP BAS networks integrated together and the necessary security measures to prevent back flow from the non-validated to the validated system. This will prevent personnel with access to the non-validated systems to have access to the validated systems, etc.

Other clients want their GMP and non-GMP networks totally separate and not connected in any way. This adds an extra layer of security because there are now two BAS systems and different access to each. This is the best approach to guarantee security and remove any doubt. A totally integrated system is very possible through correct and thorough setup. Some clients want one comprehensive system in place to have everything integrated. It is possible to have the BAS, process systems, manufacturing execution system (MES), security system, fire alarm system, etc. on one complete integrated network. This approach would utilize some form of OPC (OLE for Process Control) to connect the various systems.

The other accomplishment of this set up is that you then truly have an open system. The client is not locked into any vendor for future projects. This is really the direction the industry is heading toward because this type of system gives the client flexibility. As long as a new system to be added is OPC compatible, then that system can be added.

Process Control System

There is a general trend in the control and automation industry for the professionals in the field to be trained as electrical engineers (EEs). There are, of course, control engineers that come from other engineering disciplines, but it does make sense that EEs often fill this role since a lot of the tools used in automation are electrical or electronic devices. EEs are usually adept software people as well, which makes them good candidates for the development of the programs that run control processes. Unless the EE has lots of experience in a specific field, the decisions are best left in the hands of process engineers (civil, mechanical, chemical) who in most cases truly understand what the goal is in terms of system performance. The important point to make here is that the "process" must always come before the "control." After the process has been precisely determined, then and only then should the process engineer feel comfortable in handing the control engineers their marching orders. The "process first" approach allows the system to be a "top down" design, which will ultimately give the highest performance.

Once the process is defined then it becomes the control engineer's job to begin conceptualizing the system architecture of the automation system. At this point, control loop descriptions become critical. As the design begins, the control engineer must cross check control loop descriptions with the field instrumentation package specified in the process design. The control engineer must determine whether all the necessary system feedback will be provided to accomplish the sequence of events specified. It is not uncommon for a process engineer to request control features that cannot be implemented with the specified instrument package. When instrumentation deficiencies are found, it is wise to document them with a Request for Information (RFI) through the appropriate contract administrators and to let them make a decision on how to proceed. Frequently, some requirements will be relaxed by the process engineer to keep unexpected cost of additional instrumentation from entering the equation. The control engineer should always remember that some processes are very complex. This increases the likelihood that the Input/Output (IO) list will change during the course of the design and increases the importance of making the control design flexible so that redesign work is minimized as the I/O schedule shrinks or grows.

Control Loop Process File

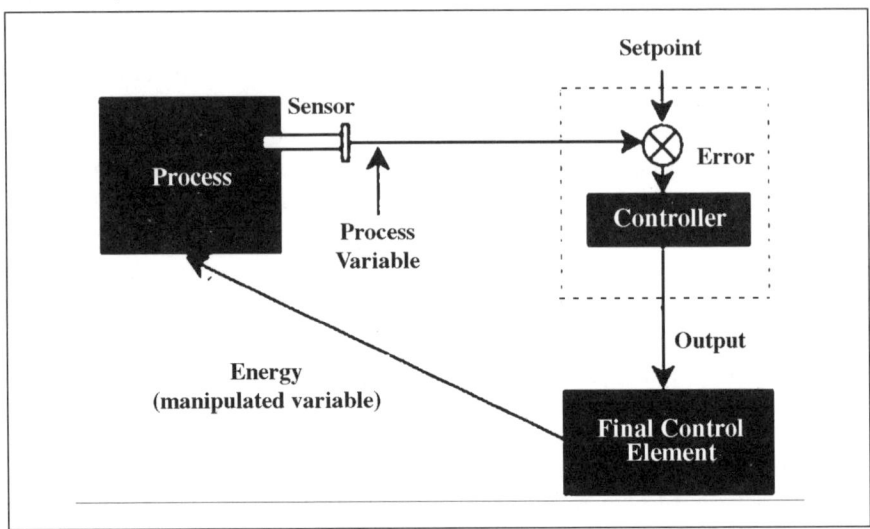

Closed Loop Process Control System

Designing Process Control Systems

Even in a design build application not every decision about control system design is in the engineer's hands. End user's almost always have some hardware and software preferences whether they were published in the specification or not. This can affect the integrators bottom line since additional training, design time, and possibly additional software licenses are needed to get the project moving. Most seasoned integrators are accustomed to this reality and will become versed in more than one manufacturer's offering of hardware and software.

Once the decision has been made about what type of controllers to use in the application, it is time to start value engineering your automation system. Very close attention should be paid to the layout of the facility and the processes being controlled and monitored. Does the application find all of your control devices in one place where a single panel can house the I/O interface? Or are there components strewn about the facility requiring some sort of distributed I/O system with multiple control enclosures? Will a single controller tied to all of your control devices be acceptable? Or will multiple CPUs be required to ensure certain stand alone processes will not be compromised by equipment failure in another part of the facility? As you might expect, consolidation of control equipment can reduce costs and is an important consideration early in the design. Spare I/O capacity is also an important feature in some systems that may be in areas where future expansion is planned. The list of design issues to sort through is large and includes:

- Network design
- Remote communication access to controllers
- Radio telemetry (fixed frequency vs. spread spectrum technology)
- I/O isolation
- Hazardous areas and intrinsic safe barriers
- Panel layout
- Rough environment equipment

It is during design that the control engineers really flex their professional muscles. There are a number of design issues, and the relationship of these issues to one another is complex.

Building Process Control Systems

There are hundreds of subcomponents typically required to build a control system of even moderate complexity—from the plastic terminal block to the 3 GHz, P-4 control and monitoring workstation equipped with the 19 inch plasma screen. Part numbers on control gear are frequently 15 characters long where the transposition of a single digit can spell disaster when it comes time to procure the equipment needed to construct your system. Lead times can be long for the more elegant electronic devices that the manufacturer may not have in inventory. In most cases it is preferable to have all of the major components for a control panel in hand prior to beginning assembly. It is almost inevitable that changes will be made by assembly technicians on the layout of control devices within a panel and having all of the parts assists greatly in decision making about the final layout. Changes to the I/O layout on a controller should be avoided if possible. After all, changes to the wiring at the control module may affect physical I/O addressing that the programmer will not be happy about after spending 400 hours writing code for a system that is now addressed differently. This, of course, leads into the importance of "as built" documentation. It is critical that the installation people have the right information for terminating signal conductors regardless of the number of modifications.

Validating Process Control Systems

Successful validation of a control system has everything to do with exhaustive preparation and has its roots all the way back to the performance requirements agreed upon in the conceptual design. From the control engineer's perspective, validation should be regarded as a tool. It is the tool that will ultimately calm the nerves of less control-savvy personnel that the automation is working and that the system will not mysteriously start misbehaving as soon as the control engineers have left the building.

Automation System Design, Build, Install/Implement, and Validate: Industry Practices and Regulations

One of the additional requirements of Automation Systems in the biopharmaceutical industry is the need to conform to U.S. FDA (and/or European or Asian) regulatory requirements. Apart from current Good Manufacturing Requirements, most automation systems are required to conform to 21 CFR Part 11, the rule that applies to omputerized systems in general.

21 CFR Part 11 regulations apply to all systems that capture, retain data, and/or are involved in a GXP environment. GXP includes Laboratory (GLP), Manufacturing (GMP) and Clinical (GCP) applications.

The rule is divided into three sections:

- Subpart A: General Provisions
- Subpart B: Electronic Records
- Subpart C: Electronic Signatures

Records are defined as "any combination of text, graphics, data, audio, pictorial, or other information representation in digital form that is created, modified, maintained, archived, retrieved, or distributed by a computer system." Electronic signatures are defined as "a computer data compilation of any symbols executed, adopted, or authorized by an individual to be the legally binding equivalent of the individual's signature."

Good Automated Manufacturing Practices (GAMP)

In order to have a common understanding and adequately meet the regulatory requirements of the FDA and other international agencies, an industry group later known as the Good Automated Manufacturing Practices (GAMP) forum was promoted. The GAMP forum is now a technical subcommittee of the industry's leading non-governmental organization called International Society for Pharmaceutical Engineers (ISPE) and has a multinational policy-making industry board. The outcome of the collective efforts of GAMP forum is a published guideline, widely accepted by the industry, called the GAMP Guide. In its fourth revision, GAMP 4 is the most widely used, internationally accepted guideline for validation of automated systems. The GAMP Guide is published jointly by ISPE and the GAMP Forum. GAMP 4 is intended for suppliers and users of automation systems in pharmaceutical manufacturing and related healthcare industries such as biotechnology and medical device. The Guide draws together key principles and practices and describes how they can be applied to determine the extent and scope of validation for different types of automated systems in view of the regulatory requirements.

GAMP 4 helps organizations (suppliers and end-users) develop:

- Validated and compliant automated systems using the concept of prospective validation following a life cycle model
- Procedures to ensure that the automated system remains in a validated state once it is validated and in operation

Advantages of using GAMP 4:

- Cost benefits by aiding the production of systems that are fit for purpose, meet user and business requirements, and have acceptable operation and maintenance costs
- Better visibility of projects to ensure delivery on time, on budget, and to agreed quality standards

- Increased understanding of the subject and introduction of a common language and terminology
- Reductions in the cost and time taken to achieve compliant systems
- Improved compliance with regulatory expectation by defining a common and comprehensive life cycle model
- Clarification of the division of responsibility between user and supplier

GAMP Lifecycle Model

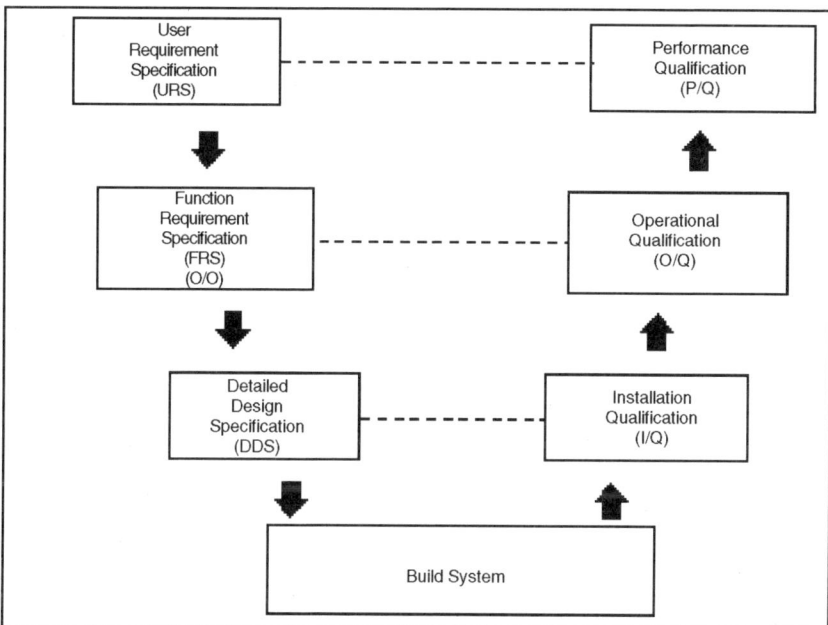

GAMP 2 File

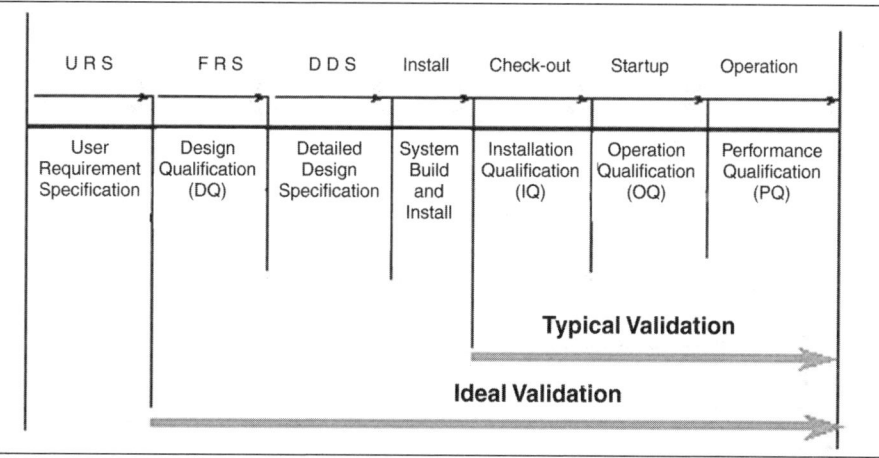

8

Validation and Facility Design

Authors: James P. Agalloco
                   Phil DeSantis

Advisors: Robert E. Chew
                   Joseph X. Phillips

INTRODUCTION

Validation is a subject that has grown in importance within the global healthcare industry over the past 25 years. During that time period, it has perhaps resulted in more changes in practices and methods, while causing more controversy than any other subject. Its relationship to facility design was not at all clear when it was first introduced in the early 1970s (1). It is now clear that validation and facility design are subjects that profoundly influence one another. One of the major concerns with any design—whether it be for a facility, a piece of equipment or a production process—is how its validation will be accomplished. Designers must now consider more carefully than ever before how their design will perform, as it must be "validated" prior to beneficial use. At the same time, validation programs must be established to facilitate the accomplishment of that very goal. A clear line of communication must be established to ensure that the operational objectives as implemented in the design can meet the validation requirements for that design. A well structured project team will mandate cooperation between designers and validators to meet the project's dual goals of performance and compliance. This chapter reviews the aspects of validation as they impact the overall design, construction, and start-up of healthcare facilities.

HISTORY OF VALIDATION: 1972–1998

Validation in the pharmaceutical industry appears to have its origins in the United States during the early 1970s. The term "process validation" was introduced to the pharmaceutical industry by Ted Byers and Bud Loftus of the Food and Drug Administration (FDA) (1). The FDA's objective was to enhance the quality of sterile drugs produced in the United States. Because validation was an outgrowth of a major regulatory crisis, firms that did not make parenterals were clearly skeptical at what was perceived to be an FDA over-reaction to a problem unique to sterile products manufacturers. Despite these misgivings, FDA pressure was such that validation activities for sterilization processes were underway at virtually all U.S. parenteral manufacturers by the middle of the decade. The definition of validation at that time did not provide clear guidance to its real intent, nor could anyone have foreseen in that definition the substantial impact validation was to have on the industry:

> *Validation is the attaining and documentation of sufficient evidence to give reasonable assurance, given the state of science and the art of drug manufacturing, that the process under consideration does, and/or will do, what it purports to do.* —Ted Byers (June 1980)

Within this context the industry began its first validation efforts. Of necessity, because the FDA utilized the FD 483 to emphasize its intentions, and the acknowledged lack of understanding of the goals of validation, almost all of these early efforts were defensive in nature. The goals of industry validation efforts in this early period were easy to understand: Keep the FDA happy, which will keep our plant operating. The rudimentary state of understanding regarding validation was such that the long-term resource requirements were unknown. The initial area of activity within the industry was totally directed toward sterilization procedures.

As firms completed their sterilization validation programs, the FDA continued to make presentations in support of validation and the industry's perspectives began to evolve. It was clear that the FDA intended to emphasize validation for some time to come and to impose it in a broad range of different areas. Validation had become a part of CGMP expectations throughout the parenteral industry. Around the same time, the FDA recognized that validation had a use in processes and products not intended to be sterile and soon began to speak about the merits of validation for the verification of process control for all types of processes. The unique role of research and development in contributing to validation were a part of the next definition that FDA proposed (1).

> *A validated manufacturing process is one which has been proved to do what it purports to do. The proof of validation is obtained through the collection and evaluation of data, preferably beginning from the process development phase and continuing through into the production phase. Validation necessarily includes process qualification (the qualification of materials, equipment, systems, buildings, personnel), but it also includes the control of the entire process for repeated runs.* —FDA Definition (ca. 1978)

By and large, validation in the pharmaceutical industry at the end of the 1970s was still primarily a regulatory exercise and remained largely isolated from the rest of the firm. The FDA's expanded emphasis on validation fostered several new areas of activity for validation: product attributes, non-sterile products, content uniformity of dosage forms, dissolution, clinical supplies, and formulation development.

In 1984, the FDA published its Guideline on General Principles of Process Validation. While there was initial opposition to the guideline's tone, there was general consensus that validation was now a way of life for the pharmaceutical industry. Within the guideline the FDA provided the following definition that clarified their expectations (2):

Process validation is a documented program which provides a high degree of assurance that a specific process will consistently produce a product meeting its predetermined specifications and quality attributes.

The industry began to recognize that validation offered advantages to the firm and implemented validation objectives that were non-regulatory and geared for the optimization of processes and systems (Table 1). The attention being placed on validation at this time led to important changes in how firms approached its implementation and should be integrated with other good manufacturing practices.

TABLE 1 Benefits of Validation

* Increased throughput
* Reduction in rejections and reworks
* Reduction in utility costs
* Avoidance of capital expenditures
* Fewer compliants about process-related failures
* Reduced testing—in process and finished goods
* More rapid/accurate investigations into process upsets
* More rapid and reliable startup of new equipment
* Easier scaleup from development work
* Easier maintenance of the equipment
* Improved employee awareness of processes
* More rapid automation

Like many other American industries, the pharmaceutical industry participated in the introduction of computers into the manufacturing environment during the 1980s. This inevitably led to FDA concerns relative to the validation of computerized system used within the industry. The pharmaceutical industry's response to the FDA's new concerns regarding validation of computerized systems was somewhat different than what had occurred previously. The Pharmaceutical Manufacturers Association established an interdisciplinary group called the Computer Systems Validation Committee (CSVC) in late 1983 to address how the industry would address the FDA's concerns. Through the creation of the CSVC, the industry began to assume a position of leadership regarding validation.

Through the auspices of the CSVC, an industry approach to the validation of computerized systems in the GMP environment was established (3). Central to the industry position, was the adoption of the "life cycle" concept as an appropriate model for managing the activities needed for the successful validation of computerized systems (Fig. 1). The life cycle approach focuses on managing a project from cradle to grave. When employing the life cycle approach, the design, implementation, and operation of a system (or project) are recognized as interdependent parts of the whole. Operation and maintenance concerns are addressed during the design of the system and confirmed in the implementation phase to ensure their acceptability. The adoption of the life cycle methodology afforded such a degree of control over the complex tasks associated with the validation of computerized systems that it came into nearly universal application within a very short period.

FIGURE 1 Stages of the Life Cycle Concept

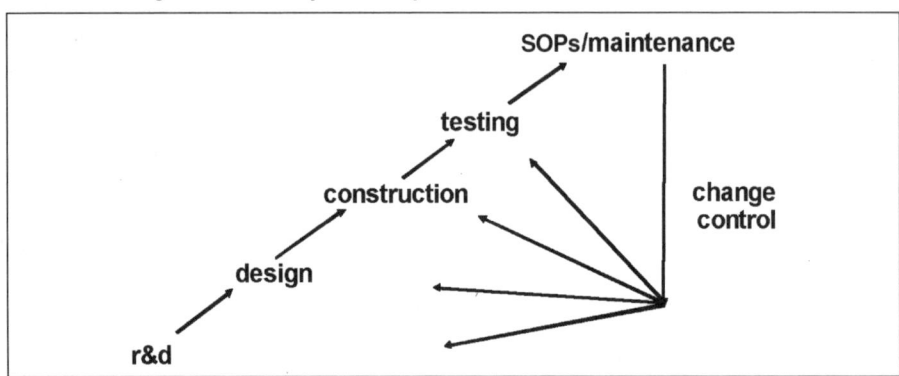

A further obstacle was the term "validation" itself. It was clearly a source of considerable confusion. During the early years of validation, the term had become synonymous with the activities focused around protocols, data acquisition, and reports. The concept of validation as a collection of related activities practiced throughout the useful life of a system that provide greater confidence in the system, process, or product came into focus. To overcome the limitations of the narrower definition of validation, many industry practitioners adopted the new term "process qualification" or "process validation" for the testing phase of an overall "Validation" program. With the introduction of this new term, the distinction between the narrower activities of "validation" and larger program "Validation" has been made evident (Table 2). Throughout this chapter, we capitalize the term validation when necessary to reinforce the distinction.

TABLE 2 Validation vs. VALIDATION

Validation	VALIDATION
Defensive	Proactive
Testing oriented	Total process control
Costly	Cost effective
Quality control	Quality assurance
Narrow focus	Diverse application

With the confusion created by the terminology eliminated, it now became possible to apply the Life cycle to the "Validation" of systems, procedures and products beyond computerized systems. Clearly, addressing "Validation" concerns during the development stage of a new facility, process or product afforded a greater degree of control over the entire project as it progressed towards commercialization than had prior efforts at organizing "validation" activities.

The use of formalized methods to control change is an integral part of the life cycle and introduces a rigor to the validation program that makes it far more useful to the firm that adopts this approach. The life cycle approach for Validation provides the pharmaceutical industry with a organizational model that makes the management of Validation activities far simpler than had been previously possible. Along with the introduction of the Validation life cycle, newer definitions of validation have come into use that are more compatible with the new ways in which validation is being performed (4).

Validation is a defined program which, in combination with routine production methods and quality control techniques, provides documented assurance that a system is performing as intended and/or that a product conforms to its predetermined specifications. When practiced in a "life cycle" model it incorporates design, development, evaluation, operational, and maintenance considerations to provide both operational benefits and regulatory compliance.
—J. Agalloco (1991)

The use of a life cycle methodology in the practice of Validation requires that validation considerations be raised early in the project. It is now commonplace to involve validation personnel with the early stages of facility design to ensure that the ultimate goals are realized expeditiously. There are continuing trends in the global pharmaceutical industry that are shaping Validation as a practice. The emergence of world class organizations in the pharmaceutical industry, along with the era of pharmaceutical mega-mergers has forced firms to review both their manufacturing and quality practices. Rationalization of facilities and relocation of equipment, products and personnel are facilitated by the application of validation principles. The utility of the Validation life cycle concept for control of products, processes, and systems is becoming increasingly wide spread. The successes realized in the proactive approach taken by the industry and industry associations in addressing regulatory and compendial issues will undoubtedly continue. The successful application of validation concepts in a range of cGMP applications will tend to place greater emphasis on Validation as a permanent fixture in our industry.

Until now, our discussion has focused on regulatory expectations as the primary impetus behind Validation as practiced in our industry. To a certain extent that is unfortunate, as it results in firms and individuals doing only that which is definitively required either by regulation or guidance documents. There are many in this industry who have found this perspective to be somewhat limiting. To those individuals, Validation is an inherently valuable activity in any project as it ensures that the end results of the design and engineering efforts will be more satisfactory. Many of the

Validation concepts employed in the healthcare industry mirror those in the software industry where (21 Part CFR 11 aside) validation is not a regulatory requirement. Our industry might be better served if we implemented validation practices for reasons of increased reliability, greater fitness for use, and closer alignment with user requirements, rather than as a required part of facility and system start-up.

The emergence of Good Design Practices is perhaps another example of how the industry has reacted to regulatory expectations. The System Design Regulations for medical devices require that the design phase of device development be accomplished in a systematic fashion. It is a logical and simple extension of this concept apply it to the facility used for the device (or for pharmaceutical and biological products), which led to Good Design Practices. Industry has led the way in this area through the many voluntary "standards" developed by the PDA and ISPE. The PDA's Technical Reports and ISPE's Baseline Guides have helped define many of the facility requirements so commonly found in our industry (5,6). Good Design Practices are nothing more than a compilation of these and other similar documents that aid the designer. They ensure that the finished facility/system will be better suited for its intended CGMP use, than if a less structured approach had been followed.

RELATIONSHIP BETWEEN VALIDATION AND FACILITY DESIGN

When practiced in accordance with the principles of the life cycle. Validation and facility design (and actually all types of design that are subject to validation requirements such as process and formulation development) are highly interactive. Each is affected by the other to a substantial degree.

Facility designs for validated facilities are profoundly altered by the additional requirements raised under the auspices of Validation. The designer must now recognize that many of the elements of the design are subject to a more intense documentation and verification requirement. The word "validatability" has been coined to express in a single term those elements of the design that are subject to validation requirements. Design engineers must now concern themselves with an independent assessment of their design concepts where the goal is to confirm the ultimate acceptability of the completed and operating system. The water system may have to be equipped with additional sample ports, temperature recorders, and flow meters, and subjected to intense scrutiny as to the specifications for the pipe (or tubing), slope of the lines, quality of the welds, and passivation of the system. HVAC systems may be rigorously reviewed to ensure that the proper particulate classification is obtained, air changes are correct, temperature and relative humidity limits are maintained, and that the system is tolerant of the disinfecting materials to be utilized. Therefore, designs must be more than merely functional; they must be capable of meeting the pre-established requirements that the firm has set for the "Validation" of the various systems.

Validation of a facility is certainly affected by the specifics of the design itself. The validation requirements must be tailored to meet the operational requirements inherent in a good design. At the same time, it must be recognized that, although designs must be flexible to accommodate varying process requirements, the

Validation approaches utilized must be tolerant of that flexibility. Designers of water systems recognize that the differences in local water supplies and process requirements will dictate the design details of a specific system. As the design varies to accomplish the removal of various potential contaminants such as silica, heavy metals, calcium, or other materials, the Validation will require the qualification of different pieces of water treatment equipment peculiar to the removal of a specific contaminant. Similarly, the process requirements for hot or cold water of various microbial qualities will dictate different distribution, storage, and sanitization methods all of which must be accommodated in the qualification and validation of the system.

To accomplish these goals, it should be evident that lines of communication must be established between the facility designers and those individuals responsible for the validation of the facility. "Throwing the design over the wall," as may have been standard practice many years ago, is the antithesis of what must be done. Designers and validators must work together to ensure that the end result of their joint efforts is a facility that meets all of the operating requirements, and that can be validated with minimal difficulty. Cooperation and effective communication between the disciplines are essential for success in project implementation.

One of the more interesting issues that must be addressed in this interplay between design and validation is the inevitable compromises that must be faced. With an infinite budget and no limitations on space and time, the "perfect design" that incorporates all of the operational requirements into an easily validated design can be accomplished. As unlimited resources are never available, there are always inherent limitations in the design where some measure of operational ease or simplicity of design is compromised to avoid excessive cost. These areas generally become points of contention between the designers (and sometimes their hidden alter egos, the project cost accountants) and the validation team (usually led by someone with a compliance background). All might agree that a hot water loop is preferable from the viewpoint of microbial control, but the project budget may be inadequate to support the increased cost associated with the installation of such a system. Rather than let the discussion grow acrimonious, it is preferable that the group consider all reasonable alternatives until agreement can be reached on a workable compromise. These types of discussions provide for balance between the design goals, which usually include consideration of project budget and schedule, and quality requirements, which are usually based upon expected regulatory concerns. In these discussions there is no right or wrong; the different disciplines are merely viewing the same operational requirement from different perspectives. Compromises between the extremes of each viewpoint that can accommodate the concerns of both are usually available. These confrontations are a normal part of the design process and ensure that the finished design is one that all concerned can acknowledge as correct for the intended purpose. When these types of discussions are not held, the finished design is likely to be skewed in favor of either extreme budget control or regulatory excess.

Having said all this, the authors will now express their personal opinion. We believe it is never desirable to institute operational constraints to compensate for inferior design. The use of a single corridor for both clean and dirty equipment, manual flushing of dead legs rather than the use of a recirculating distribution loop, and the selection of equipment based solely on price are all examples where system or facility operation (and by extension, the Validation of those systems) may be compromised by inherent flaws in the design or selection of equipment. A penny well spent may be far more cost effective than a penny saved. At the same time we recognize that there have certainly been instances where designs have been overdone. We believe that design excess is generally less prevalent and less risky in the long run, and would therefore tend to err on the side of doing more than the minimum in design to ensure the "validatability" of the final design.

Validation as a Team Activity

In the context of a capital project, it should be apparent that Validation is best executed by a well coordinated team. Depending upon the elements of the project, the number and diversity of the team may vary. The operational qualification of a water system might be best performed by individuals from engineering, with assistance from quality control to provide the required analytical support. The performance qualification of a fermentation process might be best accomplished by personnel with training in biochemistry, microbiology, and biochemical analysis. Each team needs the requisite skills to accomplish its assigned tasks, and the same system might have different team members depending upon whether it is in IQ, OQ, or PQ. The leader of each team is normally that individual who possesses the best project management skills, with the others supplying the requisite technical knowledge based upon their assigned role on the team.

Overall leadership of the validation requirements project is normally embodied in a single individual reporting into the project manager. Such individuals can come from a variety of backgrounds provided they have the right mix of technical and administrative skills.

Facility and Equipment Design for Validation

Facility design generally starts with the determination of a need for new or increased capacity, or new production capabilities on the part of the healthcare firm. In the not too distant past, that need might have been simply stated as "capable of filling 100,000,000 syringes per year" or "to produce 45 tons of bulk pharmaceutical chemicals." Today, additional needs beyond those commercial desires are included such as "to meet global regulatory requirements," or "to operate under the most stringent levels of cGMP." These broader user requirements mandate that Validation of the facility must be a major consideration throughout the design. Recognizing that the close coordination of design and validation is necessary to fulfill this objective, there are numerous opportunities to enhance both. These opportunities lie in activities carried out throughout the project design and implementation. The following sequence of events is not meant to define a rigorous step by step or document by document procedure. It is, though, a description of a project life cycle that, when the phases described below are carried out in a cooperative team environment, will result in an acceptable validated facility.

User Requirements. A written summary of the user goals that the completed facility must satisfy. While broadly stated herein, in actual practice these must be more definitive to allow for real understanding of the owner's operational needs. The user must define the approximate batch sizes, product mix, desired level of automation, inclusion of support services desired (i.e., laboratories, warehousing, office space, personnel lockers), etc. The absence of clear user requirements virtually ensures that the completed design will not satisfy the needs of the firm.

Conceptual Design. Design activity begins soon after the genesis of the need for a new facility and for large projects, may actually precede approval of the capital expenditure. It generally begins with a list of "user requirements" in which the owner (or user) of the facility states the operational goals of the finished design. These goals may be versed in two distinct and very different fashions: quantitatively and qualitatively. Quantitative goals are numerical measures indicating the size of batches, the number of vessels, the quantity of output, the number of lines, the numbers of personnel, etc. These are used to define the facility in physical terms relative to size, dimension, and layout. The second aspect of goals deals with non-quantitative attributes and include such objectives as cGMP compliance, state-of-the-art design, world class, highly automated, easily validated, etc. It should be evident to the reader that each set of goals has a profound effect on the complexity of the design and ultimate cost of the facility.

Coupled with these goals, the users must define more specifically the operational needs that the design must satisfy. To accomplish this, the following items are usually needed to develop a design concept:

Process Description. These are written descriptions that describe how the processes to be performed in the facility shall be accomplished. Batch instructions or development reports can sometimes be used to provide the information required (Table 3).

Product Description. This is a summary description of the product(s) being produced in the facility. It should include information regarding critical issues such as toxicity, safety, storage conditions, microbial control. and other aspects of the product that have an impact on the facility design (Table 4).

Process Flow Diagrams. These are simple diagrams that depict the process flow, including material and energy balances where appropriate. The diagrams can be simple blocks with written text indicating materials and conditions to be used inside. For BPC or biotechnology applications, the diagrams can be enhanced with additional blocks that mimic the process equipment. In these instances, minor pieces of equipment such as pumps and valves can be included.

TABLE 3 Process Description

- Major process steps
- Block diagram(s)
- Process flow diagram(s)
- Utilities (WFI, DI water, CIP, etc.)
- Major support equipment (sterilizers, ovens, etc.)
- Major process equipment (reactors, crystallizers, etc.)

Major Equipment List. A basic requirement is a list of major equipment items required within the facility. For dosage form facilities and pilot plants where process variation is great, this list may actually be of more use than process descriptions or process flow diagrams.

Preliminary Facility Layout. This should take into account the process flows, need for support areas (e.g., laboratories, material staging, warehousing), and required adjacency of operations.

Controlled Environment Requirements. This is a list of all controlled environments including particulate classification, temperature controls (incubators and/or cold rooms), relative humidity controls (for effervescent or other moisture sensitive materials), etc.

Process Control Philosophy. This is a brief description of any computerized process control systems to be incorporated into the facility.

TABLE 4 Product Description

- Product type(s)
- Volumes (optional)
- Batch size(s)
- Formulation (optional)
- Package(s)
- Product features (physical characteristics) (*optional*)
- Solubility
- Heat, light, air sensitivity
- Safety and handling
- Stability
- Raw materials, reactants, intermediates, processing aids

Project Schedule. A rough timetable for the project, this should include any significant milestones toward project completion.

Conceptual design, as with any of the design activities, may be done by an in-house team, but is likely done by a separate design and engineering firm. This phase allows the designers to fully understand the user's needs. Validation team input at this early stage will serve to highlight those areas where validation concerns may influence the design. This stage of the project may be somewhat lengthy as the owners and designers reach agreement on the scope, estimated cost, and functionality of the finished facility. This agreement usually is in the form of a capital appropriation to continue with design or (for smaller projects) to fund the actual construction. With the approval of these funds, the designers can now begin to develop the design and provide details required to procure equipment and actually construct the facility

Design Development

This design stage is often called Preliminary Engineering. The design engineers will develop detailed schematic drawings of the facility and systems. These drawings, called piping and instrumentation diagrams (P&ID's), depict each process, utility, and support system, including piping, instrumentation and equipment. The P&ID will include all line sizes, valve types, materials of construction, and insulation, with each item shown in the correct spatial relationship, although not necessarily to scale. In addition, this design stage usually results in a final facility layout and equipment arrangement.

These drawings should be provided to the operating personnel and validation team to review. The reviewers must assess whether the completed system will be capable of performing all of the desired functions intended. For instance the review of a process vessel must establish that the utility connections to the jacket can provide for all intended heating and cooling schemes, and that the process connections are correct for all production usages including batching, cleaning, purging, reacting, sterilizing, rinsing, etc. This is generally accomplished in a team session where each drawing is reviewed against the process descriptions to confirm its correctness for all its intended uses as defined in the user requirements.

These schematics become the key reference drawings against which systems are compared during qualification. Once the schematic drawings are approved, change management is usually imposed on them to ensure that affected members of the design and validation team are notified when a change is requested. This helps to ensure that the completed systems will meet the user requirements that originally defined the design.

As design development nears completion, enough information is available to begin the preparation of a validation master plan for the project.

Master Planning

The validation master plan has become common practice for all large capital projects within the global healthcare industry. The master plan has come into vogue to ensure that the Validation requirements for major facilities are adequately addressed. While often described as a regulatory requirement, there is in fact no such requirement in any of the world's cGMP regulations; nevertheless, its real value is as a management tool to be used to coordinate the Validation effort. For a large facility, the validation costs (which are estimated at 5–15% of the total facility cost) may well exceed several million dollars. In activities of this magnitude, the availability of a master plan that clearly delineates how the validation effort is to be executed is an almost indispensable tool. The utility of a plan diminishes with facility size and complexity, but even small projects may benefit from the structure that a master plan brings to the Validation effort.

The information needed to begin a master plan includes all of that listed previously for conceptual design plus additional items that are usually defined early in the conceptual design process. These additional items include:

Utility List. This is a list of key utilities needed to operate the facility especially any water systems used in product manufacture or cleaning.

Facility Layout. A floor plan(s) of the facility, the layout shows major equipment and controlled environments. Overlays to the basic layout including material, equipment, and personnel flows are generally prepared at the same time (Table 5).

TABLE 5 Facility Description

* Equipment layout (arrangement)
* Personnel/material/component flow
* Controlled environments
* Materials of construction
* Sketches

Instrument List. Derived from P&IDs, this list will indicate the function and range of all instruments and may be expanded to add additional details, such as vendor, material of construction, and model.

At the same time, preliminary information contained in the design concept will have been further defined and detailed to the point where Validation planning can now be carried out. Changes to the facility, as the detailed design progresses toward completion should be incorporated into the master plan document.

Reasons for Master Planning. There are numerous benefits that are derived from a validation master plan. These benefits can substantially enhance the firm's Validation posture for the project. For smaller firms building their first facility, the master plan may provide the opportunity for the firm to define its validation philosophy for the first time. A well structured master plan will:

1. Codify decisions regarding how cGMP requirements will be satisfied
2. Allow for the detailed definition of validation activities necessary for the successful operation of the facility
3. Serve as an important document in regulatory compliance and interaction
4. Serve as a communication document on the validation for use with third parties
5. Be easily converted into a Drug Master File
6. Serve as a excellent tool for audit preparation (either internal or external)
7. Define project execution through the definition of requirements
8. Help determine resource needs for personnel, materials, equipment, components and laboratory analysis
9. Ease protocol and report preparation through the definition of accepted formats
10. Be used as a bid document when soliciting bids for contract execution

Level of Detail. Master plans vary considerably in the level of detail provided. Depending upon the scope of the plan, there is a commensurate adjustment in the amount of detail provided. A plan addressing a multi-product multi-process facility will have less detail than one which addresses the qualification/validation of a new production suite for a single product. When in doubt as to the level of detail to provide, it is suggested to err on the high side. The least useful plans are those that provide only the "what to do" without insight into the "how to" and "why" of the validation effort. In the best plans, the intent of the validation is clear enough that the designers can use that information to ensure that those objectives can be realized. In certain instances it may be beneficial to provide summaries of the key acceptance criteria to be used for the various products, processes, and systems in the facility. With this, the design team has full awareness of what the expectations of the validation team are and can make appropriate adjustments to ensure their satisfaction. The validation protocols will reiterate the acceptance criteria, with expansion as to methodology, sampling frequencies and schedules, test methods, apparatus, etc.

Typical Validation Master Plan Structure. There is no standard format for master plans. The authors have successfully used the following basic template (Table 6) for plans they have developed with appropriate adaptations to suit to specific requirements of a particular project.

As indicated previously, this template can be readily modified to accommodate different project types and scales. With changes in facility type there is a corresponding change in the focus of the master plan. The following summaries delineate the major distinctions between plans for different types of facilities.

Sterile Product Facilities. The preparation of sterile products requires environments suitable for the preparation, manufacture, and assembly of materials that will prevent microbial contamination, and systems designed for the sterilization of the various items required in the processing. A master plan for a sterile production plant will place heavy emphasis on classified environments, HVAC systems, equipment utilized for sterilization, water for injection, and other key utilities. Careful consideration of

TABLE 6 Validation Master Plan Template

Introduction: Introduction to the project scope, location, and timing. Includes responsibilities for protocol, SOP, report and other documentation preparation and approval. Identifies who is responsible for the various activities. A general validation SOP or policy statement may be included.

Plant/Process/Product Description: A concise description of the entire project is provided. It will provide information on layout and flow of personnel, materials, and components; utility and support systems; description of the processes to be performed and products to be made in the facility (Tables 3 to 5). Major equipment is also described.

Computerized System and Process Control Description (If Needed): Computerized information, laboratory and process control systems are described in sufficient detail to delineate the validation requirements. This section may be omitted if the level of automation is minimal.

List of Systems/Processes/Products to Be Validated: Equipment, systems, and products are listed in a matrix format that describes the extent of validation required (i.e., IQ, OQ, or PQ) as part of the project. Additional breakout of computerized, cleaning and sterilization validation requirements can be added.

General and Specific Acceptance Criteria: Key acceptance criteria (general and specific) for the items listed in the prior section are provided. Emphasis should be placed on quantitative criteria throughout. To merely state the general requirements provides no substantial benefit to either those responsible for the validation or for those involved in the design process.

Special Issues (If Needed): Sections can be included describing in greater detail the validation requirements of an element of the project where additional clarification may be warranted. Typical subjects include automation, cleaning, containment, isolation, or lyophilization.

Protocol and Documentation Format : The format to be used for protocols, reports, and operating procedures is described. This is particularly useful in a new organization where such formats have not yet been defined. It can also be beneficial when working with an outside contractor to ensure that all documentation is in the correct format.

Required Procedures : List of SOP's (new or existing necessary to operate the facility.

Manpower Planning and Scheduling : An estimate of the staffing requirements to complete the validation effort described in the plan. A preliminary schedule of required activities is prepared to help estimate appropriate manning levels.

personnel, component, and material flow is essential to minimize the potential for microbial ingress into the classified environments. Automation of process equipment may be important given the complexity of most sterilization equipment.

Bulk Chemical Facilities. In the manufacture of bulk pharmaceutical chemicals, focus should be placed on the chemical synthesis. Validation master planning as it relates to BPC plants focuses on whether the equipment is suited for use in the various unit operations required. Identification of the critical step(s) is essential, with greater emphasis on all portions of the process and equipment that follow those steps. Automation may or may not be critical depending whether the facility is operated using an automated control system (usually a distributed control system) or not. Cleaning of the process equipment is generally of critical importance as it is generally intended for multi-product usage and is designed more for use with chemically aggressive materials and conditions rather than for ease of cleaning. Some BPC equipment such as condensors or centrifuges, by their very design, tend to be difficult to clean. Cleaning validation between campaigns of different products is essential.

Biotechnology Facilities. The manufacture of biopharmaceuticals combines the concerns for microbial control associated with sterile products with the process concerns associated with BPC plants. There is roughly equal emphasis on facility, systems, and the processes themselves. The identification of critical steps as necessary with BPCs is generally beneficial. Personnel, component, and material flows are usually important especially in the purification and fill-finish stages of the process. Automation may or may not be important and is usually restricted to bioreactors, chromatographic columns, autoclaves, and critical utility systems. Support utilities such as WFI, clean steam, and process gases will be another area of focus. Cleaning validation, especially between campaigns in multi-product facilities, is critical to success.

Solid Dosage Facilities. The blending, mixing, and dose formation steps used in tablets and capsules should receive the bulk of the attention in master plans for these products. The emphasis must be placed on the processes and products, rather than the facility. Because the equipment utilized in the production of these products is highly specialized, it must receive considerable attention during the qualification stages. If the process equipment is automated, then that too may be an important part of the validation effort. The dusty nature of the materials being processed and the manual cleaning required for much of the process equipment will require particular attention during the cleaning validation. Considerations for utilities other than process water tend to be minimal. Regulatory interest in microbial control for these types of products is emerging, but seems to have little measurable benefit to the patient.

Oral and Topical Liquids. The compounding of these formulations presents some of the same concerns addressed earlier for sterile products only to a lesser degree. The large amounts of water utilized in either the formulation of the product or cleaning of the equipment make microbial control a greater concern than it would be for oral solid dosage forms. The potential for microbial proliferation on/in either the product or equipment forces careful design to allow for easy sanitization of the equipment and facility. The water system utilized to supply the area is another area of concern.

Developmental Facilities. Pilot plants, clinical production areas, and development laboratories must be qualified and validated if they are used in the preparation of materials that will be administered to humans. The qualification of these facilities resembles that outlined for production facilities for the same product types. Product and process concerns are minimized, as there may be no defined products that can be identified at the design stage. Careful consideration of cleaning validation is essential as these facilities must be flexible enough to produce a wide range of materials.

Regulatory Interaction

There are no legal requirements that state that firms should review their proposed facility designs with regulators prior to their construction. In the past, some firms announced their new facilities to inspectors upon physical completion when they first sought approval to use them. In recent years it has become more common to hold some form of review meeting with the regulatory bodies early in the project schedule to attempt to receive regulatory approval while the design is still on paper. Where the firm has employed novelty in their design concepts, material selections, or equipment features this interaction can be beneficial in obtaining regulatory "buy-in" well before funds are committed. This type of interaction is best carried out by providing the regulatory body with copies of the conceptual design information and validation master plan some time prior to a formal meeting. The meeting is used to review the design and answer any questions regarding the facility by either the regulators or the firm. A formalized approval is not granted; the firm merely comes away with an understanding of regulatory concerns relative to the design and Validation that should be addressed prior to seeking approval to use the completed facility.

Detailed Design

This phase of the project design is the most intensive. Beginning with the schematics, the designers prepare drawings and specifications in enough detail to actually construct the buildings, equipment, and systems necessary to achieve the design concept and meet user requirements. These drawings and specifications, along with the schematics, will provide the validation team with a thorough understanding of the design from which they can develop detailed validation protocols for each system.

Enhanced Design Review

The conduct of an enhanced design review (also called Design Qualification) exercise is an optional activity that has the greatest merit in very large and complex projects that must satisfy a broad range of requirements. Enhanced design review is a formalized review of the design at selected points in the project life cycle against user requirements, company standards, and available regulatory guidance. Members of the design team will have the results of the efforts critiqued by the various project stake holders and independent reviewers to determine if the specifics of the design meet the established objectives. The design would be checked against compliance, safety, and environmental standards established by the firm and/or any affected governmental agency. After the assessment, a summary report is issued outlining the findings. The performance of an enhanced design review is *not* currently a regulatory requirement in the United States, but is required by the GMP regulations of the European Union. Its execution is recommended for projects of all sizes.

Process and Support Equipment

The following steps are those frequently encountered with the purchase of major utility and process equipment, and computerized systems. Depending upon the complexity of the item being purchased the extent of the effort may vary widely. For very simple items the only interaction between the vendor and the end user may be a purchase order. For all items, the following in some combination must be considered to adequately support the qualification effort.

User Requirements

Even the simplest of systems will fulfill a need required by the ultimate user. It is important that the procurement of equipment and systems used to operate or support a manufacturing process be driven by these needs. Clear and approved user requirements documents are strongly recommended for each major system to avoid unsatisfactory performance.

Equipment Acquisition

This activity may involve the specification and selection activities described below. For simple pieces of equipment of standard design, the specification/selection process may be compressed into a simple purchasing activity against a catalog number. In these instances, the entire process is substantially compressed and there is far less interaction between the user, designer, and vendor. Caution should be exercised: While there is nothing wrong with using standard designs (they are generally cheaper and the lead times are substantially shorter), the user requirements must be carefully considered. If an off-the-shelf item will fully satisfy the needs of the end user, then by all means it should be purchased. That purchase decision should ultimately be made by the user and not by someone unfamiliar with the process requirements.

Equipment Specification and Selection

In the course of every facility design project there will be many items of the process or utility systems that will be purchased from outside vendors. This equipment generally falls into two general categories: standard designs or custom built to fit a specific purpose or installation. In either case, these items are essentially capital projects in miniature that are just smaller parts of the larger facility project. With very complex and/or novel pieces of equipment, they may follow a design path much like that of the overall facility with all of the stages of user requirements, conceptual design, detailed design, and even design qualification specifically for a individual item. In these instances the purchaser of the equipment will be heavily involved in this entire design process. For more standard items, the approach is the same but the equipment manufacturer may have completed a similar exercise at some time in the past. In either case, the desired features of the equipment are generally embodied in functional specifications developed by the engineer in order to meet the user requirements. The vendor will propose a solution or design, including detailed specifications to be reviewed and accepted by the user. In some cases, the user may perform the more detailed design and then solicit bids from vendors for finished systems that will meet those specifications. In either case the specifications become an item for discussion and negotiation and the entire exercise should be considered one of review, negotiation, acceptance, and approval. A significant part of the interaction with equipment vendors is the detailed design drawings that the vendor provides which depict how the equipment will be fabricated. For custom equipment, the client's approval of these drawings constitutes approval to the vendor to begin fabrication.

For custom designed systems it is not unusual for the customer to work closely with the vendor. This may entail visits to the vendor during the design stages and periodically during the equipment fabrication as well. This interaction helps to expeditiously resolve the inevitable differences in understanding that exist between firms as to what the final piece of equipment will be. For automated systems, this type of interaction is mandatory or there will be little chance that the finished piece of equipment and its control system will perform as desired.

Factory Acceptance Testing (FAT)

Upon completion of the equipment fabrication, formalized factory acceptance testing (FAT) may be performed in which the completed system is evaluated for its performance. The vendor is expected to resolve any failures of the system to perform as required prior to shipment. These tests utilize vendor utilities and operating areas and, therefore, there may be slight differences between the performance observed at the vendor and the required performance. These differences must be carefully evaluated to establish whether the performance will be satisfactory after installation at the customer's site. In some FATs the customer will supply components, materials, and personnel to assist in performing the testing. Depending upon how the qualification/validation protocols are written the FAT may be an integral part of the finished documentation package. It should be recognized that a significant portion of the installation qualification for the equipment can be performed at the same time. After all, physical dimensions, materials of construction, sub-component information, and many other aspects of the system will not change as a result of shipment. Vendor notification of any changes to the equipment subsequent to the FAT must be reported to the owner as part of change management. If the client chooses to leverage the FAT in support of equipment qualification, this must be done using a pre-approved protocol and following all other client standards and procedures pertinent to equipment qualification, including documentation practices and handling of variances.

As a practical matter, the authors have had better experience in treating FATs as pre-qualification activities. They are important in ensuring that equipment and systems are ready for operation and qualification. However, because FATs involve many design details that do not directly impact product quality and because these tests often uncover problems that may need to be remediated, it is difficult to apply the documentation and variance-handling practices required for qualification.

Equipment Vendor Installation

In certain instances (lyophilizers, and sterilizers are common examples), the vendor has the responsibility for supervising the installation of their equipment at the owner's site. The inclusion of this support may be a part of the negotiated terms of purchase. The design drawings will indicate what tie-ins to the system are required. In these cases, the vendor will generally assume responsibility for making the equipment ready for use by the purchaser and would provide initial calibration, preliminary cleaning, lubrication, etc.

Site Acceptance Testing (SAT)

For large systems, especially those composed of many sub-elements such as a distributed control system, the extent of vendor installation and assembly required can be extensive. In these instances, the conduct of post assembly or site acceptance tests (SATs) may be desirable. The purpose of this test is to establish that the equipment vendors (and their subcontractors) have successfully installed a system meeting the design requirements prior to leaving the job site. The SAT documents that the system performs as required using the utilities present in the facility and in the operating environment. A formalized test procedure should be used for this purpose, and this should be reviewed with the supplier prior to its execution. If the SAT will be leveraged to support equipment qualification, this procedure should be a formal protocol, likewise subject to the owner's standards and procedures. It should be noted that the performance of an SAT is not a mandatory requirement, and for many smaller pieces of equipment that can be fully evaluated at the vendor's site may be of little, if any, value. Similar to FATs, SATs are probably best treated as pre-qualification (commissioning) for the same reasons.

Vendor Support for Validation

Throughout the preceding steps, the equipment vendor—whether for process equipment, support system equipment, or a control system—may play a major role in the qualification/validation efforts. A vendor who focuses on the healthcare industry will be better able to understand the somewhat different requirements associated with the sale of equipment to a heavily regulated industry. Many of the major vendors have well defined documentation programs that can simplify the qualification of their equipment. Vendors have been known to provide protocols for factory or site acceptance testing, installation, and operational qualification as well as comprehensive documentation on aspects of the system design and development. Depending upon the vendor, this material may be available as part of the purchase price or must be purchased for an additional fee. Wherever such vendor support is available, the purchaser may have a difficult time developing comparable quality information for the same cost, so it is usually a wise investment. The client firm should exercise caution, however, in ensuring that vendor supplied protocols or other documentation meet the standards and procedures that the firm has established.

The purchaser should indicate in their initial user requirements the extent and type of documentation required from the supplier as a minimum. The opportunity to do so should not be overlooked; vendors are better able to provide detailed documentation if they are notified of requirements for it prior to the start of their design and fabrication efforts.

For equipment that is relatively simple and follows the standard designs of the vendor, many of the items identified above will be largely transparent to the vendor. That is to say the vendor will have addressed many of these concerns internally and may have internal documentation on these activities as well. Under these circumstances, the purchaser will likely encounter some difficulty obtaining original design documentation and internal test plans and results. This should not be a cause for serious concern; equipment items that are part of a vendor's standard product offerings are likely to be fairly mature in their product life cycle and should provide reliable service despite the absence of extensive supportive documentation. As a minimum, though, the vendor should be required to provide documentation in the form of manuals and instructions adequate to operate and maintain the equipment.

Some projects will entail the design, specification, fabrication, and installation of a system that extends the vendors product capabilities such that it cannot be considered a standard item. In these instances, it will generally be necessary for the vendor to provide far more information in order to provide adequate documentation for the qualification/validation of the system. The more complex and unique the system or piece of equipment, the more emphasis should be placed on securing support from the vendor that will facilitate the qualification effort. One of the saving graces for highly custom systems is that they require increased interaction between the purchaser and the vendor, and these communications can serve as the basis for ensuring that the entire effort is documented adequately.

Construction/Field Fabrication

There are many aspects of a facility that cannot be purchased from a catalog, or even easily through a written specification. The facility itself, as well as much of the supportive infrastructure (i.e., HVAC systems, water, and other utility systems) are constructed or fabricated in the field by contractors and subcontractors. These may range from the general contractor who has overall responsibility for construction of the facility, to specialty contractors who focus on a particular type system. In these instances, the facility or system is assembled from the most basic of elements: steel, concrete, wire, glass, etc. The transformation of these items into a finished pharmaceutical plant is no simple task, and must be carefully coordinated to ensure schedule and budgetary compliance. Amid all this, the assembly of documentation supportive of qualification places another burden on the general contractor and the end user. Where contractor conformance to defined standards, reporting requirements, or procedures is required, formal agreement by the contractor to those requirements should be obtained in the commercial contracts. Failure to obtain that formal agreement will generally result in an inability to have the contractor abide by the required practices.

Construction Liaison

Once the general contractor or construction manager has been selected, the owner of the facility will find it essential to appoint a liaison to the project manager or superintendent. This individual serves as the point of contact between the owner and the builder to ensure that lines of communication are open. Depending upon the scope of the project, this liaison could be handled by a single individual, or more commonly through a group of individuals who interact with the contractors in defined areas. Their role is to ensure that the contractor complies with all of the specifications for the systems they are fabricating, while also assisting the contractors in understanding and satisfying the owner's user requirements.

Fabrication/Installation Standards

For facility features and systems that are constructed on-site rather than purchased as a pre-assembled entity, fabrication/installation standards are comparable to equipment specifications. Standards are utilized to define the specific types of materials to be employed (e.g. grades of stainless steel), the methods to be used (e.g., passivation procedures for piping), and the documentation to be provided (e.g., weld reports) upon completion. These standards may be provided to the contractors by the user (The A&E firm may assist in this effort), or supplied by the contractors subject to the approval of the owner. The standards help ensure that the construction practices employed in the field will ultimately result in a facility and/or system that satisfies the user requirements.

Enhanced Turnover Packages

A program that assists in assembling documentation on the construction of systems. It can be of benefit for systems where formal qualification is not required (i.e., city water, HVAC for un-classified environments, etc.) as a means of gathering information through the contractors.

"As Built" Drawings

The qualification of constructed/assembled systems can be greatly aided by the preparation of "as built" drawings on these systems. An "as built" drawing is prepared starting with the design P&ID drawings for the system. Trained individuals (usually working as a team) compare the system as it exists in the field to the drawing. Discrepancies between the actual system and the P&ID are noted directly on the drawing. This results in a marked up P&ID sometimes called a "red-line drawing." Once completed the red-line is critically reviewed. The owners design team will then decide whether to modify the drawing to accurately document the system "as built" in the field or to correct the system to match the original P&ID drawing. While one's initial instinct is to modify the physical system to match the P&ID, there may be little operational benefit to do so and a significant cost to make the change in the system. Whatever the decision with regard to resolution of physical system–P&ID drawing differences, what is essential is that a drawing be prepared that accurately reflects the final system as accepted by the firm from the contractor. Depending upon the extent of the changes, this may mean preparation of an entirely new drawing, or merely retention of the red-line as an accurate representation of the field installation. The decision not to update the red-line into a controlled master drawing is one that should be made cautiously. If subsequent modifications are to be made to the system, the mark-up of a red-line drawing is poor practice. Better to update (CAD is the normal method) and to certify it as accurate as soon as possible.

Material Control

For certain types of systems, primarily HVAC and liquid systems (i.e., water systems, process fluids, and gases) specialized handling of fabrication materials may be required. The control measure will ensure that storage, handling, and assembly for these materials is carried out in ways will protect its unique quality characteristics. For instance, 316L stainless steel tubing is shipped protective covering on the ends to prevent the ingress of contamination prior to assembly. The tubing must also be protected from contact with ordinary steel tools that could result in corrosion of this expensive material.

Inspection and Test Reports

These reports serve to document receiving and field inspections of materials and systems, as well as the results of any testing performed on site. The contractors should complete these reports at the time they perform the inspection or test and become a part of the construction records for the system involved.

Construction Quality Control

Many contractors that focus on serving the healthcare industry have instituted formal quality control programs that ensure that their employees, and often those of any of their sub-contractors, adhere to certain standards of performance. These standards are generally in the area of job site cleanliness, safety on the job, and completion of required documentation.

Training of Contractors

It may be necessary to provide training to contractor and sub-contractor employees to better ensure that the construction standards are adhered to. While some of the sub-contractors have employees who are aware of cGMP requirements, there will be many who may not have encountered them previously. The training helps these individuals understand the importance of proper completion of documentation and performance of their work according to the defined procedures.

Construction Audits

The owner, either directly or through their A&E firm, should conduct frequent audits of the job site to assess that the contractors are adhering to their contracted requirements. Any problems with the audited systems or the methods being followed should be reported to the construction manager as soon as possible to initiate immediate corrective action.

Start-Up/Commissioning

Once the facility/system have been completed construction and/or installation, it reaches "mechanical completion." There have been some naive individuals and firms who believe that when the facility/system installation reaches this point, formal qualification can begin. In actuality there are many activities that must be performed before qualification should be started. Some of the items are described below.

Passivation. Clean steam piping, process water systems, and process piping fabricated of 316 or higher grade stainless steel should be passivated to remove weld slag prior to filling of the system with the process fluid. In some cases, vessels and other ancillary piping may also require passivation. This should be performed and documented according to a pre-approved specification or plan.

Calibration. Critical instruments should be calibrated according to the manufacturer's recommendations and entered into the facility database. Procedures for their initial re-calibration may need to be developed if the instrument is new to the site. Calibration technicians may need training in the calibration procedures for these new instruments.

Post-Installation Cleaning. The facility and equipment should be thoroughly cleaned to remove any fabrication debris and prepare it for initial use.

Safety Requirements. Safety equipment should be installed in all designated locations. Critical safety systems may be subject to testing before the facility can receive a certificate of occupancy from the local municipality. Safety and operating signage and other hazard-related identification should be placed where necessary.

Lubrication. Lubricant levels should be checked in all mechanical drives and seals.

Electrical System Start-Up. Electrical connections should be verified as to circuits and breakers, fuses should be installed, grounding must be confirmed, pump and agitator motors must be checked to confirm that they turn in the proper direction. All of these are needed to make the systems safe for qualification.

SOP Development. Operating personnel should finalize drafts of procedures required for the operation and cleaning of the facility. While preliminary drafts may be available, there is generally some tailoring of the procedures needed to match the physical installations.

Personnel Training. Operating and mechanical support personnel should receive training on the procedures to be employed for the process equipment and facility systems.

Air System Balancing. HVAC systems for the facility must be balanced to ensure that air flow rates, air changes and pressurization within the facility match the design requirements. Any movable dampers should be firmly fixed in position after the balancing, and their locations noted.

Punch List Completion. System/facility deficiencies are inevitable with large systems, and these are often noted on a "punch list" that is provided to the vendor/contractor after the owner's inspection. These items can be either corrected or deferred providing that leaving them incomplete will have no adverse impact on the qualification effort.

On modern GMP projects, commissioning is considered to be a necessary precursor to qualification. It should be performed according to a pre-approved plan and documented according to good engineering practices. In addition to the items described above, commissioning also included the confirmation of compliance to detailed engineering specifications and drawings.

All activities related to Validation up to and including commissioning are engineering activities. They are governed by good engineering practices and not by 21CFR 210 and 211, except that facilities and systems resulting from these activities must be suitable for their intended purposes. As such, it is recommended that certain documents preceding equipment qualification be reviewed and approved by both the user group and the quality unit. These include the user requirements documentation and the enhanced design review reports. The owner's engineering representatives should approve other engineering and construction documentation, including commissioning documents.

System Impact Assessment

Systems judged to have no impact or indirect impact on product quality may be determined to require commissioning only. Those systems determined to have a direct impact on product quality require qualification.

The following is offered as a checklist to determine system impact.(7) An answer of "yes" to any of the system characteristics listed indicates a direct impact on quality and thus requires qualification.

- Used to demonstrate compliance with the registered process
- Normal operation or control has direct effect on product quality
- Failure or alarm has direct effect on product quality
- Information is recorded as part of batch record, lot release data, or other cGMP related documentation
- Direct contact with the product or product components
- Control over critical process elements that may affect product quality without independent verifications of system performance
- Used to create or preserve a critical status of the system

System and Equipment Qualification

After completion of the commissioning activities cited above, formal qualification of the systems and equipment can begin for those systems judged to have a direct impact on quality. This entails the documentation of critical installation and operating characteristics of the system that can confirm its acceptability for use in production activities. In addition the accumulated data can serve as base for subsequent change control activities. The completion of a rigorous commissioning, wherein engineering details are confirmed, allows qualification to focus on critical parameters. These parameters are usually derived from the user requirements documents and are those that truly dictate system performance as it relates to product quality. Consequently, these parameters are those that require rigorous change control.

Qualification was not a significant part of many programs when "validation" first became a required activity in the late 1970s. The focus of early papers on "validation" and much of the regulatory guidance focused only on "process validation," an activity that is sometimes called "process qualification" (PQ). Aspects of equipment and system performance were only minimally addressed in these early years. It was recognized that, in order to ensure the reliability and consistency of validated processes over time, the equipment utilized must operate in a specified and reliable manner. Measurement and confirmation of equipment and system operation could serve as a predictor of its ability to provide acceptable results in a subsequent process validation study. Thus the qualification of equipment and systems as a precursor to process Validation became a feature of a sound validation program.

Within a few years after its introduction as a supportive activity to the "process validation" effort, qualification was divided to two major activities: installation qualification (IQ), which focuses on aspects of the installation of the equipment/system, and operational qualification (OQ), which focuses on the operating parameters of the equipment/system. In some critical systems requiring the interaction of multiple units, a challenge test or an extended monitoring period, performance qualification (PQ) may be added. This division is completely arbitrary and the designation of an activity as being part of the IQ or OQ should not be considered a rigid one. Firms should not address the designation of a particular test rigidly as part of the IQ or OQ. Disputes over the correct protocol to place a particular test serve no useful purpose. Surprising, as it may seem to some, there are no regulatory requirements that the IQ be approved before the OQ can commence. Although it makes sense to ensure that the installation parameters affecting a subsequent operational test are satisfactory, the formal division of the activity into sub-tasks and their subsequent stage-wise approval are industry creations that are not beneficial to timely completion of the activity. Nevertheless, until very recently the vast majority of firms prepared separate IQ and OQ protocols and treated the final approval of each of these as prerequisites to the start of later activities.

The advent of qualification within the global healthcare industry brought about another element of change to the practice of "Validation." With the emergence of a new requirement to document equipment and systems more comprehensively, the validation service firms came into being. These firms offered their clients assistance in the validation of their facilities; however in many cases what was really offered was assistance in the qualification of standard equipment and systems. With the exception of sterilization and similar "standard" processes, these firms are rarely able to provide comprehensive support to the "process qualification" or "process validation" of a production process, whether it be for a injectable parenteral, protein purification, or chemical synthesis. These types of processes reflect the basic production technology of the owner, and are only rarely turned over to contractors for turn-key type assistance. On the other hand, water systems, HVAC systems, vessel services, sterilization equipment, and other generic-type activities could easily be given over to the validation services contractor for execution. With this division of labor came another subtle change in the way in which Validation was approached. Validation service firms recognized that the healthcare firm would only rarely rely heavily on their services for process validation activities, but would readily ask for assistance in IQ/OQ efforts. With this recognition, seemingly came what could be termed "feature creep," as IQ/OQ activities grew in size and scope with the validation services contractors subtly pushing for more and more content. This has resulted in IQ/OQ activities now far exceeding process validation (PV) activities in cost and duration. Essentially, the tail was now wagging the dog, with PV relegated to a virtually second class status, when in fact it was the reason for the IQ/OQ in the first place. As an example of the types of excess perpetrated on the industry, was a recent IQ of some 80 plus pages provided by a validation service company for a laboratory incubator! There seems to be little merit to such overblown efforts other than to increase the profits of the validation service firm. Industry is slowly becoming aware of these excesses, and a new awareness of the proper relationship between IQ/OQ activities and their contribution to the far more critical aspects of the PV is emerging. Distinctions between IQ/OQ are diminishing and perhaps in the not too distant future the industry will see a return to "qualification" as an all-inclusive term for an activity that is an element of "Validation" rather than an end onto itself. In addition, the reversal of "qualification creep" is beginning to emerge. By covering engineering details in the commissioning phase and concentrating qualification on critical installation and operational parameters the focus of the qualification activity (and its consequent cost effectiveness) is sharpened. Note well that commissioning is recommended as a valuable and necessary engineering activity. It is not done merely as a dry run to ensure variance-free qualification.

This next section addresses "qualification" within what is hoped to be a perspective reflective of the latest industry thinking, and may not reflect the emphasis placed on this subject by the majority of present-day practitioners. The authors believe that the trend in the industry will be for a reduction in the scale and scope of installation/operational qualification efforts, accompanied by a commensurate increase in the PV efforts. This is consistent with the FDA's increased pressure on PV activities as manifested by their initiatives under the pre-Approval Inspection program for increased linkage between the developmental/clinical materials and final commercial process. The financial pressures increasingly faced by all healthcare manufacturers in the late 1980s and early 1990s have also fostered a re-evaluation of Validation as a value-added activity, and bloated qualification efforts are likely to be one of the first casualties of those pressures (and, in our opinion, deservedly so).

There is no regulatory requirement that every system installed within a facility be qualified or that those that are qualified be done so to the same degree. Such a policy would raise systems /equipment with minimal influence on product quality, safety, efficacy, and purity to the same degree of criticality as those parts of the facility that directly impact those attributes. Table 7 provides some general guidance on the extent of qualification, including in some cases performance qualification, needed for a range of systems.

TABLE 7   Validation Priorities for Process and Facility Systems

High: IQ/OQ/PQ (or PV)	Moderate: IQ/OQ	Low: Commission Only
Breathing Air	Deionized water	Process drains (except biotech)
Water for injection/ purified water	Vacuum (if used in the process)	Non-process water
Clean steam	Controlled temperature rooms	Sanitary drains
Product contact gases	Process drains (biotech)	Electrical systems
Classified environments		Comfort HVAC
CIP system		Cooling water/jacket services
Solvent distribution systems		Instrument air
Process piping		

The primary objective of qualification is a critical review of the system, equipment, or facility against the design documents (especially specifications and P&IDs drawings) to confirm that the user requirements have been satisfied. Perhaps the simplest approach that can be used is a one-to-one correspondence between the individual elements of the user requirements and the qualification protocol requirements. Using such a methodology it becomes very difficult to overlook any of the essential elements of the system, and the development of acceptance criteria for the qualification is straightforward. In addition, it is permissible to add important design criteria that may not have been included in the user requirements but are judged necessary to meet these requirements.

One of the more interesting issues relative to qualification is how to select the acceptance criteria for the various tests that are performed. Consider a shelf dryer intended for use in drying of tablet granulations. The user requirements might have stated that the dryer be capable of ± 5°C for this purpose. In order to satisfy that requirement without difficulty the vendor may have provided a dryer that has a maximum variation of ± 2°C. Which criteria should be required in the qualification protocol, ± 5°C or ± 2°C? Wherever these types of situations are encountered, it is recommended that the tighter specification be included in the protocol. There are at least three good reasons for this:

1. If the system cannot meet this claim by the vendor perhaps there are other critical claims that the unit cannot meet
2. A future product may be introduced that will require a tighter range and, if confirmed initially, there is no need to retest the dryer.
3. Having paid for a dryer that can maintain a tighter range, the owner should confirm that performance.

In the qualification of equipment and systems it is generally not necessary to repeat tests more than once. If the firm feels strongly that a test be repeated, then perhaps that test ought to be part of the PV efforts. In some cases, the protocol must go into considerable detail to describe how a test is to be performed. This detail should be included in the protocol/report to enable later users of the documentation to understand how the test was performed. As qualification tests are often repeated after modification or repair of equipment and systems, details on how the original test was performed are essential if the follow-up study is to be meaningful. Qualification tests are often performed in the absence of formulations, actives, solvents, and media. This reduces the cost of the studies, and allows the tests to be conducted without any bias that might arise from the use of production materials. Placebo materials such as water (for liquids) and lactose (for solids) are used when there is a requirement that there be a material present to perform the qualification test. Results with actual production materials will likely vary slightly from those obtained using the placebo, but cost and safety concerns dictate that placebos be used. When tests must be performed with actual production materials, serious consideration should be given to placing that test into the PV effort.

There are several elements of the qualification effort that do not directly relate to the equipment or system. Standard operating procedures should be available in draft form at the start of the qualification effort. As the qualification effort proceeds these can be updated to reflect more closely the proper operating methods for the equipment. They cannot however truly be finalized until the system has successfully completed process validation (although most firms require at least an interim SOP approval before proceeding with PV), which confirms the acceptability of the sequences and set-points embodied within the procedures. In many cases, the procedures must be revised to accurately reflect the results of the PV. Typical procedures needed for equipment and systems include operation, cleaning, preventive maintenance, and calibration.

Training of Personnel

While not strictly a validation activity, personnel training is almost always an integral part of any validation effort. The installation of new equipment and systems often means that current operating practices are no longer appropriate and new skills must be acquired. It is beneficial to have operating personnel assist in the qualification of the systems and equipment that they will ultimately operate. This provides a basic familiarization with the equipment, and can be quite beneficial in the development of the necessary procedures.

Process Qualification

The conduct of studies confirm the ability of the equipment or system to successfully perform their intended function form the basis of all validation efforts. Thus blenders must blend, filters filter, and sterilizers sterilize. Moreover, this must be demonstrated with production materials on a commercial scale. In the very first programs, these efforts were termed "validation studies" and were soon renamed as "process validation" studies. More recently the term "process qualification" has come into vogue, along with its close relatives and "product qualification." For the purposes of this chapter, all of these terms are assumed to be equivalent or, at the worst, interdependent. Our apologies to those who insist that the nuances in definitions among these terms are significant; we think not and will endeavor to explain why. In a manufacturing setting, there are materials that are impacted (processed) by the equipment to effect some change in the materials (which results in a product). Neither the process nor the product exists without the other. The purpose of the process is to make the product. The product is the result of the process. Without a process, we have no product, only starting materials. Without a product, the process is only a simulation. Calling the entire activity "process qualification" or PQ wraps the product/process combination in a single term that should include consideration of both product and process aspects. The optimal approach to validation considers process parameters, product attributes, *and* their relationship. Only in combination can a process/product validation be properly addressed. A well-designed PQ protocol includes elements relating to the equipment parameters (process) and the materials (product). As examples, consider the following:

- PQ protocols for a tableting would include confirmation of press operating parameters (i.e., compression force, tablets per minute, tooling, etc.) as well as assessment of product attributes (i.e., hardness, friability, dissolution, etc.).
- PQ protocols for a chemical reaction would include equipment aspects (i.e., reaction temperature, agitation rate, etc.) and aspects of the materials (i.e., molar ratios, impurity levels, etc.).

Process qualification must balance the twin concerns of the equipment and materials to be truly complete and scientifically correct. The best protocols clearly establish how maintenance of equipment operating parameters result in product attributes that conform to specifications. The introduction of product and material consideration within the PQ effort forces greater involvement on the part of the owner of the facility. After all, the facility was built with the intent of making materials for commercial sale (or, in the case of developmental facilities, for use in experimental or clinical supplies), the expertise for which lies with the owner. The acceptance criteria included in the PQ will be driven by the expected performance of the products as measured against their specifications. Internal experts of the owner— be they pharmacists, chemical engineers or microbiologists—will dictate the PQ effort. It must be noted that it is this aspect of the overall effort that generally receives the greatest regulatory scrutiny. After all, investigators are far more concerned with the key quality attributes of the products being produced in the facility than they are with any part of the earlier qualification of the support utilities.

Change Control

Change control is one of the more important activities that are closely tied to the practice of Validation (8). The existence of a change control program is mandated in the CGMPs and must include the participation of the Quality Control (QC) unit. Change control programs ensure that the effort expended in the execution of qualification and validation provides lasting benefits, whether it be to compliance or operational performance. Undocumented and/or uncontrolled changes to qualified systems can alter the performance of the system such that it can no longer be considered to be in a validated state. For this reason, formalized change control programs are widely utilized to restrict change to validated systems. Changes may be of virtually any type and description. Validation can be compromised by changes to equipment, operating procedures or software and it is therefore necessary that the change control procedures include a means to address a variety of changes.

The basis for evaluation of changes to systems is ordinarily the documentation assembled during the qualification of the system. This is perhaps the soundest reason to organize the documentation of the system in an orderly fashion, such that evaluation of the system post-change can be readily accomplished. The evaluation might be simply a comparison of the newly installed replacement part to the one identified in the documentation. At the other end of the spectrum, the change evaluation might entail a repetition of a major portion of the operational testing of the system. The extent of the evaluation required will depend on the extent of the change. Pre-designation of changes as minor or major is possible for common changes such as gasket replacement or temperature probe calibration. This is possible because these type of changes probably occur with such regularity that the firm will have previously evaluated it thoroughly enough such that repetition of the earlier effort is considered adequate to address the current change. Where changes have not been encountered before, they must be addressed individually. In conjunction with every change control program, it is essential that the documentation associated with the system be maintained such that it remains consistent with the system as modified.

Formal change control with QC approval should be instituted at the point in the system or equipment's life when it first enters formal qualification. This ensures that the qualified systems are maintained in that state from the inception of their functional life. What of changes made to a piece of equipment or system prior to the start of qualification? These types of changes will certainly occur, and are the result of revisions or refinements to the user requirements that are identified after the initial specifications have been agreed to. To accommodate these types of changes, a less formal arrangement, sometimes called change management, is adopted. Change management mandates that changes to user requirements be documented and communicated to other parts of the design/project team.

Cost of Validation

Like any other part of the project, Validation has associated costs. The documentation activities imposed on the facility design, construction, and start-up can be significant. Estimates as to the costs of validation typically range from 5 to 15% of the total facility cost. The lower percentages are generally associated with simpler, less automated facilities, while the higher percentages are more appropriate for parenteral or biotechnology facilities where complex environmental, equipment, and utility systems generally require more extensive validation efforts.

Some caution must be raised in considering the cost of validation: Unless the basis for estimation is consistent, it can be difficult to compare costs on similar facilities. Laboratory support, training of personnel, calibration of equipment, development of procedures, and commissioning of systems are among the cost elements for which inclusion may vary from project to project.

Additionally, the cost associated with using internal vs. external resources must also be considered. For smaller projects, a firm may perform all of the required validation assignments using existing resources, while in larger projects the use of outside assistance for some or all of the tasks is more common. Other differences can occur because of a firm's relative experience (or inexperience). An existing firm will generally have a better understanding of validation requirements and may also be able to re-use existing documents from similar projects it has completed. A new firm rarely enjoys this luxury and generally has to develop everything from scratch.

CONCLUSION
Validation and facility design profoundly affect one another. As stated in the opening of this chapter: A sound design should facilitate the qualification of that very design, and the qualification effort should establish that the design is, in fact, a sound one.

Editor's Note

Formal commissioning programs are gaining popularity. Benefits include early attention to field instruction issues which can save total validation time when differences are remedied earlier in the project cycle. Preparation of compliance documents known as "Engineering Turn-Over Packages" ETOP's are also regularly prepared with good results achieved by identifying and preparing critical equipment and system documentation early and consistently during the project cycle

REFERENCES
1. Agalloco, J Validation—Yesterday, Today and Tomorrow. *Proceedings of Parenteral Drug Association International Symposium*, Basel, Switzerland, Parenteral Drug Association, 1993.
2. Food & Drug Administration, General Principles of Process Validation, 1984.
3. Harris, J., et al. Validation Concepts for Computer Systems Used in the Manufacture of Drug Products. *Proceedings: Concepts and Principles for the Validation of Computer Systems in the Manufacture and Control of Drug Products*, Pharmaceutical Manufacturers Association, 1986.
4. Agalloco, J., The Validation Life Cycle. *J Parenteral Science Technol.*, 47, (3), 1993.
5. WWW.PDA.ORG
6. WWW.ISPE.ORG
7. International Society for Pharmaceutical Engineering (ISPE). Commissioning and Qualification. *Pharmaceutical Engineering Guides for New and Renovated Facilities.* 2001;5:30
8. Agalloco, J., Computer Systems Validation—Staying Current: Change Control, *Pharma. Technol.*, 14, (1), 1990.

APPENDIX

Steam Sterilizer Qualification Protocol Outline

- General description
- System identification
- Dimensions
- Utility services to the sterilizer
    - Clean steam
    - Plant steam
    - Compressed air
    - Instrument air
    - Cooling water
    - Drains
    - Electrical service
- Materials of construction
- ASME rating
- Vacuum pump
- Heat exchanger
- System documents
- Spare parts list
- Supplies list
- Calibration of instruments

- Procedures
    - Calibration
    - Maintenance
    - Sterilization
    - Filter integrity
- Control system
    - Description
    - Capabilities
    - Electrical service
    - Printer
- Safety features
    - Door interlocks
    - Alarm check
- Controller verification
    - Cycle check
    - Controller security
- Filter integrity
- Chamber integrity
    - Vacuum leak test
    - Pressure leak test

9

Process Engineering

Author: Art Meisch

Advisors: James Laser
Stanley F. Newberger

INTRODUCTION

Process Engineering's Role in the Pharmaceutical Industry

Pharmaceuticals are chemicals that interact with living animals or humans to bring about an effect on health. There are various means used to produce the pharmaceutical chemicals and to deliver them to the patient. Production of the pharmaceutical chemicals is either by means of chemical synthesis, extraction from natural material, biological processing, or a combination of these. The primary delivery methods include oral dosage forms (solid and liquid), topicals, inhalants, and injectables.

Process engineering forms the bridge between the underlying sciences of chemistry, biology, and pharmacy and manufacturing operations. The process engineer translates the basic science and technology of the process steps into a commercially feasible production process. This task includes scale-up of the unit operations and converting them into the sizing, specification, and selection of the production equipment systems. These systems must meet the required production capacity for the selected products, while at the same time meeting capital and operating cost constraints. Along with these requirements, the Process Engineer must also consider current Good Manufacturing Practices (cGMP), safety, and environmental issues.

Relationship of Process Engineering to Other Design Disciplines

The process is at the very center of a pharmaceutical manufacturing facility. Every aspect of the facility must be focused on supporting the process operation and allowing it to function as intended. The design of pharmaceutical manufacturing facilities is a team effort, with typical teams comprised of other engineering disciplines, architects, manufacturing personnel, validation/quality operations personnel, and frequently R&D scientists and engineers. The process engineer must communicate the processing systems requirements to the other team members so that they can carry out their responsibilities to design a facility that achieves the planned production objectives.

215

cGMP Impacts on Process Engineering

Process engineering for cGMP processes starts with a well-documented scientific basis for the actual process operations and conditions. This helps ensure that, when the process is carried out under the documented conditions, the appropriate drug product results. The process (and the facility) must be designed to prevent both trace contamination of the drug product and cross-contamination from one drug product to another. Typical sources of trace contamination are production water, equipment and piping systems, and environmental particulates. The process engineer must design and specify the process equipment and piping systems to prevent contamination and to be easily cleanable, while helping to establish the room environmental conditions to help protect the product. The ISPE Baseline Pharmaceutical Guides provide an excellent resource for identifying and addressing cGMP issues.

History of Processing in the Pharmaceutical Industry

Many of the earliest pharmaceutical chemicals were extracted by the individual user from natural substances (e.g., willow leaves and bark yielded molecules similar to acetylsalicylic acid or aspirin). Early manufacturing efforts also extracted pharmacologically active chemicals from plants and from animal tissues. Animals were used to produce some of the first vaccines and antibiotics (e.g., cows were used to make the first smallpox vaccine). Beginning in the late 1800s chemists began to develop methods to synthetically produce some of the naturally occurring chemicals. Aspirin, for example, was first synthetically manufactured in the 1800s from coal tar. The trend of using chemical reactions to manufacture pharmaceuticals grew through the 1900s, especially after World War II, to become the production method for the majority of active pharmaceutical ingredients.

Key Words, Notions, and Definitions

- *API or active pharmaceutical ingredien*: The chemical entity that causes the pharmacological effect in the living body
- *BPC or bulk pharmaceutical chemical*: An API or an intermediate chemical used in the manufacture of the API
- *Final dosage form*: The drug product used to deliver the API to the person
- *cGMP*: Current Good Manufacturing Practices

ACTIVE PHARMACEUTICAL INGREDIENTS

Active pharmaceutical ingredients are produced primarily via chemical synthesis or biological processing, or a combination of both. Extraction of natural materials, either from plants or animals, falls under one or both of these two broad categories. This section will focus on chemical synthesis. (Chapter 12: Biotechnology Facilities provides a discussion of biological processing along with the facility discussion.)

Chemical Synthesis

Chemical synthesis produces the API through chemical reactions accompanied by a number of other unit operations to separate and purify the final API. The majority of chemically derived APIs are reacted in a liquid phase in organic solvents, then solid-ified and separated from the solvent and other impurities by filtration, and finally dried under vacuum to remove the last traces of the solvent. The dried API is usually milled to reduce its particle size range for formulation in the final dosage form. The primary chemical synthesis unit operations are: reaction, heat transfer, extraction, distillation, evaporation and crystallization, filtration, drying, and size reduction. API plants usually require multi-product, flexible equipment trains. A brief discus-sion of these unit operations and the equipment commonly used for such plants follows.

Typical API Synthesis Operations

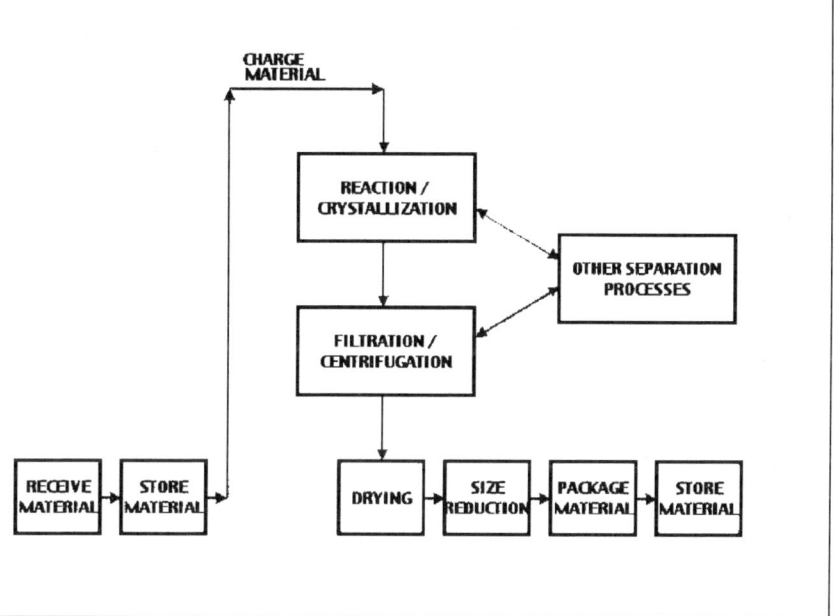

Reaction

Most reactions are liquid phase batch reactions, carried out in a pressure vessel with an agitator and an external jacket. Processes to derive the final API frequently require from three to ten separate reaction steps, depending on the complexity of the API molecule and on the commercially available intermediate chemicals. Each of these reaction steps usually requires separation and some purification. Typical reactor volumes used for production processes range from 500 to 5000 gallons. Research and development reactors generally range from 5 gallons to 500 gallons.

The reaction chemicals in API processes are frequently highly corrosive. The most common materials of construction for reactors are glass-lined steel and Hastelloy C. Associated equipment, piping, and product contact instruments must provide similar corrosion resistance. Piping materials include Teflon lined steel,

Hastelloy C, glass lined steel, and armored glass (although this is less frequently used in production plants due to safety issues).

Typical API Reactors

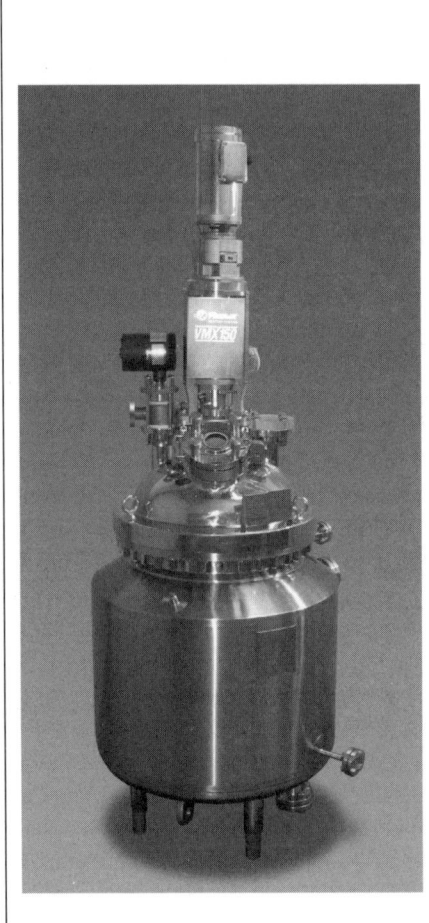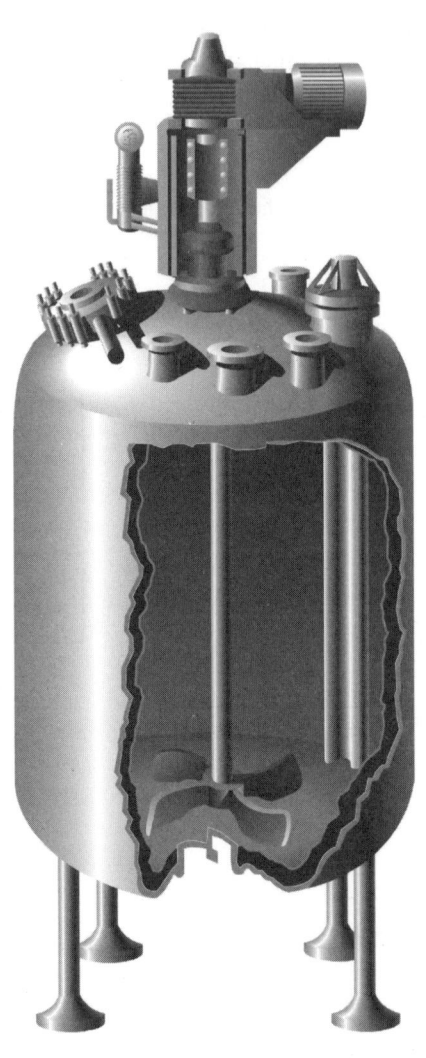

Source: Pfaudler, Inc.

Reaction pressures are generally below 150 psig, except for some gas–liquid phase reactions, which can require up to 6000 psig. Reaction vessels must also be capable of holding a full vacuum, as many operations occur below atmospheric pressure, frequently to limit the temperature exposure of the reaction product. Processing temperatures normally range from –20 C to $^+$250°C, with some reactions occurring as low as –70°C.

Typical Single Fluid Heat Transfer System Schematic

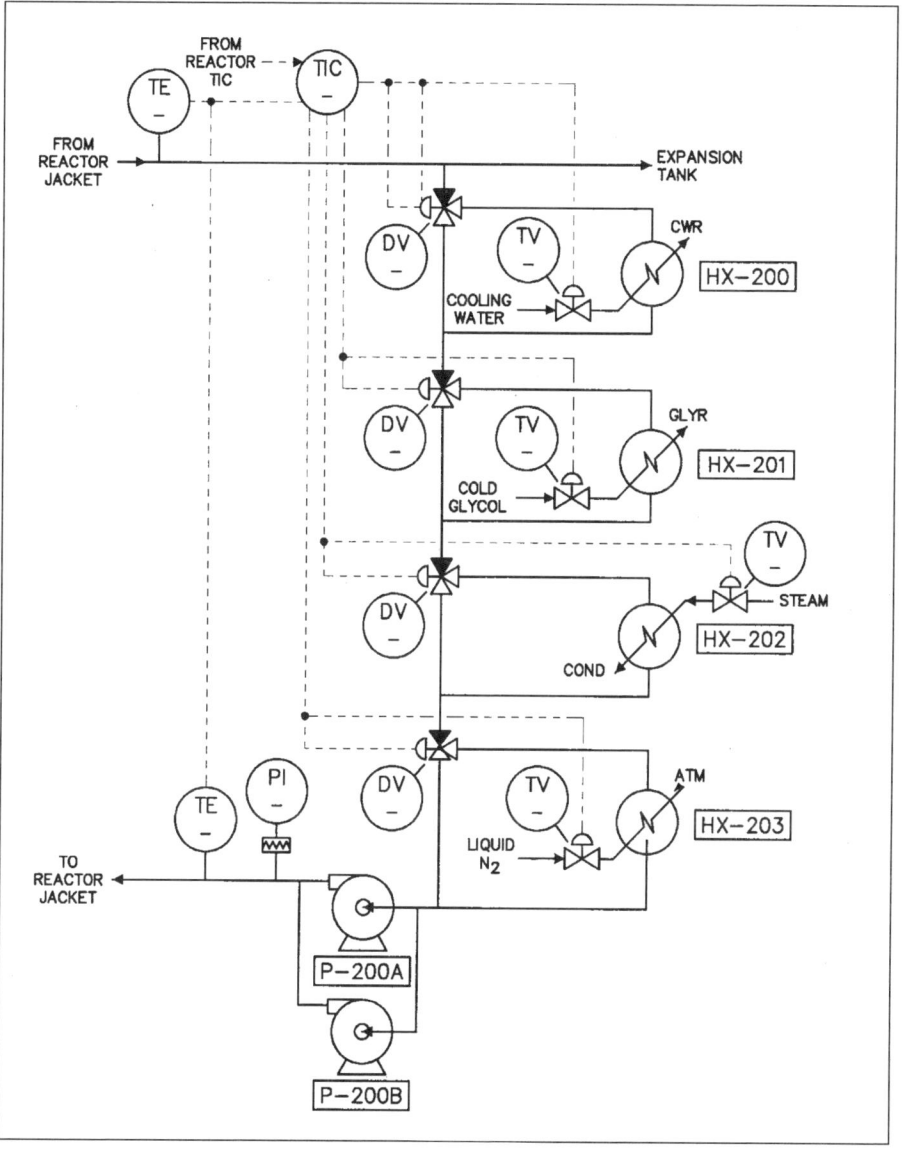

Heat Transfer

Controlling the reaction temperature is critical. Heat transfer in batch API reactors is usually done by use of an external jacket on the reactor vessel with heat transfer fluid flowing through the jacket. Unfortunately, there is an inverse proportionality relationship between the reactor volume and the relative reactor surface area; i.e. the larger the reactor, the less relative heat transfer area available. This issue is especially critical in designing reactors for highly exothermic reactions. The design tools to increase heat transfer that are available for non-pharmaceutical reactors (internal heat transfer coils and circulation of the batch through external heat exchangers) are inconsistent with cGMPs, as they create difficult cleaning problems. Therefore, the reactor size or the rate of reaction must be limited for highly exothermic reactions. The material of construction of the reactor also impacts the rate of heat transfer through the reactor wall; e.g., glass-lined reactors have heat transfer rates about one-half those of Hastelloy reactors. Furthermore, because of the potential to thermally degrade the reaction products, the maximum temperature of the fluid in the jacket must be frequently limited.

Reactor heat transfer systems most commonly use a single jacket heat transfer fluid over the entire temperature range of –70°C to +250°C. This fluid is heated or cooled indirectly using heat exchangers. In plants with fewer reactors (generally less than about 15), it is usually more economical to use independent heat exchanger modules for each reactor. In facilities with many reactors, it is generally more economical to provide a hot (around 250°C) and a cold (around –25°C) central system circulating the heat transfer fluid. In these facilities, each reactor has a jacket circulating pump and controls to bleed in the appropriate hot or cold central fluid to achieve the desired temperature. Temperatures below –25°C are achieved by closing off the reactor jacket loop from the central systems and using a dedicated heat exchanger for each reactor jacket loop, normally using liquid nitrogen to reach jacket temperatures a low as –70°C.

Extraction

Extraction is the transfer of a material (solute) from one liquid phase to another immiscible liquid phase. This is often one of the first purification steps following a reaction. Further processing is performed on the phase that is rich in the product solute. If the reactor does not have sufficient volume to perform the extraction, another agitated vessel would be used, after transferring the entire batch from the reactor. For liquid phases which are close in density and therefore difficult to separate by the force of gravity, centrifugal extractors are used.

Distillation

Batch distillation occurs as part of some reaction steps, primarily to remove an undesired reaction byproduct. The distillation is normally performed in the reactor in conjunction with a distillation column above the reactor. Most distillations are done at a vacuum to limit product temperatures and to enhance the removal of the unwanted byproduct. Some very large manufacturing facilities also have central solvent recovery systems that use distillation to recover and purify solvents for reuse in the processes.

Evaporation and Crystallization

After the desired chemical product is produced in the reactor, it is usually solidified as small particles in a slurry in order to ultimately separate it from the reaction solvent, unreacted raw materials, and unwanted byproducts, all of which remain in the liquid state. Solidification is accomplished by two means—increasing the product concentration by heating and evaporating the solvent, and/or by crystallizing the product by cooling. These operations can occur in the batch reactor, but are frequently done in a separate agitated and jacketed vessel that is located directly above a filtration device. The reason for this equipment location is to minimize the transfer distance of the slurry to avoid pipeline plugging problems and to limit the potential for breaking the solid crystals.

API Peeler Centrifuge

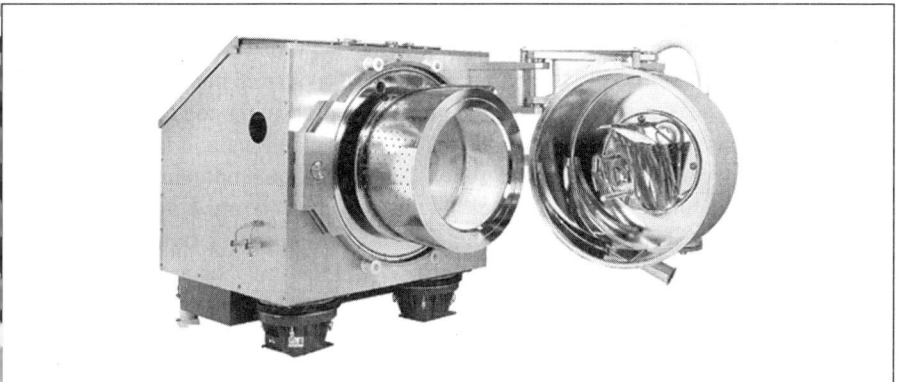

Source: Krauss-Maffei Process Technology, Inc.

Filtration

Once the slurry is formed with the solidified product, it is filtered to separate the solid product from the now undesired liquid phase components. The product is collected on the filter, while the liquid is collected in tanks for re-use, recovery, or disposal. The two most commonly used types of filtration equipment are the pressure filter and the filtering centrifuge. Recall that these items must be corrosion resistant, meaning that they must be constructed of Hastelloy or a similar metal, as fabricating the intricate parts from glass-lined metal is impractical.

When the bed ("cake") of solids is formed on the filter media, it is usually washed with cold, pure solvent to displace dissolved impurities in the still wet cake. Depending on the process, it may be practical and economical to take the initial ("mother") liquor and subject it to another evaporation or crystallization step to solidify additional product and then recover it in another filtration step. The wash liquor is generally considered a waste material.

The product cake is discharged from the filter or centrifuge and often vacuum dried. The cake is still wet with solvent and presents many handling problems. For a large volume product, the filter or centrifuge is frequently arranged to directly feed the discharged cake into the dryer via gravity flow. This arrangement eliminates most of the wet cake handling problems. However, most production plants are multi-product facilities and de-couple the filters and the dryers to increase flexibility, unless they are designed for highly potent compounds. If the filters are de-coupled from the dryers, then the cake is discharged to a lined drum or to an intermediate bulk container (IBC). These are then staged until the drying step is scheduled. Getting the wet cake out of these containers frequently requires manual intervention.

Drying

The purpose of the drying step is to remove the remainder of the solvent used during earlier processing. In order to limit thermal degradation of the product, drying is done under vacuum to evaporate the solvent at reduced temperatures. Production plant dryers are usually agitated, jacketed vessels, frequently fabricated of Hastelloy for corrosion resistance. Glass-lined rotating dryers are also used, although less frequently. Research and development facilities still use vacuum tray dryers, but they present major issues with limiting operator exposure, and they are seldom used in new production plants.

The dryer requires a heating media for the jacket, a vacuum pump, and usually a condenser and solvent collection tank for the solvent removed during the drying process. Heated water is the most common heat transfer fluid used in the dryer jacket.

The dried product is cooled and then discharged from the dryer, and then either milled or directly packed-out for shipment to the dosage form facility that will use the API.

Size Reduction

Prior to use in the final dosage form, the API must be milled to provide a uniform particle size range. Impact type mills with an internal screen are the most commonly used type of mill, with air classifying and air swept mills seeing increasing application. During the milling operation corrosion is not a concern and the mill systems are fabricated of stainless steel. An impact mill with screen is essentially a vertical flow-through device, with the mill outlet connected to the pack-out system to fill either lined drums or IBCs. Air classifying mills and air swept mills use the carrier gas (filtered, dried air, or nitrogen) to either limit the size of a particle that can leave the mill or to cause the solid particles to collide with each other to reduce particle size. These types of mills require a milled product collector to separate the solids from the carrier gas and to accumulate the product.

Potent Compound Containment

The trend in the industry is toward the production of more highly potent compounds; i.e., APIs that must be limited to operator exposure levels below 100 micrograms per cubic meter (mcg/m^3) of room volume. Compounds with exposure limits below 1 mcg/m^3 are increasingly common. Typical containment devices include isolators, split butterfly valves, downflow booths used in conjunction with intermediate bulk containers (IBCs), double lined fiber drums, disposable plastic containers, and disposable bags. Processes with potent compounds also tend to carry out multiple process steps in each piece of equipment; e.g., a filter/dryer in place of a separate centrifuge or filter and a separate dryer. (See Chapter 16 for a detailed discussion on containment issues and solutions.)

It is important to plan the API facility right from the start for potent compound handling. The containment devices require more floor area around equipment as well as more headroom above equipment. Even the basic arrangement of the equipment within the facility is different for potent compound facilities (see Facility Issues discussed below). Potent compound facilities require more floor space for the same amount of equipment as a normal potency facility. A large part of this additional floor·space is taken up by airlocks to separate the potent compound areas within the facility. A typical potent compound suite has two-stage airlocks including a personnel gowning airlock, a decontamination/degowning airlock, and a material airlock.

Process Water

Chemical synthesis operations may require USP purified water, depending on the nature of the specific step in the process. In virtually all cases, final step API processes will utilize USP purified water, however, early step processes may be performed simply with potable water or with deionized water.

Cleaning

It is difficult to clean reactors and crystallizers merely using clean-in-place (CIP) spray nozzles and a cleaning solution, due to hardened or sticky deposits that adhere to the vessel walls and agitator. Therefore, the typical cleaning method for these vessels involves "boiling up" the vessel with organic solvents to dissolve these remnant process materials. Solvent cleaning is frequently followed by aqueous cleaning using a detergent solution, with a final water rinse. This final rinse may require USP purified water, depending on the use of the vessel.

Cleaning of filters and centrifuges may also require solvents, followed by aqueous cleaning and rinsing. Mills are most commonly cleaned using aqueous solutions.

Environmental, Health, and Safety (EH&S)

Chemical synthesis processes present numerous EH&S issues due to the use of flammable organic solvents, toxic raw and intermediate materials, highly potent product materials, and the potential for runaway chemical reactions. Common health and safety measures in the design include: closed processing to contain the hazardous materials; the use of nitrogen to provide an inert atmosphere inside the process equipment; an integrated control system with extensive safety interlocks to reduce the potential for human error; overpressure relief for process vessels coupled with catch tanks to contain releases; and pressure resistant room walls coupled with pressure relief panels to direct explosion energy away from other rooms in the facility. As a secondary health precaution, operators use personal protective equipment in the event of a failure of the primary barrier between them and the hazardous materials.

From an environmental standpoint, air emission control devices are required for virtually every plant. These typically include a combination of scrubbers, low-temperature condensers and thermal oxidizers to remove organic vapors, and dust collectors to remove air-borne solid particles. Organic liquid wastes are usually classified as hazardous wastes and are segregated from aqueous wastes for off-site disposal. Aqueous wastes may be fully treated on-site at very large plants, while a more common approach is limited pre-treatment (pH adjustment) on-site followed by disposal to a publicly owned treatment works (POTW). Solid wastes are also generated, including process materials as well as filter cloths, drum liners, disposable containers, and gowning materials. Since all of these may contain some process material, they are usually classified as hazardous wastes and disposed off-site.

Facility Issues

In the United States, API chemical synthesis facilities are considered hazardous buildings. Building codes limit hazardous buildings in size, height, and number of stories, and restrict them as to how close they can be located to other buildings on the site or to the property line. Hazardous buildings are required to use pressure resistant walls and floors coupled with pressure resistant panels. Furthermore, the process equipment is highly integrated with the building in API chemical synthesis facilities. Examples of this include vessels, filters, and dryers installed through floors, and centrifuges installed through walls. The combination of cGMPs and the use of potent compounds requires the segregation of the individual process operations in separate rooms.

Typical layouts of flexible API chemical synthesis facilities for "normal" potency products usually provide reactor areas and/or rooms, filtration/centrifugation rooms, drying rooms, and milling rooms. With this configuration, the facility provides both cGMP isolation and product protection, while allowing a high degree of flexibility to run different processes at the same time in the facility. Intermediates and products are moved from room to room as required by the processing step. In potent compound facilities the trend is to include an integrated suite containing reactors, filtration equipment, and drying equipment with closed transfers between equipment. These suites frequently contain multiple floors to provide gravity flow from reactors to filtration equipment and to drying equipment. This approach reduces overall facility flexibility, since the suite and its equipment is dedicated to a single product during the operation, regardless of whether or not all of the equipment is required throughout the operation. The benefit of this approach is increased containment of the potent material.

Control Systems

API chemical synthesis facilities normally have all the controls of the process and process support systems integrated in a plant-wide control system. Control systems are based either on programmable logic controllers (PLC) or on distributed control computers (DCS) with multiple operator interfaces using graphical displays. Production facilities with well-established products and processes have full batch recipes programmed including automated addition of ingredients and process steps. Highly flexible facilities (e.g., contract manufacturing plants and pilot plants) usually do not program the entire batch recipe, but depend on operator inputs for such items as the addition of ingredients, temperature and pressure set points, etc. Since production data are normally stored in the control system, it must meet the electronic batch record requirements of CFR 21 Part 11. (See Chapter 7 for a detailed discussion on automation and control systems.)

Capital Cost Guidance/Benchmarking

Developing an accurate capital cost estimate for an API chemical synthesis facility requires significant effort in defining the process equipment needs, corresponding support equipment utility equipment needs, building and, site requirements. There is no true shortcut to obtain an accurate cost estimate. However, there is sufficient cost history with API facilities to quickly develop an order-of-magnitude cost estimate once the total number of reactors and total reactor volume are known. Benchmarking data have been analyzed to formulate a quick API chemical synthesis project estimating method that was presented at an ISPE seminar in February 2000 (1). This cost estimating method is summarized below:

- If the plant typical reactor size is above 1000 gallons, then multiply the total plant reactor capacity in gallons by $5000 to obtain an order-of-magnitude capital cost.
- If the typical reactor size is below 1000 gallons, then multiply the total number of reactors in the plant by $4.5 million to obtain an order-of-magnitude capital cost.

These order-of-magnitude cost estimates should be used with extreme caution, as the actual costs can be considerably different than those obtained by these simplified methods.

Project Schedule Implications

Because of the intense integration of the process equipment with the facility, API chemical synthesis plants are arguably the most complicated type of pharmaceutical manufacturing project. This integration limits the use of modular, fully pre-fabricated systems and, when coupled with the intensive amount of process piping, requires that the majority of the actual construction labor-hours be expended at the plant site and inside the process building. In addition, process equipment lead times after the order is placed are six months or more because of the use of glass-lined and Hastelloy equipment as well as the complexity of the equipment systems. All of this results in typical schedules for larger API chemical synthesis projects on the order of 3 to 4 years from the start of concept development through the completion of commissioning and qualification.

DOSAGE FORM PROCESSING

The usual forms by which the drug products are administered are: oral solid, oral liquid, topical, inhalant, and injectable. This section provides a brief overview of the key processing steps and equipment used for each type of dosage form. In each case, the starting point in the process is the API, produced by chemical synthesis or by biological processing. Generally dosage form processing is focused on bringing about physical changes, not chemical changes.

Oral Solid Dosage Forms

The fundamental process steps in oral solid dosage forms include: dispensing, granulation, drying, milling, blending, tableting, coating, encapsulation, and packaging. Dispensing is the accurate weighing out of the various solid and small volume liquid ingredients that constitute the dosage form that includes API(s), excipients, lubricants, disintegrants, and coatings. As corrosion is not a concern, dosage form equipment is generally fabricated from 316L stainless steel. Containment of dusts is a major issue throughout solid dosage form processing, starting with the dispensing operation. Depending on their potency, APIs may be handled in isolators, downflow

(A) Coating Pan and (B) Fluid Bed Processor

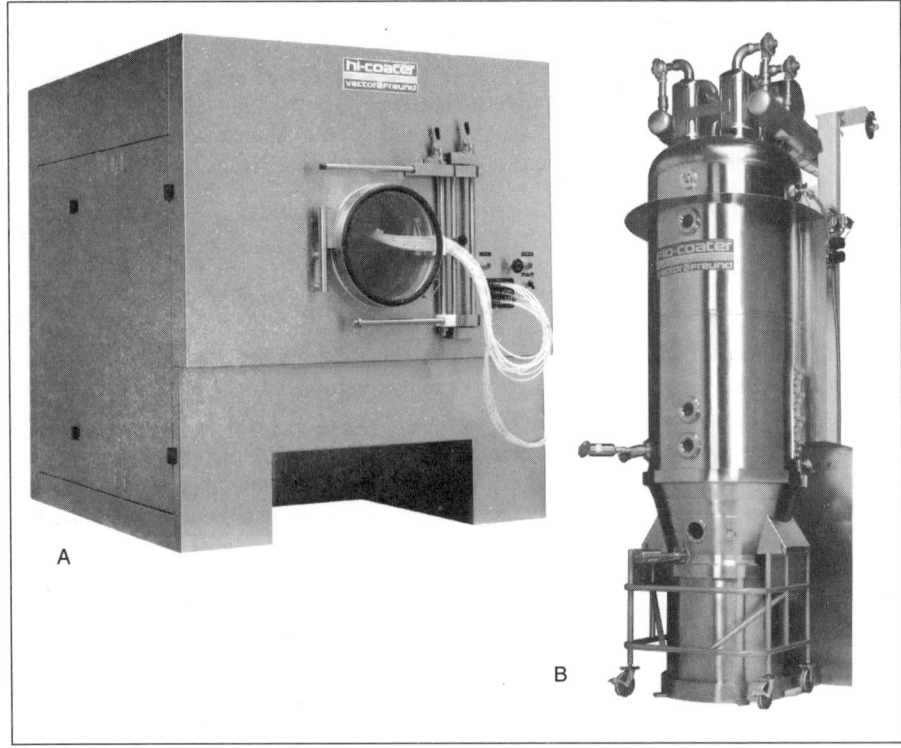

A

B

Source: Vector Corp.

booths, or simply with exhaust hoods. Non-potent materials are generally handled with exhaust hoods or a downflow booth. Once dispensed, the finely divided powders are granulated to form a larger particle (agglomerate) that contains a uniform concentration of all of the constituent solids. Granulations are frequently done using a liquid to aide in agglomeration, although for some products it is possible to successfully granulate without a liquid (dry granulation). This liquid may be USP water or it may be a flammable solvent, depending on the product. Since most APIs dissolve in water, the amount of liquid used in granulation is very small and is added while the solids are being constantly blended. Granulations are performed in a wide range of equipment including rotating blenders, agitated stationary blenders, and fluid bed processors. After a wet granulation is formed, the liquid must be dried off. If a fluid bed processor or a jacketed blender is used, then drying is done in the same equipment. Tray or truck drying ovens are still in use, but are becoming less popular because they require extensive manual handling and are difficult to contain when potent materials are processed. Microwave drying is a new and commercially proven approach to contained drying.

The dried granulation is milled with limited energy input to produce a uniform particle size for tableting operations. There is a trend toward "single pot processing" for potent compounds, in which granulation, drying, and milling are performed in a single integrated equipment train. After milling, the granulated materials are blended to develop a uniform concentration. Blending can take place in an intermediate bulk container (IBC) or in a fixed piece of equipment (commonly a V-blender or twin shell blender). The blended material is usually transported in an IBC to the tablet press, where the actual tablet is formed. Tablet presses are very complicated machines that depend on uniform flow properties in the granulation to produce tablets of uniform composition. Often, many of the ingredients in the blend are included to allow the tablet press to perform its function consistently. The tablet is usually coated, either in a coating pan or in a fluid bed coater. Coating solutions can be aqueous or solvent based, with some tablets requiring more than one coating step. Some coatings ("enteric") contain a different API from the tablet itself to provide a initial pharmacological effect before the tablet disentigrates in the digestive system. Coating solutions are prepared in jacketed, agitated tanks. The solution is usually heated slightly to promote dissolution of the solid ingredients, and then cooled to room temperature prior to addition to the coater. Tablet coaters use large volumes of filtered, conditioned air to dry the coated tablets. Occasionally when flammable solvents are used, nitrogen is used in place of air in the coating operation. In general, coating operations require large sophisticated air (or nitrogen) handling systems to support each coating pan or fluid bed unit. Coated tablets are printed with the manufacturer's product information and then packaged.

Liquid and Semi-Solid Dosage Forms

This broad category includes oral liquid, topical, inhalant, and injectable dosage forms. While there are significant differences in facility design for oral liquids and topicals vs. inhalants and injectables, basic process unit operations are similar.

Virtually all of these product types start with dispensing and then proceed to a liquid phase blending step using an agitated vessel that is usually jacketed. After the blending step, the product is filled in liquid form, and then packaged.

Generally, since the API is normally a solid, the same dispensing issues exist as discussed for oral solid dosage forms. For oral liquids, the API is usually blended either in ethanol, which is flammable, or USP purified water. Most oral liquids are blended at ambient temperature. Topicals range from low viscosity liquids to moderate viscosity lotions to high viscosity creams, and ointments. Lotions, creams and ointments frequently are emulsions formed by intense agitation of two distinct liquid phases—one aqueous based and the other oil based. Each liquid phase is first prepared in separate jacketed, agitated vessels by dissolving the required solid ingredients in the water or in the oil while heating (to aid dissolution). After each liquid phase is prepared, both the water and oil phases are combined using intense agitation (a "homongenizer") to disperse the phases and form a stable emulsion. Highly viscous topicals are filled at elevated temperature to improve flow properties during filling.

Injectables must be sterile, as they directly enter the body, bypassing the digestive tract. Therefore, while the actual process steps are relatively simple, the greatest concern with injectables is related to ensuring that the product is sterile and stable. The product is usually filled in small glass or plastic containers, and it can be either liquid or solid. Most injectables are water based, and start by dissolving the API in WFI water. After this formulation is prepared, it is normally sterile filtered through a 0.2 micron filter, prior to filling into a vial or other container. If the API can tolerate the heat, then the filled, stoppered containers are steam sterilized to assure sterility ("terminal sterilization"). Injectable liquids that cannot be terminally sterilized must be filled under aseptic conditions. Many injectable products are dried after filling using a vacuum freeze drying process called lyophilization. Vials and all items that come in contact with the sterile product must also be sterile. (Chapter 11 provides further discussion on sterile facilities.)

Inhalants, like injectables, bypass the digestive tract. They must have low bioburden, but may not have to be sterile. Inhalants require some means to provide a dose of a fixed, repeatable size ("metered dose") and a means to propel the dose into the throat. The most common method to meet these requirements has been to prepare a solution or a suspension of the API in a liquid, then fill this into the dosage container and add a propellant to pressurize the container. When used with an engineered nozzle, this assembly will provide consistent doses of the API. Processing starts with dispensing of the API and any other ingredients, then addition of the API to a liquid to form a solution or a uniform suspension. The liquid can be water, a solvent, or a compressed gas. If water is used, it is USP purified or WFI to reduce bio burden. After the blending step, the liquid is filtered and then filled into the containers. The use of solid powder inhalants, rather than the liquid solution or suspension type, is growing.

Process Water

Dosage form operations usually require USP purified water for oral and topical products, and WFI water for injectables and some inhalants.

Cleaning

Clean-in-place (CIP) spray nozzles using an aqueous detergent solution is the typical cleaning method for dosage form equipment. The final rinse for oral dosage forms is normally done using USP purified water. Equipment for injectables and some inhalants is rinsed using WFI water and steam sterilized.

Environmental, Health, and Safety (EH&S) Issues

The primary EH&S issues in dosage form processing relate to the use of combustible dusts, flammable organic solvents, and highly potent product materials. Safety measures for combustible dusts include the use of 10 bar pressure rated equipment to contain a dust explosion or the use of an explosion suppression system to limit the extent of an initial dust explosion. For flammable liquids and potent compounds, the precautions are similar to those for chemical synthesis facilities. From an environmental standpoint, dust control devices are required for virtually every plant. Dosage form facilities that extensively use organic solvent generally use thermal oxidizers to remove the organic vapors from venting gas streams.

Facility Issues

Dosage form facilities generally are not required to meet building code requirements for hazardous buildings, except for limited areas that handle flammable liquids. Therefore, there is considerably more flexibility in layouts than in chemical synthesis buildings. The manufacturing equipment is frequently integrated with the building in dosage form facilities. Examples of this include fluid bed processors installed through floors and coating pans, autoclaves, and lyophylizers installed through walls. The combination of cGMPs and the use of potent compounds requires the segregation of the individual process operations in separate rooms.

Typical layouts of flexible dosage form facilities for products that are not highly potent usually provide separate rooms for each process step; e.g. granulation rooms, milling rooms, tableting rooms, and coating pan rooms. With this configuration, the facility provides both cGMP isolation and product protection, while allowing a high degree of flexibility to run different batches or processes at the same time in the facility. Materials are moved from room to room as required by the processing step. In potent compound facilities the trend is to include an integrated suite containing granulation, drying, milling, and blending equipment with closed transfers between equipment. Tableting and coating are in separate rooms with transfers via an IBC. Often, coating does not require the same level of containment equipment as the prior process steps, as the potent active compound is "contained" by the tablet and its coating.

Control Systems

Dosage form facilities normally use an "islands of automation" approach with each equipment system having its own vendor-supplied control system. These individual control systems communicate with a plant-wide supervisory system for overall coordination and batch data storage. These systems must meet the electronic batch record requirements of CFR 21 Part 11.

TRENDS AND FUTURE DEVELOPMENTS

The overriding trend for all types of pharmaceutical processing is the increasing potency of the APIs. To date, relatively few products are highly potent, and most existing processes and manufacturing facilities are not designed to handle them. There is a current need to renovate and modify existing facilities for potent compound processing. This presents a considerable challenge, as potent compound handling generally requires more space around the equipment, more airlocks, and a means of containing wastes streams (e.g., collected dusts). As more and more potent products come to market, there will be an ever-increasing requirement for new manufacturing facilities specially designed for potent material processing. We should also see the development of new multi-functional processing equipment that will improve containment and limit the number of transfers between equipment systems. This new equipment will most likely impact the configuration of processing facilities, driving them to have more multi-story processing suites.

REFERENCE

1. Newberger, S. Planning and Benchmarking API/BPC Facilities, ISPE Seminar, Tampa, FL, February 2000.

BIBLIOGRAPHY

Baseline Guide for Bulk Pharmaceutical Chemical Facilities, ISPE, Tampa, FL, 1996.
Baseline Guide for Oral Solid Dosage Facilities, ISPE, Tampa, FL, 1997.

10
Oral Solid Dosage Facilities

Author: Ed Tannebaum
Advisor: Larry Kranking

INTRODUCTION

Meeting Industry and Market Needs

Industry and market needs have increasingly dictated the course of oral solid dosage manufacturing. Historically, solid dosage products date back to the seventeenth century in the United States. Until the 1920s, 80 % of the medicines that were compounded were produced by pharmacists in liquid, powder, and tablet form. Due to the healthcare needs of World War I's military, higher technology medicines were required to treat the injured and to cure diseases that became major health issues. The production of tablets, based on newly created drugs, became a prominent industry in the United States. Now, common definition of "solid dosage products" includes tablets, hard shell and soft gelatin capsules, and a variety of novel forms of drug delivery. These novel forms include quick dissolve, effervescent, and powdered products.

The evolution and maturity of solid dosage manufacturing in the twenty-first century have brought us to a point where significant issues pervade this arena. Issues relating to all-inclusive quality requirements, driven from both domestic and international regulatory agencies, are coupled with a "best cost" structure of products produced. Trends relating to quality and compliance, coupled with reducing the selling price of drugs, provide an ever-increasing background for the development and upgrade of solid dosage manufacturing facilities with new technology. The wide variety of product segments range from highly regulated, branded drugs to an ever-increasing variety of regulated "over-the-counter" (OTC) drugs to a major worldwide nutritional product market challenged by increasing regulatory concerns and forthcoming compliance mandates.

Drug Delivery Technologies

Drug delivery technologies are diverse for the various manufacturing operations that range from unitary, manual processes to automated, integrated processes. The technologies revolve around the processes required to produce both the physical unit dose form through to the method of active drug release. Sizes, shapes, and novel forms of delivery require increased complexity of manufacturing facilities. Alternative methodologies for immediate and sustained release characteristics for active ingredient absorption into the human system create a varied range of manufacturing environments for the finishing processes that drive solid dosage development and subsequent manufacture.

The systematic technologies required for dedicated, large volume operations differ from smaller volume, multi-product facilities. These significant differences in the scale of the production requirements are the driving force behind the strategic planning process for successful facility designs. The collaboration between the Research & Development scientists of a pharmaceutical organization with the realities of the Operations and Engineering staff in project delivery requires early intervention to secure the technologies that meet the industry and market needs of quality, compliance, and the "best cost" end result. The Technology Transfer process must consider new systems, processes, and formulation to meet facility needs now and in the future.

The Impact of New Technologies

New solid dosage technologies provide a distinct challenge to the design of solid dosage facilities. Conventional tablet and capsule dosage forms have pervaded the industry for many years, but new technologies have begun to evolve from the differing formulation matrixes being developed. The proliferation of novel drug delivery systems and/or devices has provided multiple challenges to individual manufacturing facility designs.

The addition of newly developed or emerging technologies into the design of a new or renovated facility, prior to the completion of the product's development and or regulatory approval, creates a need to provide flexibility in the design. The proactive development of "what-if" scenarios to accommodate new technologies in a facility design requires early interface between the facility design team, R & D, and Operations staff in forecasting their technology or programmatic requirements.

Regulatory Pressures on Oral Solid Dosage Manufacturing

International regulatory bodies have invoked recommendations and requirements that have "raised-the-bar" for oral solid dosage manufacturing compliance worldwide. Facility-related requirements, based on FDA, MHLWMEL, EU/EMEA, MHW (formerly MCA), TGA, and other international regulatory agencies bring a global focus to the critical utility systems, layout, and flows throughout the facility. Concerns related to filtration, purified fluid and gas or air installations, cross contamination, product mix up, processing visibility, cleaning facilities, personnel protection for high potency products, along with personnel changing (garbing) facilities, all present differing levels of concern and or compliance to differing agencies. The advent of multi-national product distribution has created this challenge of multi-agency compliance at facilities located around the world.

Branded vs. Generic vs. Contract Manufacturers

Distinctions between branded, generic, and contract solid dosage manufacturers historically had a wide disparity in their manufacturing facility designs. Cost of goods was a driving force for each of these business segments, primarily due to the total return for investment each segment was able to generate. As the level of regulatory compliance has risen worldwide, the disparity in the facility attributes has narrowed significantly. Branded drug producers have striven to streamline their operations and facilities to simplify their ability to lower the unit cost of the goods produced.

Generic manufacturers are constantly raising their level of compliance and parity with branded manufacturers. Their need to improve their image, relative to agency compliance and rapid response to aggressive ANDA product introductions, coupled with ANDA approval exclusivity, is mandated to garner market share for a limited window of commercial opportunity.

Contract manufacturers pose the greatest challenge. Their facilities must remain in full regulatory compliance, while at the same time reaching levels of compliance to meet various customer audit mandates. Combining the regulatory and customer requirements with an industry that is driven by a highly competitive cost of goods requires contract manufacturing facilities to be the most cost-effective in the pharmaceutical industry. Our expanding world of pharmaceutical outsourcing to contract manufacturers is creating a new class of facilities that must meet the majority of regulatory interpretations to satisfy all customers and service providers alike.

Branded vs. Generic vs. Contract Manufacturers Comparisons

	Branded	Generic	Contact
Single Product	■		
Multi-Product		■	■
FDA Compliance	■	■	■
Int'l Compliance	■		■
High Volume Products	■		■
Unit Processes		■	■
Automated Processes	■		
Capital Intensive	$$$	$$	$
Engineered Solutions	■	■	
Procedural Solutions		■	■
Large Eng./Op's Staff	■		

KEY CONCEPTS AND PRINCIPLES

The Effect of Sales Forecasts on Optimization of Manufacturing Equipment

Sales forecasts are the baseline capacity requirement for most oral solid dosage facilities. Sales forecasts are based on data driven by anticipations of hospital, physician, and consumer usage, along with the realities of competition. The forecasts are initially based on timelines relating to regulatory approvals and projected launch dates. Many, many factors impact the accuracy of the sales forecasts; thus, great care must be exhibited in utilizing these data at face value.

Facilities professionals, chartered with the task of quantifying the relationship between the dosage unit requirements and the sizing of the manufacturing facilities, must understand the assumptions of the forecast baseline requirements. This understanding is vital in producing a consensus as to the quantification of the manufacturing equipment needed and the overall optimization of the facility design. The company philosophy related to batch sizes, equipment sizing, capacity utilization, change over, and cleaning ability all play a major role in the development of a manufacturing equipment strategic plan.

Optimization of manufacturing equipment, upon acceptance of a sales forecast by management, is a balance between operations, quality assurance, quality control release, and/or actual order receipt or inventory requirements. The sizing and optimization of equipment is calculated based on a downstream evaluation of increasing run capacity to minimize bottlenecks and maximize the output of the entire process. A typical optimization model is illustrated by the static simulation graph for a typical tablet product.

Typical Capacity Analysis

Lots per Room	2003 139 No. of Rooms Required	Utilization %	2004 203 No. of Rooms Required	Utilization %	2005 266 No. of Rooms Required	Utilization %
791	1	18%	1	26%	1	34%
718	1	19%	1	28%	1	37%
718	1	19%	1	28%	1	37%
856	1	16%	1	24%	1	31%
242	1	57%	1	84%	2	55%

Sample CT Percent Contribution

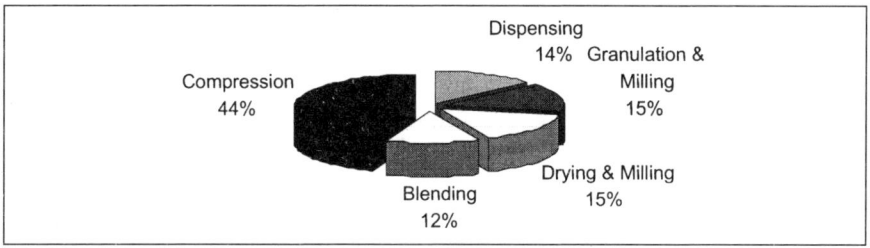

Similar models are performed for multiple products, with simultaneous manufacturing operations.

Management Preferences

Branded manufacturers develop products for both large-scale production and smaller, niche market products. Each of these widely divergent markets requires significantly different types of facilities to optimize manufacturing and maintain the lowest cost of goods produced. Larger, branded manufacturers, with large volume products, traditionally have made larger capital investments in their facilities. Larger investments are usually directed at creating automated, higher throughput facilities, increased yield rates and a reduced labor cost per unit produced, thus minimizing risk in achieving the major financial objectives for the drug. Smaller volume, niche market-focused branded drugs are traditionally manufactured in older, less automated facilities, with unit operations. The concerns for volume throughput and major financial objectives relegate this segment of branded manufacturers to their "dog and cat" operations. While these products are not the "flagship," blockbuster drugs of tomorrow, the smaller volume products are important segments of a company's market penetration strategy, especially if it is for unmet medical needs.

Generic manufacturers focus on a product mix that is usually driven by a specific segment of drugs—oncology, hormone replacement, cardiology, beta-blockers, gastroenterology, dermatology, etc. Their choice in selection of drug types can relate to the complexity of its manufacturing level of difficulty to reduce potential competition or simplified compounds, requiring shorter ANDA approval schedules or the specific branded competition resistance to potential patent challenge litigation. These manufacturers of ANDA drugs traditionally utilize unitary processes due to the financial viability and life cycle of their products. Multiple product plants are commonplace and require a level of investment that keeps their profit margins at the very highest level possible. Modest capital investment in facilities and overall facility overheads are also commonplace in this arena. Manufacturing equipment for generic manufacturers and the overall level of regulatory compliance have risen over the past decade to a level equivalent to branded manufacturers.

Contract manufacturers are a growing resource to both branded and generic manufacturers. Whether it is to be the outsourced, single outsource manufacturer, an overflow resource, or the expert in specific processing/drug delivery or packaging technologies, the primary focus is on speed to market and cost of goods.

Unitary capabilities, with a high degree of product cross-contamination controls, are a requirement that is paramount. The manufacture of multiple customer products, in directly adjacent spaces, creates the need for facilities with validatable HVAC and critical utility systems that ensure the compliance with each of their customer's quality concerns. Quality and regulatory compliance are"givens" and mandated in each of these distinctly different manufacturing segments.

Single Product vs. Multi-Product Environment

Single product facility design provides a platform for the innovations that enable a branded producer to maximize throughput, without the restrictions created in a multi-product plant. Manufacturing equipment selections are driven by product transfer capabilities that maximize equipment utilization and reduce down time. Special material handling issues, related to potent and cytotoxic compounds, are more readily achieved in a single product plant due to the clear definition of a single process. Manpower and personnel protection issues can be dealt with in one, well-thought- out method, thus minimizing risk. The multi-product plant environment is one that must deal with competing needs on a regular basis. Cross contamination, product mix up, and cleaning issues are a few of the issues that must be addressed through a combination of engineering and procedural solutions. The life of a multi-product facility design is ever changing and requires an adaptable layout, a set of critical utility systems (HVAC, purified water and gases, steam and hot water) that can meet changing capacities and distribution needs. Quality assurance concerns for this changing work environment are vital components of a design solution that assists in maintaining regulatory compliance.

Production Technology—Yesterday, Today, and Tomorrow

Drug manufacturing processes have made a gradual transition over the past century. The basic end products—a tablet, coated or uncoated; hard-shell capsule with powder or bead fill; and liquid filled as well as soft gelatin capsules—have been the principle dosage forms for many years. Newer solid dosage forms have evolved including quick dissolve tablets or wafers, along with film technologies for rapid drug solubility. The changes that have taken place include alternative methods of rapid drug solubility, sustained-release, and other nuances to the end product's ability to deliver an active chemical into the body.

Technology is primarily divided into the following categories:

- Sampling/Dispensing/handling of active solid and liquid chemicals and excipients
- Alteration of particle size, granulating, mixing, drying, and milling
- Compression, encapsulation, coating and printing, along with primary and secondary packaging

Manufacturing Flows

An increased concern has evolved in developing facilities with distinctive flows to minimize cross contamination and meet the intent of cGMP attributes for separation of products and activities. Flows related to personnel movement and personnel changing facilities; materials management, waste removal, and cleaning have become major components of pharmaceutical facility design. The level of concern for these definitive flows combined with procedural requirements is not equivalent to current regulatory mandates for sterile manufacturing. *The flows that are mandated for sterile manufacturing flows should not be equated to the design of solid dosage facilities.* The design of flows for solid dosage facilities should be weighed against specific project concerns related to cross contamination and product mix up and maintaining the physical environment for each specific project. The relative throughput of the facility must be a governing factor in the design of all solid dosage facilities. The actual "traffic" of materials, personnel, and waste should dictate the degree of concern for crossing of flows and the risk that is present during day-to-day operations.

Personnel/Employee Health and Safety Considerations

Personnel protection requirements have evolved from both governmental agencies and the individual pharmaceutical companies. The design challenge presented in solid dosage projects for health and safety concerns is significant and increasing in importance. Due to the nature of the processes with their usage of dry powders, significant employee exposure concerns have been raised. The level of experience and docu-

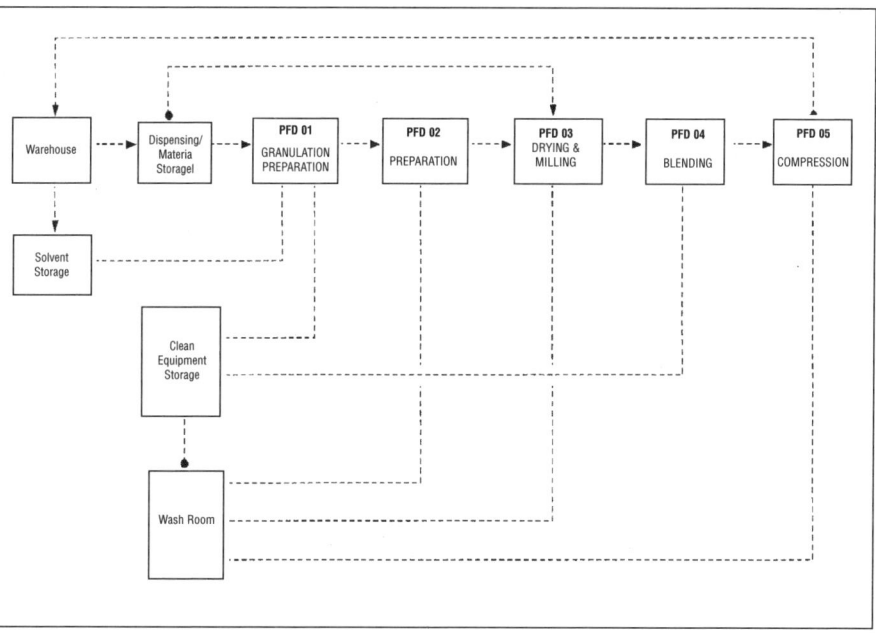

mented research on the short- and long-term health concerns that were present in the past and will be present in the future have evolved into differing levels of design solutions. Engineered and procedural solutions are commonplace, coupled with specific employee health and safety policies, tied to human resource management. Determining the hazard levels present, either through physical testing and/or empirical modeling, has provided a matrix as to the level of risk that must be addressed. The determination of the policies and procedures, coupled with the physical facility design, is one of the most important aspects of sold dosage facility design now and in the future. The issues relating to the employee health risks will grow with each year of experience in the manufacture of yesterday's, today's, and tomorrow's drug products.

Challenging Preconceptions

Preconceptions of the mandated requirements for solid dosage manufacturing facilities have exceeded the practical requirements for facility design. Concerns related to regulatory compliance have created facilities well in excess of practical needs. Specific areas of concern are related to layout, critical system specifications, and scope of required validation, all of which have exceeded true regulatory compliance. *The thoughtful balance of interpretive procedural compliance vs. "bricks and mortar" solutions can provide sound methods of preserving precious capital resources.* Thus, balance in challenging preconceptions is a major risk management issue that should be discussed, analyzed, and determined early in the design process. This is one of the largest cost issues to be dealt with in determining the scope of a solid dosage project.

New Greenfield vs. Expanded or Renovated Facility

Most major solid dosage projects face the dilemma of this decision. The cost and schedule implications of this decision are irrevocable. Determining the "right choice" is a challenge to each organization. Do I plan for today, next year, or the long term? Strategic decision making must bypass personal agendas.

Identification of a realistic short-range, mid-range, and longer-term business plan must be prepared and receive buy-in and support by senior management. Part of the plan will be based on current manufacturing issues; some will be based on forecasts and a long-term vision based on the organization's strategic plan. Accepting such a plan is a decision based on an organization's capital spending resources or philosophy, or it may simply be a vision. Looking beyond the practical horizon of a business plan can expend resources that could be directed at other, shorter-term profit opportunities.

Flexibility for Tomorrow and Beyond

Designing a facility that meets the initial requirements for production capability, cost, schedule, and compliance is paramount. The design of facilities that provide the flexibility to adapt to the changing product types, product capacity needs, personnel protection needs, and increasing regulatory regulations is a task that requires experience, vision, and a clear understanding of the direction of the industry—a difficult goal to achieve, yet a goal worth exploring.

KEY CONCEPTS IN FACILITY DESIGN

Production Requirements

Planning a solid dosage facility begins with the drug product or products forecasted for current or new products inclusion into the facility. Correlation of a production forecast with the reality of a production environment requires a strategic plan specific to the facility. Production requirements range from high volume, large batch size products, to small volume, small batch size products. The facility design philosophy requires a direction modeled on the volume and batch size parameters. This production order of magnitude sets the platform for the manufacturing equipment quantification, facility staffing, materials management capabilities, and support requirements necessary to initiate a scope of the facility needs. The "domino effect" of the production requirements initiates a large group of design variables that determine a cause and effect that will create a unified approach to meeting the production requirements.

Manufacturing Equipment

Manufacturing equipment requirements are primarily driven from research and development of a drug product. The process is primarily developed on equipment selected by the product development team. Engineering and operational staff is encouraged to participate in the equipment selection. This participation and interaction, during a product's development, are dependent on the drug manufacturer's internal philosophy of collaboration. The collaborative effort ranges from full involvement to very little involvement. The arena of internal politics is an area that can produce valuable insights into equipment selection, the ease of manufacturing, quality assurance issues, and the all-important cost of goods produced. Upon resolution of the process, it is incumbent on the facilities' professionals to determine an "equipment train" that maximizes the product output, through balancing the overall throughput of the multi-step process. This balancing process is dependent on the equipment's rate of production, the batching philosophy, the cleaning and changeover logistics/timing, and the quality assurance/quality control constraints that are imposed at each step of the process. The actual manufacturing equipment utilizes both dry and wet processes. Dry processes offer a containment challenge for dust migration, while wet processes require purified water and/or solvents to achieve their desired processing step.

The following types of equipment constitute the primary means of solid dosage manufacturing:

Step 1: Delivery and Measurement of Active Chemical Ingredients, Excipients, Liquids, Fillers, etc.
Manufacturing Equipment: Dispensing, Weigh-Off, or Pharmacy Areas or Rooms.

- Material handling devices, both horizontal and vertical for dispensing.
- Scales: Pit or surface-mounted for larger quantities; pedestal models for mid-range quantities; bench top, balances for small quantities

Step 2:   Milling, Blending, Mixing, Granulating, Compacting, Drying, and Gelatin Preparation

Manufacturing Equipment: Production rooms can be separate or combined for individual pieces of equipment, depending on the batching philosophy, volumes of products produced, material transfer technology, and transport container type.

- Material handling for all steps may be performed utilizing a mechanical device, gravity fed from an elevated platform or floor above, or by a manual device. The means and methods depend on the quantity of material, its particle flow characteristics, the ergonomic/personnel issues, or ability to meet a validated cleaning process. Lift trucks, pallet jacks, drum dumpers (portable or fixed) handling "super sacks," drums (lined fiberboard, stainless or a polymer), along with metal or polymer tote bins are the primary mode of transport and container. This is typical for the following manufacturing steps.

- *Equipment:*
  Milling: Sifters, comills, separators, comminuters, etc.
  Blending: Twin shell "v" or cone, ribbon, tote blender, axial, etc.
  Granulating: Low/high shear, fluid bed, interplanetary, kneader, etc.
  Compacting: Roller compactors, tableting compaction
  Drying: Fluid Bed, Ovens, Microwave, Vacuum, etc.
  Gelatin Preparation: Tanks, mixers

Step 3:   Compression, Encapsulation, Specialty Drug Delivery Unit

Manufacturing Equipment: Primarily equipment is housed in individual rooms to limit cross-contamination and product mix-up.

- *Equipment*:
  Compression: Multi-station, single or layered tablets, equipped with de-duster, check-weigh, or other quality or discharge devices
  Encapsulation: Hard capsule powder and liquid fill, equipped with discharge device
  Gel-tab: Tablets that have a liquid gelatin coating to simulate capsules
  Soft gelatin capsules: Liquid filled soft gelatin capsules

Step 4:   Coating, Printing, and Inspection

Manufacturing Equipment: Primarily, equipment is housed in individual rooms to limit cross contamination and product mix up. Equipment utilizes dedicated air-handling systems.

- *Equipment*:
  Conventional rotating coating pans, utilizing aqueous- or solvent-based coating solutions
  Cylindrical, perforated, revolving coating pans
  Fluid bed coating utilizing internal coating column, utilizing aqueous- or solvent-based coating solutions
  Printing equipment, inkjet, laser, or other marking systems. Inspection can follow that utilize a wide range of techniques from random visual inspection to automated vision systems.

Step 5:   Packaging

Manufacturing Equipment: ranges from hand-packaging operations to fully integrated filling, bottling and blister lines, with cartoners, case-packers, and palletizers.

- *Equipment:*
  Bottling Lines: Bottle unscrambler, blow/vacuum, accumulation tables, desiccant loader, slat filler or photo eye counter, cottoner, tamper evident sealer, capper, retorque, labeler, leaflet inserter, cartoners, case packer, case sealer, bar code printer or labeler, palletizer and stretch wrapper
  Blister Lines: Blister former, filler, foil sealer, card applicator, cartoner, leaflet inserter, case packer, palletizer, and stretch wrapper

MANUFACTURING FLOWS

Flows through solid dosage facilities are categorized into the following types:

- *Material:* Incoming raw mterials–packaging components; sampling; work in progress; finished goods
- *Personnel:* Change/uniform facilities; manufacturing (operations/quality assurance); Materials management; Support (maintenance); Administration; Quality control
- *Cleaning—Equipment/Parts:* Dirty equipment staging; cleaning; inspection; assembly; validation; equipment-part storage
- *Waste Material—Liquids/Solids/Trash:* Waste neutralization; holding; removal disposal recycling

It should be noted that the once-through, non-crossing flow patterns are an ideal situation within a given design. *The reality of operational flows typically does not warrant the total "once through" philosophy.* Analyzing the actual material through-put in terms of pallet counts, per shift or hour, for raw materials, work-in-progress, finished goods, and waste flows rarely creates instances of extensive traffic within solid dosage manufacturing areas. Modeling of the concurrent material quantities flowing through a solid dosage facility will provide a more "common sense" approach to the level of segregation of flows that is truly required.

Quality Assurance Requirements

Quality assurance is an all-encompassing design consideration in a solid dosage manufacturing facility. The facility-related quality assurance or regulatory compliance design inclusions relate to many of the facility's physical attributes, from flows and layout to specific employee change philosophy, sampling/testing locations, label storage/distribution, to office/workstation space. Requirements also revolve around critical utility design parameters for temperature, humidity, pressurization differentials, and other vital validation criteria.

Standard operating procedures (SOPs), and their link to the physical design, provide vital information that should be formulated at the inception of the project to gain the greatest advantage during the design process. Traditionally, many SOP considerations are not developed until the design is far along or the facility is actually under construction. This proactive approach can generate many collaborative ideas that can simplify the design and eliminate the needs for compromise and concessions determined late in the project delivery process.

Physical Manufacturing Environment

The physical manufacturing environment can vary greatly, depending on the nature of the business, the philosophy of the manufacturer, and the capital resources that are available. Compliance is not directly proportional with the magnitude of the investment or the sophistication of the facility. The balance of creating the ideal manufacturing environment is a point of discussion that should occur very early in the planning process.

The short- and long-term goals for each facility require analysis of many influences including:

- New or an existing facility; life span of facility need
- Single product vs. multiple product output
- Volume of products to be produced
- Hazard level of products to be manufactured
- Breadth of regulatory compliance: FDA and/or MHLW (formerly MCA), EC

The attributes that affect the complexity of the design include:

- Flexibility in its long-term use
- Risk tolerance to meet manufacturing criteria; level of regulatory compliance
- Staffing philosophy; projections for supervision; and level of daily operations

Special Product Considerations

Special product considerations can range from personnel protection to the physical ability to manufacture in a given space. Potent compound requirements from simple Category 1 product exposures to High Hazard, Category 5 exposures and Cytotoxic compounds require an analytical approach to the facility design. This is a major component of the risk assessment that is required by a manufacturer of solid dosage drug products. The ever-increasing legal liability for the manufacture of these types of drug products, on all parties involved, is a consideration warranting senior management buy-in and legal opinions at certain times to ensure the correct course of action is taken. The FDA and other regulatory concerns for cytotoxic drug cross contamination also merit an analytical approach to defining the true hazard vs. the implied hazard and determination of separate facility requirements. Special product considerations should be determined by fact, not speculation. Gaining data relating to the specific product hazard level or difficulty to manufacture must be determined early in the design process. Testing of the special product effect on the facility design is critical in developing a common sense approach to meeting the stated level of manufacturing capability required. Personnel Protection Equipment (PPE) affects the level of safety for personnel. Combining specific equipment capabilities with the recommended exposure period and the limitations on personnel mobility and productivity requires careful analysis. Respirators, breathing air systems, laminar flow masks, and barrier type garb are examples of individual PPE.

Engineered solutions for particle containment are limited to HVAC solutions, equipment isolation devices, and material transfer devices and each has an impact on the facility design. Water misting and air showers are additional engineered solutions that limit the migration of particles to non-classified space. Combining the engineered solution with the proposed PPE solution can work hand in hand to create an overall, realistic approach to a cost-effective and safe design.

CLEAN DESIGN: DETAILS

Implications for Performance and Compliance

Risk Analysis: Facts vs. Perceptions

Architectural solutions to clean pharmaceutical design is an area of differing perspectives on the ideal solution. Clean details can be very costly to design and install. The materials and finishes also can be expensive and play a vital role in the cleanability. Solid dosage projects tend to be in facilities with varying degrees of dust accumulation due to the processes contained within areas, or the dust containment (collection) systems employed.

The true risk associated with "clean" detailing is a balance between the actual clean detail and the SOPs for the actual room housekeeping. Flush details improve the ability to keep a vertical or horizontal surface clean. The SOPs for the scheduled cleaning procedure can be the true test for the extent of the flush or ledge-free detailing. Frequent quality cleaning procedures are the vital link in the quality assurance program for housekeeping, thus a more important fact than the detail itself. (Examples of "clean detailing" are presented within the Architectural Considerations chapter of this book.)

Assigning Proper Level of Design to the Appropriate Solution

The level of solution, in great part, is in proportion to the level of Quality Assurance Protocols and Procedures that are set forth by the facility operations. The cost of capital vs. the cost of cleaning labor and validated cleaning requirements conformance is a delicate balance that requires economic analyses. *Determining the proper level of physical solution and ensuring that it is appropriate is a risk assessment of the highest consideration on every project and is a product-to-product analysis.*

The level of engineered solution in most cases is proportional to the capital resources available. There is no right or wrong decision in terms of any engineered solution. The burden of right or wrong rests in the overall engineered solution, combined with standard operating procedures leading to the quality assurance and regulatory compliance of each product produced.

Value-Added Solutions

Examples of value-added solutions for solid dosage manufacturing facilities can include:

- Equipment selections that utilize the fewest numbers of equipment to produce the largest volume of product
- Capacity modeling that provides data to maintain output level going downstream in all steps of the process and to yield de-bottleneck alternatives, unitary operations, and a consistent throughput at all stages of operation
- Layouts that reduce the overall number of personnel required to operate a facility
- Material handling systems that maximize throughput, diminish operator ergonomic issues, and minimize opportunities for dust migration and cross contamination
- Solutions that provide containment of product particulate matter within each processing room
- Installation of an adequate quantity of vision lights into manufacturing rooms for supervision and for regulatory observation of operations
- Design and installation of Part 11 compliant, validatable Building Automation Systems (BAS) that control and monitor critical utilities

Common evaluations that are performed during the design of solid dosage facilities:

- Building Automation Systems (BAS vs. manual documentation of critical utilities that utilize independent magnehelic gauges. These gauges are visually read vs. automated, integrated differential pressure sensors, integrated to the BAS for control and monitoring.
- Flush, double-glazing vs. sloped sills that require scheduled SOP housekeeping to maintain dust-free surfaces
- Wash down manufacturing rooms vs. dry wipe/vacuum of particulate matter
- PPE protection of manufacturing personnel with "once through" HVAC systems vs. recirculating HVAC systems
- Electronic, interlocked "magnetic-locks" for air locks vs. red light/green light SOP-focused operation of interlocked air-lock doors

PROJECT MANAGEMENT ISSUES: COST, SCHEDULE, AND QUALITY

Appropriate Level of Capital Investment

At an early point in a project's life, a determination of the funding limitations, scheduled completion, and level of quality expectations must be established by senior management. This level of funding can set many of the variables that must be selected to quantify an overall facility philosophy. The philosophy can be a determination between "first cost" vs. "long-term cost" of the capital investment.

Typical decision points relative to this determination include:

- Sizing of utility systems for future capacity
- Levels of redundancy of critical and non-critical engineered systems for chilled water, steam, compressed air, electrical systems, etc.

- Overall sizing of the individual space components of the facility for future growth and flexibility
- Quality of materials, finish selections, types of doors, extent of vision lights, and flush details

As stated earlier, in this chapter, there are no correct or incorrect answers to these decisions. Determining the level of acceptable risk combined with the available capital is a decision that becomes the baseline criteria that set a facility's long-term standard for flexibility, space, finish, and capability.

The Reasonable Level of Quality for the Desired End Product

Quality is an attribute that can range from the life expectancy of facility-related equipment such as air-handling units, to the durability of wall, floor, and ceiling systems. Quality can be dictated by corporate standards, plant standards, or industry standards. Again, there are no right or wrong answers to the primary quality standards of any facility. SOP conformance can help achieve levels of serviceability that can also be attained by procurement of more sophisticated designs. The overall determination of quality must be determined on a system-by-system basis, or the attributes of a specific material of construction.

Examples of typical quality ranges can include:

- USP Water piping, Ranging from polypropylene to polished stainless tubing
- Flooring materials from painted epoxy-to-epoxy terrazzo with integral base
- Wall coatings, water-based epoxy coatings to heat-welded pvc materials
- Active pressure control HVAC systems, with supply and return variable air volume boxes, to hard balanced, damper-controlled HVAC systems
- Integrated BAS for control and monitoring to unitary control systems on each air-handling unit with a freestanding environmental monitoring system not connected to the system controls
- Variable frequency electric drives to fixed frequency drive motors

The benefit for each quality decision can be determined independently or in the context of an overall facility design philosophy.

TRENDS AND FUTURE DEVELOPMENTS

Reducing the Cost of Products Produced

Reductions in the costs of goods produced can lie in many realms surrounding a solid dosage operation. Many of the reductions lie outside the design parameters of a solid dosage facility.

The areas of cost savings that result from the design process include:

- The energy efficiency of the utility-related engineered systems
- Reductions in the physical layout adjacencies to reduce travel distances for material, personnel, and waste in both GMP/non-GMP areas
- Standardization of equipment and procedures.

International Compliance

Individual pharmaceutical regulatory agencies vary in their depth of compliance for solid dosage facilities. Their concern for regulating specific design parameters is primarily focused on cross contamination, product mix-up, and facility cleanliness. FDA guidelines, (listed in the Federal Register (for facility design are very general, while international agencies, such as the MHW, set specific thresholds for design. Care must be taken to ensure that the design for each facility meets the intent of the country or countries for which the manufactured product is destined, for distribution and or sale.

Regulations for controlled substances, such as those of the U.S. Drug Enforcement Agency (DEA), set highly specific design standards. These standards deal with the handling, manufacture, and short- and long-term storage of controlled substances. The standards, in the case of the DEA, are categorized by drug classes, from Class 1 to 5. Storage may vary from locked rooms to cages to vaults. Technically specific specifications are contained within these regulations in the Federal Register.

Outsourcing to Low-Cost Providers

The manufacture of solid dosage products is frequently outsourced to contract manufacturers. The contract manufacturers can be either independent contractors or major branded manufacturers with excess production capacity. As the concern for the cost of goods increases, the pressure on all manufacturers is to seek out their best option to improve their bottom line, without creating risk for their brand.

Facility design for contract providers is subject not only to the regulatory bodies, but also to the quality audits of the firmss potential customers. In many cases, the potential customer requirements can exceed the requirements of the regulatory bodies. This increase in facility scrutiny creates a need for designs that at times exceed industry standards to meet the customers' quality and risk avoidance standards.

Challenging the "Mores" and Preconceptions

A fundamental strength of an experienced solid dosage facility designer is challenging a manufacturer's operation. This challenge will provide the dialogue necessary to test the validity of current manufacturing practices, facility flows, and SOPs. The ideal separation of GMP and non-GMP zones of activity requires detailed discussion related to material handling from receipt of materials at the loading dock though all of the manufacturing steps to finished drug product departure from the loading dock. Personnel flows, including garbing, transitioning between differing zones of cleanliness, and their interface with the actual manufacturing process all require challenge to determine the most reasonable solution for the specific project.

Benchmarks to Other Industries

Solid dosage manufacturing has some comparison to the food industry in terms of unitary processes, standard of care, and ingestion of products by humans and animals. The primary differences are the lack of validated processes and creation of a regulated environment that ensures the long-term quality of the products produced. The regulatory statutes mandated by each country are the crux of the framework for the faculty's design and operation. The regulatory scrutiny and enforcement placed on the pharmaceutical industry by individual countries provides a much higher level of compliance than virtually any industry that affects human welfare on a continuous basis. The nuclear industry is the only other highly regulated industry. The primary difference is protection of the public welfare through the physical environment versus the manufacture of a consumable product.

Comparisons/Contrasts to Other Technologies

Solid dosage drugs are delivered through ingestion and absorption into the body's system of organs or absorptive surfaces such as the tongue. Compliance concerns relate to cross contamination. Manufacturing concerns revolve around particulate control through containment and cleaning procedures.

Aseptic or non-sterile liquid drugs are delivered via direct injection through the skin, directly into the bloodstream, through trans-mucosal transfer or direct contact with absorptive surfaces such as the eye. These drugs can be delivered in either single or metered dosage delivery systems.

Compliance concerns are highly stringent in terms of personnel garb, air filtration, positive pressurization, microbial control, and air changes, tied to regulatory "grade" definitions. Manufacturing concerns include air lock separation of cascading "grade" areas, cleaning procedures, and stringent monitoring of all environmental and product specifications.

Compliance concerns relate to the technology that permits consistent delivery of the active drug product from the patch into the dermatologic membrane or the rate of absorption with topical application. Manufacturing concerns primarily relate to the uniform method of drug application. Manufacturing issues can relate to the high quantity of solvents required to compound the active drug products that may create safety issues for the facility or personnel involved with the manufacture. Solid dosage drugs are among the simplest to manufacture, deliver, and provide consistent quality.

RECOMMENDED READING

ISPE Baseline Guides for Solid Dosage Manufacturing

GMP Regulations: U.S. FDA / EU-EMEA / MHW (formerly MCA) / TGA

DEA Guidelines: Controlled Substances Security Manual; Controlled Substances Act of 1970.

11
Sterile Manufacturing Facilities

Author: George Wiker

Advisor: Brian Lange

INTRODUCTION

This chapter reviews key concepts and principles in the design and development of a sterile (aseptic) processing facility project. It reviews the development of sterile injectable products as well as describes some broad and underlying principles in practice today. Comparisons are made between open and closed process unit operations, typical engineering discipline practices, as well as implications of compliance on projects and operations. Finally, key elements and considerations in the development of a sterile manufacturing facility are presented, along with commonly accepted terms, ideas, and future trends.

This chapter, in conjunction with others in this book and other readings, will enable the facility professional to be better informed and better prepared to design, build, and qualify sterile manufacturing facilities. A strong and educated facility professional will be equipped to successfully execute fully operational and licensed sterile manufacturing facilities.

Filling Equipment

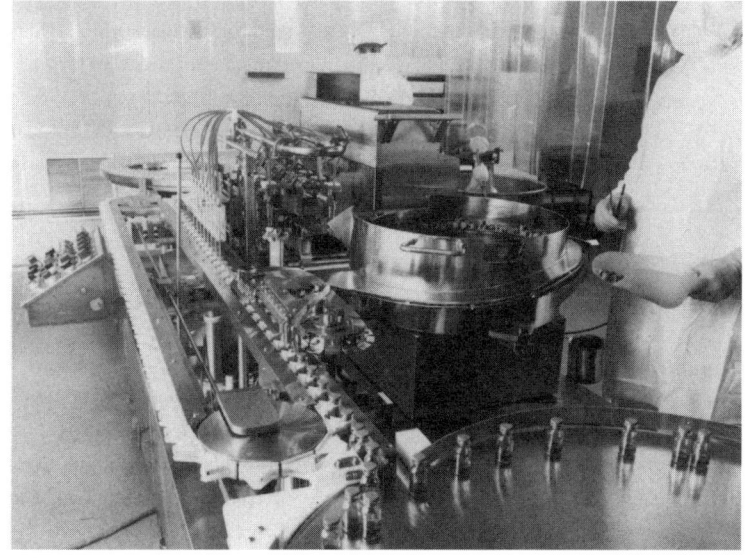

WHY IS THIS IMPORTANT?

Sterile injectable products typically function by targeting specific regions or indications within the body. Such drugs like vaccines, genetic therapeutics, and other more delicate drug matrices must be introduced directly into the bloodstream to be most effective, since these drugs are often unable to pass through the body's natural defense mechanisms when ingested.

Thus, by introducing the drug directly into the bloodstream, it can respond much faster and with much more intensity than other dosage forms. Therefore the dosage must be sterile and free of any by-products that may adversely affect the body (1). Also, many sterile products have limited stability, so the shelf life and storage conditions are critical elements to the product's effectiveness

GMP CONNECTIONS, HISTORY, AND BACKGROUND

GMP Connections

Sterile products are manufactured worldwide and, for this reason, agencies governing the development and manufacture of these products have been established for major regions. These regions have adopted guidelines for the development and operation of sterile manufacturing facilities. Table 1 provides an overview of regions, along with the governing agency.

TABLE 1   Table of Regulatory Authorities

Region	Agency
United States	Food and Drug Administration (FDA)
Europe	European Commission (EEC)
Europe	World Health Organization (WHO)
Europe/United States (pre)	International Organization for Standardization (ISO)
China	State Food and Drug Administration (SFDA)
Australia	Therapeutic Goods Administration (TGA)
Japan	Ministry of Health and Welfare (MHW)
India	Ministry of Health and Family Welfare

*Editor's Note:*_____
This table will be the foundation for many design decisions, so keep it readily available.

History and Background

Sterile injectable products have been used in medicinal practice for decades. In Western medicine it first began in 1796, with Edward Jenner's vaccination for smallpox (2). Use of sterile products expanded to include delivery of anesthetics, transfusions, and a wide variety of delicate drug matrices. Processing of sterile products expanded over the decades, and in 1987, the U.S. Food and Drug Administration (FDA) issued a Guideline on Sterile Drug Products Produced by Aseptic Processing. This guideline was issued under the U.S. Code of Federal Regulations 21 CFR 10.90 and, while it did not set legal requirements for aseptic processing, "it states the principles and practices of general applicability . . . acceptable to the Food and Drug Administration" (3). With new and more delicate drug matrix developments came a surge in the use of sterile injectables as a method of effective drug delivery into the human body. Today, sterile injectable products represent a significant portion of the total prescription drug delivery methods, and are regulated by agencies all over the world. As the distribution of drug products broadens to a more global basis, the regulatory trend is moving toward "harmonization" of regulatory guidelines and practices, particularly for European and U.S. bodies.

Examples of Sterile Containers

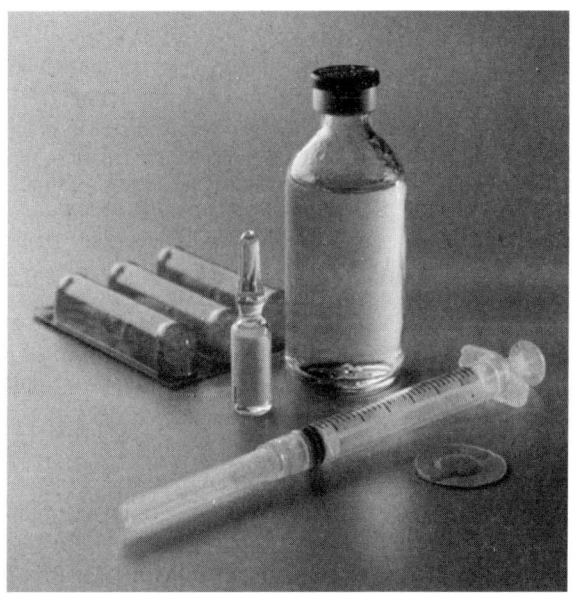

Sterile products come in a variety of primary package forms, including:
- Ampoules
- Vials
- Syringes
- Bottles
- Bags

Other products, such as inhalants and medical devices, may be processed in a similar manner as injectables to maintain a high level of integrity and protection. Thus, some of the principles and ideas presented in this text may also be considered for those products.

KEY CONCEPTS, PRINCIPLES, AND DESIGN CONSIDERATIONS

Key Words, Notions, and Definitions

The following provides a brief overview of the key elements for sterile manufacturing facilities, and focuses specifically on filling and finishing of sterilized products.

Sterile Manufacturing Operations

This chapter focuses mainly on the final formulation filling, and finishing of sterile products. Major sterile manufacturing operations include:

- *Component Preparation*: In ultrasonic sinks, autoclaves, and other wash and preparation equipment
- *Compounding*: Mixing and formulation in either fixed or portable tanks
- *Filling*: Ranging from hand-fills in a hood, to a fully automated high-speed container filling system
- *Freeze Drying (Lyophilization)*: Removing water from a drug dose for greater stability and longer shelf life.
- *Inspection*: Ranging from a manual inspection by operators, to a fully integrated multi-functional inspection system.
- *Process Utilities*: "Direct impact" systems that support manufacturing, including water-for-injection (WFI) and clean steam generators, as well as the supply of sterile air/gases and other product contact utility supply systems

Governing Bodies and Guidelines

A foremost consideration in the design and operation of a sterile manufacturing facility is the identification of which regulatory bodies will have jurisdiction. This is decided by determining where the final product will be distributed on a global basis. Since most products are distributed to the United States and Europe, the FDA and the European Commission (EC) are widely recognized as leading agencies with jurisdiction over the review, qualification and inspection of sterile manufacturing facilities.

Technology Background

Sterile manufacturing facilities have been in operation for decades. Principles and approaches to cleaning and sterilization are the centerpiece of technological development, evolving from manual operations recorded on paper (by hand), to fully automated cleaning and sterilization systems with compliant electronic recording devices.

Sterile manufacturing technologies have been influenced by developments in the processing of biologics and dairy products, where product and system sterility is essential. In these types of manufacturing industries, the design, construction, validation, and operation have greatly contributed to the success of pharmaceutical sterile manufacturing facilities today.

Product filling containers also have played a significant role in the technological development of sterile manufacturing facilities for filling and finishing. Typically, final sterile product is filled into containers, which are then closed, sealed, and inspected prior to secondary packaging.

DISCUSSION

Designing a sterile manufacturing facility requires careful consideration of basic engineering principles and details, particularly in rooms containing critical process operations. It also requires particular focus and attention to not only each design discipline, but also to considerations in construction, qualifications, and operation of the facility. Critical GMP design elements include:

- Room Finishes: Hard and easily cleanable, minimal/no crevices
- Material and Personnel Flows: Unidirectional in critical environments
- Equipment Placement and Ergonomics: To maintain product/process integrity and operator safety
- HVAC, Controls, Zoning, and Pressurization: To protect product, control contamination, and keep people comfortable
- Air Flow: Unidirectional in critical operations to protect product exposed to the room environment
- Risk Assessment, Management, and Mitigation: Control risk by procedural or engineering solutions in order to make the sterile product safe for the marketplace

*Editor's Note:*_____

Strong technical coordination drives a successful project, so assign a person(s) to be accountable here.

This section discusses common concepts, principles, and design considerations for the following major design disciplines:

- Programming
- Process
- Process architecture
- Architectural
- Mechanical
- Electrical
- Plumbing
- Instrumentation and Controls

This list also indicates the general order of involvement for each discipline. Good Design Practices require each discipline to address specific concepts and principles and, in an iterative manner, each discipline should review and understand its effect on the ability to successfully construct, qualify and operate a sterile manufacturing facility.

Programming

The participating facility professional requires clear direction (and agreement) regarding the basic concepts, principles, and considerations that directly effect the outcome of a project. From the very beginning of a project, a team must work through a series of discussions, identifying the drivers of a project by answering a series of questions that begin at a very broad perspective, and then focusing particularly on vernacular drivers that relate specifically to a project.

Developing Project Drivers and Objectives

When a project begins, usually a new team is assembled to deliver the project. They must meet and discuss the drivers, goals, and objectives of the project. This is typically achieved during intensive kick-off sessions, where everyone in the group participates by identifying the basic components in the project, as well as understanding and agreeing to general ideas, terms, and expectations.

This approach should flush-out basic decisions and factors in the project, including:

- Purpose of the project
- Concerns about the project
- Basic goals and objectives
- Functionality
- Compliance requirements
- Cost
- Schedule
- Quality

*Editor's Note:*_____

Keep these principles handy, and review them periodically over the course of the project to better ensure success.

Project Philosophies

At the beginning of a project, the team will also develop basic project philosophies, which are brief statements about each major project factor. These philosophies become part of the basis of design (BOD), which serves as the record and source of team and project scope information.

Editor's Note: _____

FDA is pushing for the use of new technology in draft guidance on aseptic processing. The agency emphasizes the need for a well conceived design as well as deployment of new technologies and a strong commitment to GMP's make an ideal combination for successful aseptic processing. *Gold Sheet—9/03*

Some examples of philosophies for a sterile manufacturing facility include:

- *Processing:* Determine process operating conditions and approaches, such as whether the process is "open" or "closed," primary or secondary containment, multi-product or single product, integrated or stand alone processing operation controls, as well as campaign or concurrent batch processing.
- *Operational/Functional Zoning:* Define the general GMP zones and critical functions in a project. This will effect the scope of the project and the general composition of the layout, as well as basic environmental design principles.

- *Materials/Product Flow and Management*: Develop basic logic for the general flow of critical and noncritical materials throughout the facility, as well as how the overall project flows will integrate into the surrounding environment.
- *Personnel Flow and Gowning*: Define how people enter and exit operating areas, as well as move from street clothes to critical sterile operations. The logic developed here should be consistent with similar operations within the company's domain.
- *Cleaning*: Develop a simple logic as to how product and nonproduct contact surfaces will be cleaned. This philosophy will also review ideas such as cleaning in place (CIP), cleaning out of place (COP), the use of prepared/disposable items, as well as the general flow during cleaning conditions.
- *Sterilization*: Define the boundaries of sterilization, as well as the general criteria for sterilization, in a simple and basic manner. A well-developed sterilization plan is essential to good facility operating practices.
- *Waste Management*: Identify how the waste will be managed in a sterile facility operation.
- *Constructability*: Develop the execution approach for how the project will be built from a cost, schedule, and quality perspective; also define basic ideas of modularization, facility lifespan, and how any adjacent operating areas will be managed during project delivery.
- *Commissioning and Validation*: Develop a realistic validation master and execution plan, clearly describing "direct" and "indirect" systems and boundaries, as well as agree to basic performance requirements, acceptance criteria, definitions, and terms.

Developing a project philosophy will provide a platform for future project decisions and, over the lifespan of a sterile operation, assist operators to comply with inspections as well as modify and maintain the facility.

Process Design

With the philosophies, drivers and project goals identified, the design may begin. The design effort commences with the development of core process functions and in an iterative manner, progresses from process systems, to primary environments, secondary support mechanisms; and finishes with the project support components.

Types of Sterile Processing Operations

Generally, there are two main types of processing operations within a sterile manufacturing facility: primary bulk processing of the drug substance, and secondary formulation, filling and finishing of the drug product into its final dosage form. Testing of diagnostic kits, medical device assembling, and in-process product testing are examples of other types of operations carried out in a highly controlled manner.

The primary drug substance is made from either a biological or chemical process, producing a bulk approved pharmaceutical ingredient (API). (Discussion of biological and chemical processing can be found elsewhere in this book.)

Table 2 below outlines the major steps for the secondary processing of the drug product and shows typical room cleanliness classifications in European Commission standards. Controlled not classified (CNC) designates rooms with a good level of environment control, but will not validated.

TABLE 2   Table of Room Functions

Function	Compounding Operations	Filing Operations	Typical Room Cleanliness Classification
Lyophilization		✔	Grade A local, Grade A or B background
Capping		✔	Grade B local, Grade B or C background
Terminal Sterilization		✔	Grade B/C
Inspection	✔	✔	Grade D
Packaging		✔	CNC
Cleaning and sanitization	✔	✔	(Performed in functional rooms)
Gowning	✔	✔	Varies to support functional room
Staging and Storage	✔	✔	Varies, best to locate outside core area, Grade D at most
Raw Materials Staging	✔	✔	Controlled Not Classified (CNC)
Materials Dispensing/Weigh	✔		Grade C/D
Component Preparation		✔	Grade D
Equipment Preparation	✔	✔	Grade D
Product Preparation and Transfer	✔	✔	Grade C/D
Filling		✔	Grade A local, Grade A or B background
Sampling and Testing	✔	✔	(Part of other functions)

Primary Processing of Drug Substance. Compounding is the basic preparation of drug product for final filling. This includes the formulation of a product through the dilution, concentration, or other preparation of a mixture of approved pharmaceutical ingredients into a bulk quantity. This process can range from a simple one-step dilution, to a multi-step process of homogenization or emulsification. During this process, the batch is sampled and when the process is complete, it is then quarantined, tested, and released for final filling and finishing.

Drug product filling in a sterile facility consists of the transfer of a bulk formulation (prepared in the same facility or elsewhere) into a dosage form for patient administration. Dosage form containers typically consist of bags, vials, and syringes, and the final product may either be in liquid form or lyophilized (freeze-dried) if required.

Processing Scales

When developing a facility program, the intended scale of manufacturing drives many decisions that impact design and operational methods and approaches. For example, in a developmental scale, design solutions may call for more manual operations and procedural solutions, rather than fixed, automatic, or complex engineering solutions. In a commercial scale facility, designs may lean more toward automatic operations and engineered systems, including redundancy and robustness.

In general, there are four main scales of processing of products:

1. *Developmental Scale*: A processing scale developing the drug or drug matrix from the bench scale to a measured quantity. Considerations of eventual scale-up to larger volumes are essential. Many processes are carried out manually, so having a firm grasp on standard operating procedures (SOPs) is prudent. Careful consideration of drug toxicity is also critical here, since the process may need to be highly contained to protect operators. In this case, creating a contained process which is also scaleable is highly recommended.

2. *Clinical Scale*: The manufacture of product for integrity and patient testing. Processing is still relatively manual and controlled through procedures. Engineering systems and controls are more employed, especially for critical steps and data collection. Some automatic features may also be included as the process develops through clinical trials, along with tighter controls in practice. The scalability of the process is further developed, so that when the product reaches agency approval, the process capacity is scaleable to meet market launch demand. As the product progresses through clinical trials, the process moves toward a more uniform, consistent, and repeatable operation.

3. *Launch Scale*: Once a regulatory body has approved a product for commercial use, larger quantities are needed to satisfy product launch into the marketplace. Launch-scale quantities are often made from the clinical scale facility. Typically, as a product moves through Phase III clinical trials, sourcing decisions are made to either build their own facility or contract with another company for larger scale manufacturing capacity. Some companies have operations set up specifically for new products being introduced into the marketplace, while a full commercial-scale facility is being prepared for operation.

4. *Commercial Scale*: A full-scale process operation is designed to meet marketplace demand for one or more products. Here, the process operations are well defined and developed, with automatic/engineered methods of processing being employed. The facilities are substantially larger and more expensive, providing high reliability with risk managed through complex engineered solutions, along with operational procedures.

Process Equipment

Sterile manufacturing operations are highly scrutinized for integrity and consistency. Accordingly, the process equipment supporting or controlling sterile operations is designed to meet strict regulatory guidelines and design requirements.
Major design considerations in process equipment include:

- Operability and ergonomics
- Cleanability of the system
- Ability to sterilize the system
- Drainability
- Smooth, hard, and crevice-free finishes of all product contact surfaces
- Fully controllable, consistent and repeatable functions (manual or automatic)
- Closed vs. open process systems
- Ability to control the manufacturing environment to a prescribed level

Editor's Note: _____
Purchase texts for reference during projects—the cost is minimal, but the information is essential.

Materials of construction for sterile manufacturing equipment typically is comprised of 316L grade stainless steel, designed for cleanability, strength, durability, and especially sterilizability. Stainless steel product contact surfaces often meet very high standards, consistent with interior surface finishes as defined in Part SF, Stainless Steel and Higher Alloy Interior Surface Finishes, *Bioprocess Equipment, An International Standard* (7).

Process Design of "Open" vs. "Closed" Systems

Issues related to "closed" vs. "open" systems will significantly effect the development, size, cost, and operation of a sterile manufacturing project, and as such becomes a top priority in the design of a process.

While closed process systems require greater design and operational integrity to function consistently in a controlled manner, "open" systems often require more "real estate" in a facility, so a comparative understanding of each approach is very important in the development and operation of a facility.

A "open" process system is a system that is exposed to the background environment in a processing facility. Such examples include final filling into dosage forms, loose connections in a process system, testing of samples, as well as open transfer of product.

An "open" system processing an injectable product that cannot be maintained in a closed state is typically located within a Grade A or Class 100 environment. This approach requires rooms and functions to support this critical operation. For example, a closed process system occupying 500 square feet may grow to as much as 2,000 square feet to accommodate support and background features for an open system.

Editor's Note: _____
Closed process systems are more difficult to design, but generally reduce environmental requirements and capital cost.

A "closed" system is commonly defined as a process that has no potential exposure to the surrounding environment. This system may be comprised of multiple or single unit operations. A closed system can be opened initially for cleaning and/or product/parts change over, but then is intrinsically closed and sterilized-in-place (SIP) prior to use in a process operation.

If a system can be operated and maintained in a closed state, then it is viewed that the background environment may be significantly downgraded. In most cases, however, the background is maintained to a determined level regardless of a closed process state due to conservative design practices (engineering solutions over procedural solutions) and conservative risk management considerations.

Primary and Secondary Containment Considerations

Every process operation in place today essentially has a primary and secondary level of containment. The most common type of primary containment is a process equipment/system (ideally closed); the process room and surrounding environment is a secondary level of containment. Examples are listed in Table 3.

TABLE 3   Table of Containment Levels

Line	Primary Containment Mechanism	Secondary Containment Mechanism, Surrounding the Primary Mechanism
1	Process System	Process Room
2	Process Room	Background GMP Rooms
3	Process System	Isolation System
4	Process System	Process System
5	Isolation System	Process Room

When targeting an efficient cost structure for a project, a review of the background environment (the secondary containment) should be done first, since often this costs more than the process equipment (the primary system) while offering no more manufacturing capacity. For example, in a typical sterile manufacturing facility, the process equipment consumes 10–35% of the total cost of the project, compared to 30–60% for the background environment. Any reduction in the background environment is significant to the overall cost of the project, while not affecting process capacity.

In some cases, the secondary containment element (the room and/or local protection) is often required to perform to a certain level, since the primary containment system may require an opening or break in the system during a process run, or if the product has a containment/exposure limit requirement. In this case, the secondary containment element becomes an important line of protection to maintain product integrity, protect operators, and/or contain a product within a certain boundary.

Processing in Barrier and Isolation Systems

Barrier and isolation systems represent a growing trend in the design and operation of sterile facilities. Benefits to these technologies include:

- Protection of product
- Containment of potent and/or cytotoxic compounds
- Protection of personnel
- Potential ability to reduce the environmental classification level of the background environment

Barrier Isolation Technology

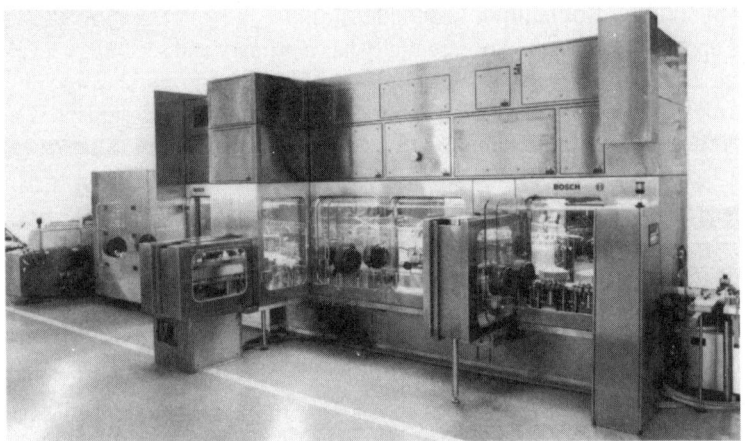

Since process systems and unit operations often require a variety of interventions during an operational run, understanding the benefits, limits, and risks of barrier and isolation systems is important during early conceptual design and development. The integration of a barrier or isolation system with process equipment often requires the process equipment to be fabricated and then sent to a vendor specialist to locate a process component into a barrier/isolation system. Consideration of schedule and cost should be made here when considering process equipment vendor options. (Further discussion on barrier, containment, and isolation systems can be found in Chapter 15: Containment/Isolation.)

Cleaning, Sanitization, and Sterilization

Any equipment, materials, or systems that offer product contact surfaces in a sterile manufacturing facility must be free of all forms of viable microbial organisms on or in inanimate surfaces (5). To achieve this, any contact surfaces must be thoroughly cleaned and sterilized. Consistent and thorough preparation of product contact surfaces represents a great challenge in a sterile manufacturing facility, therefore intensive design efforts are required to achieve a fully qualified operation. Common terms used in the preparation of equipment include clean-in-place (CIP) and sterilize-in-place (SIP). To mitigate risk or achieve an economic advantage, a company may opt to purchase rather than produce certain sterilized raw materials and disposable products.

Editor's Note:

Use sterilized disposable and prepared materials to reduce capital cost and simplify operations.

Cleaning Process Equipment

While non-product contact equipment, such as tables, racks, carts, etc, are cleaned at intervals, product contact equipment, such as tanks, pumps, piping, etc., must be cleaned more frequently (typically between product batches or change-overs). Product contact equipment also consists of fixed and portable equipment. Fixed equipment is disassembled with some components removed from the room for cleaning out of place (COP) in a purpose-built room. This also includes the removal of portable equipment for cleaning, typically at the same location as fixed equipment. Remaining components are cleaned in place (CIP) by flushing the system with a series of solutions and rinses while the system is closed. Control of these fluids is managed by both the process equipment and a CIP system (typically a skid) control units. COP typically consists of further disassembly of equipment, where it is cleaned with an ultrasonic-type or detergent flushing cleaning cycle (semi-automatic or automatic). A final rinse and drying step complete the cleaning process. Cleaned equipment is then reassembled (if required) and may be placed into a container or bag for protection and sterilization. As the equipment moves through the cleaning process, the surrounding environment increases in cleanliness to correspond with the state of the equipment being cleaned. This typically means that the room(s) will be designed to meet a Grade D/C environment, with local Grade B/A areas as required.

Sanitization

Sanitization, in comparison to sterilization, is the "process of substantially reducing or destroying a number of microbial organisms to a relatively safe level." Sanitization "generally requires a 99.9% or greater reduction of a test organism." The "test organism should be agreed upon with the inspecting agency" prior to completion of the design and validation of the process (8).

Sterilization

Product Sterility During Processing. In general, most agencies, designers, QA personnel, and operators prefer that a product be rendered as sterilized toward the end of a process cycle (bioburden is controlled throughout the process). This is typically known as *terminal sterilization*, in which filled containers of product pass through a prescribed process, sterilizing the product at a fixed range of parameters.

Diagram of Sterility Point

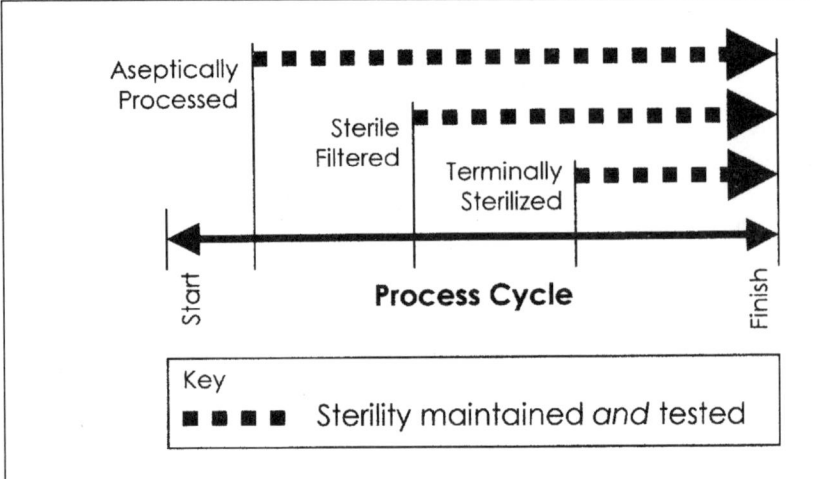

Editor's Note: _____

Use terminal sterilization whenever possible, to reduce the background environment and capital cost of a project.

Some products, though, cannot be terminally sterilized as they might degrade due to the high heat temperatures. Two examples of are aseptically processed and sterile filtered products. Aseptically processed products are those that reach a sterile level early in the process cycle, since the drug matrix cannot be filtered or heat sterilized.

Basic solutions, that can be filtered but cannot be terminally sterilized, are often sterile filtered just prior to the filling operation. Sterile filtration typically consists of a bulk solution passing through a sterile filter just prior to filling into containers.

Equipment Sterilization. In the development of a sterile facility and operation, understanding the meaning of a term and the effect of declaring it in a GMP environment is extremely important since, once that term is declared, it must be maintained. One such declaration is the need to declare a system either "sterilizable" or "sanitizable."

Once a process room and equipment have been cleaned, product contact components and other critical items are sterilized. To claim that a system or unit operation is sterilized or sterilizable, one must prove that the system can consistently and repeatably "destroy all forms of viable microbial organisms on or in inanimate surfaces." Sterilization is required usually for the following reasons:

A Sterile Filter Assembly Located in a Facility

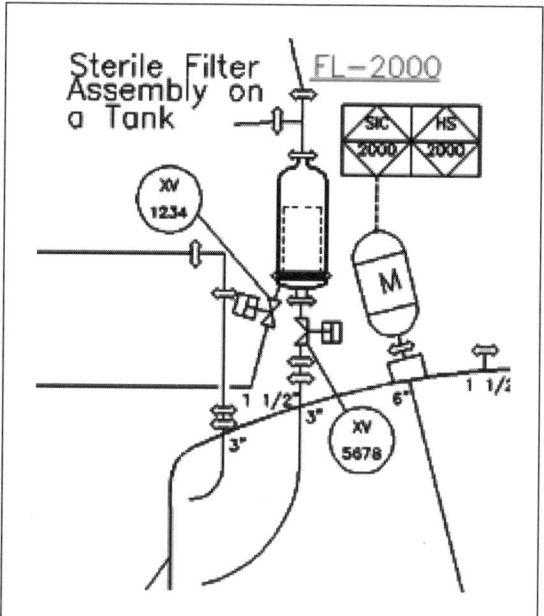

- Prevent contamination
- Protect the product
- Protection of the patient
- Ensure that only a certain product is present (9)

Sterilization is achieved typically via one of the following methods:

- Moist heat" Transfer of energy through contact with water or water vapor to cause the protein in the microbial organism to coagulate
- Dry heat: Transfer of energy through contact with air to cause the protein in the microbial organism to oxidize"
- Chemicals in vapor form: Contact with a chemical that causes biological activity in the microbial organism to cease
- Radiation: Mainly used for the sterilization of heat sensitive materials and products

Critical design factors for sterilization are the material compatibility with the sterilization method, as well as the design elements of time, environmental conditions, and temperature (or chemical contact) (10).

Equipment sterilized in place (SIP) is typically achieved through the introduction of pure steam in a closed system for a prescribed interval of time and temperature. Equipment and components that cannot be sterilized in this manner must be removed from the system and installed in a Grade A environment prior to a process operation. These types of components typically consist of silicon or plastic materials for disposable tubing, containers, and other types of components, and can either be chemically sterilized, irradiated, or purchased as being sterilized.

Once a level of sterility has been achieved in a typical injectable operation, that level must be maintained from that point forward. Thus, having a clear understanding of why, when, and how a product in a process is to be sterilized is very important.

Monitoring of Sterility

Once a product is rendered as being "sterilized," that level of purity must be maintained and tested to ensure product integrity, so a clear understanding should be made early on in the development of a project as to the method of monitoring batch integrity.

The QA Team will verify that a process room has been cleaned through testing prior to commencement of a process operation, through the sampling of surface areas in a room as well as the measurement of microbial organisms and particles. This is typically in accordance with the environmental table of classifications (Table 5).

Sterilization of Utilities Used in Processing Sterile Products

In a sterile manufacturing facility, process utilities, such as water, steam, air and other gases are rendered as pure or sterile so that the product integrity is not compromised during processing.

Design Considerations for Operations Interventions. A manufacturing process typically has materials introduced to and/or taken from the product area during an operation. These activities include:

- Initial materials additions
- Materials additions made during a process operation
- Sampling of in-process product
- Transfer of product from one system to another, as well as
- Integrity testing of a process system batch

While these activities may at times seem insignificant in the overall manufacturing effort of a sterile product, any intervention like those listed can destroy the integrity of a product batch if not designed and operated properly.

Sampling of product and utilities also represents a significant portion of a daily operation. Routine sampling requires careful design consideration to afford the operators reasonable access while preserving the integrity of the process. A review of sampling requirements and locations should be conducted prior to the commencement of construction.

Process Utilities

Process utilities are those systems that directly support manufacturing and also come in contact with product. According to the ISPE Baseline Guide to Commissioning, these systems are considered "direct impact" systems, and therefore need to be validated in GMP operations (11). These systems must provide a utility supply that does not contaminate or damage the integrity of a sterile product in manufacturing.

Editor's Note: _____

Use text references and other precedents to assess what is "direct" and "indirect," rather than an opinion.

Process utility systems are generally expensive; therefore, careful design is required to balance demand of capacity as well as cost to the project. On smaller projects, alternative considerations to developing a process utility within a project include the purchase of prepared products, as well as the more extensive use of disposable processing products. This is typically done in smaller scale operations, such as developmental and clinical manufacturing.

Examples of Process utilities include:

- United States Pharmacopoeia (USP) Water for Injection (WFI)
- Clean steam
- Process gases
- Process vacuum and extract systems (in product contact conditions)

Applicable regulatory guidelines and engineering texts should be considered when designing these systems, such as those listed in the reference section. Also, sampling of utilities and maintenance must be considered prior to the completion of the design.

Process Architecture

Flow of Materials and Personnel

In sterile manufacturing facilities, the flows of materials and personnel are very influential on product integrity, and agencies and quality personnel will often scrutinize these flows. This is particularly true in rooms involving product contact and critical operations. In these cases, unidirectional flow of personnel and materials is very important to minimize risk of product contamination. This principle is applied from room to room as well as within the room whenever possible.

Proper material and personnel flows are essential in pharmaceutical operations. Good flows efficiently manage and control the movement of people and materials through processing operations, minimizing risk of contamination whenever possible.

Flow patterns to be addressed typically include:

- People entering an operation
- People exiting an operation

Diagram of Flows

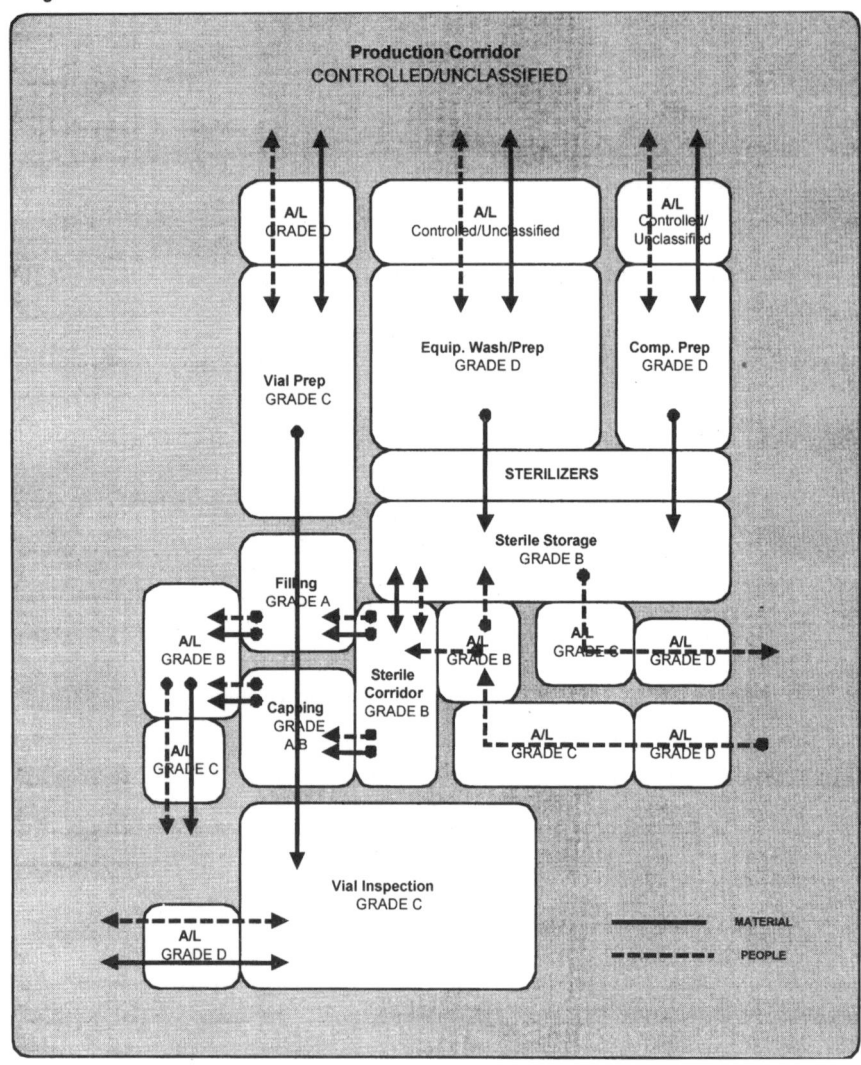

- Clean equipment entering an operation
- Equipment returned for cleaning
- Raw materials and components supply
- Prepared equipment for processing
- Materials in process
- Finished goods
- Waste materials

Room Layout and Facility Configuration

Since operator and maintenance personnel in a critical operation represent one of the more significant sources of contamination, careful consideration must be made to minimize risk through good ergonomic design and operation of a sterile process.

When developing a program for a sterile facility project, careful consideration is required for the placement of equipment and people within segregated process operating rooms. In a critical operation, the location of the supply and return air grills with equipment locations and operations since is essential so that the clean air stream flows in a unidirectional pattern across the critical operation without interference from people or other obstructions.

Room Volumes. The footprint of a room affects the capacity of an HVAC system. Additionally, even though the height of a room does not affect the number of air changes per hour in a room, it does affect the capacity of the heating and cooling system required to maintain a set range of temperature. Thus, a facility professional should drive a coordinated effort to minimize the height of a ceiling in a processing room.

A Fill Room

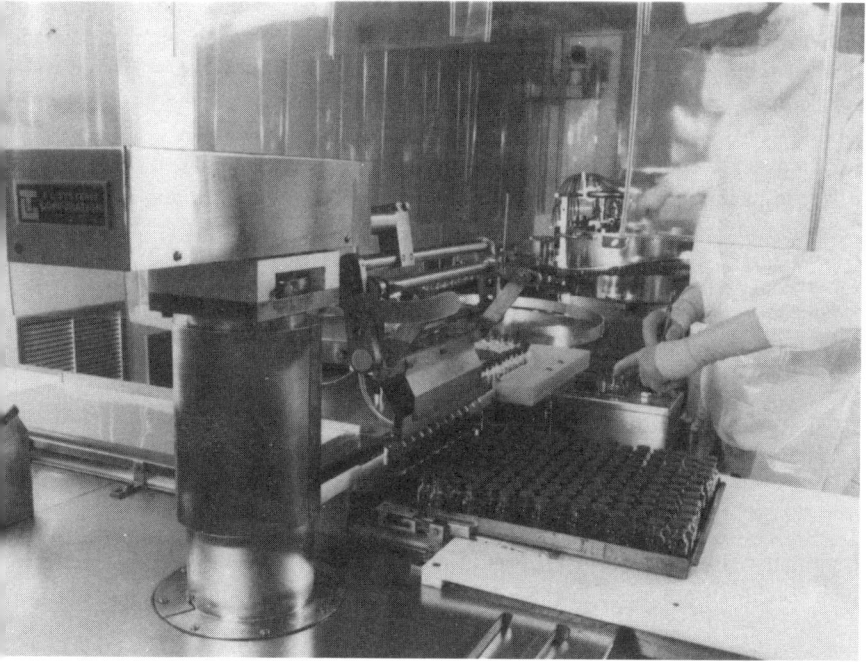

Room Geometry. When designing a room for a critical operation where unidirectional airflow will be included, the design and layout of the room should carefully balance process equipment and ergonomics, as well as the ability for the critical environment to meet design airflow. For example, designing a room 16 feet wide by 22 feet long will more likely perform better than a room 22 feet by 22 feet. Also, the more simple the room footprint (i.e., a rectangle), the easier it is to design the HVAC system. The variation of the geometry for an air filters should be considered, so that only one or two sizes of replacement HEPA filters will be required.

Editor's Note: _____
    Layout process operation rooms efficiently and simply, keeping the geometry and size economical.

Architectural Design

The design of surfaces in cleanrooms requires careful attention to detail, construction methodology, smooth and hard surface characteristics, as well as the ability to withstand frequent cleaning with chemicals.

In the *Guidance for Industry, Sterile Drug Products Produced by Aseptic Processing—Current Good Manufacturing Practice, Draft Guidance*, we see that:

Cleanrooms are normally designed as functional units with specific purposes. A well-designed cleanroom is constructed with materials that allow for ease of cleaning and sanitizing. Examples of adequate design features include seamless and rounded floor to wall junctions as well as readily accessible corners. Floors, walls and ceilings are constructed of smooth, hard surfaces that can be easily cleaned (211.42). (12).

In general, epoxy coated materials and stainless steel dominate the finish types in sterile manufacturing facilities. Common materials of construction exposed in cleanrooms typically include:

- Epoxy paint on gypsum board and steel studs for walls and ceilings
- Epoxy terrazzo or resinous flooring on concrete
- Epoxy-coated suspension grid system, with smooth ceiling tiles sealed to the grid
- Epoxy-coated steel for doors and frames, with stainless steel hardware
- Stainless steel for doors, frames, panels, and escutcheon plates
- Glass and plastic for vision panels and barriers
- Modular panel systems

While most of these items are readily available, the challenge is to integrate these materials in such a manner as to minimize joint failures and other crevices. Such conditions are prone to cause microbial and other contamination problems.

Editor's Note: _____
    Thoughtful and consistent integration of systems in a sterile facility project creates attractive facilities at a good value.

Image of Detail

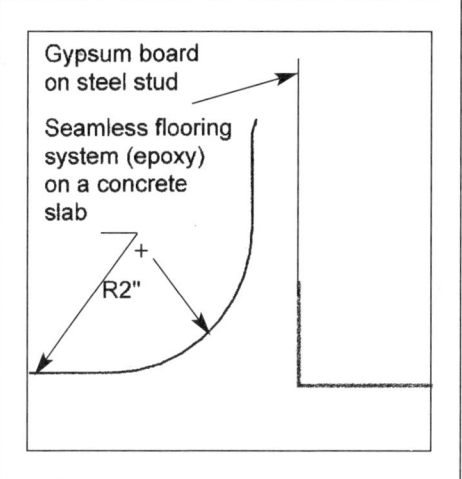

Gypsum board
on steel stud

Seamless flooring
system (epoxy)
on a concrete
slab

+

R2"

The designer must also understand that as construction progresses to completion, the construction tolerances become much tighter. From a construction standpoint the ability for an architectural system to accept and absorb these tolerances, while minimizing/eliminating joints and seams, is essential to a successful completion of a cleanroom fit-out.

Image of Detail

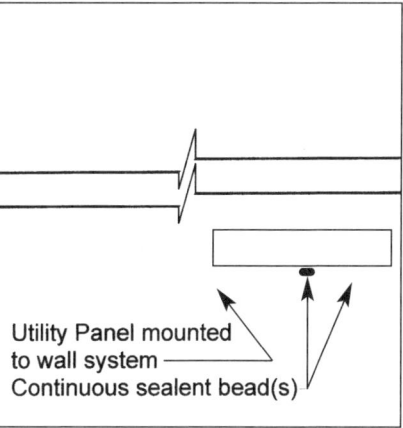

Utility Panel mounted
to wall system
Continuous sealent bead(s)

Failure of surface finishes typically stem from:

• Lack of integration of process equipment into architecture
• Varying tolerances of systems (+/–1/8 inch epoxy on +/–1/2 inch concrete)

- Improper installation/application of materials
- Impact of architectural finishes on other systems (inability to balance a room air pressure due to air bleeding through tile and grid ceilings)
- Different material types expanding/contracting at different rates, causing cracks and crevasses
- Inadequate attention to materials and surface connections
- Degradation of surfaces due to chemicals in cleaning
- Lack of understanding of basic design ideas

There are many ways to complete architectural details in cleanrooms, but only through good communication (vis à vis, good documentation and communications between the designer and builder) can the systems be completed successfully.

Room Finishes

The level of cleanroom finishes vary for room functions and particular conditions. In general, one could consider the following table of room grades as a starting point when developing a sterile manufacturing facility:

TABLE 4   Table of Room Finishes

Room Grade	Flooring	Walls	Ceiling	Other
Controlled Unclassified	Seamless vinyl or epoxy	Epoxy painted gypsum board	Tile and Grid	Field epoxy painted steel doors/frames
Grade D	Epoxy	Epoxy painted gypsum board	Tile and Grid	Field epoxy painted steel doors/frames
Grade C	Epoxy	Epoxy painted gypsum board	Tile and Grid	Field epoxy painted steel doors/frames
Grade B	Epoxy	Epoxy coating system on gypsum board	Gypsum board	Factory coated or stainless steel doors/frames Integral corner coving
Grade A	Epoxy	Epoxy coating system on gypsum board	Gypsum board	Factory coated or stainless steel doors/frames Integral corner coving

Modular Wall Systems

Modular wall and ceiling systems may be considered in place of "stick-frame" construction materials and methodologies, especially when quality control and speed are essential. Modular wall systems have developed significantly to provide factory-built panels and systems of high quality and performance and can be installed very quickly.

Room Design Considerations

Sterile manufacturing facilities consist of an intensive design array of utilities, environmental controls, and access requirements. At the conceptual design stage, careful consideration is given to access to mechanical system serving cleanrooms. Whenever a GMP spatial envelope is broken to provide access to utilities, the room must be re-established per approved SOPs prior to commencement of the next operation. Thus good access design, while maintaining the GMP envelope and ongoing operations, can be achieved through the inclusion of such items as technical spaces, walkable ceilings, and controlled unclassified peripheral spaces to afford necessary access to mechanical systems.

Editor's Note: _____

Start a design with equal parts of mechanical to operational space to afford realistic access to and performance of mechanical systems.

Modular Panel System

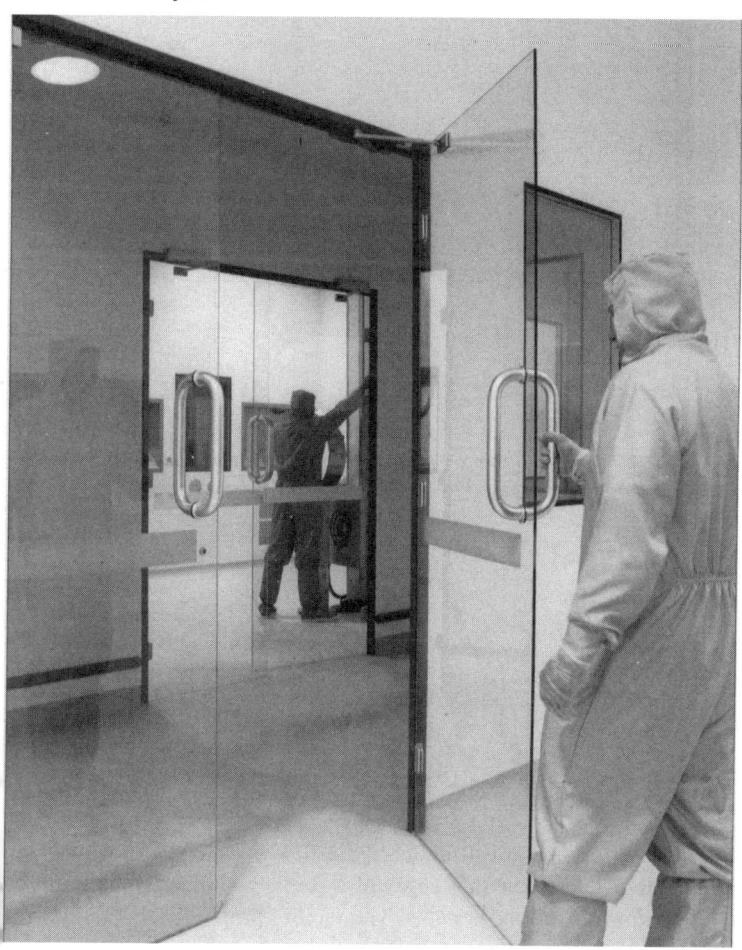

Modular Panel

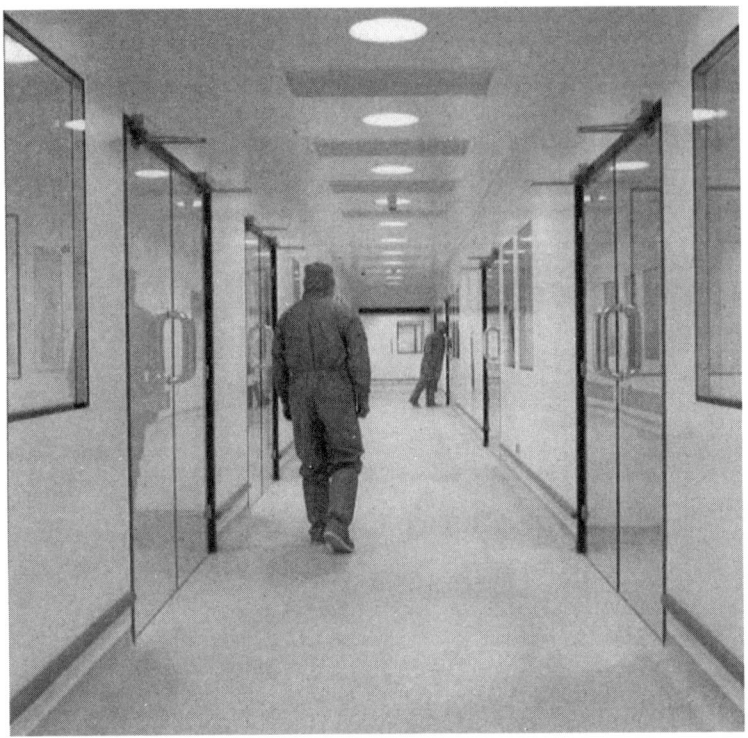

Mechanical Design

Plant Utility Systems ("Indirect Impact" Systems)

Utilities supporting process and facility systems that do not come in direct contact with product are considered "indirect impact" systems. These systems typically include:

- Plant utilities
- Process water
- Plant steam and hot water
- Chilled water
- Potable water
- Compressed air
- Lubricants
- Water pretreatment

Design of Utility Systems ("Direct Impact" Systems)

One of the significant development challenges of a sterile manufacturing facility is the design of "direct impact" utility systems. The facility professional should drive the design to be as simplistic as possible, by utilizing readily validatable technologies as well as proven off-the-shelf skidded systems provided by qualified vendors.

A "direct impact" system can fail qualification because the design is not coordinated with expectations. Early design activities should establish clear objectives and criteria for systems, with proper documents of these basic decisions collected into User Requirement Specifications (URS). This approach will increase the probability of success through clearer communications and development.

Utility Systems Documentation
When developing "direct impact" systems, the facility professional must account for and document all of the components and characteristics of a system, as typically found in the following progression:

- Utility capacity and demand calculations
- Process and Utility Flow Diagrams
- User Requirement Specification
- Equipment Arrangement Drawings
- Process and Instrumentation Diagram
- Piping Plans, Sections and Isometrics
- Functional Requirement Specification

Editor's Note: _____

Remember that good construction documentation must tell builders the ideas and methods for construction.

Systems should be developed and documented consistently, and the engineer should understand what level of documentation the client and qualification personnel expect prior to completion of the design. The engineer should also drive a coordinated effort to document each item only once, to minimize duplication and confusion if changes should evolve. Lastly, when possible, the engineer should consider the "black box" design approach in which certain unit operations or systems are packaged and developed separately by another engineer or vendor to expedite the design schedule and reduce cost. In this approach, only the general service loop and connections are shown on a diagram, and this diagram references another diagram for information within the "black box."

HVAC

Control of Room Environments and Pressurization. "Design of a given area should be based upon satisfying microbiological and particle standards defined by the equipment, components, and products exposed, as well as the particular operation conducted in the area" (6). When the product is exposed or opened to the surrounding environment, the room must designed to meet substantial mechanical performance minimum, to satisfy regulatory agency guidelines such as Class 100, Grade A and/or ISO 5.

Achieving a compliant sterile manufacturing operation requires the use of increasing levels of environmental cleanliness, or "zones." Utilizing a design with increasing quality levels of zones facilitates the ability for product and people to enter and exit the facility.

Editor's Note: _____

Keep the process closed and reduce the background environment condition whenever possible.

The diagram below illustrates a typical zoning overlay, along with a typical air pressurization cascade from critical to noncritical zones. In noncritical peripheral areas a design can be downgraded to a Controlled Not Classified (CNC) state, where the room is designed to meet Grade D performance parameters but is not typically validated. CNC room classifications should be utilized whenever practical in a sterile manufacturing facility.

Pressurization. Room pressurization and pressure differentials are usually a highly scrutinized element in design. This is the case since there are times when basic design philosophies may contradict each other, or when followed rigidly, may put the design into an impractical design/operational state.

Room pressurization in a sterile manufacturing facility is controlled typically by the difference between the pressure in a particular process room and a fixed atmospheric point outside the core processing area. Through this approach, the HVAC system is more likely to remain stabilized in normal operating conditions since all monitoring points are tied back to a single reference datum.

Room pressurization values are generally determined through the analysis of clean room zones and process functions within a conceptual floor plan for a manufacturing environment. Typically, air will "cascade" from the cleanest and most con-

Zones

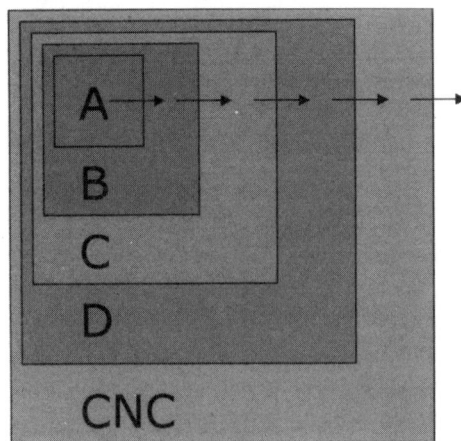

trolled operating environment to an uncontrolled area. Exceptions to this approach stem mainly from the requirement to contain a process environment due to potency, containment of an open process (such as dispensing of powders), or other operator exposure limitations. In such a case, an additional airlocking level or zone is included to achieve the design objectives.

The challenge in designing a pressurization scheme is to balance practical design with published regulatory guidelines. For example, if a designer were to rigidly follow the FDA's 1987 issue of the *Guideline on Sterile Drug Products Produced by Aseptic Processing,* then the facility professional designs for a minimal and relative pressure differential (between two different area classifications) of 0.05 inch of water (13). Compounding this instance is that the QA group may also refer to the same text body and require that the differential should never go below that value. This approach compounds itself into the following diagram:

Thus, with a typical cascade effect from a Grade A room to an uncontrolled space, the resultant pressure value for the Grade A room may be 0.31 inch of water to meet a minimal operating differential of pressure between areas of 0.05 inch of water.

Our recommendation here is to first balance a realistic design with good procedures and operations, to achieve a good pressure regime at a reasonable value.

Editor's Note: _____

Understand the effect of a QA requirement on a design, and be realistic about a system's capabilities and system recovery.

Air Filtration and Airflow Movement. In order to achieve the various grades of spaces, it is necessary to filter the incoming air supply to remove airborne particu-

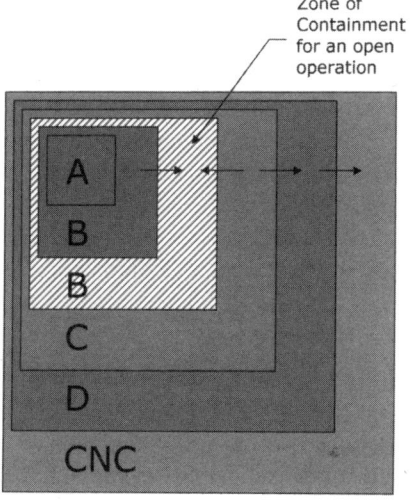

Diagram of Air Pressurization Conditions

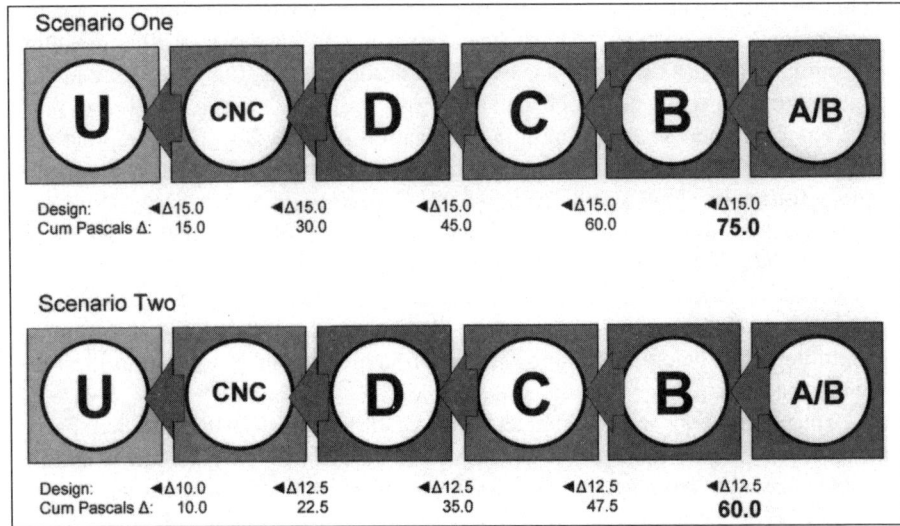

late and microbial forms. Most regulatory texts offer guidelines for airflow and filtration that represent a good starting point for design. In Grade A spaces, for example, airflow should be high efficiency particle arrestor (HEPA) filtered, unidirectional as well as moving at a higher velocity at the working elevation, especially when sterile product is exposed to the room environment.

Supply Air. Most of the supply air in a sterile facility operation is high efficiency particulate arrestor (HEPA) filtered. Only nonclassified and uncontrolled areas should be considered for supply air less clean than HEPA air, provided there is no significant adverse risk put on the system(s) or operations.

Airflow Control over a Surface of a Supply Grill. Part of the qualification of a critical environment includes the measurement of airflow over an entire area of supply. With a plenum supply design, airflow may vary over the total surface, which at times can cause problems due to a perceived (and at times real) inconsistency. To achieve an acceptable design, the facility professional must decide on the design and operational tolerances for the rate of supply. Additionally, a design may include an airflow control device, such as an adjustable baffle plate, to create a more uniform and consistent rate of airflow over an entire surface.

Recirculating vs. Once-Through Air. Typically in a sterile facility project, the room environment air conditioning is recirculated, mainly to reduce utility demand and operating cost. Only in exceptional circumstances, such as open potent or biological processing operations open to the room environment, should a once-through air system be considered for part (or all) of the HVAC design.

Velocity of Air at the Working Elevation. For a Grade A critical process, the desired unidirectional airflow at the location where product is exposed to the environment is generally in the range of 90 feet per minute (0.45 meters per second). To achieve that level of an airflow at a working level, a higher velocity of air is often required at the face of the supply air discharge point, reaching as high as 120 or more feet per minute (0.60 meters per second). These levels should be considered a starting point in design development, and the actual level should be raised or lowered to satisfy the particular design condition for a project.

An HVAC Module

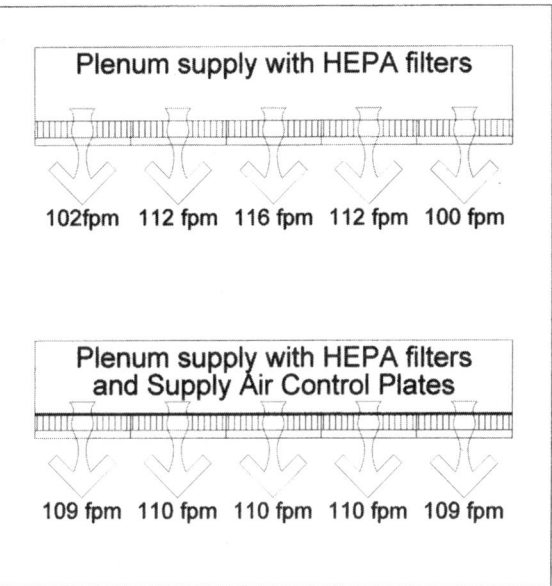

Editor's Note: _____
Reduce velocities whenever possible to ease performance requirements and reduce capital cost.

Prefabricated HVAC Modules. Prefabricated airflow modules offer a good solution to achieving local Grade A or B conditions at a good value. These units can be designed to fit a certain operating condition, or purchased as a standard size and set-up. The boundary between this local Grade A environment and the surrounding area is typically achieved with a plastic curtain or prefabricated transparent partition barriers commonly referred to as Restricted Access Barrier (RABS).

These units typically utilize a large plenum box where fan and filter unit(s) are located. Return air is typically brought from within the room where the unit is located, and filtered through the unit to supply clean, laminar flow air necessary to achieve a Grade A operating condition. Access for maintenance to the unit is neces-

Fill Room Section 1

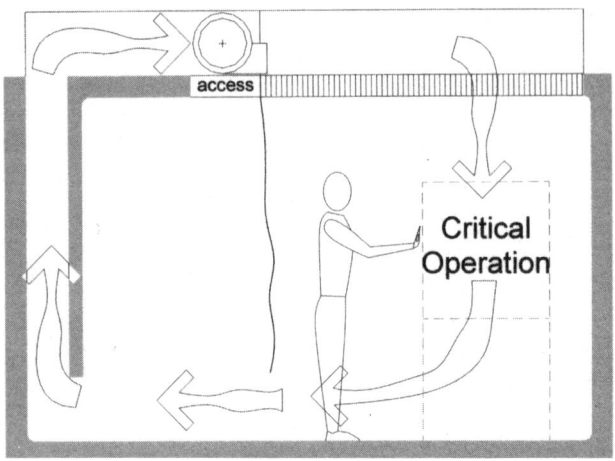

sary, as well as the need to provide space for filter monitoring devices and an electrical service disconnect.

Return Air. Low wall returns are used in Grade A spaces to achieve unidirectional airflow, and are typically used for Grade B spaces as well to maintain proper airflow turbidity. Grade C and D spaces typically utilize ceiling returns, but may also use low wall when required for a particular operation or circumstance.

Fill Room Section 2

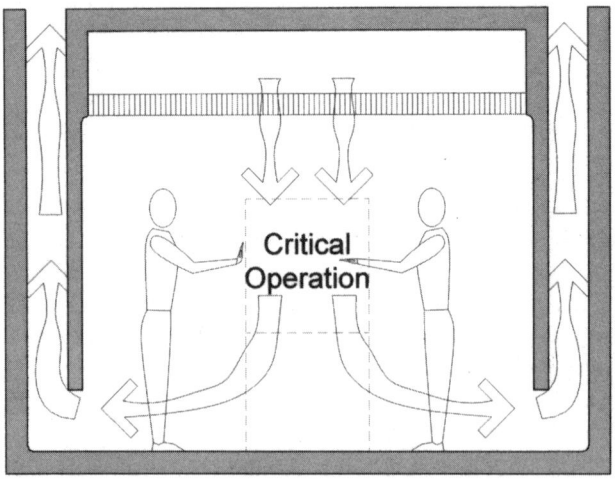

Editor's Note: _____

Keep parallel walls free of penetrations, and allow up to 30% additional room area for return chases.

Low Wall Return Chase Design. Since Grade A spaces with unidirectional airflow move a tremendous amount of air, the amount of low wall return area required to meet the desired air change rate is significant, often occupying two entire sides of a process room.

Electrical Design

The electrical service in a sterile manufacturing facility is a service that is not usually readily visible in an operation but is always relied upon. Critical process and building functions rely on consistent power to keep process equipment PLCs and building management systems working properly. Any glitch in the quality of the power supply can significantly affect an operation.

Fill Room Plan

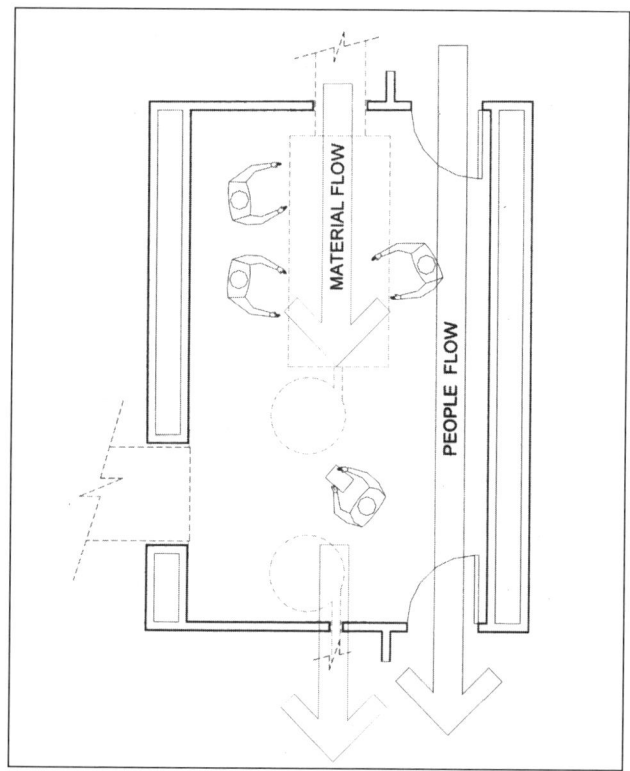

When power must always be available for certain electronic recording devices or controls equipment, the facility professional may decide to utilize Uninterrupted Power Supply (UPS), with emergency power backup. These two utilities in combination can keep a critical operation functional until the operators can properly and safely shut it down. These systems can be expensive, so a clear understanding of which items should receive these services and the associated cost should be reviewed and agreed upon early in the design of a project.

Editor's Note: _____

Consider utilizing UPS only to save data on a PLC to reduce capital cost, and develop an SOP to minimize product loss in a potential power failure.

Lighting for operators in process rooms is typically designed for 70–100/candle watts at a working elevation. Consider this measurement as a starting point, and then adjust the level to suit real operating conditions and applicable codes.

Lighting systems in critical process rooms, classified as Grade A, are typically integrated into the HVAC supply system, since that system occupies most of the ceiling surface. These lights are gasketed and sealed, and typically are either fluorescent or LED. Lighting in Grade B and lesser-controlled areas typically consists of fluorescent tubes in a sealed prefabricated housing that is then inserted either into a ceiling tile and grid system, or a gypsum board ceiling. These light fixtures must be cleanable and designed for minimal crevices, as well as resistive to the cleaning agents used in process rooms. Good design coordination is required to achieve proper lighting levels, as well as locations for other services in the ceilings of process rooms.

Electrical devices in process rooms typically consist of power connections to equipment, as well as any electrical control/supply boxes located in walls. As with all other materials and surfaces, these items need to comply with basic design guidelines for GMP process rooms.

Items that require electrical service include:

- Door interlocks
- Automatic doors
- Safety devices
- Telephone and intercom
- Clocks

These systems must comply with applicable regulatory guidelines and codes. While purchasing these devices for clean rooms has been difficult in the past, vendors have now developed complete product lines designed exclusively for clean room applications.

International power requirements can be an issue when process equipment for a project is purchased from different countries. A careful understanding of CE, ISO, UL, and local/state code requirements is essential to a successful design of a system. An electrical engineer should review the type of power required for each process system (volts, hertz, etc.) as well as process equipment specifications and design criteria prior to final development and procurement.

Power for manufacturing equipment typically is supplied locally to the equipment, either from a disconnect switch or a control panel. Connections to freestanding components in rooms are often made from overhead, with a flexible line connecting directly into the equipment. The cleanability and safety of flexible connections must be considered prior to the completion of design and engineering.

Instrumentation and Controls

Instrumentation

In the design and construction of sterile manufacturing facilities, instrumentation components and controls systems (I&C) have developed significantly. Developments in I&C include:

- The establishment of Good Automated Manufacturing Practices (GAMP)
- A better understanding of direct (GMP) and indirect (non-GMP) instruments and controls
- The availability of electronic batch records and recording devices
- Better software and hardware designs affording greater control capability and quality

In a facility, instrumentation components will monitor systems in operation to verify that the system is performing as planned. In a variety of manners, instruments typically will monitor:

- Particles
- Microbial levels
- Pressure
- Temperature
- Humidity
- Flow
- Volumetric levels
- Mechanical settings and status conditions

These monitor points are essential in order to monitor and trend the performance and quality of product, process utilities, process manufacturing, and room environments.

Editor's Note:

Expect intensive design coordination of instrument locations and coordination in the field during construction.

Control Systems

Control systems will collect the information gathered from the instruments and then will monitor, record, and control the systems to meet prescribed performance settings and requirements. Within a sterile manufacturing facility, there typically are control systems set up for Direct Impact operations, such as control of process equipment and GMP room environments, as well as Indirect Impact operations, such as plant steam, potable water, chilled water, etc. The level of complexity for control systems can vary greatly, but typically a company will opt to separate GMP controls from non-GMP controls. This approach enables a programmer to manipulate non-GMP system programs more freely than a change-control managed GMP system modification. An additional consideration here is to create a mirror image of the controls software for each system. This will allow programmers to "tweak" the software more easily in the non-GMP system, and then they can very quickly make the proven modifications in a GMP system under change control.

Diagram of Controls System Hierarchy

Factor	Fully Integrated System Characteristic	"Islands of Automation"
Control Unit	Central active control module with local passive module	Local active control module
Data output	Electronic, for a total batch run	Electronic or manual, local to unit operation
Data Recording	Centralized compliant "hard drive" data collection	Typically a hard copy output, no hard drive data storage

Editor's Note: _____

Separate GMP from non-GMP controls. It may cost more initially, but will ease and simplify operations of the long term.

Data Recording

Data recording in GMP operations is a topic of much discussion. When a company decides to include electronic data recording for batch records and trending, much work must be done to prove the integrity of the data collected and stored. Books like the ISPE Baseline Guide to Good Automated Manufacturing Practices (GAMP), provide excellent information and guidance for the development of such systems. When the "islands of automation" approach are used, data is typically printed out at the completion of each process unit operation and collated into the process batch record. All data is subsequently erased from the controller the next time it is used.

Islands of Automation vs. Integrated Controls Systems. Depending upon the scale and complexity of a sterile project, the team must decide whether to develop and operate a fully integrated controls system, or to develop stand-alone islands of automation. A comparison table below reviews both approaches:

Plumbing

Plumbing systems in sterile manufacturing facilities typically consist of domestic cold and hot water and waste drainage. While these systems are widely used in non-

Controls System Hierarchy

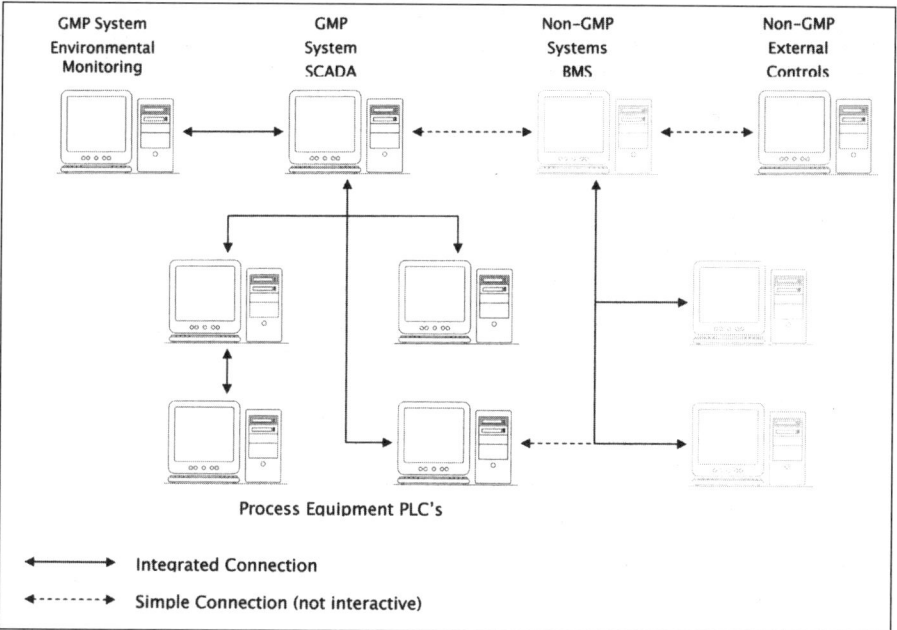

controlled environments such as utility rooms, wash rooms, and cleaning stations, they are not typically used or exposed in a controlled environment due to risk of contamination. Often, when a drain is required in a GMP operation, it is limited to Grade C or D spaces, and is designed to be a contained connection with the proper air break to comply with codes. Alternatively, drains can also be located in adjacent technical spaces to manage risk.

Many drainage system designs are specialized for sterile manufacturing facilities, since the liquid introduced may be very hot, slightly corrosive from cleaning materials, or mineral deficient. Such considerations as specialized pipe materials or quench (or "flash") tanks can be used to render the waste safe for disposal into a common waste system.

Any water for use in general cleanup in non-critical areas is typically treated, while water used in critical operations rooms is sterilized.

DETAILS/IMPLICATIONS FOR PERFORMANCE/COMPLIANCE

Points for a Project Manager to Consider

Balance Engineering with Procedural Solutions. Throughout the development of a sterile facility project, many issues surface that must be addressed. Solutions to these problems generally fall into two categories: Engineering and procedural. Engineering solutions are solutions that mitigate processing risk through the inclusion of physical elements or engineering controls. Procedural solutions manage risk through the development of standard operating procedures that require an operator or process to work in a certain manner. The facility professional must strike a balance between engineering and procedural solutions, since engineering solutions can drive the cost of a project up significantly, and procedural solutions may be more scrutinized in certain situations.

Know Where You're Going Before You Get There. Organize a core team comprised of personnel representing all aspects of the project to develop a program and execution approach for the project. This team should describe in simple form the essential goals for a project.

Design for the Most Sensible Compliance. Understand the importance and limits of compliance in a project, and establish a group within the facility professional to monitor and ensure compliance in a GMP project. Also, connect the design team to the importance of compliance to better ensure a successful qualification and operation of a facility. Lastly, develop a sensible approach to compliance by understanding first what compliance is, and second what level of compliance is necessary for a given project.

Develop a Matrix Comparing Design and Operating Ranges for Systems. Often the validation group may use design ranges to qualify a facility, when a broader operating range is certainly acceptable. Take time early on in the design to develop a matrix comparing design ranges to acceptable operating/qualification ranges for regulated systems.

Editor's Note: _____

> Develop room layouts in the concept phase that show all elements in a room, and how it is intended to work.

Put Engineers in the Patients' and Operators' Shoes. Create a better product and operating facility by connecting the design team to the aspects of product quality and facility operability.

Connect Designers to the Cost, Schedule, Quality, and Compliance Drivers in a Project. Many times the designers and engineers are not "connected" to the project. They need to be connected, not only in terms of understanding the drivers, goals, and particular conditions within a project, but also in terms of understanding the effect of a design decision on a project. The management team should maintain a consistent connection of project drivers to the design team.

Design to the Project Execution Approach. When sterile filling equipment takes a year to be delivered to a project site, design the project so this equipment can be successfully installed and connected at the site, by working with the management team to understand the project execution sequence.

Editor's Note: _____

> Remember, if you can't build it on paper, you probably can't build it in the field. So take the time to develop a realistic design to avoid cost and schedule overruns.

Drive Quality Management Through the Project. In many respects, good quality management in the development of a sterile facility operation drives the successful completion of a project.

Design, Build, and Qualify for Cleaning and Changeover. With every additional surface introduced into a critical process room comes the need to clean frequently and maintain it. Every exposed surface must be accessible for routine cleaning, so every effort should be made to minimize the amount of surfaces through the relocation of nonessential components to an area outside the room, as well as the concealment of components in cabinets and panels. Cleaning equipment and the formulating/dispensing of cleaning solutions consume a significant amount of space in a sterile facility. Careful consideration should be made to include space allocations in the program for these operations. In larger scale operations, a dedicated cleaning system or area may be designated specifically for the preparation and storage/staging of cleaning components.

Understand the Differences Among "Green Field," "Brown Field," and Renovation Projects. Agencies understand that the basic context of a project effects the solutions generated for a project. It is essential, therefore, to document "why you did what you did" so a representative may better defend a position taken in the project. Sometimes, for example, space limitations may require an airlock regime or process flow to be nonstandard, relying more on standard operating procedures for control of product integrity.

Processing Risks and Issues

Contamination Sources. People represent the single most significant source of contamination in a sterile manufacturing operation. This is due to particle shedding, microcontamination, as well as airflow disturbance due to movements by operators. Proper gowning, the minimal presence of operators in critical rooms, as well as proper training for the movement of operators is necessary.

Unvalidatable Systems. Process systems are often unvalidatable because the major phases in a project are not properly coordinated. For example:

- A design may be developed without an understanding of how it will be managed, cleaned, and inspected, creating significant challenges to the construction, qualification, and operation team.

- Documentation is not properly maintained over the course of a project's development, leaving significant voids in the document trail of a project.
- A construction team may not install the equipment as designed, creating significant challenges for the commissioning and validation team.
- A validation team may attempt to force a system to perform within unreasonable ranges as well as qualify parameters that do not need to be validated, because the team was not properly engaged and managed.

Thus, develop a "System Approach," that connects the front-end ideas to the back-end licensing and operation of a sterile manufacturing facility.

PROJECT MANAGEMENT ISSUES: COST, SCHEDULE, AND QUALITY

In today's economy, pharmaceutical clients demand a high quality sterile manufacturing facility at a low cost and on a fast-track schedule. For a facility professional, balancing these three points can be difficult. It is therefore essential that the project management team connect the design and execution team to the particular cost, schedule, and quality drivers in a project.

Triangle Diagram of Cost, Schedule, and Quality

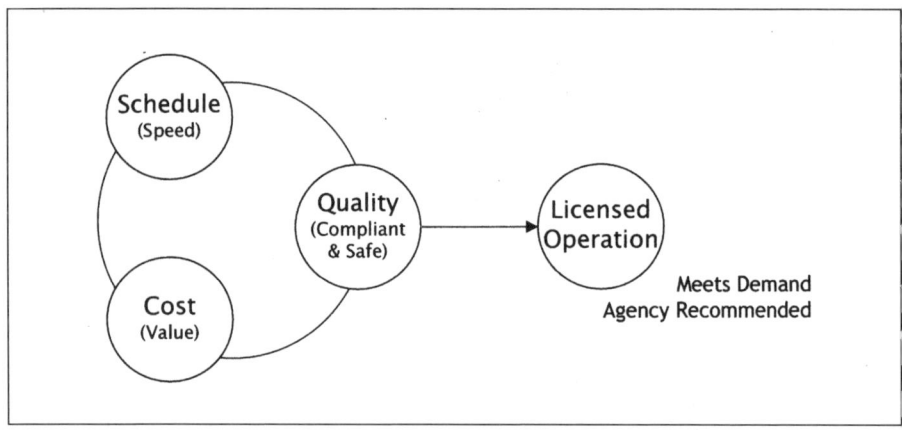

Cost

Sterile manufacturing facilities represent a significant portion of high-cost facilities. The direct facility cost alone can be $400 to $600 per square foot, and the process equipment can cost millions more. Add to these costs the allowances for indirect service costs and contingencies, and the total cost can be significant. The table below is for sterile manufacturing facility projects built in the United States, and provides examples of what one could expect to pay for these types of projects.

The profiles of the projects referenced above are diverse, so before a comparison can be made between any facility projects, a clear understanding of the factors that drive the cost must be understood. Particular considerations in the review of a sterile manufacturing facility cost include:

- Separately identify facility, process, and indirect services costs
- Green field, retrofit, vs. renovation projects
- The project execution approach (integrated or phased execution)
- The scale of the project (some economies with larger scale projects)
- The location of the project (availability of skilled labor, cost of materials and labor)
- The targeted speed of the project completion
- The extent of modularization
- The sophistication of the facility and process design
- Product containment requirements (potent, cytotoxic, etc.)

Only when a project is broken down into its components, can a team understand the significant design factors that drive the ultimate cost of a project.

Editor's Note: _____

Continually connect the design team to the project drivers to better ensure success.

Schedule

Sterile manufacturing facilities are complicated projects, and therefore typically take a significant time to design, build, and qualify. For a green field project, the duration for a new sterile manufacturing facility may take as long as 48 months to fully complete and qualify. Since many clients seek to complete a project as fast as possible, the facility professional must develop an execution approach that balances schedule targets with cost and quality.

Schedule is particularly driven by the project execution approach. When a fast-track project schedule is essential, then the client may choose an integrated engineering, procurement, construction management, commissioning, and validation (E/P/CM/C/V) execution.

Schedule is also greatly effected by the delivery of long-lead equipment. Typically, the long-lead equipment is the core of the sterile manufacturing operations, and they can also be the most difficult to install. A filling system alone can take one year to design, fabricate, test, and deliver to a project site for installation. In this case, select equipment packages may be ordered very early in the project schedule, and the surrounding components then designed to fit the purchased equipment configurations.

As with cost, it is essential to connect the entire team to the importance of schedule so the team may account for schedule drivers in the design of a sterile manufacturing facility.

When accelerating a project schedule, one should consider using some level of modularization as an element to deliver a project faster than a conventional stick-frame approach. This notion assumes, though, that the project may be broken into parallel tracks in which process, utility, and facility components are

A Project Schedule

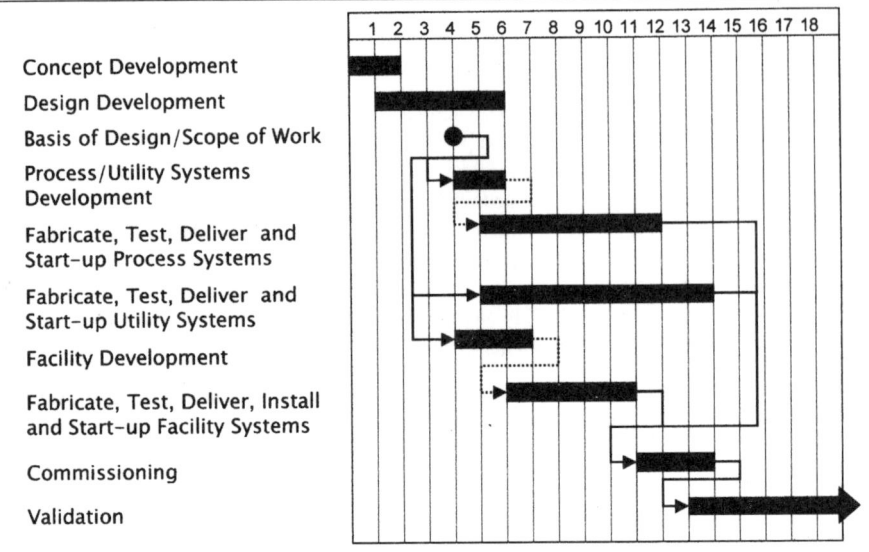

designed by vendors into skids, fabricated in a controlled facility environment, and tested prior to delivery to the project site. In fact, some of the testing done in the factory may help accelerate the qualification process at the site. Meanwhile, the main facility components can be constructed at the site. When completed, the modularized systems are then delivered and installed in the facility.

Lastly, when a project schedule is accelerated significantly, completing all the preferred paperwork such as User Requirement Specifications (URS) may be difficult. Consider developing an execution approach utilizing interim (draft) documents, that capture the essence of a system, with additional and more particular information to follow.

TRENDS AND FUTURE DEVELOPMENTS

Trends
Over the last two decades, trends in sterile manufacturing facilities include:

- Potent/biological drug matrices
- New filling techniques
- New sterile container types
- Improved environmental system controls
- Virtual modeling of the project
- Modularization
- Harmonization of regulatory bodies

New and More Potent Drug Matrices

As biotechnology and more sophisticated approved pharmaceutical ingredients (APIs) are developed to target specific regions in the body, the need to deliver the drug directly into the body is imperative to its efficacy. Many of these new products, however, are either very delicate or potent and as such require engineers to be far more cognizant of their design for sterile filling of these products. Isolation technologies, highly controlled filling systems, more robust room environments/controls, and better trained operators are but a few of the implications of such new drug developments.

New Filling Techniques

Filling techniques and container types have dominated new trends in sterile manufacturing facilities. New and more accurate filling methods, such as pressure-sensitive filling and syringe filling, have enabled pharmaceutical companies to safely fill vials and containers with new and more delicate drug matrices.

New Sterile Container Types

Additionally, advances in plastics and other material technologies have allowed companies to sterile fill complex bags and containers, as well as actually form and fill a container in one step (referred to as blow-fill-seal).

Improved Environmental System Controls

Minimizing contamination of product exposed to the environment has always been an issue. With the advent of more reliable and sophisticated controls capabilities, the designer is better able to create a system and facility that will work reliably and effectively. Since the actual operating environment is also difficult to predict before it is built, new software developments have enabled designers to create virtual simulations of an actual room condition through computational fluid dynamics (CFD). This technology allows engineers to review how airflow, temperature, and humidity within an environment are projected to behave. This allows designers to make adjustments to the design before it is built, thus improving the chances for a successful operation. This, in combination with more robust and reliable environmental controls systems, has helped to produce more reliable and consistent sterile operations.

Modularization

Applying various levels of modularization in the development of sterile manufacturing facilities has become an increasing trend. Vendors and designers have responded to this trend by developing process unit operations within a skid, as well as offering a modular wall and ceiling panel systems and fully functional process operating modules. From skidded systems to fully developed process

A CFD Image

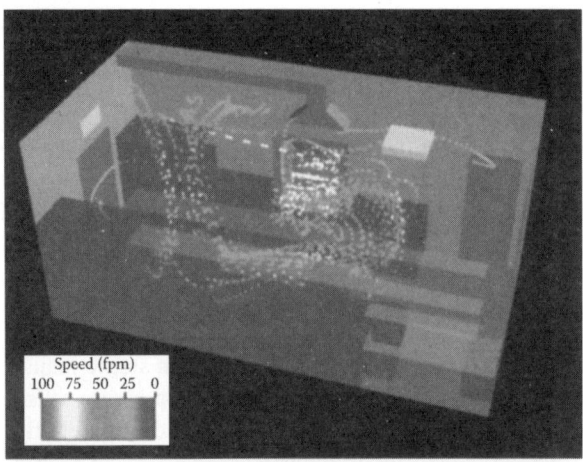

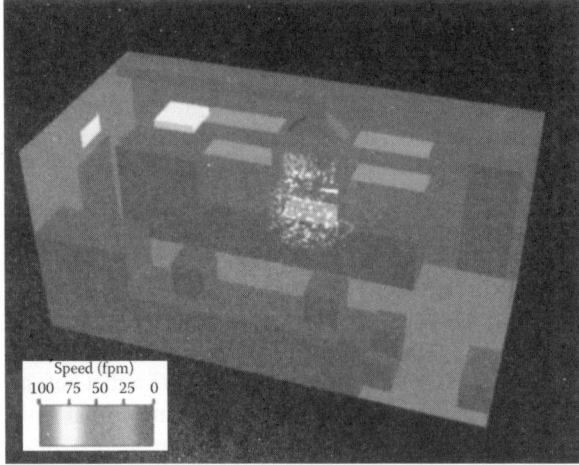

environments, pharmaceutical companies are looking to modularization as a means of improving quality, performance, and even cost and schedule for the development of projects.

Harmonization of Regulatory Agencies

In the past, pharmaceutical companies have typically developed sterile manufacturing facilities to meet only local regulatory compliance guidelines. As product demand broadens across multiple regions, the demand for a sterile manufacturing facility to comply with a variety of different agencies is increasing. Over the past few years, a concerted effort has been made by regional agencies, particularly in the FDA and by the European Commission, to work toward a more unified set of guidelines for sterile manufacturing facilities.

Future Developments

Modularization

As new sterile manufacturing facilities are constructed globally, applying modular concepts will improve the success potential of projects. Where experienced and skilled labor is at a shortage, or where material availability is an issue, modular facility systems provide an excellent solution to a real problem.

· Skidded systems will tend to grow in size, and pharmaceutical companies will continue to look at this idea as a means of leveraging skilled labor working in a more controlled environment to produce a better system. Also, these skids will be better qualified and tested prior to installation in the field, thus improving completion time of a total project.

Standardization

As pharmaceutical companies have grown and expanded operations, some companies have developed different practices and techniques for manufacturing sterile products. This is an issue with regulatory agencies, especially as products are further distributed to many global regions. The need to harmonize operations from location to location will become even more important, since regulatory agencies will look for more consistent operations and practices in sterile manufacturing operations.

Editor's Note: _____

Keep it simple, engage equipment vendors in a project, and utilize proven technology whenever possible.

Harmonization of Regulatory Bodies

The trend for harmonization of regulatory is already in process. Continents like North America, Europe, and others recognize the importance of creating a more unified basis for sterile manufacturing operations, since many products are distributed globally. This trend should continue into the future in order to make new drug products available throughout the global market.

Risk-Based Approach and Risk Management

To assist in the approval process of new drugs and new facility operations, regulatory agencies (particularly the FDA) will employ a new risk-based approach to GMPs. Pharmaceutical companies will become more able to modify a process, or enhance a process at their own risk. Proof of equivalency, safety, and compliance is still necessary, but with this growing trend, companies will be better able to capitalize on new trends in processing and operating technologies.

CONCLUSION

The reality of our profession today is that most people learn how to manage and design a sterile manufacturing facility project through on-the-job training. In this regard, consider this chapter as a starting point for learning the basis practices, guidelines, and drivers behind the development of sterile manufacturing facilities, as well as identifying some of the key issues that must be dealt with in earnest as the project develops. We recommend that this chapter be reviewed in conjunction with the references in the following pages, and particularly:

BIBLIOGRAPHY

Pharmaceutical Engineering Guides for New and Renovated Facilities, Volume 3, Sterile Manufacturing Facilities, First Edition, ISPE Baseline Pharmaceutical Engineering Guide, January 1999.

Guidance for Industry, Sterile Drug Products Produced by Aseptic Processing—Current Good Manufacturing Practice, Draft Guidance, U.S. Food and Drug Administration, August, 2003.

Good Manufacturing Practices for Sterile Pharmaceutical Products, Annex 6, WHO Technical Report Series, No. 902, 2002, World Health Organization.

Bioprocess Equipment, An International Standard, ASME BPE-2002 (Revision of ASME Bpe-1997), The American Society of Mechanical Engineers, 2002.

12
Biotechnology Facilities

Author: Daniel Mariani

Advisor: Jim Dougherty

INTRODUCTION

The fundamentals of biotechnology have been around for a long time. The Egyptians used biotechnology in 4000–2000 B.C. to leaven bread and ferment wine. In 1663, Hooke discovered the existence of the cell. In the mid 1800s proteins and enzymes were discovered and labeled. Penicillin was discovered as an antibiotic in the 1920s. In 1953, Watson and Crick described the double helical structure of DNA, which marked the beginning of the modern era of genetics.

The development of genetic engineering and monoclonal antibody technology started in the early 1970s. It has led to the introduction of a large number of new products with applications in many different areas. The emergence of recombinant DNA, monoclonal antibody, and other such technologies have challenged engineers and scientists to develop the methods and facilities required to manufacture on a commercial scale. Biotechnology encompasses many steps to synthesize, isolate, and formulate the products. There is a great deal of diversity in methods, equipment, and facilities to accomplish this.

In 2002, more than 325 million people worldwide benefited from more than 230 biotech drug products approved by the FDA. More than 350 biotech drug products and vaccines aimed at treating more than 200 diseases are currently in clinical trials.

The field of biotechnology encompasses a wide spectrum of areas such as:

- Large molecule (protein) development and manufacturing
- Vaccines
- Medical diagnostic tests
- Genetically modified agricultural products
- Bio-pesticides
- Environmental products utilizing pollution eating microbes
- Enzyme-based cleaning products
- Human Genome
- DNA fingerprinting

This chapter focuses on the manufacture of large molecule bulk biologics.

REGULATORY OVERVIEW

The US Food and Drug Administration did not approve any biologically derived products between 1975 and 1981. Between 1982 and 1994, there were an average of four product approvals per year. To reverse this trend, an increased focus was placed on development and clinical trial activities resulting in a tremendous increase in FDA approvals.

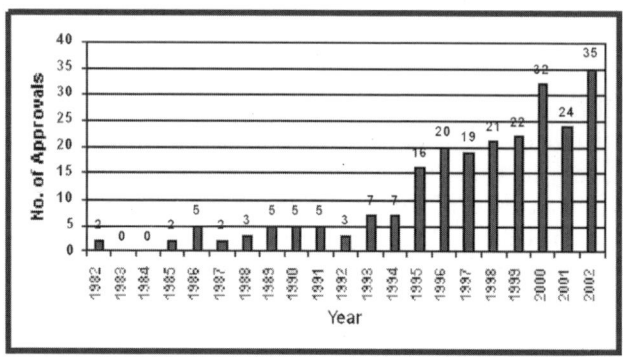

From 1995 to 2002, the average approval rate was 24 products per year. It is expected that in the coming years, more than 50% of therapeutic products will come from biological sources.

The International Society for Pharmaceutical Engineering (ISPE) is in the process of finalizing the *Baseline® Guides for Biologics*, which is intended to guide the industry in the design, construction, and validation of biological facilities. The basic GMP requirements are still governed by the FDA regulations and guidelines that include:

- Umbrella GMPs, 21CFR210 and 211
- Biologics GMPs, 21CFR600 series
- FDA's *Points to Consider for Biologics*
- NIH guidelines for containment

The ISPE *Baseline Guide* is intended to supplement and interpret FDA requirements in terms relevant to the design and operation of biologics facilities. The 1997 Modernization Act of the FDA had a major effect on the design of biological facilities. In an effort to streamline the approval process, the Center for Biologics Evaluation and Research (CBER) abolished the Product License Application (PLA) and Establishment License Application (ELA), and replaced these applications with a single Biologics License Application (BLA). In general, this has two major implications for biologics manufacturing. First, the commercial license is now attached to the product rather than the facility. A product can now be developed in one location and be manufactured in another provided that the manufacturing process remains unchanged. Second, the overall approval process is shortened considerably by eliminating the lengthy and time-consuming ELA filing.

As the biotechnology industry has matured, so has the FDA's treatment of "well characterized" products. Since most biologic products are made by methods that are not as precise as those in chemical synthesis, the FDA has exercised great caution toward approving changes in process, equipment, or manufacturing location. This has stifled innovation and efficiency improvement because the FDA has always required rigorous proof that manufacturing changes have not altered the product in any way. The FDA has agreed to treat some "well characterized" biologics that have been on the market for a long time similar to drugs, particularly small molecule biologics, allowing for flexibility in design. These changes have been positive for the industry; total design, construction, validation, and product delivery time have been reduced.

KEY CONCEPTS AND PRINCIPLES

Materials

According to the Code of Federal Regulations (21 CFR 211.80), raw materials and components used in pharmaceutical manufacturing must be received, stored, and handled in a manner designed to prevent damage, contamination, and any other adverse effects. Incoming materials must be treated and handled according to approved written procedures and current industry standards. Batch integrity must be maintained from beginning to end, and record keeping begins with the Certificate of Analysis delivered with each shipment. All incoming materials and components must be treated as "quarantined" until proper sampling, inspection, testing, and release can be carried out by in-house personnel. For this reason, receiving and warehouse areas must be designed with adequate space and security measures to separate quarantined materials and materials under test from those released for use.

In order to facilitate raw material sampling, it is recommended to include a Sampling Room adjacent to the warehouse with a laminar flow curtained area and stainless steel workbenches. Quality Control personnel can then take representative test samples in a controlled environment without having to move large material containers to an appropriate testing lab.

In addition, most biotechnology production facilities include an area for storage of their Master and Working Cell Banks. These cell banks—the most valuable raw material in any facility—are stored in several liquid nitrogen dewars or ultra-low temperature freezers. Daily monitoring of nitrogen levels and/or freezer temperature is required, and access is limited. Elaborate alarm systems and video surveillance of the cell bank storage area maintain a high level of security 24 hours a day.

Inoculation

At the start of a production run or campaign, material is taken from the Working Cell Bank and thawed. These cells are slowly and carefully re-suspended and cultured in the laboratory until there is sufficient cell density to scale-up to spinner flasks. These spinners are then transferred to an inoculum prep room in the production area, to prepare for large-scale fermentation operations. Inoculum prep rooms universally require controlled access, bio-safety hoods, incubators (supplied with CO_2 if necessary), and adequate bench space for manual operations. The cell growth patterns are characterized and their volume is increased until enough material is available to inoculate a small production-scale bioreactor. Seed bioreactors can be 5% to 30% of their large-scale counterparts, and are usually purchased as a skid system with self-contained controls and hose connections for utilities. Depending upon the cell line, one or two seed reactors (with increasing volume) are necessary to grow the cells to sufficient density for production scale operations. Inoculm generation is labor intensive and many commercial operations are operated on a semi-continuous mode to alleviate this step for every batch.

Fermentation/Bioreactor

Large-scale production is accomplished in large bioreactors, a term that is often used synonymously with fermentor. Industry convention dictates that the term "fermentation" be used for cultivation of single-celled organisms (bacteria and yeast), while "cell culture" is reserved for bioreactor batches of multi-cellular organisms (plants, insects, and mammals).

Mammalian cells are very delicate and typically larger than their microbial/bacterial counterparts. They are heat and shear sensitive, requiring the bioreactor to have strict temperature and agitation control. Low shear equipment must be employed when mixing or moving broth from once vessel to another as care must be taken to avoid destruction of the organisms. Many installations employ nitrogen overpressure when transferring live cells from seed to production reactors to avoid the potential destructive effects of pumps. However, peristaltic pumps are proven to be a mechanically effective means of fluid transport with little danger of contamination. Bacterial cells, in contrast, are very hardy and can withstand vigorous agitation and pumping forces. Rather than strict temperature control, heat removal is the problem, and must be properly accounted for when designing fermentor jackets and temperature control mechanisms. Also, tight control of parameters such as pH, gases (oxygen, carbon dioxide, nitrogen, etc.), nutrient feed, etc. are required.

The growth rate of mammalian cells is very slow compared to bacteria. Depending upon the cell line, it can take more than ten hours to double the number of mammalian cells in culture compared to approximately one-half hour for bacteria. Cell culture runs can be from ten days up to several months. Because mammalian cells express their products outside the cell walls, it is possible to run cell culture in continuous perfusion mode. Cells are kept and regenerated inside the bioreactor while product is continuously withdrawn for several days, weeks, or months.

3000 L Bioreactor

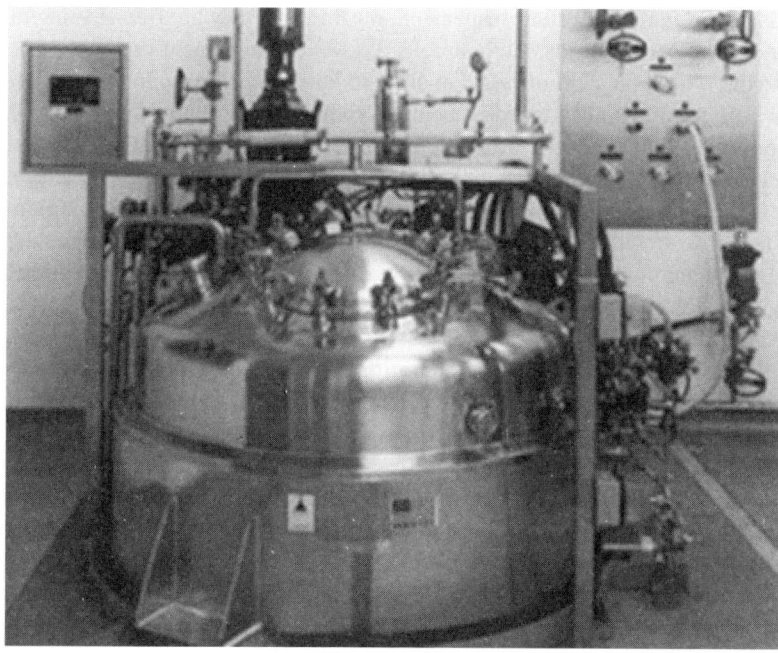

Specific measures must be taken in the bioreactor design when operating in the perfusion mode. For example, perfusion reactors usually withdraw product from the top of the bioreactor where the cell density is lowest. They often contain or utilize proprietary settling devices to keep the cells contained within the reactor as product is withdrawn. Continuous perfusion presents the most technically complicated design scenario, as the equipment must be maintained in sterile operation for many weeks, and the product harvest vessels must be kept within the sterile boundary. Many details must be considered when designing for continuous perfusion vs. batch mode.

Stirred Tank Reactor

Cell culture has occurred in stirred tank reactors in a batch mode for years. Stirred tank reactor technology for mammalian cell culture has benefited from the experience and knowledge gained from the traditional and reliable fermentation industry. Stirred tank reactors are typically used in a batch, semi-continuous, or continuous (perfusion) mode. In batch mode the entire contents of the bioreactor is sent to harvest/capture each batch. In the semi-continuous mode, most, not all, of the contents of the bioreactor are sent to harvest leaving a portion of the batch to re-inoculate the next batch. The continuous mode usually utilizes a perfusion system. These systems are based on techniques that retain the cells inside the reactor while continuously perfusing fresh medium into the reactor and continuously harvesting product and spent medium at a similar rate.

Roller Bottles

Some cells do not function well in suspension, regardless if they are free-floating or attached to micro-carrier beads. Certain cells, known as attachment cells, must be attached to the wall of the culture vessel in order to function properly. In these cases, bioreactor cell culture is abandoned in favor of roller bottle culture. Small (1 to 2 liter) roller bottles, with serrated walls to maximize the wall surface area, are used as mini-bioreactors and function much the same way. Unique to roller bottle culture, however, is the lack of controls for automated gas sparging and nutrient addition. Each bottle must be manipulated manually (or by automated robot) to change out the harvest supernatant for fresh media. Here, cells continue to grow and multiply, having their own "doubling time," and the number of roller bottles may increase 16-fold as the run progresses.

Facility design for a roller bottle operation differs from a large-scale bioreactor facility only in the layout of the fermentation area. Large scale bioreactor suites are replaced by warm-rooms in which to keep the racks of bottles and robots (if desired) to manipulate the bottles during a campaign. Downstream purification operations can be treated similarly for each of the two designs; however, roller bottles tend to yield fermentation products requiring more purification steps.

T-Flask Cell Culture

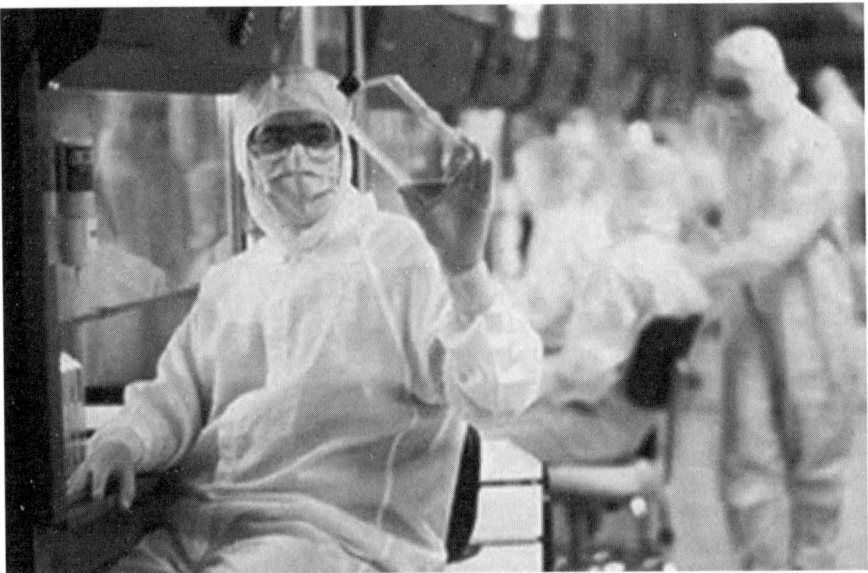

Harvest /Filtration

Harvest and filtration operations occur immediately after fermentation. Harvest vessels are the first step in separating the product from all of the other materials in the bioreactor. Impurities such as carryover cells, cell debris, and nutrient media components are removed through various filtration and centrifugation methods, depending on the product. The figure below illustrates a typical biologics unit operation and details the difference between mammalian cell culture (extracellular) and bacterial fermentation (intracellular). With most products derived from bacterial fermentation, the products are intracellular, remaining trapped within the bacterial cell walls. In order to obtain and purify the product, the cell walls must be ruptured via the use of homogenization or other techniques. Separation of the desired product from the broth then becomes more difficult because of the cell wall debris. Fermentation via cell culture, although inherently more difficult due to the delicate nature of mammalian cells, is much easier in downstream processing because the products are expressed outside the cell walls.

Typical Biologic Unit Operation

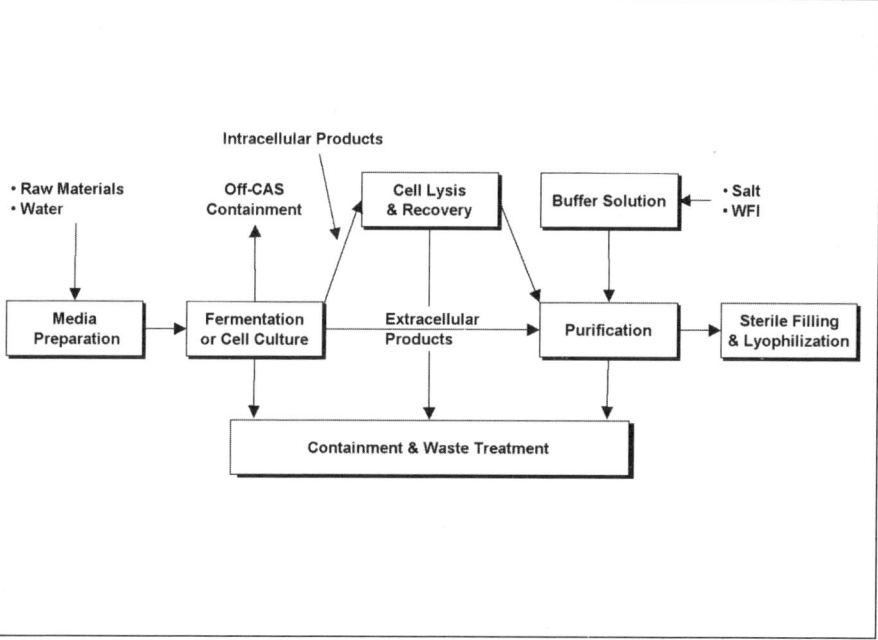

The product undergoes primary and sterile filtration steps between harvest and capture vessels in order to establish a baseline starting point for downstream purification operations. Centrifuges, homogenizers, micro-filtration systems, dead-end filters, and chromatography unit operations are utilized to achieve the initial recovery step. Often, product material is stored and frozen to await sterility, purity, and other testing prior to release for downstream processing.

Purification

Most products in a biotechnology facility are proteins, which are heat sensitive. In order to minimize potential degradation problems, and minimize product bioburden, purification operations are carried out between 4°C and 8°C. These temperatures are achieved by processing in cold rooms or in jacketed vessels.

Purification operations normally involve concentrating the product as well as purifying it. Concentration is most easily achieved via high pressure ultrafiltration (UF), which can result in a 10X concentration with very little loss of product. Other common purification steps involve pH adjustment and buffer exchange through diafiltration. Microfiltration (MF), UF, and diafiltration are generally used as preparatory steps for column chromatography. Column chromatography, whether via size exclusion, ion-exchange, or affinity methods, purify the products by either binding it or the impurities to the column resin. The bulk product can then be eluted off the column or rinsed through the column into appropriate containers to await final formulation and finishing.

There are several considerations for the proper design of a purification system:

- Design for sterile and pyrogen free product
- Sanitary design of equipment and piping
- Controlled environment rooms with specific particulate calssifications
- Heat and shear sensitivity of product requiring 4°C rooms and low shear pumps and agitators
- Support systems (WFI, buffer solutions, CIP)

There are many different types of purification systems including:

- Ultrafiltration, microfiltration, and diafiltration
- Gel filtration chromatography (based on size)
- Ion exchange chromatography (based on charge)
- Affinity chromatography (based on affinity or "lock and key")
- Hydrophobic chromatography (based on hydrophobic nature)
- Sterile filtration to obtain sterile bulk product

Bulk Fill

Many biotech facilities produce only bulk materials and ship the product to another facility for formulation and dosage form preparation. Due to the high cost of filling equipment and the high value of the product, special care must be taken when designing a filling suite. Operations are carried out under laminar flow, in Class 100, fully HEPA-filtered processing suites. Access to the room is limited during filling operations to minimize disturbance in the air flow patterns and to minimize contamination risk from personnel. Protein products are heat and shear sensitive and cannot be terminally heat sterilized; therefore, they must be sterile filtered. All components including tanks, lines, filters, and filling equipment must be separately heat sterilized. The components that are exposed to the product are assembled under laminar flow. The product is filled in vials in filling machines and partially stoppered with special stoppers, ready for lyophilization.

Media and Buffer Preparation

When considering the design of a large-scale manufacturing facility, support functions such as media and buffer preparation are critical. There are many factors to consider when designing the support spaces for these critically central operations. If large-scale vessels are to be used, their size and number will depend greatly on the number of required solutions. If the facility is multi-product, a greater number of different mixtures are likely to be required than for a single product facility.

Additionally, in a multi-product facility, there are likely to be many different permutations of the production schedule creating variable demand for these services. The media and buffer support functions cannot be a bottleneck for continued facility operation, and must be designed with flexibility in mind. An adequate number of vessels must be available at all times for solution preparation, sterile filtration, and storage, allowing for adequate turnaround time to clean and sterilize between batches. Solutions cannot be stored indefinitely, and the media/buffer preparation schedules must be coordinated so that sterile solutions are used before they expire.

Small-scale production facilities may choose to purchase ready-to-use media and/or buffers in bags in lieu of the capital investment. This approach is only practical when the number of different solutions required is few. The capital equipment expenditure on stainless steel vessels and filters is eliminated; however, the facility operating and raw material costs are increased. Rather than space for cleaning, storage, and operation of support vessels, cold room space must be designed for long-term storage of media and buffer bags.

FACILITY DESIGN

Biotechnology operations have changed dramatically over the last ten years. Biological operations have gone from being performed in small batches in bioreactors of 1000 liters to continuous operations with bioreactors of 20,000 liters and larger. Along with this transformation has been the gradual movement from all processing spaces being in controlled/classified environments, to maximizing the use of non-controlled or "gray" space.

The design of large-scale bulk biopharmaceutical manufacturing facilities requires the integration of fully developed processing operations with an appropriate environment ensuring compliance with all applicable building, safety, hygiene, and environmental regulations.

Layout and Adjacencies

Product, personnel, and material flow are important issues in any facility design. In cGMP pharmaceutical facilities, they are critical. Every step of the process must be analyzed to ensure unidirectional flow and eliminate any potential possibility of cross contamination. The facility conceptual layout must be carefully considered to mirror the flow of materials and product, and to allow personnel to access the process and exit the area without retracing their own footsteps, as shown in a typical people and material flow diagram. Strict gowning protocols must be adhered to and material must be placed in pass-through airlocks and wiped down before continuing into clean areas. Strict care must be taken so that incoming raw materials and exiting waste products do not cross paths with final product leaving the building. In addition, all products must be strictly segregated to avoid potential contamination mishaps. Step-by-step detailed flow diagrams are an integral part of all submissions for FDA, CBER, and CDER facility reviews.

Material storage and warehousing issues become increasingly more important as the processes are scaled-up and the quantities of raw materials increase. A well-planned biopharmaceutical facility must take into consideration all of the various materials that will be maintained in inventory and the various methods of storage required. Incoming raw materials must be isolated and tested for quality control before being released for general use. Some materials have specific temperature sensitivity that require refrigerated storage or freezers. Large quantities of flammable liquids must be isolated in separate storage areas that meet the requirements of the building and fire codes. In addition, waste solvents must also be contained, isolated, and potentially stored for pick-up by a waste removal company.

Final product storage must allow for quarantine and release areas for final quality testing and provide security for the product as well. A local quality control testing lab is required if the warehouse is remote from the general laboratories of the facility. Also, a large general storage area for the hundreds of small items required to support the process and the gowning/cleaning protocols must be included. Finally, sufficient office space must be provided for warehouse personnel and for Quality Assurance to handle the volumes of paperwork generated by the controlled tracking of all these materials.

Product and material flow provide the foundation for detailed facility design. Key layout design criteria associated with the developed material flow and building layout include:

- Adequate staging and access
- Containment (for both product and personnel)
- Direct and sequential flow, minimizing unnecessary rerouting, movements, and distances
- Minimal material handling steps

Along with an efficient process, an efficient facility design is also very important. Some of the general design considerations for a facility are as follows.

- Layout
- Airlocks
- Building codes, e.g., Americans with Disabilities Act (ADA)
- Clean and dirty corridors
- Gowning and degowning areas
- Material handling

- Mechanical/utility rooms
- Process suites–functional areas
- Shipping/receiving
- Support areas (toilets, locker rooms, etc.)
- Vertical or horizontal manufacturing
- Warehousing

Cost effective space utilization and minimization of classified areas:

- Unidirectional people and material flow
- Allocation for access of future equipment
- People circulation for good interaction
- Architectural finishes for controlled areas
- Surface finishes to be smooth, cleanable, and impervious to sanitizing solutions
- Surface material to be resistant to chipping, flaking, and oxidizing
- Floors to be sloped, coved, and sealed
- Floor material can be epoxy or terrazzo
- Windows and doors should be flushed to the inside of room
- In heavy traffic areas (e.g., corridors), bumper guards should be installed on the walls
  Waste flows
- Hazardous wastes
- Non-product wastes
- Product wastes

Ease of Maintenance

Ease of maintenance is a key component of any facility design. Many of the same issues that affect the design of a product development center are even more important when applied to the design of the manufacturing facility. An FDA-regulated facility presents special challenges in operations and maintenance because of restrictions in the movement of personnel in and out of classified areas, gowning requirements, and interference with operations in clean rooms. Some of the considerations for maintenance design are as follows.

Interstitial Space

Clean rooms have interstitial space above the room to house large volume HVAC ducts. By providing walkable ceilings and increasing clear height so that personnel can stand erect, this space can be used for a number of maintenance functions such as the changeout of HEPA filters and the service of piping and valves without disruption to the clean space below. Also, instruments can be housed in this space to get them out of the process areas where possible. The benefit of utilizing interstitial space is that maintenance personnel access this area without special gowning.

Gray Area (Service Chase) Maintenance

For a highly piped area such as a solution prep room, an adjoining room can be designated as a non-classified area in order to house the piping valves, control valves, and instruments that are not required for operation in the clean room (below). A gray space/corridor running along the processing area can house a large amount of distribution piping above as well. This reduces clutter inside the clean rooms and allows maintenance from outside the clean environment.

Gray Area Maintenance

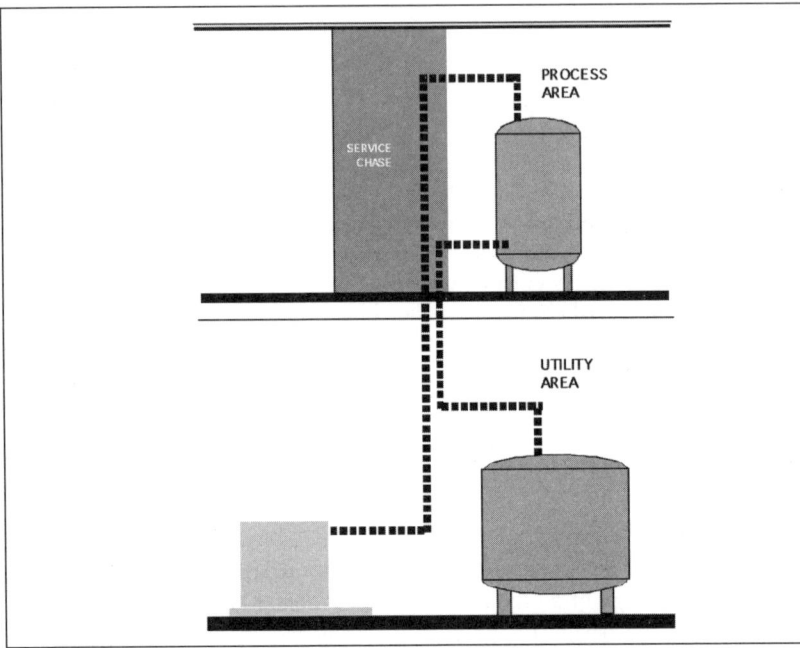

Finishes

Wall materials must be washable and durable enough to withstand years of cleaning regimens with various industrial disinfectants. Appropriate materials may include PVC, descoglass, epoxy paint on plaster/gypsum board, and stainless steel for wet areas (washing and steaming). Ceilings materials may include epoxy paint on plaster/gypsum board or suspended systems with mylar-faced ceiling panels, heavy aluminum grid, and gaskets to hold room pressure. Floor material may include epoxy terrazzo systems, troweled on epoxy, or sheet vinyl systems. Windows and doors should be flush to the inside of room. In heavy traffic areas (e.g., corridors), bumper guards should be installed on the walls.

HVAC System Design

The most critical parameters for process rooms are temperature, humidity, and airborne contaminants. HVAC cGMP requirements for room pressurization, particulate control, dilution ventilation, recovery time from upset, relative humidity, cooling and heating, and direction of flow between rooms are critical.

The cost associated with cGMP compliance of HVAC may be reduced by the use of other technologies such as containment isolation or utilizing closed processing systems. Other technical concerns regarding HVAC systems are:

- Dust collection
- Cross contamination via air handling systems
- Monitoring for both particulate and organism growth
- Ventilation for hazardous environments
- Recirculated vs. once-through air systems
- Ductwork
  Leak tight
  Materials
  Pressure rating
- Filtration
- Cleaning and maintenance

HVAC strategies are a critical component of technical facility design. Strict control of the air flow in and out of the process and research areas is required to maintain verifiable quality control and eliminate the possibilities of cross contamination. cGMP guidelines require classified clean room conditions and control for the pharmaceutical process. HEPA filtered air must be provided to reduce air borne contaminants. The table below indicates the various typical clean room classifications required.

Required Clean Room Classifications

Specific Process Step	US 209 E 1992	Room Classification EEC cGmp 1989	ISO EN 14644-1 1999
Fermation & Upstream			
Processes including Media and Buffer Prep	Class 100,000	D or C	8
Purification	Class 10,000	C	7
Product Filling and Lyophilization	Class (at rest)	B	5
Actual Point of Fill	Class 100 (at work)	A	5

During filling operations, Class 100 laminar flow clean air is required because the product is at its most exposed point in the production process. HEPA filters directly above the filling station direct air downward, and the air is removed from the room at floor level to prevent air borne contaminants.

A variety of air pressure strategies are used to isolate areas and processes depending on the design intent of the facility.

For cGMP compliant pharmaceutical facilities, the intention is to eliminate cross contamination of the product. Therefore, the highest air pressure is used in the process or production spaces. Lower air pressure in the airlocks and corridors ensures that the air flow is always away from the product thereby guaranteeing a high quality environment for the production spaces.

In biotechnology or high potency/toxic applications, the design intent is often to isolate a particular biohazard to protect laboratory and operations personnel. In this case, it is important to keep the actual process area negative to all surrounding areas to eliminate the possibility of spreading the hazard. Higher pressure in the surrounding airlocks and corridors effectively contains the hazard to the production space in the event of leakage. In some cases, isolation chambers may be employed to further isolate personnel from the hazards.

For these situations, these two opposing requirements are often at odds with each other. It may be necessary to both protect the product from cross contamination and protect the occupants from exposure to the product or process. In this case, it is the intermediate airlock that is given the highest pressure so that air flows toward the corridor to reduce airborne particulate contamination and toward the process areas to eliminate hazardous contamination of the adjacent spaces. Again, process isolation chambers can further reduce the risks for critical processes.

DETAILS AND IMPLICATIONS

Principals of Segregation and Flow

The design of a biotech manufacturing facility is highly dependent on the method of operation the facility is expected to perform. Many facilities are designed for a single product and are optimized around a single set of operations. Many facilities are designed for multi-product operation. Within the single product vs. multi-product operations issues there lies a need to determine the level of segregation. Within this section, the design implications of each scenario are addressed.

Basic Biotech Manufacturing

The basic processing flow for a biotech manufacturing facility is shown in Figure 1. As shown, raw materials enter through a warehouse and then flow through the process via solutions preparation, upstream processing, downstream processing, and, ultimately, exiting through the controlled warehouse.

Single Product/Minimal Segregation

Figure 2 depicts a single product facility layout where minimal segregation is required. As shown the entire upstream processing (inoculum preparation, cell culture,. Harvesting, Recovery) rare performed in a one common area. This concept provides for very efficient use of space, but requires cleaning of the entire suite before the inoculum for the subsequent batch is prepared. Similarly the downstream processing area (crude and final purification, bulk formulation) is performed in a common space. This too is a highly efficient use of the space, but has its drawbacks for the processing more than one batch at a time.

FIGURE 1 Basic Processing Flow

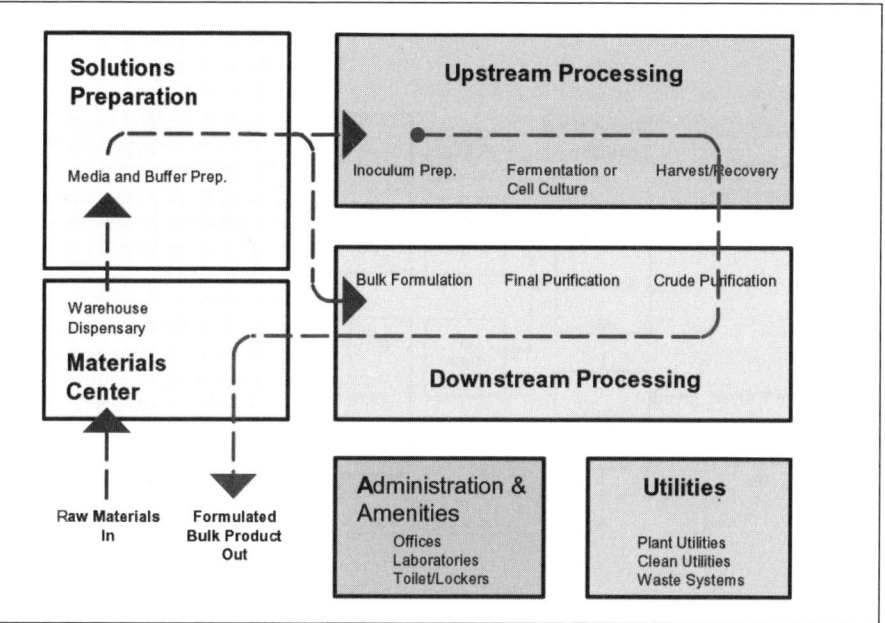

FIGURE 2 Single Product/Minimal Segregation

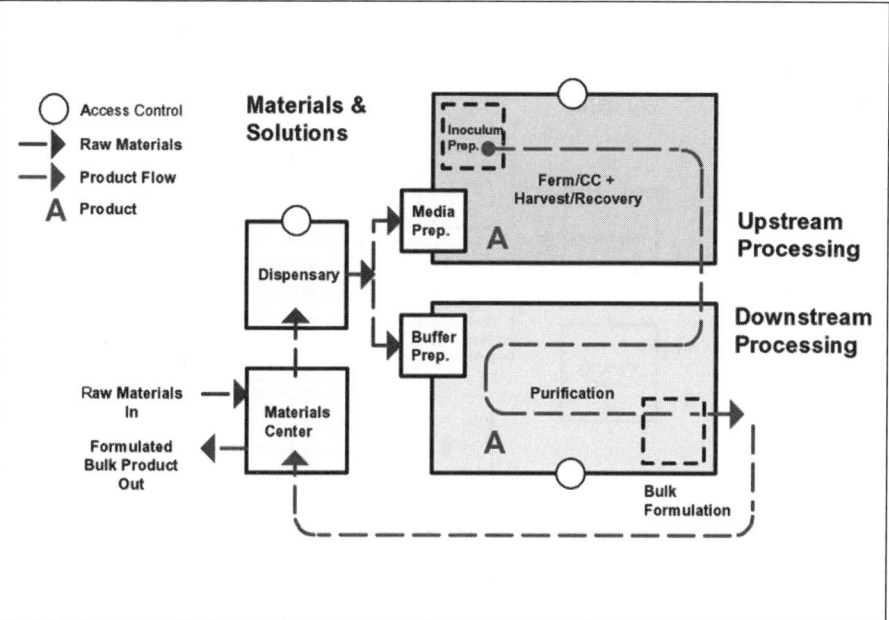

FIGURE 3   Multi-Product/Minimal Segregation

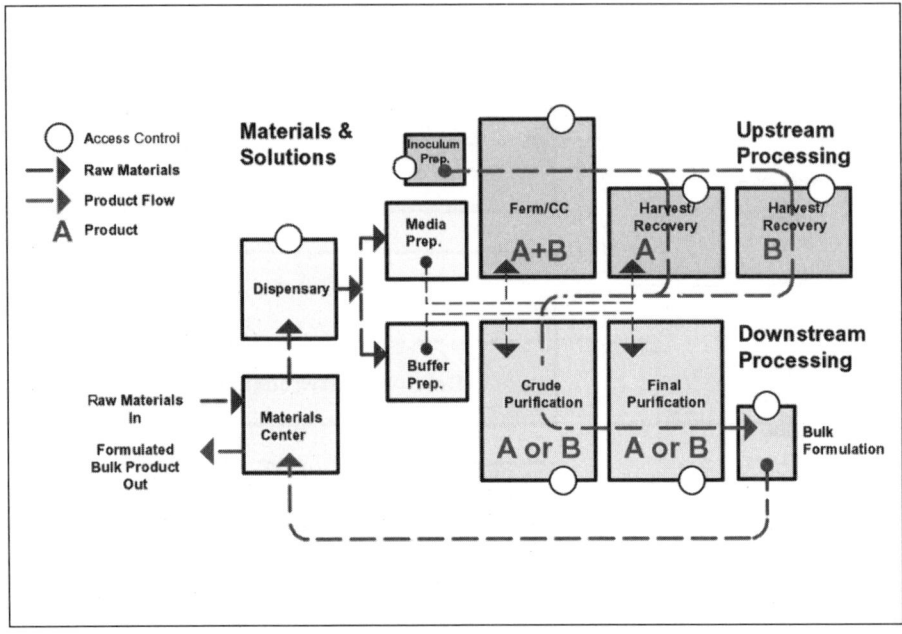

FIGURE 4   Separate Upstream and Downstream Processing

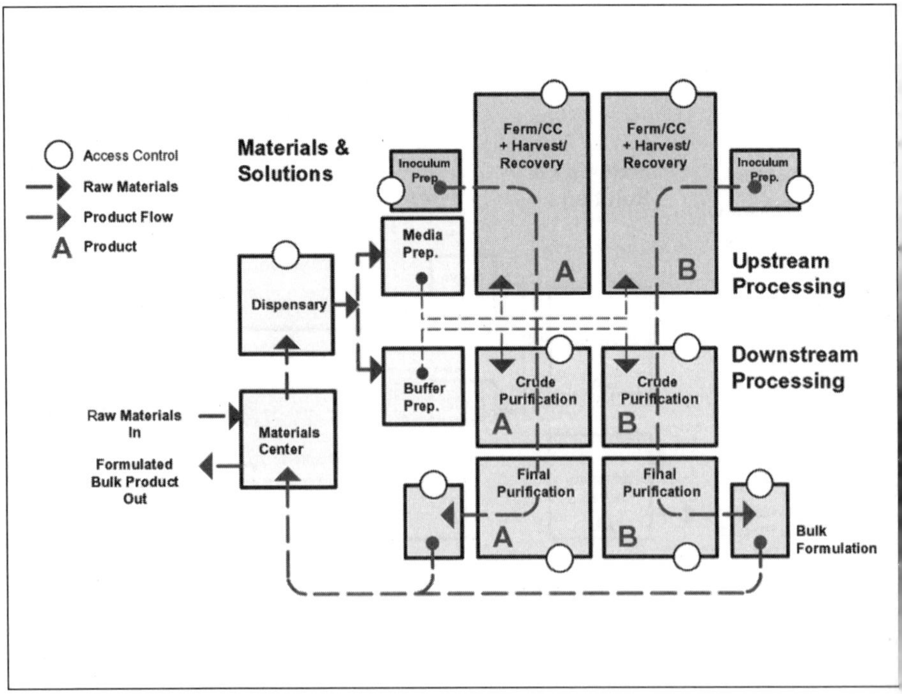

FIGURE 5 Common Fermentation/Cell Culture Areas

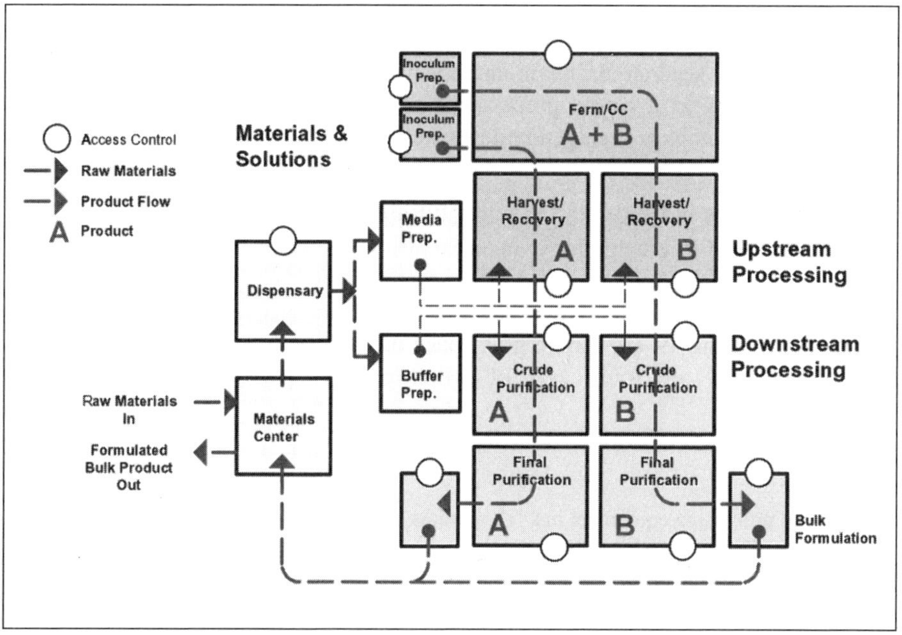

Single Product/Moderate Segregation

In a moderate segregation scenario, there are some key differences to the minimal segregation scheme. Within the upstream processing area the inoculum preparation area is segregated from the upstream area. This allows the inoculum preparation to be performed for the next batch while a current batch is in process. In the downstream processing area, the key differences are with the segregation crude and final purification as well as bulk formulation. The dedicated areas for these operations with separate personnel access allows the operation increased flexibility, as well as operation of each area during different batches.

Multi-Product/Minimal Segregation

Many new facilities require the flexibility to operate within a multi-product environment. This flexibility poses segregation challenges to the facility designer. The challenge is to segregate the different product manufacturing. Even minimal segregation involves a much more complex layout with multiple areas or suites. In this layout, the fermentation is performed in a common area with the assumption that this operation is performed in a closed system and therefore does not require segregation (Fig. 3). Harvesting will require segregation to give multiple product flexibility to the downstream processing. The downstream processing can be common, similar to the single product moderate segregation mode, since the downstream processing typically is performed in a less time per batch than upstream.

Multi-product/Moderate Segregation

A multi-product/moderate segregation has common support functions such as media and buffer preparation, but completely segregated production trains (Fig. 4). Some systems entirely separate upstream and downstream processing; others have slight variations where, in a closed process, the fermentation/cell culture areas can be common with complete segregation downstream.

Closed Systems in Controlled Manufacturing Space

As the cost of biotechnology manufacturing facilities have increased, the industry has been moving toward incorporating more "gray space" into facility layouts. Gray space is defined as space where operations can occur in non-controlled environments. Designing gray space into facilities is not always straightforward. Below are four cases of utilizing gray space, from minimum to maximum.

Case 1
- All processing equipment in a "clean room"
- Sampling of vessels performed in "classified" environment
- All equipment subject to cleaning, maintenance, and changeover is within a "gowned" environment

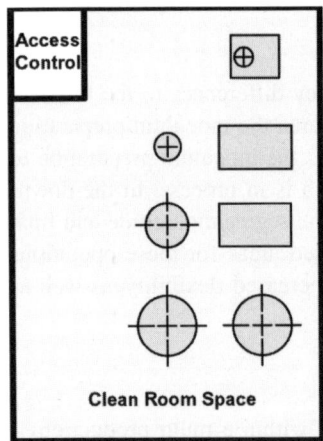

Case 2
- Most processing equipment in a "clean room"
- Sampling of vessels performed in "classified" environment
- Most equipment subject to cleaning, maintenance, and changeover is within a "gowned" environment

- Some "closed" equipment in "controlled unclassified" space
- Clean room envelope is reduced, architectural finishes and life cycle cost of environmental maintenance reduced

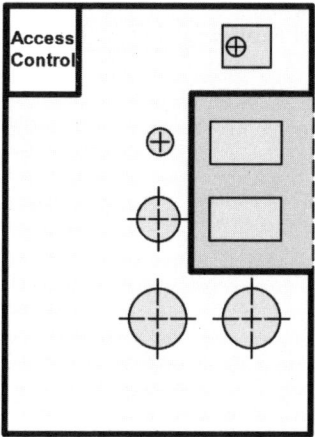

Case 3

- Some processing equipment in a "clean room"
- Sampling of vessels performed in "classified" environment
- Most equipment subject to cleaning, maintenance, and changeover is outside the "gowned" environment
- Most "closed" equipment in "controlled unclassified" space
- Clean room envelope is reduced, architectural finishes and life cycle cost of environmental maintenance reduced

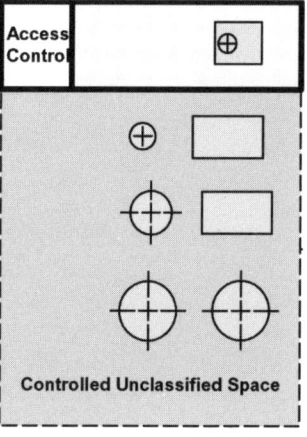

Case 4

- Minimum processing equipment in a "clean room"
- "Closed" sampling of vessels performed in "controlled unclassified" environment
- Most equipment subject to cleaning, maintenance, and changeover is outside the "gowned" environment
- All "closed" equipment in "controlled unclassified" space
- Clean room envelope is greatly reduced, architectural finished and life cycle cost of environmental maintenance is greatly reduced

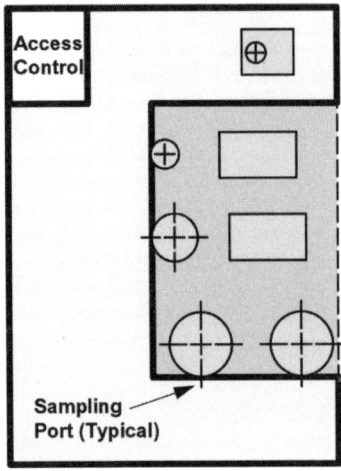

TRENDS

The biologics industry is an ever evolving as the industry matures. Some of the more recent areas/technologies to watch for are: bag/disposable reactors, larger cell culture reactor sizes, flexibility, and gray space.

13

API Facilities

Authors: David Barr
                Miguel Montalvo

Advisors: John Dubeck
                Eric Sipe

INTRODUCTION

What Are APIs?

Active pharmaceutical ingredients (APIs) are defined as:

> Any substance or mixture of substances intended to be used in the manufacture of a drug (medicinal) product and that, when used in the production of a drug, becomes an active ingredient of the drug product. Such substances are intended to furnish pharmacological activity or other direct effect in the diagnosis, cure, mitigation, treatment, or prevention of disease or to affect the structure and function of the body. (*ICH Q7A*)

In reality APIs are chemicals or biochemicals that are used to improve health, reduce pain, sustain life, or perform a medical diagnosis. These materials are produced by chemical or biochemical processes in non-contaminating equipment and/or systems. These chemicals or biochemicals are used to produce final dosage form pharmaceutical products such as tablets, capsules, sterile liquid-filled vials, sterile powder-filled vials, sterile fluid-filled bottles, therapeutic ointments and balms, etc. The quality and properties of APIs can have a significant impact on the successful manufacture of final dosage form pharmaceutical products; therefore, the creation and purification of these chemical entities is regulated by the Food and Drug Administration (FDA) and requires adherence to current Good Manufacturing Practices (cGMPs). Additionally, the manufacturing and purification processes for these materials must ensure that the API product is not contaminated or otherwise adulterated. Excipients, non-active chemicals, and non-active biochemicals are also used in the production of final dosage form drug products and thus their manufacture may also be regulated by the FDA and require adherence to cGMPs.

Under the Federal Food, Drug, and Cosmetic Act, a drug (which includes the final dosage form as well as APIs and excipients) is considered adulterated if the

313

facilities or controls used for its manufacture, processing, packing, and holding do not conform to cGMPs. [a]However, it was not until early to mid-1990s that GMP regulatory requirements began to be effectively focused and applied on bulk pharmaceutical operations and production of APIs. Within the last decade, we have seen the development of various regulatory guidance documents and, most recently, the International Conference on Harmonization (ICH) Q7A Guidance for Industry. With the establishment and discussion of the industry's standard practices, the topic of API facilities design and construction is now becoming an important area of interest.

The quality and attributes of an API can have a critical effect on the quality of the finished drug product, therefore, it is not surprising that the focus has been shifted to include the predecessor processes and the production of the bulk APIs. The design and construction of the API manufacturing facility will have a substantial impact on the capability to produce a product that will "consistently meet its predetermined specifications." Aspects such as environmental controls, personnel and equipment flow, maintenance and cleaning feasibilities, utility systems service quality, location and distribution of piping, and process separation/product segregation must be considered during the design of such facilities to ensure quality and efficiency and avoid unnecessary complications.

In addition to ensuring the production of quality drug products, facilities for the production of APIs must also be designed to ensure that the appropriate environmental regulations are met by properly treating and disposing of solid, liquid, and gaseous waste byproducts from the API manufacturing process, and by preventing spills and other possible contaminations. The design must also ensure the safety of the personnel who work in API manufacturing facilities by providing ergonomically sound work processes, adequate walking and working areas, suitable means of egress, suitable means for materials handling and storage, suitable guarding of machinery, an appropriate work environment for the various operations being performed, and appropriate fire and explosion protection.

There are many different of types of API facilities. The makeup of an API facility will depend on each of the following: 1) the type of API product; 2) the manufacturing process associated with the API product; 3) the type and configuration of the process equipment; 4) the unit operations required to synthesize, purify, dry, and size the API product; and 5) the required API quality attributes and other API properties such as corrosivity, flowability, bulk density, etc. This chapter discusses the different types of facilities and the design, construction, commissioning, and qualification implications for each. This chapter, discusses those related to the areas identified in the ICH Q7A Guidance for Industry as the buildings and facilities used "in the receipt of materials, manufacture, processing, packing, labeling,

---

[a]In order to prevent API products from being considered adulterated the API manufacturer must have a defined and defensible process for manufacturing, testing, packing, and storing each of these products and must continuously prove compliance and adherence to these defined processes. In developing defined and defensible processes, the API manufacturer will be well served by looking at the viable risks to the API product or its precursors throughout the manufacturing process and by implementing safeguards into the manufacturing proceess to ensure that any viable risks are avoided.

quality control, release, storage, and distribution of APIs." We also include the requirements for areas used for the sampling and testing of APIs and related materials, as well as areas used for the cleaning, maintenance and or storage of manufacturing equipment.

Regulatory Background

While the production of APIs are, to a degree, the manufacture of chemicals, there are considerable additional regulatory burdens imposed on the production of APIs as they are an integral part of pharmaceuticals and there must be strict controls over the potential of contaminants and cross-contaminants in the API. Therefore the design of an API facility must not contribute to any potential contamination of the API. This often includes the use of physical barriers and the use of area controls to create various levels of protection for the materials being manufactured. API manufacturing is pervasively regulated by local codes, EPA effluent and exhaust limitations, OSHA concerns, and by the regulations promulgated by the Food and Drug Administration (FDA).

Under the Food, Drug, and Cosmetic Act (FDC Act), the manufacturing of APIs must be in conformance with "Current Good Manufacturing Practices" The FDC Act does not provide specifics on what cGMPs require; however, the FDA promulgated regulations defining cGMP requirements for pharmaceutical dosage forms in 1962 and in 1978 (see 21 CFR §§210, 211). In the preamble to the 1978 cGMPs, the FDA stated that these regulations should also be used as a guideline in the manufacture of bulk pharmaceutical chemicals (BPCs), a term which includes both APIs and excipients. Subsequently, the FDA issued several draft guidelines on cGMPs, which addressed the manufacture of BPCs and APIs. The ICH issued its GMP guidance for the manufacture of APIs in 2001, [Q7A Good Manufacturing Practice Guidance for Active Pharmaceutical Ingredients (ICH Q7A)]. ICH is an international collaboration; members include the United States FDA, the Pharmaceutical Inspectorate of Japan, the European Medicines Evaluation Agency (EMEA), and the corresponding industry organizations of these regions including PhRMA. The ICH Q7A was adopted as an official FDA guidance document in the Federal Register, Vol. 66, No. 186 in September 25, 2001. From a pragmatic standpoint, ICH Q7A is currently the primary document providing guidance on cGMP requirements for APIs. This document, like the other cGMP guides before it, has sections that speak directly to facilities as well as sections that address the activities within the facilities.

The key concept to remember in designing API facilities from a cGMP standpoint is that pharmaceutical facilities, processing systems, and packaging equipment must be protective of the drugs manufactured, packaged, labeled, held, or distributed within them. They must be designed to minimize the potential for contamination, alteration, or adulteration of APIs and must use materials of construction that are compatible with the drug products manufactured. They must provide adequate space for the various operations performed, including sufficient space for the cleaning and maintenance of the facility and equipment.

KEY CONCEPTS AND PRINCIPLES

Key Terms

The industry and FDA utilize a number of terms in API manufacturing. Many of these terms reflect the production stage and many refer to the regulatory status of the material. A few of these key terms are listed below:

API Starting Material: "A raw material, intermediate, or an API that is used in the production of an API and that is incorporated as a significant structural fragment into the structure of the API." (*ICH Q7A*)

Intermediate: "A material produced during steps of the processing of an API that undergoes further molecular change or purification before it becomes an API. Intermediates may or may not be isolated." (*ICH Q7A*)

Raw Material: "A general term used to denote starting materials, reagents, and solvents intended for use in the production of intermediates or APIs." (*ICH Q7A*)

Bulk Pharmaceutical Chemical (BPC): An older term that encompassed all chemicals used in the production of pharmaceuticals, including APIs as well as excipients/inactives.

Integrated Design: An approach to plant or process design that ensures that all of the API process or facility design is coordinated to achieve the desired business goals, cGMP compliance, environmental regulation compliance, safety regulation and code compliance, and operability and maintainability criteria.

Integrated Project Implementation: An approach to project implementation that ensures that all capital project activities are synergized and coordinated in order to achieve best case financial, schedule, deliverable, operating, and long-term maintenance goals.

Excipients/Inactives: Excipients and inactives are chemicals used in the manufacture of pharmaceutical dosage forms. Excipients are those non-API chemicals that are used in the dosage form's formulation to provide specific chemical and/or physical properties that directly affect the dosage form's activities (e.g., dissolution). Inactives are substances that aid in the manufacturing process itself (e.g., glidants). For the purposes of this chapter, these two terms shall be considered synonymous.

Good Engineering Practices: A general term used to denote commonly accepted practices for designing, installing, and commissioning equipment and systems, and the documentation associated with these project activities. API manufacturing facilities and processes should be built according to industry accepted best engineering practices.

Good Manufacturing Practices (GMPs): A set of rules and guidances that set forth an appropriate system for managing the quality of materials produced. The GMPs applicable to APIs are stated in the ICH-Q7A document.

Process Train: A term used to denote a collection of equipment employed in the manufacture of a stage or process step for an API or Intermediate. A typical process train might consist of a raw material mixing and feed tank, a batch reactor with supports systems, a centrifuge or filter, a dryer, and sizing equipment.

Flexibility: A term used to denote the versatility and interconnectability required in API facilities that produce multiple products in multiple process trains.

Overview of the Design Process
During the design of an API manufacturing facility, the following aspects must be considered:

- Type(s) of API production
- Basic unit operations
- Process configuration(s)
- Equipment requirements
- Process utility requirements
- Waste treatment/environmental system
- Risk analysis: Contamination sources and operational conditions/controls
- Facility requirements: Location, utilities, lighting, building materials, and ventilation
- Facility layout
- Flow of personnel/materials/equipment/wastes
- Maintenance and cleaning access

Design Tools
The API plant or process design team will likely find these tools helpful in navigating the design process for an API capital project:

Corporate or Industry Design Standards; Applicable Industry Codes and Regulations; Process Material and Energy Balances; Reaction Kinetics Data; Process Cycle Time Data; Process, Material, Equipment and Personnel Flow Diagrams; Piping and Instrumentation Diagrams (P&IDs); Floor Plan(s) or a 3-Dimensional Model of the proposed API process or plant; Piping And Conduit Plans, Elevations, Details or a 3-Dimensional Model of the proposed API process or plant; Ductwork and Fire Protection System Routing Drawings or a 3 Dimensional Model of the proposed API process or plant; Facility Electrical and GMP Classification Drawings; Process or Facility Basis of Design Document; Equipment and Facility User Requirement Specifications; Equipment and Facility Functional Requirement Specifications; Vendor Equipment Installation Drawings; Equipment Operating and Maintenance Requirements; Equipment Utility Requirements List; Instrument Location Plans; Equipment List; Instrument List; Valve List; Piping Specialty List; Piping Specifications; Process and/or Facility Hazard Analysis; Commissioning

Master Plan and Commissioning Protocols; Equipment Data Sheets; Instrument Data Sheets; Specialty Valve Data Sheets; Equipment Sizing Calculations; Project Implementation Schedule; Project Cost Estimate/Cost Control System and the Document Control System.

DESIGN OF API FACILITIES

Defining Your Process

Types of API Production
The first step in any design project is to define your process or processes and determine what types of operations will be performed in and be appropriate for your facility. The different types of API manufacturing processes and the key features of the facilities used for these processes are compared below.

Chemical Synthesis and Purification
Chemical synthesis is the creation of a new molecule or chemical entity by means of a series of controlled chemical reactions. A typical chemical synthesis begins with the addition of the "starting materials" and other materials such as solvents to a closed vessel where the first reaction will occur. Subsequent steps may involve the transfer of materials, addition of other chemicals, heat-ups and cool downs, solvent extractions, reactive and solvent distillations, purification steps such as filtering or centrifuging, drying, milling and particle sizing, and final packaging into bulk containers. The reaction steps in the process are usually numbered and once the API molecule is synthesized a series of purification steps generally occur.

Biological Manufacturing
The starting materials for a chemical synthesis may be created by the fermentation of microorganisms. These may be traditional fermentations utilizing various strains of bacteria, yeasts, molds, etc., or may utilize biotechnologically modified strains. Typically, the process is to provide the optimal conditions for the organisms to live and create the appropriate molecules. Nutrients and gases to support their metabolism must be supplied in the fermentation chamber and waste products removed. Often light, temperature, and pressures must be controlled. The biologically produced molecule may reside within the organism or in the nutrient materials in which the organism is living. These molecules may then be removed (recovered) from the fermentation, and may undergo purification steps and may be subjected to chemical synthesis.

(See Chapter 12: Biotechnology Facilities chapter for information on facilities for fermentation and other steps.)

R&D, Development, and Clinical Materials
Research and development of new APIs often includes a suite of early development laboratories in which bench top and/or small scale processing takes place. These

facilities are often on the scale of 20L batches and may rely heavily on glassware for processing. Such facilities require full safety controls and cGMP controls as the materials produced may be utilized in early clinical trials. These facilities should be designed to perform a wide variety of chemical processing unit operations at varying conditions on a small scale. Further, these facilities should be designed so that critical operating parameters can be determined and documented for inclusion in a chemical entity's product development file and possible hand-over in a future technology transfer package. The development work done in these facilities should include the identification of applications for the use of Process Analytical Technology (PAT) or continuous process quality assurance practices. These facilities can be used to generate scale up data such as reaction rate data, perform sensitivity analyses on unit operations within the evolving process, and determine preliminary mixing and utility requirements.

Large Scale R&D Production

Research and development production generally approaches the same scale as commercial production once the clinical testing enters into the Phase 3 multi-center trials. The facilities utilized at this stage are generally typical base units for API production.

Sterile API Facilities

From a regulatory perspective, the FDA treats the production of sterile APIs the same as the manufacture of sterile products. Typically, API chemical entities intended for use in sterile drug products are manufactured under aseptic conditions so they can be supplied as sterile product and or a product with a low pyrogen content specification. (See Chapter 11: Sterile Facilities.)

Commercial Multi-Product Facilities vs. Dedicated Commercial Facilities

Commercial production facilities generally are multiuse facilities designed to accomplish the synthesis of a variety of chemicals within the same equipment. These facilities may have the capabilities for the production of 40 or 50 different API chemical entities. Some of the issues facilities of this nature face are as follows:

1. The prevention of cross-contamination from one API or its intermediates to another API product.
2. Cleaning process development and validation are necessity to obviate the potential for cross contamination from residues within the equipment
3. Supplying utility systems with broad capabilities to accommodate a wide range of processing scenarios.
4. Supplying process piping systems with multiple transfer capabilities that prevent incorrect product transfers and are cleanable.
5. Handling and processing hazardous materials safely and in a cGMP-compliant manner.
6. Properly treating and/or disposing of byproducts of chemical reactions.

When an API is needed in sufficient quantities, an API facility may benefit from one or more equipment bays designed and designated for dedicated use. To be effective, dedicated equipment trains will also require the inclusion of features that accomplish the prevention of cross contamination between bays. However, the cleaning validation for dedicated systems will likely be less burdensome because cross-contamination pathways are minimized by the equipment and facility design. In dedicated process systems, residues that may degrade or become microbiologically contaminated are the main concern for product adulteration.

Basic Unit Operations

Most APIs are produced by chemical synthesis or, as for biotech drugs, purified/finished by chemical processing. (Further information on bioprocessing can be found in Chapter 12.) This chapter focuses on the unit operations for chemical processes. Figure 1 gives a graphical depiction of a typical API manufacturing process. Of special note is that API chemical processes are typically are accomplished in flammable organic solvents. Thus, these processes usually require equipment or other system components to be inerted prior to and during materials processing.

The typical chemical synthesis process consists of the following material handling steps or unit operations:

FIGURE 1   A Typical API Manufacturing Process

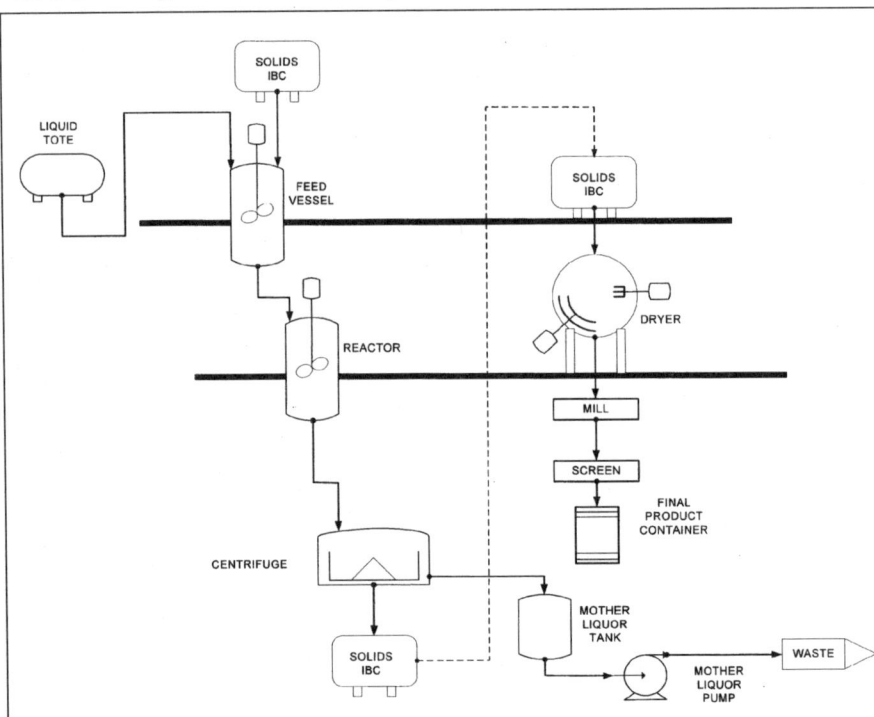

Raw Material Preparation, Material Transfer, and Charging Steps. Solid materials are usually employed in the manufacture of APIs. These materials must be introduced into and transported through the API manufacturing process in a manner that does not introduce contaminants into the process or pose a hazard to operating personnel. A variety of systems and technologies exist today to aid API manufacturers in the preparation and charging of solid raw materials. These systems and technologies will be discussed in the next section entitled Equipment Requirements.

A Reaction Step or Steps. This unit operation usually encompasses charging and mixing of raw materials, distillations, heat-ups, cool downs, and possibly solvent extractions. Reactions may be heat generating or heat consuming and thus require some type of reliable and accurate heat transfer and control system. The heat transfer system for a reactor must be able to maintain the specified reaction temperature within acceptable limits to ensure that the chemical formulation progresses as intended. Additionally chemical reactions may have other critical operating parameters such as pressure or pH. Therefore, instrumentation and controls are necessary for monitoring and documenting that these parameters are being maintained during a chemical synthesis. Based on the FDA's new initiative to promote the use of process analytical technologies to achieve continuous process assurance, companies should look at using online analytical instrumentation to provide constant confirmation that their validated chemical manufacturing process is producing good product. Companies implementing new processes or process modifications should also consider the use of online analytical instrumentation to provide constant confirmation that other API unit operations such as crystallization, drying, centrifugation, etc. are progressing as intended so that they yield the desired end product.

A Crystallization Operation. This is a unit operation in which dissolved solids in a supersaturated solution are forced out of solution by cooling or evaporation of the solvent. The crystallized solids are usually recovered as crystals in a slurry. Crystallization operations are heat generating and thus require some type of reliable and accurate cooling and control system. This heat transfer system must maintain the specified crystallization temperature within the crystallizer inside acceptable limits to ensure that the crystal formation progresses as intended. Additionally, crystallizations may have other critical operating parameters such as pressure or pH that must be controlled reliably and accurately. Therefore a crystallization system will need instrumentation and controls for monitoring these parameters and documenting that they are being maintained within established limits during a crystallization operation.

Purification Operation(s) (Filtration, Extraction, or Centrifugation). This is typically a separation operation in which liquid materials are passed through a filter media and the unwanted materials are rejected. The solids collected during a filtration or centrifugation operation frequently are washed with an appropriate solvent in order to remove residual impurities or collect residual product. Filters and centrifuges can be used to collect either the solids retained on the filter media or the mother liquors that pass through the filter media. Solvent extraction is another form of separation operation that may be used in the purification of an API product. When this separation operation is employed, it is typically combined with an additional separation operation such as filtration or centrifugation.

A Drying Step. This is an operation where solvent (aqueous or organic) is removed from a crystal or amorphous solid by evaporation or sublimation (vacuum freeze drying), leaving solid materials for further clarification or use. Drying operations in the API industry are typically performed under vacuum. They are heat consuming and require some type of reliable and accurate heat transfer and control system. The control system must be able to maintain the specified drying temperature and pressure within acceptable limits to ensure that the drying operation is progressing as intended.

Final Particle Sizing Prior to Packaging into Bulk Containers. This operation consists of milling or size reducing the bulk API product followed by sieving to remove any oversized particles.

Equipment Cleaning. This operation happens at the end of a production campaign for a specific product. This operation seeks to remove impurities from the entire manufacturing process train so that it can be used for production of another product.

Editor's Note:

Equipment/System Inerting

In order to accomplish inerting, equipment or system components are purged with nitrogen or another inert gas prior to the introduction of flammable materials. Once the initial equipment or component inerting is accomplished, the inert environment is maintained by supplying a continuous maintenance flow of nitrogen through the system. For unit operations such as centrifugation where a special risk of spark generation exists, a continuous oxygen monitor may be employed to ensure that the equipment and any associated system components are inerted throughout the process.

Equipment Requirements

Each of the unit operations mentioned in the preceding section of this chapter usually comprises a single piece of process equipment or a single process system. These are:

Solids Preparation, Weighing, Transfer, and Charging System Components. These devices consist of containers and other solids handling system components that receive, pre-package, pre-weigh, and charge raw materials into API manufacturing processes. The current state of cGMP evolution dictates that these operations are done in a manner that prevents contamination of the raw materials. The preferred method for accomplishing this cGMP goal is to use closed systems to accomplish these raw material handling operations. Some of the apparatus available for performing closed system raw material handling operations are as follows:

- Enclosed bag dump stations
- Intermediate bulk containers with discharge stations
- Intermediate bulk containers with rapid transfer ports or split butterfly valves
- Barrier isolators with rapid transfer ports of split butterfly valves, such as a glovebox isolation (Fig. 2)
- Solids transfer chutes
- Vacuum conveying systems

FIGURE 2   A Typical Glovebox Isolator

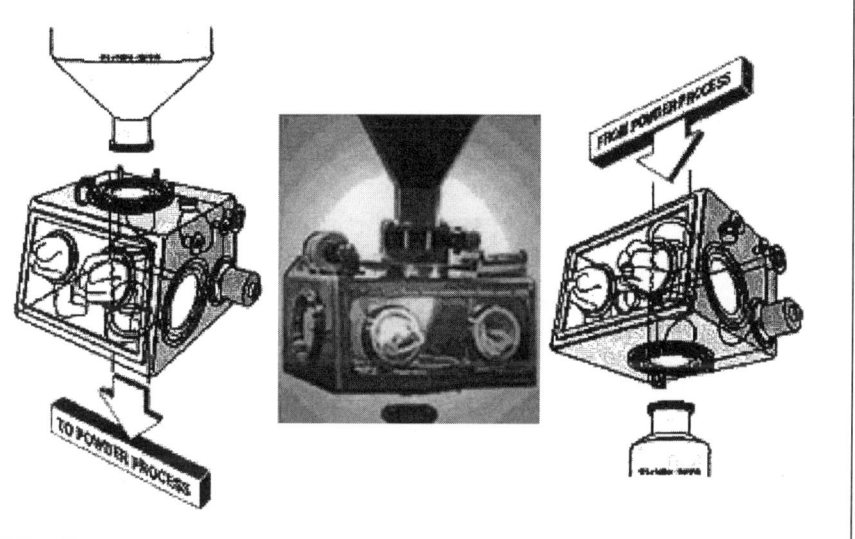

The process designer must be cognizant of how solids will be charged, transferred and otherwise handled within an API manufacturing facility. Equipment and the facility itself must be designed to accommodate the use of any special solids handling systems or solids handling components. Equipment may need to be specially designed in order to attach a barrier isolator, discharge station or vacuum conveyor. The facility may also need special features to be able to incorporate these specialized material handling systems.

Reactor. This is the process vessel in which chemical reactions take place. The reactor is usually a pressure and vacuum rated jacketed vessel with an agitator. The reactor is usually supported by a temperature control system, a condenser, a solids charging system, a raw material mixing tank, and a distillate receiver. Chemical reactors are usually fabricated from 316L stainless steel or glass-lined carbon steel. Equipment vendors currently supply GMP style glass lined vessels for use in the manufacture of APIs (Fig.3). Sometimes special alloy (Hastelloy) pressure vessels are used to carryout chemical reactions involving highly corrosive materials (Fig. 4).

FIGURE 3   GMP Style Glass-Lined API Reactor

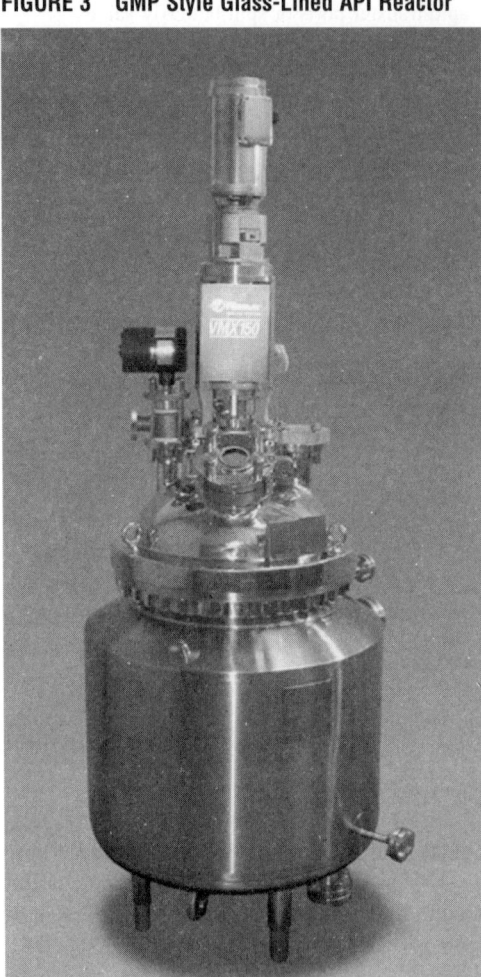

Source: Pfandler, Inc.

The API chemical reactor is typically attached to a condenser via a vent pipe. Condensers employed in API manufacturing plants are typically constructed of graphite, 316L stainless steel, or tantalum.

The heat transfer system for a typical API reactor uses a series of heat exchangers for controlling the temperature of a heat transfer fluid that is supplied to the jacket of the reactor (Fig. 5).

FIGURE 4   Standard Glass-Lined API Reactor

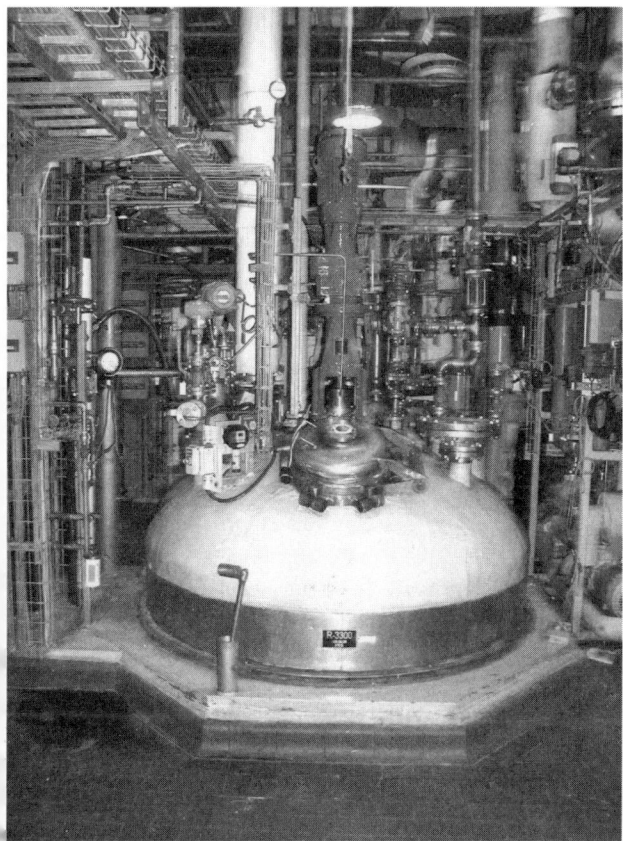

Source: Lonza, Inc.

Crystallizer. The process vessel in which crystallizations take place. This is usually an agitated vessel with cooling capabilities and it may have a conic bottom discharge for discharge of the crystals. This unit operation may be performed in a dedicated crystallizer or evaporator but sometimes this unit operation is performed in the reaction vessel in an API manufacturing facility. Crystallizers are typically fabricated from 316L stainless steel or glass-lined carbon steel. The 316L stainless steel vessels may be supplied with enhanced surface finish for wetted parts and other components to facilitate solids discharge and cleaning. As with reactors, special alloy (Hastelloy) vessels are sometimes used to carryout crystallizations involving highly corrosive materials (Fig. 6).

Filter/Centrifuge. This equipment is used to separate solid materials from mother liquors or waste. Filters and centrifuges are typically fabricated from 316L but can be fabricated from special alloys such as Hastelloy or plastic-lined carbon steel or

FIGURE 5   Chemical Control Module

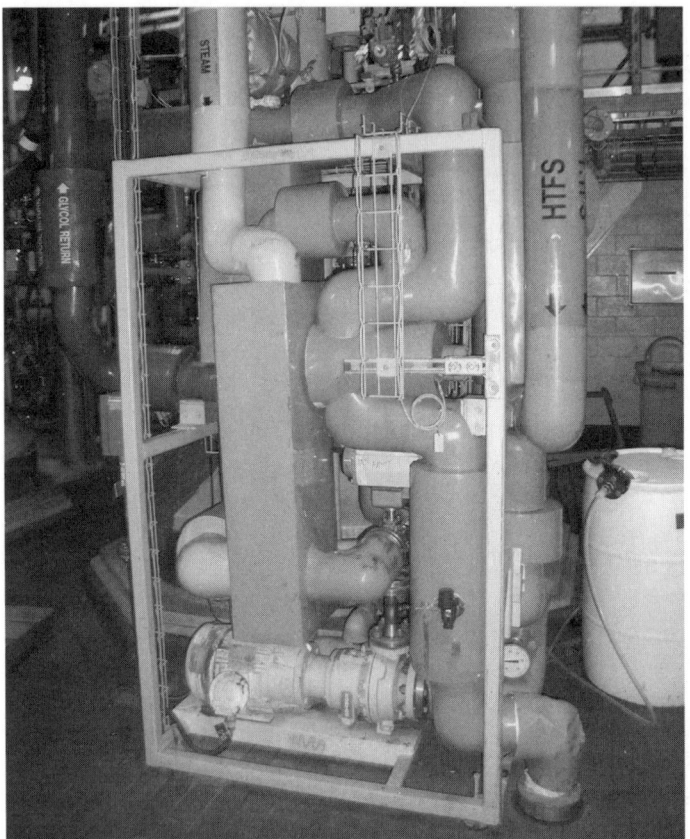

Source: Lonza, Inc.

stainless steel components. The 316L stainless steel and special alloy filters and centrifuges may be supplied with enhanced surface finish for wetted parts and other components to facilitate solids discharge and cleaning (Fig. 7).

Dryer. A dryer reduces the solvent or water content of an API before further processing or packaging. Dryers are typically fabricated from 316L stainless steel or glass-lined carbon steel. The 316L stainless steel dryer may be supplied with enhanced surface finish for wetted parts and other components to facilitate solids discharge and cleaning. As with reactors, special alloy (Hastelloy) vessels are sometimes used to carry out drying operations involving highly corrosive materials (Figs. 8 and 9).

Mill/Sifter. A mill is the device that reduces the API product to the necessary particle size by means of direct impact, or impingement, and segregates out any oversized API product prior to bulk packaging.

FIGURE 6 Typical API Crystallizer

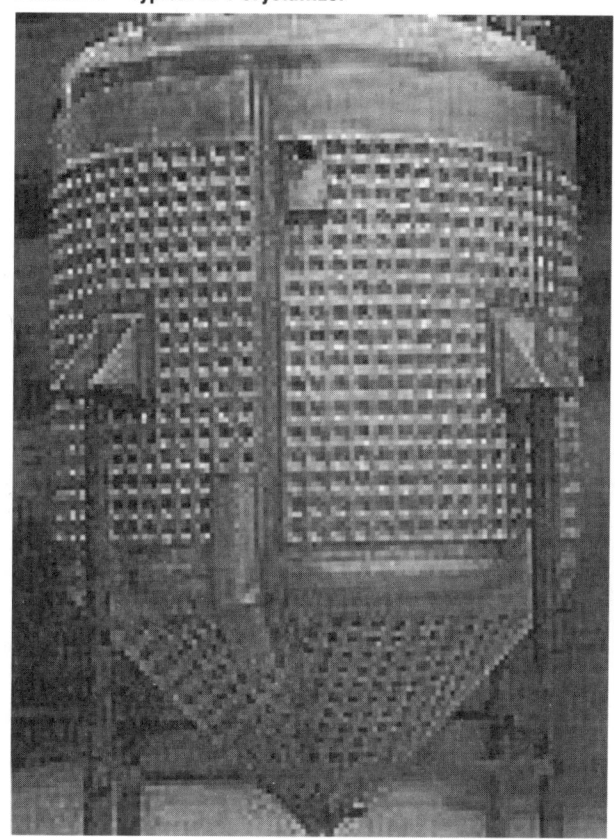

Source: Triangle Components.

Cleaning Equipment/CIP Systems. Cleaning equipment consists of devices that effect the cleaning of the components of an API manufacturing process train. Cleaning equipment may be portable, integral to the API manufacturing equipment, or part of a centralized cleaning system. Typical devices used for the cleaning of API plant process equipment are sprayballs or high pressure nozzles. These devices may be connected to a portable or centralized liquid supply system.

Editor's Note: _____

Materials of Construction

In many cases the process equipment or process system is a permanent installation within the facility. Therefore it is necessary to determine that the equipment is not reactive with the full spectrum of material being produced. In one instance a firm synthesized a number of APIs under contract for a firm that was producing several new drugs. In one shipment of APIs, it was discovered by the customer that a variety of particles contaminated the API. One API was contaminated with blue and black particles and obvious pieces of metal. An investigation revealed that the reactor utilized had gasketing material that reacted with the material produced and broke down causing the black particles. The other contaminants were due to inadequate maintenance—blue particles from broken sight glass and metal from loose nuts which had fractured.

FIGURE 7   Typical API Centufuge

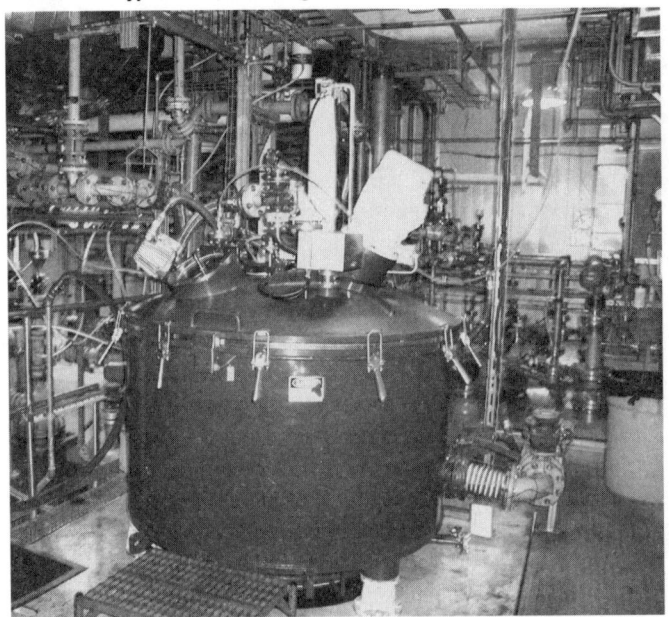

Source: Lonza, Inc.

FIGURE 8   Typical API Dryer

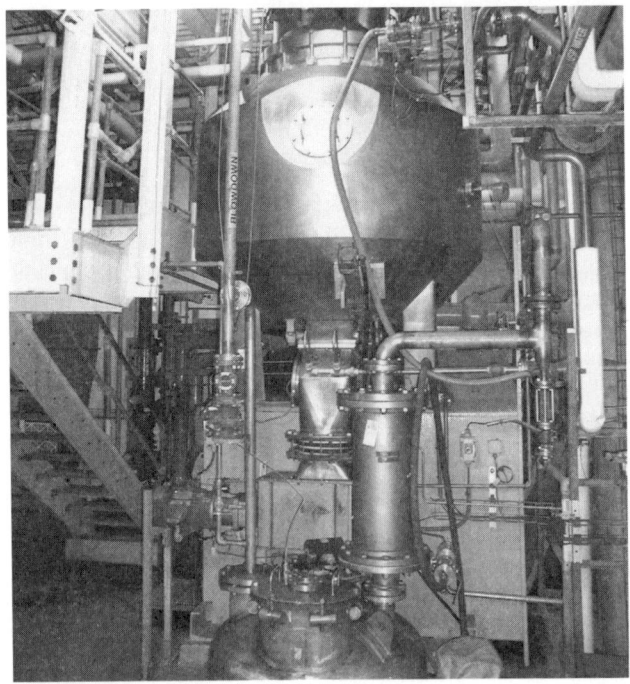

Source: Lonza, Inc.

FIGURE 9   Typical Filter/Dryer Used in API Manufacturing

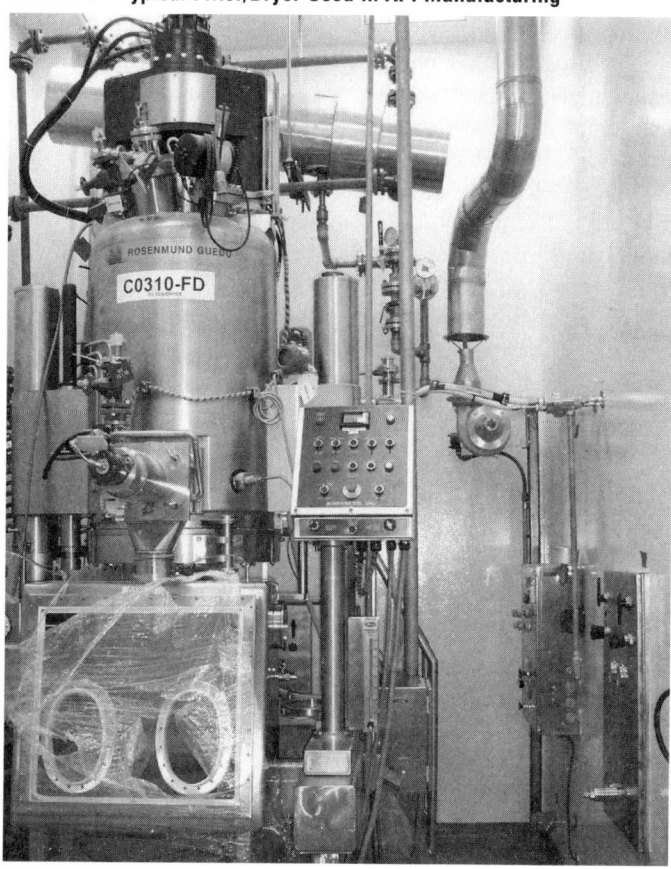

Source: Pfandler, Inc.

Editor's Note: _____

Skidded Equipment, Systems, and Plants

Many equipment manufacturers currently supply completely pre-assembled skids containing a major process equipment component or series of components and all of the necessary supplemental equipment, piping, instrumentation, and support structures. Some manufacturers will even assemble pre-fabricated, pre-piped, and pre-wired modular API plants. These pre-manufactured skids or plants can typically be tested at the factory by connecting them to the appropriate utilities. This type of factory testing (known in the pharmaceutical industry as Factory Acceptance Testing) can provide the benefit of identifying manufacturing defects, operational issues, documentation issues, etc. at the factory where they can more easily be corrected, thus optimizing project cost and schedule compliance. Additionally, when these pre-fabricated systems are brought onto the API plant site they can be easily and quickly dropped in place and connected to the necessary utilities. A further benefit of these types of systems is that they can be pre-commissioned and pre-validated at the factory when the completed skid is available. These pre-commissioning and pre-validation activities can potentially be leveraged to expedite the completion of onsite commissioning and validation activities.

Process Configuration(s)

The equipment that comprises the basic unit operations of an API manufacturing process must be connected together via piping systems and/or equipment movements in order to create an actual manufacturing process configuration. A process configuration should accomplish the safe, efficient, cGMP compliant and cost effective manufacture of a quality API product. The process configuration must take into consideration the safe and efficient movement of materials, equipment, personnel, waste, samples, and product. The process configuration should also be integrated with the facility configuration to produce an effective API production facility. A multi-product API facility may need to have several process configurations installed and set-up within the manufacturing facility at one time. Therefore all of these process configurations must be designed to fit into the API facility and designed to prevent cross contamination, product adulteration, or other undesirable alterations of products being produced simultaneously within the plant.

Piping/Ductwork Requirements

An API manufacturing facility, especially a multi-purpose or multi-product plant will have an extensive and complicated network of piping and ductwork systems. These piping systems must support chemical synthesis and purification operations while at the same time upholding the cGMP requirements involved in API production. The level of piping required in an API facility is vastly greater then that found in a typical final dosage form pharmaceutical processing facility but less then that found in a typical petrochemical processing facility. However, the sophistication of the piping in an API plant may be greater then that found in a petrochemical facility due to the flexibility of fluid transfer required in an API manufacturing process. Thus, it is advisable to prepare a 3-dimensional model of the equipment, piping, walls, electrical conduit and cable trays, structural steel, ductwork, etc. in an API facility project to prevent interferences or other space problems. The piping networks in an API manufacturing facility include both process and utility piping systems. The ductwork includes supply and return air networks for accomplishing ventilation, and temperature and humidity control within the facility. Some of the piping and duct networks or runs that are found in an API facility are as follows: product transfer, solvent transfer, vacuum, process vent, process water, potable water, USP water, Highly Purified water, Water for Injection, steam, chilled water, chilled silicone oil, nitrogen, compressed air, instrument air, tower water, dust collection, HVAC air, liquid waste transfer, pressure relief vent, clean in place, and clean steam.

Due to the large number of cross connections between equipment required in an API manufacturing facility the design engineer may look at installing manifold stations near major equipment and at other strategic locations within the facility. These manifold stations provide flexibility to facilitate the transfer of product between processing units within the facility. Much thought and planning should be expended to ensure that the correct transfer pipes are built into an API manufacturing facility. Additionally, if portable equipment is employed or if connections to equipment in a GMP style room need to be done neatly, then the design engineer should consider designing and installing piping hook-up panels. These panels allow piping

FIGURE 10   API Facility Hook-up Panel

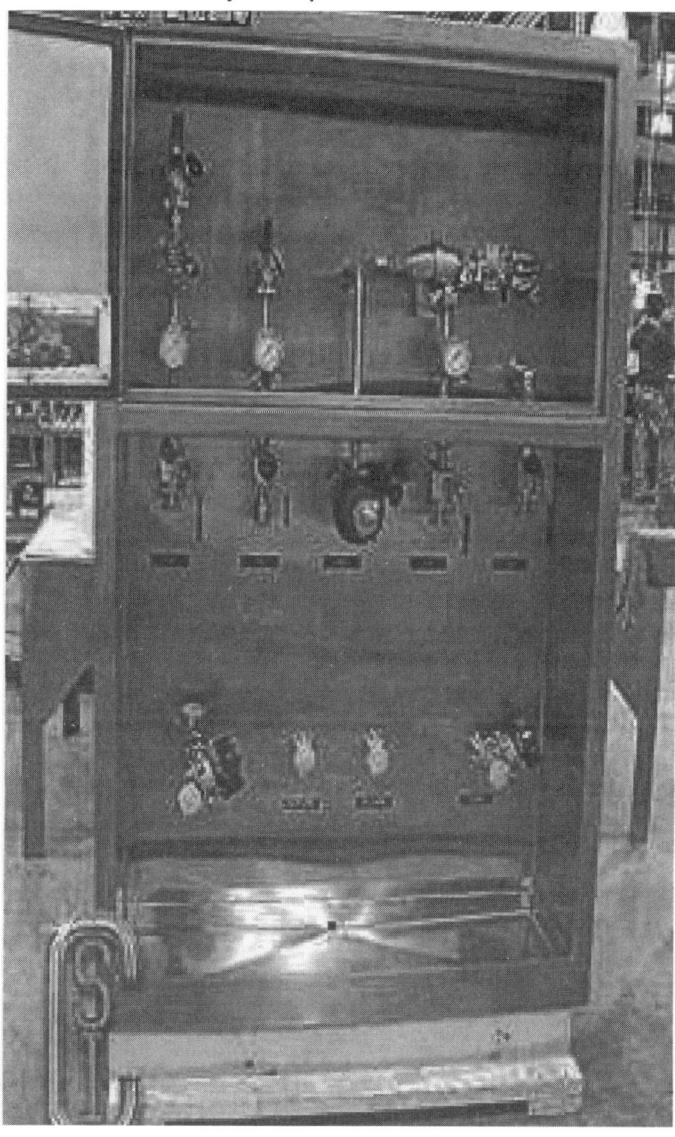

drops to be installed near installed equipment with the piping system remaining behind a wall or closed off pipe chase (Fig. 10). When dealing with water or other liquids that may act as media in supporting microbial growth, it is usually necessary to avoid piping configurations that permit pools of standing media. In a number of cases microbial contamination of APIs has resulted from these pools. These conditions have resulted in recalls of APIs and of the finished pharmaceuticals subsequently manufactured. Dead legs and inadequate slopes often result in this condition. Therefore the process piping designer must pay special attention to the routing and sloping of process piping systems by preparing piping isometric details or a 3-dimensional model of critical piping system for contractors to use for construction.

Refer to the ISPE Baseline Guide and ICH Q7A for more information on appropriate piping system design for API facilities.

Process Utility Requirements

The process equipment in an API manufacturing facility is designed to perform various unit operations on the API starting materials and subsequent API chemical entities. These unit operations consist of heating, cooling, distilling, condensing, transferring, separating, drying, grinding, and size classifying API intermediates of finished products. A great diversity of process utilities are required to support the operation of the equipment that perform these unit operations. Listed in Table 1 are the typical utilities that might be required to support the equipment installed in an API manufacturing plant.

TABLE 1 API Plant Utilities

Utility	Function/Service	Special Design/Engineering Considerations
Plant steam	Heating: Process and facility	Adequate condensate collection points and transfer system
Chilled water	Cooling: Process and facility Dehumidification: Facility	High point vents and low point drains, system balancing components
Chilled silicone oil	Cooling: Process	Special surface finish flange fittings and special gaskets
Tower water	Cooling: Process, facility, and utility systems	High point vents and low point drains, system balancing components
Nitrogen	Inerting: Process systems Pressurization: Process systems Product transfers Pipeline blowing	Consider special filters, pharmaceutical grade pipe and sample connections for API contact nitrogen. Consider enhanced surface finish for inside of pipe. Consider documenting piping system with material certs, weld maps/piping isometrics
Compressed air	Pressurization: Process system Operation of pneumatically Operated equipment and Devices Agitation/sparging: Process systems	Consider special filters, pharmaceutical grade pipe and sample connections for API contact air. Consider enhanced surface finish for inside of pipe. Consider documenting piping system with material certs, weld maps/piping isometrics
Vacuum	Vacuum distillations and drying, product transfers, vessel evacuation for inerting, product containment	Adequate sloping, insulation and knock-out capabilities built into piping system

(Continued)

TABLE 1 *Continued*

Utility	Function/Service	Special Design/Engineering Considerations
Scrubbing system		Compatible with wide variety of process off-gas streams
Vent gas extraction and treatment	Venting and purifying: Process equipment	Compatible with wide variety of process off-gas streams, properly sloped and insulated, provisions for condensed liquid removal, LEL monitoring and control. Consider explosion venting or mitigation
USP water	Chemical synthesis, API purification, equipment cleaning	Loop system, no dead leg design. Sanitizable. Sampling capabilities at each use point
Water for injection	Chemical synthesis, API purification, equipment cleaning	Loop system, no dead leg design. Sanitizable. Sample capabilities at each use point. Consider enhanced surface finish for inside of pipe. Consider documenting piping system with material certs, weld maps/piping isometrics
Potable water	Equipment cooling, steam generation, facility washdown	Backflow prevention
Liquid waste collection and treatment	Collect, store and treat waste liquids generated by API manufacturing processes	Piping system capable of handling flammable solvents and solids containing liquids
Dust collection system	Extract and collect dust from solids handling operations	Explosion venting or mitigation for hazardous dust transport systems
Blowdown system	Collect vents from process relief devices	Compatible with wide variety of process off-gas streams, properly sloped, provisions for entrained liquid disengagement, provisions for condensed liquid removal, separation of vent lines from different systems
Clean in place system	Provides cleaning fluids to fixed equipment	Loop system, no dead leg design. Consider enhanced surface finish for inside of pipe. Consider documenting piping system with material certifications, weld maps/ piping isometrics
Clean steam	Provides sterilization fluid to fixed equipment for steaming in place	Adequate condensate collection points and transfer system, finish proper sloping, sample capabilities at appropriate use points. Consider enhanced surface for inside of pipe. Consider documenting piping system with material certifications, weld maps/piping isometrics

Generation, processing and/or storage equipment and supply networks or distribution systems for all of these utility systems must be designed into the layout of an API manufacturing plant. The location of the equipment for these utility systems and the routing of the piping of these utilities should be designed so that they will be effective and efficient but not have a negative impact on product quality. The clean utility systems such as nitrogen, USP water, and WFI that may have direct contact with product should be designed, installed, commissioned, and validated in accordance with accepted industry practices. The ISPE Baseline Pharmaceutical Engineering Guide on Water and Steam Systems can be used for guidance in defining and designing "clean" water generation and distribution systems.

Process Hazards/Safety Systems

API manufacturing processes are inherently hazardous due to the use of flammable, corrosive, or toxic liquids; flammable, corrosive, or toxic gases; and combustible organic powders. Some liquids, powders, and gases used in API processes also pose extreme short- and long-term health risks to plant personnel. Therefore, all ingredients of an API manufacturing process must be evaluated for potential risk to personnel, equipment, and facilities. Further, certain safety systems or features will likely need to be designed into process equipment, process systems, and piping systems to prevent unacceptable property loss and/or harm to personnel. Material Safety Data Sheets should be collected and reviewed for all ingredients to determine what safety features or measures need to be included in the process or facility design to minimize the likelihood of the occurrence of an unsafe event.

Chemical reactions must be evaluated for the potential to get out of control or run away, and proper safety devices or systems must be evaluated and then employed in the process or facility design to prevent these events or to neutralize their occurrence. This evaluation may involve the sizing and design of safety relief valves and venting systems, reaction quenching systems, explosion venting or mitigation systems, as well as reliable and effective heat removal systems and safety control devices and systems.

Powders and dusts must be evaluated for their explosivity and toxicity, and proper safety devices or protective systems must be evaluated and then employed in the process or facility design to prevent harm as a result of an explosion or release of a toxic compound.

API process operations such as vessel charging or emptying, product or material transfer, etc. must be evaluated for safety risks.

The aforementioned safety risks and other safety risk are best identified by a team of experienced API plant personnel while performing a structured process hazard analysis such as a Hazards and Operability review (HAZOP). Process and facility safety analyses are discussed in more detail in the Risk Assessment section of this chapter.

Waste Treatment/Environmental Systems

Several types of waste treatment/environmental systems were listed with the utilities in Table 1. These systems are the vent gas extraction and treatment system, the liquid waste collection and treatment system, and the solid waste collection and treatment system. A brief description will be given below for each of these waste treatment/environmental systems:

Vent Gas Extraction and Treatment System. This system collects all of the contaminated gaseous discharges from an API plant and treats the gas stream so that the contaminants are not discharged into the atmosphere. The vent gas treatment system typically consists of a licensed thermal oxidizer or a low temperature condenser. A scrubbing device alone usually does not suffice to remove organic constituents included in a vent gas stream. All thermal oxidizers are required to comply with the MACT standards promulgated by the U.S. EPA.

Liquid Waste Collection and Treatment System. This system collects all of the hazardous or contaminated liquid discharges from an API plant and treats them so that the contaminants are not discharged into the environment. The liquid waste treatment system typically consists of a licensed thermal oxidizer, a stripper/evaporator, and/or a wastewater treatment up to and including tertiary water treatment system. All thermal oxidizers are required to comply with the MACT standards promulgated by the US EPA. Liquid waste treatment for an API manufacturing plant alternately may consist of collecting the waste and sending it to a certified and licensed offsite facility for proper treatment and disposal.

Solid Waste Collection and Treatment. This system collects all of the hazardous or contaminated solid discharges from an API plant and treats or processes them so that the contaminants are not discharged into the environment. A solid waste treatment system may consist of a licensed thermal oxidizer or offsite handling and disposal of the solid waste by a certified and licensed waste processor. All thermal oxidizers are required to comply with the MACT standards promulgated by the U.S. EPA.

Risk Analysis

During all stages of the design of API manufacturing facilities, a risk analysis must be performed. This risk analysis must include evaluations in terms of the following items.

Differences Between Manufacturing APIs and Other Materials Such as Excipients. The risks involved with the manufacture of a particular material will depend on what final drug product the material will be used in. For instance, an API produced for the purpose of being utilized in the manufacture of a sterile drug product will usually need tighter controls over HVAC air and process water quality, as these APIs generally have strict limits on microbial load and pyrogens.

The Q7A Guidance document and the Draft FDA Guidance documents were not prepared with a focus on the manufacturing of excipients but "much of the guidance provided may be useful" for such processes. The International Pharmaceutical Excipients Council has also issued a Guideline for the Manufacture of Excipients, which may be useful in determining the design of an excipient manufacturing facility.

The risk levels will help determine the instrumentation and equipment required for the control of critical parameters, the documentation level for such operations, the quality requirements in terms of testing and monitoring, and the overall management level appropriate for the type of product.

Conditions for Receipt, Storage, Handling and Processing of Starting Materials. Starting materials may be purchased from a supplier or produced in-house. If purchased, then controls must be established in terms of storage, sampling, release testing, handling, and use of such materials. If the starting material is produced in-house, it should be remembered that the processing steps before the introduction or development of the "starting material" will represent less risk to the end product than the steps occurring after the starting material is present. Once the starting material is present, the levels of controls on the process must be more stringent. Therefore, more attention must be given to the facility and utility systems controls, cleaning and sanitization procedures, the flow of materials and personnel, the quality requirements in terms of sampling, testing and monitoring, the documentation level for the operation, and the overall management level and attention.

Differences in Levels of Control for Starting Materials, Intermediates vs. Final API Product (Including In-Process Testing, Cleaning Requirements, and Product Handling). Production may take over in-process testing under quality assurance approved procedures. Therefore, the production facility may be an appropriately designed and equipped laboratory facility near the production floor in order to accomplish the necessary in-process testing.

As the process moves closer to the final API, the control requirements must be more stringent including the cleaning residues criteria and the documentation related to the process steps.

Definition of Critical Steps and Parameters
Critical steps may occur throughout the manufacturing process; therefore, all steps and their sub-operations must be evaluated for risk. However, as the process moves closer to the final API, the critical steps and parameters must be clearly identified, defined, and documented; specifications must be clearly stated, and the controllers in charge of the critical parameters must be more reliable to ensure that the parameters remain within the pre-established ranges. During these steps it may be useful to employ some type of continuous process or product analysis instrumentation and controls (PAT).

Definition of Critical Instrumentation and Required Controls/Automation
The company must have a calibration/instrumentation procedure that clearly defines which instruments are critical. This determination should be based on the applica-

tion of each instrument and the effects (both direct and indirect) of a failure of the instrument on the both facility operation and the process itself. With the technological advancements of today, automation of the controls for the facility and utility systems is advantageous for facility operation but it is critical that procedures be established for how to work with the systems, the testing to qualify such systems, and the maintenance required. This includes software maintenance and back-up procedures.

Levels of Protection

Once an evaluation of the process(es) to be utilized is conducted, an evaluation of the potential exposure of the intermediate or finished API must be conducted to ascertain the level of protection necessary. An intermediate, which is fully enclosed within a reactor, will generally not require any level of protection from the building as the equipment itself provides this protection. Wherever the material being produced is potentially exposed to the environment a level of protection must be provided. The levels of protection are generally defined as:

- *Level I: General*: Normal housekeeping and maintenance
- *Level II: Protected*: Various steps such as restricted personnel entry and use of gowning and foot covers are set to protect exposed intermediates and APIs.
- *Level III: Controlled*. Environmental control levels such as air particles are set and monitored.

The level of protection is set based on the sensitivity of the intermediate or API to contamination (this sensitivity may be based on the chemical compound or the ultimate use of the material) and the probability and degree of exposure. For instance, a material that is maintained within a reactor without environmental exposure may be reasonably maintained in a Level I area. Where the intermediate or API may be exposed to the environment when the reactor is opened, Level II protection should be employed. This Level II protection may be achieved through procedural controls— e.g., the use of procedures to ensure that multiple reactors are not opened simultaneously to prevent the potential of cross-contamination. In an area where the API is unloaded for transfer or further manipulation, Level III controls are generally utilized.

In addition to providing protection of the product, an API facility design must also incorporate protection of employees. This is especially true when potent compounds are being processed. Potent compound should be processed in closed systems such as barrier isolators or closed piping and duct systems whenever possible. These closed processing systems should also be supplemented by a secondary means of containing the potent compound in the case of a failure of the primary containment system. Closed processing rooms with an associated air lock are one means of providing the required secondary containment. Localized dust collection hoods are another means of providing secondary containment. For extremely potent compounds the designer may need to consider the inclusion of a tertiary means of potent product isolation or containment. Some factors to consider when defining equipment or system approaches to personnel protection are: type and quantity of personnel protective equipment, potency classification of the potent compound, cost, cleanability of barriers and isolators, etc.

(Refer to Chapter 16 of this book or the ISPE API Baseline Guide for more information on containment system design for API facilities.)

API Process Risk Assessment—An Example

Process and Facility Safety Analysis

As part of the design of an API facility or process the design team should perform a process and facility safety analysis. The design team can choose to perform any one of several structured process hazard analysis procedures for analyzing the safety of the process or facility. If extremely hazardous processing will be performed in the facility, then the design team should choose a structured

API Risk Assessment Flow Chart

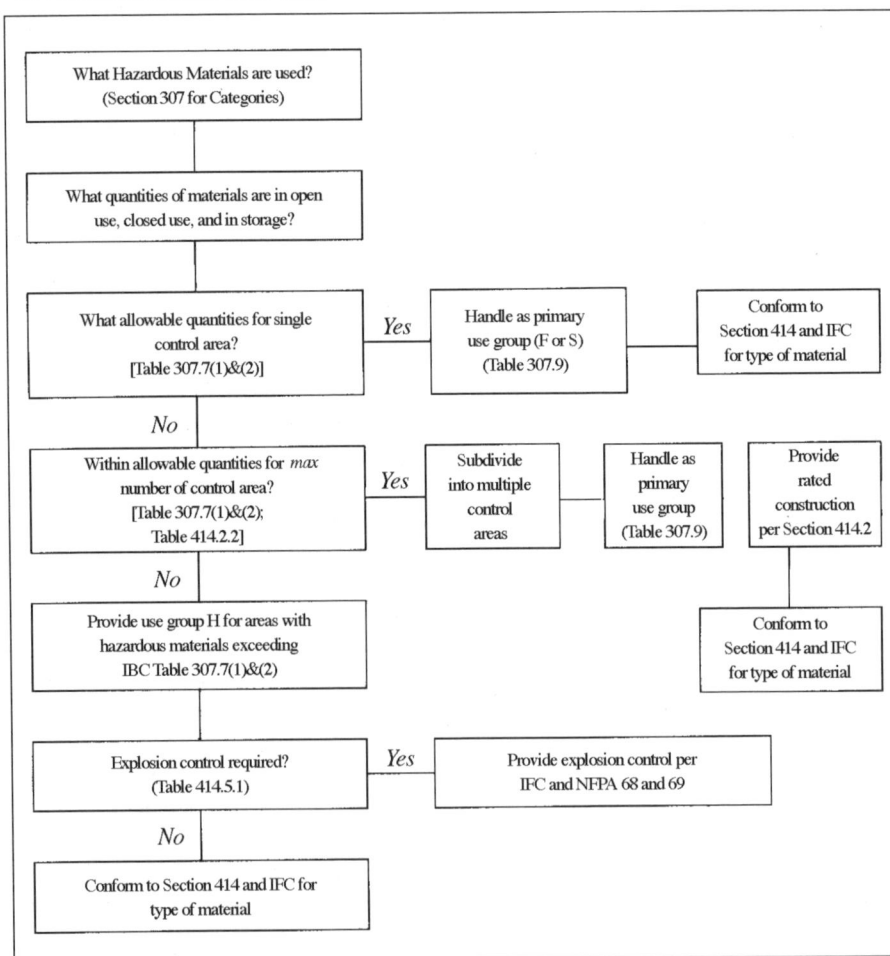

and detailed hazard evaluation procedure such as a Hazard and Operability (HAZOP) study to perform a line-by-line or operation-by-operation safety evaluation of the new process or facility. The design team may opt to perform a failure modes and effects analysis on high risk operations or equipment. If a less structured and disciplined safety evaluation can suffice then the design team may opt for performing a "what if" safety evaluation. (See Chapter 16 for further details on Process Safety Management and Process Hazard Analysis Techniques.)

In addition to a performing a process hazard analysis the design team will needs to review any process or facility upgrades with the insurance provider to guarantee insurability. Such a review should focus on proper identification and application of area electrical classifications. Further, this review with the company's insurance provider must look at code compliance for the methods identified for storing and handling flammable and hazardous compounds.

Site Requirements/Considerations

The site for an API facility must have all of the necessary attributes required to support the functioning of a chemical processing plant. The site will need to have adequate real estate to contain the API processing facility as well as any infrastructure required to support the operation of this facility. A typical API plant site will need real estate for the following non-production entities: Raw material and waste storage tank farms; liquid, solid and gaseous waste processing facilities; office space; maintenance shop and maintenance stores area; inside and outside storage areas for non-process items; central utility facility for steam generation; compressed air generation; process water generation and storage; chilled water generation; chilled silicone oil generation and storage; nitrogen storage; tower water generation; fire protection water storage; fuel storage; etc. Additionally, the grounds need to be suitable, securable, and properly zoned. Consideration should also be given to parking and vehicular access to the facility.

Facility Requirements

Location and Size

The size of the building must allow adequate space for the proper operations to be performed including receiving, storage, and staging of all materials, manufacturing, maintenance and cleaning, analytical testing, process development, and administration. It must provide accessibility to equipment and ensure appropriate and efficient flow of personnel, portable/auxiliary equipment, materials, samples and waste to avoid product contamination.

The location must consider aspects such as environmental conditions; water, natural gas, electricity, waste water treatment availability; constraints and cost; and proximity to residential neighborhoods, office buildings, shopping centers, industrial parks, schools, emergency services, and other manufacturing facilities.

Building Materials and Features

The materials used for construction must be appropriate for the product/process being considered. Materials should also be adequate to address safety considerations in terms of fire hazard and explosion-proof materials. Materials should also be durable and cleanable. The International Society of Pharmaceutical Engineering (ISPE) Baseline Guide for Bulk Pharmaceutical Chemical Facilities is an excellent resource for these considerations and has specific recommendations on materials for use in the construction of facilities, depending on product exposure, etc.

An enclosed API manufacturing facility must also contain provisions for blowout panels within building walls. These blowout panels must be adequately designed and sized in order to mitigate the worst case potential explosion within the facility. This explosion mitigation system shall be designed in accordance with applicable codes and regulations.

An API manufacturing facility must also contain a properly designed fire protection system, fire separation walls, appropriately designed and installed trenching or piping system to carry hazardous and flammable liquid waste streams to a suitable storage system.

Electrical Systems and Classification(s)

The prevalent use of organic solvents and other combustible materials in the manufacture of APIs dictates that special consideration be given to the type of electrical equipment and components, lighting fixtures, wiring and cabling systems, motors, and instrumentation and controls that are installed within an API facility. If organic solvents or other combustible organic materials have the potential of becoming exposed within certain areas of the API manufacturing facility then electrical equipment and fixtures will need to be fabricated and installed in accordance with the NFPA/NEC requirements for hazardous areas. Further, equipment and piping system bonding and/or grounding must be given special consideration where organic solvents or other combustibles are processed.

If portable equipment is employed in an API manufacturing facility or process, then special electrical adapters may be needed to connect equipment to an electrical power source.

The facility designer must consider what equipment or systems need to be connected to an emergency power source for cGMP compliance or to ensure plant/facility/personnel safety. The designer also must ensure that all necessary utility systems such as plant/instrument air, chilled water, etc. are also connected to emergency power so that crucial instruments and controls remain active when emergency power is applied to critical equipment or systems.

The facility designer must also consider where uninterruptible power supplies need to be instituted in order to maintain the operation of controls of the API facility or process equipment as well as the receiving and storage of critical process data from the facility and processes.

Process Utilities

Any substance (liquid or gas) that comes in contact with the API, intermediates, or the equipment/facility product contact surfaces must comply with the required company defined specifications and must not be a source for contamination or adulteration of the materials being produced. This includes:

Direct Contact Steam Systems and Boilers. These systems interact directly with the product raw materials or with equipment that comes in contact with raw materials introduced into the API manufacturing process or equipment that comes in contact with cleaning solutions introduced into API manufacturing equipment. These systems produce and transmit steam used by the API process for sanitization or sterilization operations. They must be designed to prevent API product contamination or adulteration and should be capable of periodic steam quality testing to verify the quality of the steam being generated, especially to confirm the absence of contamination with boiler additives or other residues.

Compressed Gases. These systems consist of process raw material gases such as hydrogen, chlorine, ammonia, etc., or may be process support gases such as nitrogen, air, or carbon dioxide. These gases act as product raw materials or purge gases, or interact with equipment that comes in contact with raw materials introduced into the API manufacturing process. Therefore, these gases must comply with specifications developed by the API manufacturer through consideration of the types of process and products being manufactured.

Water Generating and Distribution Systems. These must comply with USP Purified Water standards if used on a product intended for parenteral product. Otherwise, water used in processeses must comply with internal company specifications. This will apply even if the water is used solely for cleaning of the equipment. Potable water must comply with WHO and/or Federal Standards for Drinking Water. If water is treated to maintain a consistent level of chlorine, then it should be treated as generated water and must comply with the company established specifications and tested to meet such standards.

Cleaning Solutions/Agents. These agents must be suitable for the cleaning application(s) and capable of being removed from process equipment after cleaning so that they do not pose a contamination risk to the manufactured API products. Cleaning solutions or agents may consist of hot or cold water or solvents, high pressure water, surfactants, enzymes, or other pressurized and directed fluid streams. Alternatively, equipment may be filled with water or other solvents and operated in order to effect cleaning. Whatever method of cleaning is chosen, the process must be validatable.

Product-contact utility systems must be qualified to demonstrate adequate design, installation and operation. Engineering drawings must be available and verified to show the systems as "as-built" conditions. System distribution piping must be properly identified including the direction of flow. Drains must be adequately located and designed to avoid back-flow and, therefore, potential contamination.

Systems for substances that will not come in contact with the product and/or equipment must be be designed, installed, and tested to verify that they perform as expected. However, the systems for producing such substances are not required to be qualified, although at the least, a commissioning document should be prepared to show that the system has been installed properly and functions as desired.

The design team for a new process or facility needs to ensure that utility systems have adequate capacity and component redundancy in order to ensure cGMP compliance, and reliable and cost effective operation of the production process(es) supported by these utility systems.

Lighting and Ventilation

Lighting must be adequate to facilitate proper execution of manufacturing, maintenance, cleaning, and testing procedures.

The design for ventilation must take into consideration the environmental conditions that have been established for the process and related equipment. The comfort of personnel working in these areas also needs to be considered to allow them to adequately perform their assigned tasks. Special considerations must be provided for those products that require low levels of microbiological contamination. In addition, equipment controls and instrumentation must be considered when establishing environmental conditions for the areas to ensure their consistent operation and calibration.

Normally, environmental parameters such as temperature and humidity often need to be controlled during API operations. Additional controls are necessary to reduce microbiological loads on the final API (if required), such as pressure differential controls, higher velocity profiles, and a higher level of air-filtration efficiency.

While air recirculation is allowable and may be utilized, the trend in the industry is to provide fresh-air systems to avoid any possibilities of cross-contamination between products or other materials such as intermediates or other formulation components.

The ventilation/air conditioning system must be qualified to demonstrate adequate design, installation, and operation. Engineering drawings must be available and verified to show the system's "as-built" conditions.

Environmental Conditions

Environmental conditions in the areas should be kept so as not to adversely affect the products or materials within the area. Determination of the appropriate environmental conditions within a particular area will depend on several factors including the process steps performed in the area, the level of product exposure, and other process and product characteristics (i.e., is the level of endotoxins in the product controlled or not?). If the API is sterile, the FDA will view it, for regulatory purposes, as if it were a finished product rather than as a bulk API. Temperature is usually not a critical parameter unless the product is stored or exposed for significant periods of time. For areas where this applies, the temperature requirements will depend on the product characteristics.

Humidity may affect final products that are sensitive to it, e.g., and liquid products may lose moisture if exposed to low humidity for extended periods of time. For aseptic processes, lower humidity is generally desirable to reduce possible microbial growth. Again, the appropriate relative humidity for an area will depend on the specific product requirements and the level of product exposure.

Control of air particulates will also depend on the product characteristics and level of exposure. For example, in areas with entirely closed process systems, no air filtration is necessary, whereas exposed aseptic production areas may require Class 100,000 or 10,000 room classifications.

Layout

Equipment Type and Placement

Equipment must be designed and/or purchased as required by the processing steps. The facility design should provide sufficient space as needed for the type and size of the equipment and appurtences required for such operations. There must be sufficient space surrounding the equipment to allow proper access for cleaning, maintenance, and other process related operations associated with the system. There must also be room for the proper handling during manufacturing operations, including installation and removal of auxiliary equipment such as piping or pumps. In addition, consideration must be given to the installation of required utility systems for each piece of equipment and the accessibility of these utilities. Therefore, the location of the equipment within the facility or area becomes a critical factor during the design phase.

Since API manufacturing processes include many operations and sub-tasks, it is advisable to do a detailed review of the intended manufacturing process when preparing the equipment layout. This time spent at the beginning of the design process will prevent rooms or areas from being undersized or badly arranged. All operations and sub-tasks should be visualized and evaluated in light of the floor plan at each stage of the design process.

Areas

Production/Manufacturing. The production area will generally utilize the largest portion of the facility. This area is comprised of all equipment relevant to the manufacturing process, space in which any portable equipment may be cleaned, and area for personnel gowning.

Storage. Adequate space must be provided for storage of materials including segregation of those items that have been rejected or quarantined, or that are undergoing further testing. Materials include received components/ ingredients, intermediates, APIs, or any other related item purchased for the manufacturing process.

These materials must be stored under the conditions specified by the supplier or manufacturer. These normally include temperature, humidity, and accessibility controls for certain materials (when applicable). In some occasions, such conditions involve the availability of cold rooms and other types of controlled environments.

Material storage areas should have controls to prevent product mix-ups and contamination. This includes defined areas or other controls for the following:

- Receipt, identification and storage of materials (raw or in-process) prior to their release for use
- Holding of rejected materials prior to disposition
- Storage of released materials
- Storage of quarantine materials prior to release

These areas should be separated from the manufacturing/ processing areas, and the environmental conditions in these areas should be maintained to ensure that the quality of the materials will not be adversely affected. The design should incorporate controls to ensure that rejected and quarantine materials are stored in a manner to prevent use in manufacturing or processing. Rejected and quarantined materials should be maintained in a controlled area accessible only to authorized personnel.

Sampling Areas. The design should consider:

- Permanent sampling rooms vs. moveable sampling rooms
- Sampling of raw materials in warehouse
- Storage of sampling utensils
- Environmental controls (temperature and relative humidity requirements)
- Sample storage: Testing samples, reserve samples, stability samples

Defined/adequate areas for sampling of materials and components must be available within the facility. These areas could require environmental controls and safety equipment availability when applicable for those raw materials and other chemicals, which could be hazardous to the employee. The main concern must be the proper sampling of material while avoiding contamination of the material being sampled or cross-contamination with other materials.

Packaging and Labeling. There must be areas assigned for packaging of the product and labeling of the containers as specified for the material being stored. These areas must be segregated to avoid cross-contamination and possibilities of a mix-up of different materials. Utilities must be available for the proper operation of the necessary equipment and the layout must be designed considering the space to perform the operation and the handling of the containers, including the inspection of the packaged material.

Laboratories. There must be defined areas for laboratory operations, which normally will be segregated from the manufacturing areas. In the case of in-process testing, these are allowed to be close to or inside manufacturing areas, provided the operation does not affect the accuracy and operation of laboratory instrumentation.

Various types of laboratories as shown below may be incorporated into an API facility or on the site of the API plant: Analytical testing laboratory for raw materials, intermediates, and the API product; raw material use testing laboratory; process development laboratory; microbiological laboratory; and environmental testing laboratory.

Laboratory operations must follow the same guidelines applied to manufacturing areas in terms of accessibility to equipment, utility systems, cleaning/sanitation and minimization of contamination.

Locker and Restroom Facilities. Locker rooms and restroom facilities should be physically separated from the laboratory and processing areas by a room, corridor, or other intermediate space. Physical separation is particularly important when the processing area is one where the product is exposed to the environment or is aseptic. Such facilities should have adequate space and should be sufficiently equipped for facility personnel. All facilities should also meet the applicable building code requirements.

Gowning Areas. Gowning areas should be used when exposure to the product or materials could put personnel at risk and when it is necessary to prevent product contamination. Where gowning areas are needed, such areas should meet the same architectural material requirements as for the production areas to which they connect. Controls should be in place to ensure that the gowning and degowning are not potential sources of contamination. For instance, the facility should prevent personnel from simultaneously gowning and degowning—gowning areas in facilities producing very potent APIs may require separate gowning and degowning areas. The degowning areas for API plants processing potent APIs may also need to be equipped with decontamination showers or other decontamination facilities.

Flow of Materials and Personnel in the Facility

Material Flows

Material flows should be designed to provide easy movement of materials yet prevent product mix-ups, cross-contamination and contamination from the environment. This is especially true for multi-product facilities. One-way flows, while not required, are an efficient way to achieve these goals. Other options include controls to prevent simultaneous flows or the use of simultaneous flows with specific controls to prevent cross-contamination. However, simultaneous material flows should not be used in aseptic facilities.

The design should also adjust flow patterns when exposure to materials or products may place personnel at risk. Controls should prevent flow between areas with open containers and prevent unprotected personnel from entering areas where they could be exposed. Appropriate protective equipment should also be provided in the areas where personnel could be exposed to the material or product.

Material flow diagrams should be generated and used to facilitate the evaluation of the potential impact of material flows on personnel and API processes, as well as raw materials and API products.

Personnel Flows

The design and equipment layout should allow adequate room for personnel access for routine and non-routine maintenance. The layout must also allow for sufficient room for personnel flows in compliance with the applicable building codes. Personnel flows should be designed to prevent contamination to products and materials and to ensure personnel safety. Again, this is especially true with multi-product facilities, where extra precautions may be necessary to prevent cross contamination. In aseptic facilities, controls to prevent simultaneous personnel flows should be in place if necessary to prevent product contamination.

Personnel flow diagrams should be generated and used to facilitate the evaluation of the potential impact of personnel flows on API processes as well as raw materials and API products.

Cleaning/Maintenance

The facility must be designed to allow proper maintenance of the equipment, utility systems and the facility itself. Sufficient space must be available to access the equipment or utility system without requiring dismantling critical parts or components during normal preventive/repair maintenance.

The design of the facility should be done with an eye toward cleanability. The layout of equipment and the materials of construction for both equipment and the facility itself should be chosen to increase ease of cleaning. These decisions will be dependent on the product and process characteristics, as well as the operational issues for the facility.

For process equipment, product contact surfaces should be smooth. Crevices and other hard-to-clean areas should be eliminated to the extent possible. Areas in the process system where material may accumulate and become difficult to clean out (i.e., dead legs) should also be eliminated.

For facilities, flooring and walls should be made of materials that can be easily cleaned. Epoxy paints, although expensive, can last a long time and are easily cleaned. All areas that would normally be dust collectors (i.e., open areas over side wall cabinets) should be closed in.

Aseptic areas require utmost and meticulous cleaning and maintenance. Materials should be carefully selected to ensure minimization of contamination.

The decision on whether to use automated or manual cleaning will be dependent on the facility operations. While automated cleaning provides several advantages, including reproducible results and better process control, automation is less desirable for processes that are only to be run a few times. Manual cleaning may be more appropriate in these situations.

For larger pieces of equipment, clean in place (CIP) procedures may be desirable, therefore the layout of the equipment must allow for access for cleaning. If clean out of place procedures are to be used, adequate facilities for cleaning (e.g., designated wash areas) should be available and the design should minimize the potential of re-contamination of the equipment after cleaning.

Other Considerations

Automation/Controls

When designing a facility, a decision must be made in terms of the level of automation to be included. This decision will have an effect on the initial cost, the operational cost, and the long-term maintenance cost for the facility. More automation normally implies more initial cost and a higher on-going maintenance level/cost. The advantage of automation is on the precision/accuracy of the control over the selected parameters and the elimination of manual controls that can result in errors or even quality problems with the API being manufactured. This becomes a risk assessment that must be made to determine which parameters/areas/systems will require more automation than others.

The API manufacturer must evaluate and decide upon a suitable control system architecture and installation plan for control system components early in any API project. The manufacturer needs to decide what type of process control system will be employed to accomplish the control objectives for the API project. Additionally, the manufacturer needs to decide what type of field devices will be used and how they will be installed and wired in the field. All instruments and control devices must be suitable for the environment in which they will be installed. If instruments will be installed in a hazardous area then, they must be intrinsically safe or explosion proof rated. Another field wiring consideration related to field devices for the API facility or process designer is the extent of use of distributed wiring, field bus wiring, and hard wiring of individual devices. Many DCS systems and PLCs offered by vendors today have processors that can communicate with input/output modules mounted in the field near the equipment via a two wire cable. Additionally, fieldbus technology exists that allows field instruments to be daisy chained together in the field. These field bus systems not only reduce the amount of field wiring required for field devices, but they also have the capability of communicating a greater amount of information to the main processor at high speeds. (See Chapter 14 for a more detailed discussion of DCSs, PLCs, and input and output wiring practices for these modern process control systems.)

API manufacturing processes usually involve multiple unit operations performed in succession in order to produce a usable chemical entity. These multiple unit operations are typically performed in a series of interconnected pieces of process equipment—what is called a process train. The activities associated with the manufacturing process and the operation of the process equipment systems are usually quite complicated and therefore need to be monitored and controlled by a process controller such as a DCS, PLC, process computer, or some combination of these devices. Additionally, since APIs are considered pharmaceutical starting materials, the process control system will need to provide some type of secure data collection and storage. All of the various activities and operations of a manufacturing process constitute the batch recipe for a particular product. The many API processing activities and operations can typically be broken down into discrete tasks or phases. These tasks or phases can then be linked to API manufacturing unit operations and specific equipment in a batch recipe in order to accomplish an API manufacturing process. Table 2 shows some typical phases that may be established for controlling the manufacturing processes in an API facility.

TABLE 2   Process Phases

Phase	Description
Liquid addition	Charge a liquid to a vessel
Inerting	Reduce oxygen content in vessel below LEL
Pressure hold test	Confirm acceptable leakage rate for vessel when pressurized
Vacuum hold test	Confirm acceptable leakage rate for vessel when under vacuum
Heat-up	Apply heat to a vessel or system to bring the contents up to a defined temperature

Editor's Note: _____

The S88 Batch Control Standard is a document that can be used to assist the API process designer in developing efficient, modular, and organized control system programs for implementing batch recipes and process operation phases. S88 provides a framework for defining and detailing batch process operations and their control within a process controller. This process control tool should be consulted when developing the process control system for an API manufacturing process.

Closed vs. Open Equipment

Closed equipment is preferred to minimize the probability of contamination. If open equipment is used, the facility must be designed to control the sources of possible contamination so that the product is protected. Additional levels of "containment" may be required for specific materials and these requirements must be considered during the facility design.

In addition to the decision to use open or closed equipment, the designer must also consider whether the equipment will be installed in an open processing area or within a closed room. As mentioned previously, closed rooms are preferable for equipment processing potent compounds. Further, closed rooms are also preferable for equipment where the API product is at risk due to open equipment operations.

DESIGN IMPLICATIONS IN TERMS OF PERFORMANCE AND COMPLIANCE

Quality Implications

Proper design of an API facility can mean less opportunity for errors and quality concerns. Some of the typical problems with facility design that have been observed and may have an impact on the product quality are:

- *Access to facility/equipment is not adequate for cleaning/maintenance.* If the procedures for cleaning and maintenance are difficult, these will have an effect ultimately on the product quality.
- *Necessary utilities not considered as part of the design.* Some companies still use drums to carry water and other components between areas and for storage, increasing the probability of contamination for the API product.
- *Open vs. closed processing.* Facilities not designed for open processing of the API could cause the product to be contaminated. They must provide the proper environmental controls to eliminate the possibility of contamination when the product is exposed to the environment. Closed systems could be considered as a separate facility, even if they are physically within the same area. Clean environments are normally required for the final API process steps.

Safety

Safety is a matter of the highest priority in the design of a facility. In most pharmaceutical environments, the chances of hazardous conditions occurring must be considered, monitored, and prevented. Safety issues are most apparent when the chemicals used are potentially bio-reactive (including carcinogenic, explosive, and/or corrosive chemicals), but should still be a top priority even where non-hazardous chemicals are used. In facilities where the materials and processes are known, the design of the facility may be tailored to its needs; however, the future potential for additional processes or changes in the processes should be considered.

The design of the facility must also be in compliance with local, state and federal (OSHA) safety and building codes.

Waste Disposal/EPA Issues

Waste disposal is a major area of concern in API facility design. Aside from the usual sewage waste facilities, there must also be systems capable of handling chemical waste materials "dumped" from manufacturing equipment and laboratories, as well as systems for disposing of unwanted, expired, or degraded materials. Systems must be in place to accommodate solid, liquid, and gaseous wastes. Most wastes are considered pollutants and therefore the systems must comply with local, state, and federal requirements. Federal requirements include compliance with the Clean Air Act and the Clean Water Act and related regulations.

Depending on the type of production, some firms may need to consider on-site bio-containment systems in order to denature, degrade, or alter the pollutants before discharging them into local systems. If the site produces DEA controlled material, then additional controls will be required to ensure security. (Refer to Chapter 20 of this book for further guidance on EPA concerns regarding API manufacturing sites.)

Flexibility

The design of an API facility should incorporate elements of flexibility commensurate with its intended processing needs. API facilities that will produce multiple products simultaneously or perform multiple types of API manufacturing processes require significant elements of flexibility such as solvent distribution networks, standardized equipment system design, standardized process unit control templates, manifold stations/transfer panels, shared utility networks, communication between and control of different processing units via a master control system, etc. It must be ensured, however, that any elements of flexibility do not compromise the intended purity of the API product.

Standardization

The design of an API facility or process improvement should seek to provide standardized equipment, instrumentation, electrical system, etc. as appropriate to reduce spare parts and training costs.

Expansion and Bottleneck Concerns

The design should take into consideration potential bottleneck concerns. Bottlenecks are process specific and may occur for a variety of reasons such as equipment scheduling issues and maximum batch size constraints. An evaluation of the processes should be performed to determine where bottlenecks are likely to arise. Allowances should also be made for expected growth. The layout should include space for additional equipment to meet future growth and expansion requirements as appropriate.

The effects of future expansion should be considered for all areas of the facility design. For example, the designer should consider allowing room for additional piping, increasing the capacity of utilities, and providing adequate space and facilities for additional personnel.

PROJECT MANAGEMENT ISSUES

Project Approach

An API manufacturing company has a variety of options available for implementing a new facility project or a plant renovation project. If available the API manufacturer may choose to implement the project with in-house personnel. If in-house personnel are not available to implement the project, then some or all of the following functions may be outsourced to an outside firm or firms: engineering and design, procurement, construction management, equipment inspection, commissioning, and validation.

In the late 1990s a major API manufacturer performed two significant plant renovation projects, each using a different approach to implementation. One of these projects was implemented entirely by an in-house staff of engineers and contractors. The second project was implemented entirely by an outside firm from the detailed design stage through to the commissioning stage. Both of these approaches yielded successful API plant renovation projects.

Project Scheduling: Milestones

It is critical to prepare a project schedule for the definition, design (including design review and qualification), construction, start-up, commissioning, and validation of the facility. It is also imperative to involve all applicable functions throughout the entire process as necessary. The Quality Control and Assurance and Validation groups must be involved during the design review and qualification to confirm that the process/equipment/compliance considerations are being included during these steps. Environmental personnel should also be involved during all facets of the project definition and design effort to ensure that environmental compliance is achieved via appropriate waste treatment strategies and practices. Milestones must be established for each major section of the schedule. Design logic should be incorporated into the report process. To be successful, a description of each of the unit operations is required. This should highlight conflicts before they affect any timelines. Figure 11 provides a generic timeline for the activities to be performed during an API capital expansion or renovation project. Many standard and specialized programs exist for developing project schedules. These projects can be used to identify, track, and report the resources required for a project as well as track the progress of the project. Additionally, a well maintained electronic project schedule can be useful in identifying critical path project tasks throughout the project so that resources can be appropriately assigned to ensure the timely completion of these activities.

It is often a good approach to visit the local FDA District Office with the proposed plans to seek their advice and input.

Resources Allocation

As explained above, it is imperative to involve all appropriate functions during the entire design/construction process, especially the Quality and Validation departments. Resources must be identified and committed for these activities. The probable cost of not involving and considering these needs as early as possible are exponentially higher than selecting and committing the appropriate resources at the right time.

Good Engineering Practices (GEPs) Throughout the Project

The application of the GEPs will support the overall GMP level of the design, construction, and start-up procedures and documentation so that the quality and validation functions will have a higher probability of success during the actual review of the design and qualification of the facility. The application of GEPs recognizes that

FIGURE 11   Timeline for API Expansion or Renovation

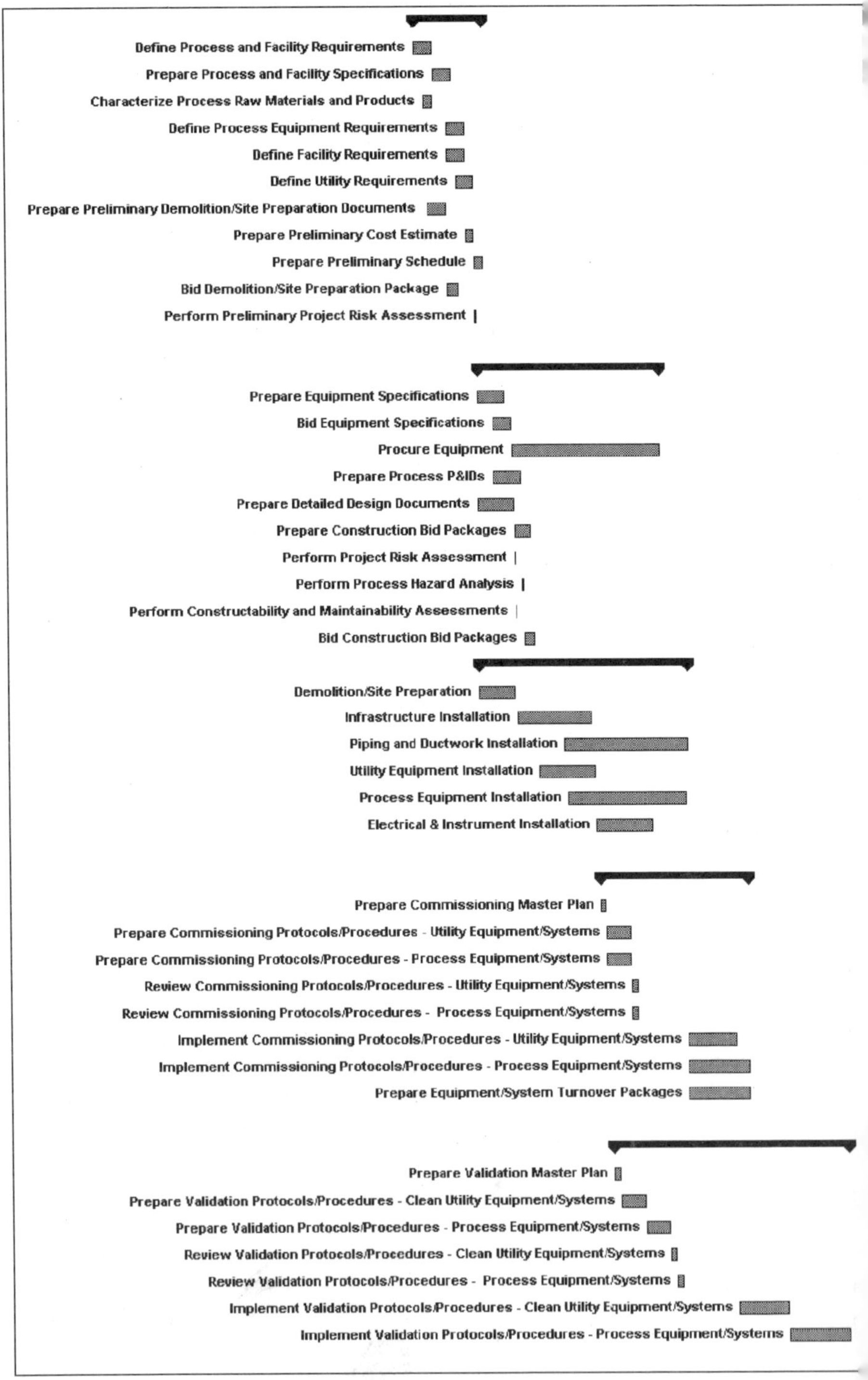

Define Process and Facility Requirements
Prepare Process and Facility Specifications
Characterize Process Raw Materials and Products
Define Process Equipment Requirements
Define Facility Requirements
Define Utility Requirements
Prepare Preliminary Demolition/Site Preparation Documents
Prepare Preliminary Cost Estimate
Prepare Preliminary Schedule
Bid Demolition/Site Preparation Package
Perform Preliminary Project Risk Assessment

Prepare Equipment Specifications
Bid Equipment Specifications
Procure Equipment
Prepare Process P&IDs
Prepare Detailed Design Documents
Prepare Construction Bid Packages
Perform Project Risk Assessment
Perform Process Hazard Analysis
Perform Constructability and Maintainability Assessments
Bid Construction Bid Packages

Demolition/Site Preparation
Infrastructure Installation
Piping and Ductwork Installation
Utility Equipment Installation
Process Equipment Installation
Electrical & Instrument Installation

Prepare Commissioning Master Plan
Prepare Commissioning Protocols/Procedures - Utility Equipment/Systems
Prepare Commissioning Protocols/Procedures - Process Equipment/Systems
Review Commissioning Protocols/Procedures - Utility Equipment/Systems
Review Commissioning Protocols/Procedures - Process Equipment/Systems
Implement Commissioning Protocols/Procedures - Utility Equipment/Systems
Implement Commissioning Protocols/Procedures - Process Equipment/Systems
Prepare Equipment/System Turnover Packages

Prepare Validation Master Plan
Prepare Validation Protocols/Procedures - Clean Utility Equipment/Systems
Prepare Validation Protocols/Procedures - Process Equipment/Systems
Review Validation Protocols/Procedures - Clean Utility Equipment/Systems
Review Validation Protocols/Procedures - Process Equipment/Systems
Implement Validation Protocols/Procedures - Clean Utility Equipment/Systems
Implement Validation Protocols/Procedures - Process Equipment/Systems

all systems in the facility routinely undergo some form of commissioning. Most of the engineering specifications require levels of documentation, inspection, and field-testing which must be appropriate and acceptable to regulatory officials. GEPs also recommend that facility management engage all applicable functions as early as possible in the planning, design, construction, start-up, and commissioning of each plant system. This can result in the elimination of redundancy on the documentation of such steps by using these documents during the actual qualification activities. Change control will also be an integral part of the application of the GEPs, which is extremely important during the validation efforts.

Some of the important elements of GEPs that must be applied throughout the project lifecycle are as follows: routine constructability, maintainability, and operability assessments; equipment factory inspections; factory acceptance testing; equipment history tracking and documentation; project risk assessment and management; multiple discipline design coordination; design document updating; etc.

Compliance and Validation Concepts: From Project Definition Through Design, Construction, Start-Up, and Commissioning

The application of quality, validation and general GMP compliance concepts during the project definition and design stage are key to the success of the entire project to get the facility into operations quickly, effectively, and within compliance. GMP design must be built in and cannot be added afterward. Steps such as a documented design review and design qualification are concepts extracted from the 21 CFR §820, Quality Systems Regulations for Devices, that have been applied to other industries, and the trend shows that they are effective tools that will be, in the future, required for pharmaceutical and API production facilities. These steps are normally included in a quality plan document. In this document, the necessary functions involved with the facility project are involved in its development, review, and approval. This plan should include the following:

- Project definition/objectives/purposes
- References: Regulatory documents, company policies, definitions
- Definition of responsibilities
- Design basis
- Specifications: User requirements, functional requirements
- Design process: Reference to GEPs, handling of drawings and specifications (change control)
- Design review and qualification requirements
- Start-up and commissioning requirements
- Facility qualification requirements
- Audit/monitoring of the plan

This Quality Plan is not a Validation Master Plan but a predecessor to it.

The selection of the vendor/supplier for the equipment and materials of construction must, of course, consider their capability of providing the specified materials/equipment, but also the necessary documentation, installation, service and guarantees. It is desirable to work with vendors that are certified to be ISO-9000 compliant, and the user must verify the availability and implementation/effectiveness of procedures and internal controls even before making the decision of purchasing the material/equipment from them. This is usually completed through a vendor audit. The probability of performing a Factory Acceptance Test is also desirable. These criteria must also apply to the designer/construction contractors, who must provide adequate documentation of the work performed and change control procedures during the design and construction phases.

Project Documentation

Any project related to an FDA-regulated facility of process requires a substantial amount of documentation. It is expected that the API manufacturer will establish and document their process(es) and facility as well as the rationale used to define the process(es) and facility. These design documents then become the basis for validating the suitability of the process(es), facility, equipment, and support systems of the API facility or process renovation. Many of the documents mentioned earlier willl be required to be maintained and verified for correctness as part of the commissioning and/or validation of the API process project.

TRENDS AND FUTURE DEVELOPMENTS

Biotechnology: Vaccines Manufacturing, Virus, and DNA Removal Facilities

The design of biotech facilities should incorporate controls to prevent or minimize possible contamination to the product. The level of environmental controls depends on the process step involved and the level of exposure of the product to the environment, etc.

- Descriptions and diagrams of the facility must include air intakes and outlets. The planning of air handling systems should take into consideration prevailing wind direction. Information must be available as to proximity of animal facilities or animal housing (including farms). Air handling units of in-house animal facilities must be separate from units of environmentally controlled areas.
- Planning of the production area must include appropriate traffic patterns for personnel and equipment. Critical areas must be controlled for access. For example, unauthorized and untrained personnel must not be allowed into critical areas. Personnel control may be affected by physical means, such as key-cards. All personnel must be trained on controlled entry.
- Layouts of multi-use facilities must be designed so that cross-contamination among substances, components, or an intermediate does not occur. Air handling and the environment of component preparation and compounding must be designed and controlled to assure the absence of cross-contamination.
- Cleaning procedures must be established and validated in all areas of storage, preparation, and production.
- Air handling must be designed to prevent cross-contamination among drug substances, intermediates, and components.

R&D and Clinical Material Manufacturing: Facility and Equipment Requirements for Validation and Regulatory Compliance

The industry standard practices have applied the GMP qualification requirements to the facility and equipment used for R&D and clinical material manufacturing processes. More and more companies are having their facilities for R&D and clinical material manufacturing qualified under the same requirements as for the processing of commercial product. The reason is to be able to justify that their R&D and clinical materials were manufactured with "qualified equipment/facilities" and to provide a higher level of assurance in terms of the product success and consistency of operation, not only to the regulatory officials but also to company management.

Further Controls to Eliminate Cross Contamination: Physical Barriers Between Equipment/Processes

The appropriate level of protection is determined based on the following factors:

- *Exposure of the substance to the environment.* This will be dependant on whether the process is performed in an open or closed equipment/system. For open systems, the concern is more critical than for closed systems where the substance is not exposed to the environment.
- *Phase within the synthesis.* This includes initial intermediates vs. final intermediates, or crude BPC vs. final purification. As the process moves closer to final product, more controls must be in place.
- *Risk of contamination*: Perform a risk assessment of the possible sources of contamination and the probabilities of each of them to occur.
- *Impact of trace quantities of contamination.* This will be specific for the process or product.

The ISPE Engineering Guide recommends the establishment of three levels of protection: Level I: General; Level II: Protected; and Level III: Controlled. Each level includes certain requirements based on the contamination impact and the other aspects listed above. The company must establish their own levels and guidelines and include them on their Quality Plan described on Section V(d).

Process Analytical Technologies

In designing new API facilities, manufacturers may want to consider the use of process analytical technologies (PATs). PATs are "[s]ystems for analysis and control of manufacturing processes based on timely measurements, during processing, of critical quality parameters and performance attributes of raw and in-process materials and process to assure acceptable end product quality at the completion of the process." The FDA has recently taken a particular interest in the use of PATs in pharmaceutical manufacturing recognizing the potential benefits, such as increased process efficiency. The FDA is encouraging manufacturers to propose submissions for the use of PATs in their processes and is willing to work with companies through the development process and answer questions as they come up.

When evaluating the potential use of PATs in a process, manufacturers should ensure that the PAT is suitable for the intended use and that it is equivalent or better than the corresponding traditional product test.

BIBLIOGRAPHY

ISPE. Pharmaceutical Engineering Guide, Volume 1: Bulk Pharmaceutical Chemicals.

ICH. Q7A Good Manufacturing Practice Guidance for Active Pharmaceutical Ingredients.

FDA. Guidance for Industry: Manufacturing, Processing, or Holding Active Pharmaceutical Ingredients.

PDA Technical Report No. 29, Points to Consider for Cleaning Validation, 1998.

Petrides, D., Koulouris, A., and Siletti, C. Throughput Analysis and Debottlenecking of Biomanuacturing Facilities, *Biopharm.* August 1992, pp. 28–34.

Brocklebank, M.P., Deo, P. V., GMP Issues for Bulk Pharmaceutical Chemical Plants. *Pharmaceutical Engin.*, Jan/Feb. 1996, pp. 8–26.

S88. Batch Control Standard.

RESOURCES

Synthetic Organic Chemical Manufacturer's Association (SOCMA)
International Society of Pharmaceutical Engineers (ISPE)
American Institute of Chemical Engineers
Chemical Engineering
Pharmaceutical Engineering
Design Institute for Emergency Relief Systems (DIERS)
World Batch Forum (WBF)
Instrument Society of America (ISA)

14

Building Code Compliance

Author: Eric Bohn

INTRODUCTION

This chapter provides an overview of the building and zoning codes and associated standards and regulations that impact the design and construction of pharmaceutical manufacturing facilities. Local municipal and state governments are the primary authorities promulgating these codes. However, there are also additional agencies at the federal level promulgating regulations and standards that impact facility design and construction. Examples of these include the Americans with Disabilities Act (ADA), Occupational Safety and Health Agency (OSHA), and many specialty concerns such as the Nuclear Regulatory Commission (NRC) for control and use of radioactive materials, and the Drug Enforcement Agency (DEA) for controlled substances.

Codes represent the minimum requirements required by local, state, and federal governments to legally construct a facility. A design for a new facility, as well as renovation of an existing facility, must be based on the codes that apply to the particular circumstances and then be constructed to meet them. As will be demonstrated, compliance with codes represents an extraordinary amount of information that must be incorporated into a design. Fortunately, on any given project, the responsibility for code compliance is divided between the numerous specialty designers engaged, such as the architect and civil, mechanical, electrical, pumping, fire protection, and environmental engineers.

In the United States, all levels of government have a constitutional mandate to protect the health, safety, and welfare of the public. All codes are an outgrowth of this mandate. During the course of the early twentieth century, the public's health, safety, and welfare has increasingly been interpreted to include minimum requirements for the construction of buildings and structures. This interpretation has largely been the result of large disastrous events. One of the earliest events was the Chicago Fire of 1871, after which the city required all construction to be masonry. In the twentieth century, regulations to protect the public health, safety, and welfare relative to construction spread until it became almost a universal requirement in communities all across the nation. Interestingly, many of the events that encouraged code development were fires where large numbers of individuals were killed. The public outrage that followed such events lead to a belief that government has a role to play in guaranteeing minimal, consistent levels of safety in building construction. A current example of this historical process is the tragedy of September 11, 2001. The World Trade Center terrorist attacks are being aggressively researched and debated within the code community. This will, no doubt, result in new and more stringent code requirements for the design and construction community.

The first building codes were simple and direct, such as the Chicago Building Code of 1875 that was in response to the fire of 1871 mentioned earlier; the Code mandated the use of masonry construction in an attempt to prevent devastating fires. An example of the intent of a modern building code is the following excerpt from the International Building Code:

> The purpose of this Code is to establish the minimum requirements to safeguard the public health, safety and general welfare through structural strength, means of egress facilities, stability, sanitation, adequate light and ventilation, energy conservation, and safety to life and property from fire and other hazards attributed to the built environment.

The first zoning ordinance was adopted in New York City in 1916. This was a revolutionary set of land use laws that were a response to the intense development occurring in lower Manhattan after the turn of the century. The zoning code initially established height and setback controls to ensure that neighboring properties had access to light and air. Also, the code separated what were considered to be functionally incompatible uses; thus, factories were excluded from residential neighborhoods.

While building codes ensure public health, safety and welfare within individual properties, which is to say the buildings themselves, the intent of zoning codes is to ensure the health, safety, and welfare of entire communities. The concern here is how multiple properties interact with each other and what impact they have on the overall community. Zoning concerns include:

- Encouraging appropriate land uses for the community
- Safety from fire, flood, panic, and other natural or man-made disasters
- Establishing appropriate population densities, thus preventing overcrowding of land
- Providing all properties with access to adequate light, air, and open space
- Convenience and coordination of transportation routes
- Encourage efficient expenditure of public funds by coordination of public development
- The conservation of property values

Besides building and zoning codes, there are numerous additional guidelines and standards that impact the design and construction of buildings. These generally fall into two groups. There are technical standards that are specifically referenced by the building codes and thereby supplement and extend the technical precision of the code. These include standards by organizations such as American Society of Heating, Refrigeration and Air Conditioning Engineers (ASHRAE), American National Standards Institute (ANSI), American Society for Testing and Materials (ASTM), Factory Mutual (FM), and National Fire Protection Association (NFPA). The second class of standards are specific federal ordinances that apply to special and specific aspects of a building, especially manufacturing facilities. These include regulations from the following government agencies Occupational Safety and Health Agency (OSHA), Environmental Protection Agency (EPA), Drug Enforcement Administration (DEA), Nuclear Regulatory Commission (NRC), and the Americans with Disabilities Act (ADA).

KEY CONCEPTS

Codes are a legal minimum for the design and construction of any facility. Codes cannot be avoided. They must be embraced, understood, and integrated into every facility design. There is a legal obligation to follow the code minimums; however, exceeding the codes is sometimes appropriate and may be in the owner's best interest.

The sheer number of codes that relate to facility design is daunting. In order to proceed in an effective manner, it is necessary to be familiar with all the codes and know when and where each is applicable. In this way one can narrow the pursuit and make compliance a manageable endeavor.

There are many codes and even more standards. Continual updates and new editions of the codes are common. It is crucial to follow the codes that are adopted and enforced in the jurisdiction where a building is being built. This is not necessarily the most recent code. Sometimes it is assumed that the new codes are "better" and therefore more appropriate. However, it is only the legally adopted code that has legal standing and a legal basis for enforcement. Not following the adopted code can easily result in non-compliance.

Codes are not presented in a linear manner. This is particularly true when you consider the many different codes that must be researched and addressed. However, it is also true within the individual codes themselves. A thorough code review is an interactive process, requiring one to work back and forth between the various parts of the code and testing the various options available, before settling on an approach beneficial to the owner.

The language of codes tries to be precise. However, when applied to real world situations the code does not always provide a clear answer. At such times it is necessary to seek an interpretation of the code. The local code official is typically charged with the legal authority to make final interpretations of the code. However, the design professional makes code interpretations as a matter of course in development of every design and has a responsibility to provide a design that is code compliant.

Zoning Codes

Local codes addressing building construction are split between the issues of overall land use and of the building itself. These are, respectively, zoning codes and building codes. Zoning codes regulate general land use and development issues for individual properties. They provide specific restrictions on the use of individual properties from the perspective of the "greater good" of the community. Zoning and land development is an open, public process. Depending on the specifics of a project, public hearings are often necessary. When changes or variances are being sought for a specific property the public hearing process is usually measured in months. Large projects covering many acres can take a year or more before approval is granted and very large projects involving perhaps hundreds of acres may take several years. In many jurisdictions, especially for commercial and industrial development, it is prudent to have legal representation. Occasionally, establishing the limits of the individual property owner's rights vs. the governing authority is adjudicated in the courts.

The fundamental component of land use regulations is the zoning district. Every acre of land within a community is categorized for uses that are acceptable. In general these districts are categorized as residential, commercial, retail, and industrial. Often these categories are further subdivided into "levels" or densities of use, such as industrial and light industrial. Also, special "mixed use" districts can be created that combine several of the traditional uses. The zoning code details the uses that are allowed for each particular district and establishes specific design standards and regulations. Besides the main or primary uses that are allowed, each district usually includes certain other special uses. These are typically called "conditional uses" and are considered compatible with the main use or are allowed under certain specific circumstances.

The regulations pertaining to each zoning district is described within the text of the municipality's zoning code. Historically there have been no nationally recognized "model" zoning codes that are ready-made for adoption by local communities. However, the International Code Council has recently begun to publish such a model code. Most existing zoning codes have been developed by the individual jurisdiction and is specific to that locale. Also, local zoning codes usually evolve over time allowing communities to modify and change in response to the changing needs, concerns, and circumstances of the community. The zoning codes for different municipalities vary greatly and must be consulted for each project.

Building Codes

Since the early part of the twentieth century, three regional organizations have developed the model codes that have dominated the building industry throughout the United States. These are the Building Officials and Code Administrators International, Inc. (BOCA), International Conference of Building Officials (ICBO), and the Southern Building Code Congress, Inc. (SBCCI). While regional code development has been effective and responsive to the needs of the country, in time it became apparent that a single set of codes, applied across the country, could be beneficial. It was believed that uniform codes would allow consistent and efficient code enforcement, encourage greater commerce across state lines, and result in consistent and higher construction quality. In 1994, the three model code organizations came together and created the International Code Council (ICC) and developed the International Building Codes (IBC). These codes are currently in the process of being adopted by many local municipalities across the country.

A second model building code has recently been introduced and is attempting to challenge the current perception of dominance by the IBC. NFPA 5000^{TM} Building Construction and Safety Code^{TM} has been developed by the National Fire Protection Association (NFPA). There is merit in much of the rational behind the development of NFPA 5000^{TM}, and in many respects it is similar to the IBC. At first glance however, it seems unlikely that NFPA 5000^{TM} will supplant the IBC across the country. The International Code Council, which develops the IBC, is a national organization dominated by code officials. Because code officials are the primary advocates and enforcers of codes, they are naturally inclined to support their own organization—an organization established to facilitate and reflect the concerns and demands of their profession. However, in the fall of 2003 NFPA 5000 Building Construction and Safety Code and NFPA 1: Uniform Fire Code™ was approved for adoption by the State of California. It will be interesting to see how this competition develops.

In this chapter, we focus on the International Building Codes assuming that these represent a more general set of standards at this time. The IBC is not just a single building code but a complete set of coordinated codes designed to accommo-

TABLE 1 International Model Building Codes

International Building Code
International Fire Code
International Mechanical Code
International Plumbing Code
International Code Council Electrical Code
International Energy Conservation Code
International Fuel Gas Code
International Property Maintenance Code
International Residential Code
International Private Sewage Disposal Code
International Existing Buildings Code
International Zoning Code
International Urban-Wildlife Interface Code
ICC Electrical Code Administrative Provisions
ICC Performance Code

date the complete code needs of all municipalities and jurisdictions. These model codes are listed in Table 1.

There also exist several other specialty model codes. These are often adopted in conjunction with the other model codes. Prime examples of these are the National Electrical Code, which is a popular electric code developed by the NFPA, and the National Standard Plumbing Code, developed by the National Association of Plumbing–Heating–Cooling Contractors. Both these model codes can be used and frequently are used in place of the corresponding ICC codes listed above. Very often, the total package of model codes adopted by a jurisdiction are a mix from these and other agencies. As an example see Table 2 that lists codes adopted statewide by the State of New Jersey as of 2005. Note in the table that there are a series of model codes from different years or "code cycles," as well as from different agencies. Also, there are two specialty codes written by the jurisdiction itself.

TABLE 2 Construction Codes Adopted in New Jersey (2005)

Code	Originating Agency
International Building Code (2000) with amendments	International Code Council
International Residential Code (2000) with amendments	International Code Council
CABO Energy Code/ (1995)	International Code Council
ASRAE 90.1 (1999)	American Society of Heating Refrigerating and Air Conditioning Engineers
International Mechanical Code (2000) with amendments	International Code Council
International Fuel Gas Code (2000) with amendments	International Code Council
National Electric Code (2000) with amendments	National Fire Protection Agency
National Standard Plumbing Code (2000) with amendments	National Association of Plumbing–Heating–Cooling Contractors
Rehabilitation Subcode	State of New Jersey
Barrier Free Subcode	State of New Jersey
ANSI A117.1 (1998) with amendments	International Code Council

Model codes are designed to be adopted as is. However, usually there are administrative modifications and additions. In some cases, for example New York State, the jurisdiction modifies the technical content of the model code and effectively publishes their own code. In all cases, each jurisdiction adopts the codes they deem appropriate. Therefore, it is important to verify the codes that are enforced for each given location. Also, the model codes change over time. The ICC is on a 3-year cycle with yearly supplements. Therefore, it is important to determine if a jurisdiction has recently changed or is planning to change their adopted codes to a more recent edition.

Beyond the specifics of the building code itself are the requirements set forth in the other codes. Most of these are specific to the various trades and cover code minimum technical requirements for the engineered building systems including plumbing, mechanical, electrical, fuel-gas, and private sewage disposal. In addition, the Fire, Energy Conservation, Property Maintenance, and Residential Codes cover areas of construction of special concern that can not be adequately covered in the other codes. Depending on the scope of the project some or most of these codes may apply. Fortunately, on any given project, the responsibility for code compliance is divided among all the specialty designers.

Other Standards

In addition to the building codes listed above, there are numerous standards and regulations that must also be addressed. The IBC itself devotes 19 pages to standards from 50 different organizations that are specifically referenced in the text of the code. Many of these standards are specific to the use and design of particular materials and systems like those from the American Concrete Institute (ACI) and the National Fire Protection Association (NFPA).

The referenced NFPA standards include many that are typical for all types of construction, such as NFPA 13: Installation of Sprinkler Systems. However, due to the use of hazardous materials so common in pharmaceutical manufacturing facilities, the following are also of special importance:

- NFPA 30: Flammable and Combustible Liquids Code
- NFPA 69: Explosion Prevention Systems
- NFPA 654: Prevention of Fire and Duct Explosions in the Chemical Dye, Pharmaceutical and Plastics Industries

Additional codes and standards deserving special note are as follows:

Elevator Code. ASME A17.1 Safety Code for Elevators and Escalators is a standard referenced in the building code. However, because historically the elevator was recognized as posing a potential life and safety danger before the advent of most building codes, the individual states usually mandate compliance with their own elevator code. Often this is ASME A17.1, but frequently the states add special, detailed requirements.

Factory Mutual (FM). Factory Mutual Standards Laboratory has developed many construction related standards. A few of them are referenced in the building code. However, if a company is insured by Factory Mutual then compliance with these standards must be explored. In any case, it is always important to check with the insurance carrier that will insure a facility whether they have special requirements that will impact the facility design and construction.

Occupational Safety and Health Agency (OSHA). A portion of CFR 29, Part 1910 addresses design of buildings and structures. Usually, the building codes cover the same ground and are often more stringent. However, in practice there are times when the building code does not cover a particular situation. It is not unusual to find such conditions when developing the layout of mechanical rooms and equipment platforms. At those times when the building code is not applicable, it is necessary to look to OSHA as a minimum standard.

Drug Enforcement Agency (DEA). When narcotics or other controlled substances are present in a pharmaceutical facility the DEA provides guidance. These provisions usually focus on security of the controlled substances and include the need and special criteria for the design of vaults.

Americans with Disabilities Act (ADA). A unique regulation that impacts the design and construction of pharmaceutical manufacturing facilities is a federal law entitled the Americans with Disabilities Act. This is a federal *civil rights* law that intends to guarantee accessibility to the public realm for all people with disabilities. As such it extends well beyond building design and construction, addressing such issues as hiring, firing, and the working conditions of disabled employees and potential employees.

This civil rights law addresses the design and construction of public and commercial buildings with a set of design guidelines. The Americans with Disabilities Act Design Guidelines were based on an old edition of the ANSI handicapped standards. Although these design guidelines are not dissimilar to other existing handicapped design standards and are familiar to construction and design professionals the ADA Design Guidelines supplement existing local codes and carry the weight of a civil rights law. The implication of these design standards as a civil rights law means that they would likely to be resolved in a court of law if an accusation of discrimination has occurred. It should also be reiterated that this law goes well beyond the design guidelines for a facility and may impact a company's hiring and other operational considerations.

Environmental Protection Agency (EPA) and State Department of Environmental Protection (DEP) Permits. When working with development of a site there can be environmental restrictions and guidelines for its development that must be followed. These issues can effect how a building is sited on the property and often concerns the presence of adjacent wetlands and, in some locations, endangered species. Also, the various discharge potentials for a site, such as sanitary waste and storm drainage, may be an issue that must be carefully considered. The air discharge for a facility, if it contains potentially dangerous substances, may also be an environmental issue. In more urban areas these issues are sometimes addressed locally, but there are locations where permits are required at the state or even federal level.

Code Interpretation

Reading and understanding the various codes is an involved and intricate process. While much of the codes are reasonably clear, inevitable there are areas and situations requiring interpretation. Because the origin of codes arises from the government's duty to provide for the public's health, safety and welfare, interpretations must be objective and not just made in favor of the building owner. Enforcement and interpretation of codes for the public good are provided through the building plan review and building permit process. It is a long established principal that the local code authority responsible for enforcement is the final authority and arbiter of any code. This is clearly stated in the International Building Code. However, it is not appropriate or practical to look to the local code official for continuous code input during design. Likewise, it is the design professional that holds the legal responsibility for a code compliant design. By necessity the design professional provides code interpretations whenever they develop a design and can be called upon by the owner to consider various options and implications vis-à-vis the codes. When an unusual or particularly difficult situation arises that is outside the design professional's experience or expertise, it is possible to hire a consultant who specializes in code interpretation. Finally, the model code organizations provide code interpretation services for individuals and firms who are members. In fact, design professionals often take advantage of such interpretive services as a normal part of their design work.

To summarize, there are four primary sources for code interpretations:

- The design professional
- Specialty code consultants
- The model code organizations
- The local code official

Role of the Design Professional

As a profession licensed by the individual states the design professional has a legal responsibility to provide designs that meet the codes enforced within that state. On a daily basis the design professional deals with the codes and their design implementations. Their experience dealing with the codes, the code officials and the resulting impact on design can be extensive. As a result, they are usually the best first source for interpretations, especially when dealing within their areas of expertise.

Role of the Specialty Code Consultant

Due to the complexity and potentially intimidating quality of codes, a code consultant industry has developed. For these professionals, working with the code is a daily endeavor. Due to the intensity and singular nature of their practice they are capable of acquiring an extraordinary depth of knowledge about the details of the codes.

Role of the Model Code Organizations

As noted before, the ICC and the NFPA are the primary organizations responsible for the two competing groups of building codes. Both organizations have procedures designed to help the design professional and building owners interpret their codes. These include informal interpretations via the telephone as well as formal, written interpretations.

Role of the Code Official

The code official is the public entity entrusted with enforcement of the code and has the legal authority to make code interpretations. Section 104.1 of the IBC states:

The building official shall have the authority to render interpretations of this code and to adopt policies and procedures in order to clarify the application of its provisions. Such interpretations, policies and procedures shall be in compliance with the intent and purpose of this code. Such policies and procedures shall not have the effect of waiving requirements specifically provided for in this code.

The normal procedure is for the final construction documents to be submitted to the code official for review and approval, and is a prerequisite for issuing a building permit. Only when there is non-conformance does the code official make a statement about the code. Typically, the code official requests changes be made to bring the design into conformance with specific code citations. While this is the formal procedure, it is often advisable and appropriate to request an informal meeting or even a number of meetings with the code official. These meetings should be used to review code issues early in the development of the design and perhaps again during the construction documents.

As with any opportunity for interpretation, agreement among all parties is not assured. Sometimes the design professional and the code official will not agree on a particular interpretation. When this occurs the owner can choose to accept the code official's interpretation or to work with the design professional to change the code official's opinion. Sometimes this is as simple as asking the code official to use the text of the code to demonstrate the basis and logic of their interpretation. At other times, such situations amount to a negotiation. In those situations it is always advantageous for the owner to state how the code official's interpretation may cause hardship or injury to the owner. Also, it is necessary for the design professional to use the text of the code to demonstrate the logic of their counter interpretation. Providing the code official with an interpretation from an appropriate model code organization can also be a powerful argument. Although the code official, as the local authority with jurisdiction over interpretations, has no obligation to accept the model code organization's interpretation, it is hard to refute the opinion of the organization that actually developed the code. And finally, some jurisdictions allow for the appeal of rulings by the building official. At such times a third party panel is empowered to resolve the conflict.

A different case is when a clear conflict arises between the owner's needs and the requirements of the code. In cases where this conflict is clear, the only means of resolution is to apply for a variance. It is advisable to meet with the code official prior to a variance application and use this opportunity to understand, from the code official's view, what the issues are and the potential for awarding the requested variance. As with all forms of interpersonal interaction, it is also possible to reduce the variance process to a negotiation. In such a case, the building owner may be required to provide certain additional measures beyond the letter of the code in order to mitigate what would otherwise be a non-code compliant condition.

PROJECT MANAGEMENT ISSUES

The code issues that effect the management of a construction project are primarily time and schedule. Understanding what reviews, public meetings, and variances are required and then allotting enough time for them is key. Establishing an effective sequencing of activities that moves the project forward, but does not expose the owner to project redesign, and therefore unnecessary financial expanse, is also important.

The land development process is complex. It includes formal and informal submissions and reviews (often from several public agencies) as well as public meetings. It is common for the land development process to take a minimum of 3 months. While a simple project can be submitted and approved in as little as a month, 2 or more months is a more reasonable estimate especially when considering the time for initial contact and discussions with the jurisdiction. Affecting this too, is that the schedule for public meetings is usually monthly. As a consequence, when a submission date is missed by one day, the schedule is setback an entire month.

Large or complex projects almost always take more time. Large complex projects on a new site can easily take a year or more. And there are cases where the owner has opted to take the community to court instead of accepting the jurisdiction's decision. Due to the public nature of the review process, when the project is controversial within the community the public meetings can become difficult, emotionally charged, and highly political. Identifying such potential very early in the project and perhaps avoiding sites and communities with this potential should be taken into consideration by the project manager. On top of all this, there is the variance process. The same considerations hold for a request for variance, and additional time should be allocated. Therefore, except for the most simple of projects, it is best to allow at least 3 months for land development review.

The plan review/building-permit process is not a public review process. Because this process is essentially administrative, the duration for submission, review, and issuing of building permits is usually measured in weeks. However, in jurisdictions that are experiencing rapid development, the building official's backlog of work can greatly slow the process. Understanding such local dynamics can be crucial for developing an accurate schedule. Of course, as with land development, variances will take longer. In some jurisdictions the body responsible for granting variances meets monthly.

Another project management concern is developing a strategic concept for the facility vis-à-vis the codes. This is necessary in order to align the desired result with the requirements of the building code. Such early conceptual work can facilitate optimization of the building size, allow for effective future expansion, and increase the flexibility in the use of the facility, especially regarding the use of hazardous materials.

TRENDS AND FUTURE DEVELOPMENTS

Today, codes are a fact of the construction industry. During the twentieth century, codes became a prominent factor and represent the minimum standard of health and safety for building design and construction. Codes will continue to be influenced by major building disasters that result in loss of life. Also, research into every aspect of facility design is becoming more commonplace and our knowledge of the optimum use of materials and building systems is increasing. As the original code issues of egress and fire resistant construction become highly refined and deeply entrenched in the construction industry, the other less obvious areas of the code come to the fore. Some examples include the relatively new and changing developments in accessibility standards and the accommodation of hazardous materials.

A clear future trend, then, is the refinement of the codes resulting in more precise definition of their requirements. Greater and clearer definition of the codes results in fewer questions; however, it usually simultaneously expands their restrictions. As we demonstrated in the introduction of the chapter, this is a historical trend that shows no sign of changing. A good example is the World Trade +Center disaster of September 11, 2001. As research and debate over the details of this disaster draw to a conclusion it is anticipated that the findings will prove to be a major influence on future code upgrades. Also, as more research is developed on the technical topics of materials and construction, the codes will be revised when found inadequate.

Since the adoption of the ADA in the early 1990s, accessible design has been vigorously embraced. However, due to the nature of the Act as a civil rights law vs. a technical design standard, when and to what extent the ADA Design Guidelines is applied is not completely clear. Over the last ten years there have been a number of lawsuits that have begun to define these limits. These sometimes unsettling developments will continue until the law is more clearly defined or the courts provide that definition. There is also debate about the adequacy of some of the detailed requirements commonly found in the current accessibility standards and more research will, undoubtedly, lead to more effective and appropriate design standards.

Over the last ten years there have been many changes to the hazardous material portions of the codes. With the introduction of the IBC a major step has been taken in clearly defining these requirements, especially regarding the need for explosion control. However, this clarity has also resulted in more restrictions. Due to the highly variable chemistry of hazardous materials in a room environment, facility design for hazardous materials is a particularly difficult endeavor. The physical characteristics of the particular material, the details of the handling and/or processing of that material, and the particulars and environmental conditions of the room itself all contribute to the potential hazard and mitigation of hazard. These highly variable circumstances seem to leave a lot of room for more code precision. Therefore, it seems likely that further changes are possible here, too.

An interesting development to watch over the next few years will be the competition between adoption of the International Code Council codes and the NFPA codes. The original intent of the ICC was for the three, regional code organizations to combine and create a unified, comprehensive building code system. This was thought beneficial because of the potential to standardize the design and construction of facilities all across the country. Such standardization would greatly simplify the building process when working in more than one state. However, with California adopting NFPA 5000™ this potential is greatly compromised. Given the size of California and its economy, other jurisdictions will likely give NFPA 5000™ consideration, especially the surrounding states. The progress of code adoption by the various states has just become an interesting, if not entertaining, event.

There has been much discussion through the years about the prescriptive nature of the building codes, and how this stifles creativity and denies alternatives to both designers and owners. In Europe performance-based codes are common and represent an opposing approach. The ICC and NFPA are both researching and experimenting with performance-based codes as an alternative to their code prescriptions. It remains to be seen whether this approach will catch on, but the discussion is far from ended.

Sustainable design is another potential trend. In the construction industry the development and codification of "green" design is becoming part of the mainstream. Many public and private organizations have embraced green design including various branches of the U.S. government, many with responsibilities for a great amount of construction. While sustainable design seems to be here to stay, it remains to be seen if any sustainable features will be taken up as a legal requirement by the individual states and the construction codes. While such changes in the code may seem unimaginable at this time, be aware that, in Europe, sustainable design has been a part of the building requirements for many years.

SPECIAL DISCUSSION: HAZARDOUS MATERIALS

Hazardous materials are common in the pharmaceutical industry, both in manufacturing and research. The ICC codes address facility requirements for the storage and use of hazardous materials with the intent of mitigating the potential for dangerous conditions.

When dealing with hazardous materials the precise materials or chemicals must first be identified. In identifying chemicals it is necessary to categorize them per the definitions provided in Section 307 of the IBC. The Department of Transportation hazard classifications easily found on MSDS data sheets do not usually have a direct correspondence to the code categories. Instead, the physical properties of the material must be reviewed and compared to the code in order to determine their proper definition. For instance; isopropyl alcohol is a liquid with a closed cup flash point below 23°C and a boiling point above 38°C. These criteria define a Class IB Flammable Liquid. Table 3 gives a list of the categories of hazardous materials defined in the IBC.

Next, the maximum quantity of each material that will be used must be determined. Current and accurate information of this sort should already be available within the company since OSHA, as part of its employee safety mandate, requires that a detailed hazardous material inventory be maintained. However, this informa-

TABLE 3   Hazard Classifications

Material	Class
Combustible liquid	II
	IIA
	IIIB
Combustible fiber	Loose baled
Consumer fireworks (Class C, common)	1.4G
Cryogenics, flammable	
Cryogenics, oxidizing	
Explosives	
Flammable gas	Gaseous
	Liquefied
Flammable liquid	1A
	1B
	1C
Combination flammable liquid (1A, 1B, 1C)	
Flammable solid	
Organic peroxide	UD
	I
	II
	III
	IV
	V
Oxidizer	4
	3
	2
	1
Oxidizing gas	Gaseous
	Liquefied
Pyrophoric material	
Unstable (reactive)	4
	3
	2
	1
Water reactive	321
Corrosive	
Highly toxic	
Toxic	

tion must be further categorized in terms of its use. There are three categories of use; storage, open use, and closed use.

Table 307.7 of the IBC establishes a threshold below which materials can be allowed in the building without changing the primary use group. That is to say, the amount of material that can be maintained in an F or S use group. This threshold corresponds to what the code terms a "control area." A control area is a portion of a building that is enclosed in fire rated construction. A building can contain more than one control area. Table 414.2.2 of the IBC defines the maximum number of control areas allowed per floor of a building. When floors occur above or below grade, Table 414.2.2 also reduces the quantity of material allowed. Maximizing the use of control areas is often all that is necessary to accommodate hazardous material in a facility.

Regardless of the quantity of hazardous material, the codes establish certain basic requirements that must be followed. Chapter 4 of the IBC covers general requirements for the use of the various types of material. In addition, the International Fire Code (IFC) devotes entire chapters to the various types of material covered in the code and establishes more detailed requirements. Therefore it is important to review both the IBC and the IFC when coming to terms with hazardous materials.

When the quantity of hazardous material exceeds those listed in IBC's Table 307.7, the use group must change to the appropriate high hazard use group. The most common high hazardous use groups found in the pharmaceutical industry are H-3 and H-5. H-3 corresponds to the hazard classification of the majority of solvents used in the pharmaceutical industry. H-5, which used to be referred to as a special HPM (Hazardous Production Material) use group, is a unique use group that was originally designed to accommodate electronic fabrication facilities. However, it can be utilized where appropriate, for pharmaceutical facilities especially when hazardous materials are piped throughout the facility Under all high hazard use groups the allowable building areas are greatly limited per Table 503 of the IBC. This, in turn, limits the final size of the building even when it is a mixed-use structure. The alternative approach is to make the facility an Unlimited Area building. However, once again, high use hazard use groups are greatly restricted within an unlimited area building. In the end, it is clearly the intent of the code to restrict the size of High Hazard uses to a "manageable" size. In fact, an H-1 use is not allowed to be "mixed" with any other use group. An H-1 use is dedicated to detonation hazards and must be in a completely separate building. However, H-1 is a non-typical use for the pharmaceutical industry.

Whether a material is in storage, being dispensed, or used in open or closed processes are also important considerations. The code has specific requirements for each of these uses and again the code must be consulted for the particulars. When it comes to the dispensing and use of flammable materials the need for special electrical classifications must also be considered. Chapter 5 of the National Standard Electric Code refers to Hazardous Locations Class I, II, and III. Here the parameters of each class are clearly defined and relate directly to the conditions of the materials used.

A critical issue that must be reviewed when the quantities of hazardous material exceed those listed in Table 307.7 of the IBC, is that of explosion hazards. When an explosion hazard exists, explosion control must be provided. Under the code explosion control systems are defined as barricade construction, deflagration venting, or explosion prevention systems. NFPA 68: Venting of Deflagrations and NFPA 69: Explosion Prevention Systems provide the full requirements for explosion control. IBC Table 414.5.1 indicates where these controls are required. The IBC, IFC, and the appropriate referenced standards such as NFPA 68 and 69 must be consulted when dealing with explosion hazards.

The need for explosion control is not just triggered by the quantity of hazardous material. A process itself can be an explosion hazard even when the quantities of hazardous materials are below the threshold values of IBC Table 307.7. Therefore, if those responsible for a process know or believe that an explosion hazard exists,

TABLE 4   International Building Code Hazardous Material Decision Tree

What Hazardous Materials are used? (Section 307 for Categories)			
What quantities of materials are in open use, closed use, and in storage?			
What allowable quantities for single control area? [Table 307.7(1)&(2)] — *Yes*	Handle as primary use group (F or S) (Table 307.9)	Conform to Section 414 and IFC for type of material	
No			
Within allowable quantities for *max* number of control area? [Table 307.7(1)&(2); Table 414.2.2] — *Yes*	Subdivide into multiple control areas	Handle as primary use group (Table 307.9)	Provide rated construction per Section 414.2
No			
Provide use group H for areas with hazardous materials exceeding IBC Table 307.7(1)&(2)	Conform to Section 414 and IFC for type of material		
Explosion control required? (Table 414.5.1) — *Yes*	Provide explosion control per IFC and NFPA 68 and 69		
No			
Conform to Section 414 and IFC for type of material			

regardless of the quantities, then code complaint explosion control must be provided. Of course, this determination is outside the expertise for most construction design professionals. Usually individuals trained in chemistry and industrial hygiene are capable of analyzing such situations.

The IBC and IFC reference several NFPA standards in regard to hazardous materials. All such standards need to be reviewed when they are referenced. For example, NFPA 30: Flammable and Combustible Liquids Code regulates the distance from a building that bulk tanks for hazardous material storage must be located.

Table 4 presents a decision tree that outlines a logical sequence that can be helpful when reviewing the code requirements for hazardous materials.

BIBLIOGRAPHY

International Code Council Codes including:
* International Code Council *International Building Code* 2000 Ed. Falls Church, VA.: International Code Council, Inc., 1999.
* International Code Council *International Fire Code* 2000 Ed. Falls Church, VA.: International Code Council, Inc., 1999.
* International Code Council *International Mechanical Code* 2000 Ed. Falls Church, VA.: International Code Council, Inc., 1999.
* International Code Council *International Plumbing Code* 2000 Ed. Falls Church, VA.: International Code Council, Inc., 1999.
* www.iccsafe.org

NFPA Codes including:
* National Fire Protection Association *NFPA 30: Flammable and Combustible Liquids Code.* Quincy, MA: National Fire Protection Association, 2000.
* National Fire Protection Association *NFPA 68: Venting of Deflagrations.* Quincy, MA.: National Fire Protection Association.
* National Fire Protection Association *NFPA 69: Explosion Prevention Systems.* Quincy, MA: National Fire Protection Association.
* National Fire Protection Association *NFPA 70 National Electric Code*, 1999 Edition, NFPA, Quincy, MA: National Fire Protection Association.
* www.nfpa.org

Other:
* New Jersey Department of Community Affairs *New Jersey Administrative Code Title 5:23 Uniform Construction Code.* Trenton, NJ.: New Jersey Department of Community Affairs
* Occupational Safety & Health Agency *29 CFR, Part 1910, Occupational Safety & Health Standards* Washington, D.C.: Occupational Safety & Health Agency.
* www.osha.gov
* Sabatini, Joseph N. *Building and Safety Codes for Industrial Facilities.* New York, NY: McGraw-Hill, Inc., 1993.
* Yatt, Barry D. *Cracking the Codes, An Architect's Guide to Building Regulations.* New York, NY: John Wiley & Sons, Inc.

15
Containment/Isolation

Authors: Julian Wilkins
David Eherts

Advisors: Denise Proulx
George Petroka
Hank Rahe

INTRODUCTION

Containment has increased in importance in the pharmaceutical industry over the last decade. The reasons for this are not hard to find. Active pharmaceutical ingredients (API) have increased in activity dramatically as more targeted drug delivery systems have emerged. Pharmaceutical companies' pipelines have moved from a position where potent entities were a minority, to the current position where they are the majority. Some companies now have 80% of their pipelines as potent, and this trend shows no signs of diminishing.

Containment is not just about protecting the operator and the environment; increasingly it is about avoiding cross contamination. Traditionally potent materials once were handled by dilution as the solution to pollution. Fume hoods and similar devices simply diluted the problem and sent it elsewhere. Not until the rapid development of nuclear power in the post-World War II period did the concept of isolation in a segregated and separated environment begin to emerge. Similar techniques were used to develop chemical and biological weapons, but it was not until the 1970s that the concept started its slow cross-over into pharmaceutical production. Since then it has developed at increased speed. Now containment is a major subject.

This chapter looks at the crucial topics that must be considered when dealing with potent pharmaceutical entities. What is potent? This is a difficult question. Typically bands 3, 4, and 5 are considered potent. The names of the bands and the limits of the bands vary from company to company. However, some processes challenged by volume and unit operation in band 2 can be a greater risk than the smaller volumes and less challenged processes of more potent entities. The industry generally accepts $10\mu g/M^3/8$ hr and lower as potent.

A list of general definitions and abbreviations is given in the Appendix at the end of the chapter

Because containment minimizes product loss there is now a trend to use the technique to minimize the loss of expensive non-potent substances to dust collectors, where they become a disposal cost. Increasingly, regulators worldwide are treating potent compounds differently in terms of contamination, cross-contamination, and mix-up, in some cases requiring dedicated and segregated processing.

OCCUPATIONAL EXPOSURE BANDS (OEBs) AND LIMITS: DEFINITIONS

Effective and efficient hazard communication concerning the relative degree of toxicity and/or pharmacological activity of active pharmaceutical ingredients, intermediates, purchased chemicals (e.g., excipients and solvents) and other chemicals is an important component in ensuring employee health and safety. Use of Occupational Exposure Bands (OEBs) 1 through 5, in conjunction with additional designations (i.e., R, S, or Cor; Risk, Skin sensitive, or Corrosive, respectively) provides a common and understandable "language" to accomplish this communication. As there is no clear consensus in the industry, it is that much more important to understand the principles.

Additionally, the 1 through 5 categorizations serve as the "keystone" for Safe Handling Guidelines" describing typical safe handling methods and degree of containment that should be achieved when handling or processing pharmaceutical actives. So that these designations can serve both as a means of effective hazard communication and a means to communicate the recommended control technology, administrative procedures and/or PPE are necessary to safely handle each product at each typical process step.

OEBs are established qualitatively (as will be explained in more detail later in this chapter) and quantitatively based upon the resulting Occupational Exposure Limits (OELs) (if one exists). OELs are the airborne limit concentrations of compounds that are believed to safeguard the health of employees. Industrial hygienists conduct monitoring to assess employee exposures relative to these levels. Many functions, including occupational health, engineering, and management utilize the results to make important decisions to ensure on-going protection of employee health.

For solvents and other liquids, OEBs will be designated by a preceding "V" and, based upon the OEL (with units of ppm), assigned R phases and vapor pressure. A specific range (in ppm) is assigned for each category of OEB.

Typical Banding

OEB	Range of OEL (mcg/m³)	Toxicological/Pharmacological Properties
OEB 1	1000–5000	Harmful and/or low pharmacological activity
OEB 2	100–1000	Harmful and/or moderate pharmacological activity
OEB 3	10–100	Moderate toxic and/or high pharmacological activity
OEB 4	1–10	Toxic and/or very high pharmacological activity
OEB 5	< 1	Extremely toxic and/or extremely high pharmacological activity

Note: This table is now codified in Europe and most companies are modifying their bands accordingly.

OEBs for Solvents and Liquids

V-OEB	Range of OEL (ppm)	Toxicological Properties
V-OEB 1	>1000	Harmful and/or low activity
V-OEB 2	100–1000	Harmful and/or moderate activity
V-OEB 3	10–100	Moderate toxic and/or high activity
V-OEB 4	1–10	Toxic and/or very high activity
V-OEB 5	< 1	Extremely toxic and/or extremely high activity

OEB ASSIGNMENTS FOR APIs

Default OEB Assignments: Exploratory Studies and Candidate Identification Stage

During the early discovery phase, limited data are available for a compound. During this period, research compounds are assigned to Default OEB 3, unless a structure–activity–relationship (SAR) analysis of the molecular structure or other indicators (such as therapeutic class or compound class) suggest potential for high to extremely high toxicity or pharmacological activity. Especially of concern are mutagenicity and/or carcinogenicity structural alerts. In these cases, the compounds are provisionally assigned to Default OEB 3, 4, or 5, depending on the evaluation of the alerts by an SAR expert. A description of the alerts and their corresponding OEB assignments is shown in Appendix D. In any case, SAR analysis and any necessary genotox screening must be completed prior to the first pilot plant, including process usage by oriented research and development facilities. Normally this will require SAR to be completed 6 months prior to planned initiation of pilot batches. For example, if there is an SAR alert and not enough time for completion of genotox tests, the compound must be handled as OEB 4 in the pilot plant in the meantime, referred to as the default.

Preliminary OEB and Preliminary OEL (EDC Decision Point)

During team discussions, the Chemistry Dept. gives an overview regarding structural characteristics and possible implications on physico-chemical and biological properties (solubility, log P, vapor pressure, etc.). They also provide possible toxicity and predicted pharmacokinetics and metabolism characteristics, rationale for the drug design to increase activity, metabolic stability, and bioavailability.

The Pharmacology Dept presents data on the degree of activity and comparisons with related drug products for which an OEL already exists. Results from in vivo studies should be considered as more suitable for evaluation and allocation to a preliminary OEB. Toxicology presents preliminary data from in vivo studies.

Based on all these data and according to the guidelines, a preliminary OEB is assigned; if sufficient data are available, a preliminary OEL is also assigned.

A draft Criteria Document summarizing all pertinent data about the molecule and the rationale for the preliminary OEB/OEL (P-OEB/P-OEL) is produced. All relevant data about the compound are included in the Criteria

Document including chemical, physical, pharmacological, and toxicological data. A hazard assessment is conducted and a determination is made as to which OEB is the "best fit." Team members collectively apply their expertise in industrial hygiene, toxicology, pharmacology, occupational medicine, and clinical medicine to review the data for the pharmaceutical active ingredient and make the OEB assignment. This is the ideal; review of many MSDSs show this is not normal for outsourced AP.

Both acute and subchronic data are considered and the assignment relies on the professional judgment of the team and reflects the assessment of the compound's characteristics. To assess the potential acute effects, both the toxicity and pharmacological activity of the compound are evaluated. The type of pharmacological effect(s) expected, the mechanism of action, and the dose required to produce these pharmacological effects are important considerations. The severity of acute (life threatening) effects is assessed. An important aspect of the assessment is a determination of whether emergency medical intervention might be required and how rapid the response must be if an occupational overexposure occurs. Results of acute toxicity studies in animals also provide information on the likelihood of the compound to produce immediate adverse effects. These may include median lethal dose (LD50), for example. Compounds with a high order of acute toxicity and poor or delayed warning properties are of greater concern.

Often the OEL assignment is conservatively based on the most sensitive effect endpoint, especially when there is potential for life-threatening or disabling, irreversible chronic effects.

ASSIGNING OEBs FOR ISOLATED INTERMEDIATES

In addition to the decision points for active ingredient development, chemical and process development have their development timeline, that includes transfers from Research to pilot and then to production. During the first development phases, the isolated intermediates that are presumably active and which have not yet been investigated are assigned a default OEB. Available information based mainly on the structure-activity relationship and the comparison with known products could predict a default OEB 3–5; the decision logic is the same as for APIs. As soon as the synthesis route is relatively fixed and the isolated intermediates are identified, the appropriate tests should be performed. Genotoxicity tests (in vitro micronucleus and ames) should be performed as soon as possible if structure-activity analysis yields any mutagenicity or carcinogenicity alerts, followed by the remaining tests from the prescribed battery.

At the very latest, when transferring from the pilot plant to production, all isolated intermediates must have been assessed and classified.

Assigning OEBs for Raw Materials, Solvents, and Other Purchased Materials

When assigning V-OEBs to pure substances, an existing regulatory or authoritative exposure limit is the primary determinant in choosing the band. In the case where multiple authoritative or regulatory limits exists for the same substance, the lowest existing major country limit will be used for assignment of the V-OEB. When no valid regulatory limit exists, data taken either from the supplier or from the literature may be used in determining the OEB for a purchased chemical, according to Annex C. A comparison with similar chemicals or product classes may also be performed as well as SAR. In some cases, such as custom-manufactured starting materials, toxicity testing may be conducted to assess the chemical and determine the appropriate OEB.

FACTORS CONSIDERED IN ASSIGNING OEBs

Active pharmaceutical ingredients are intended for administration in human patients normally through the oral or parenteral routes. Consequently, experimental toxicological data are developed in laboratory animal species using these routes of administration. However, the important routes of exposure for humans during production and manufacturing are inhalation and dermal/mucosal contact to the aerosols.

For dusts, particle size is an important consideration. In general, small particles penetrate deeper into the bronchial system, which enhances the opportunity for absorption and systemic exposure and, therefore, toxicity. For exact extrapolation, toxicokinetic studies or toxicology studies using the inhalation route are necessary. Where such data are not available, lung absorption is assumed to be total (100%). Possible local effects on lung tissues must be considered separately. Where toxicokinetic data or specific inhalation toxicity data are available, this information is valuable in the determination of an OEL.

When an OEL (or equivalent) is available, this would drive the OEB. However, when this is not the case, especially in the early development phases, the OEB should be assigned after considering physicochemical, toxicological, and pharmacological data available.

Therapeutic Daily Dose

The therapeutic daily dose should be considered as a rough tool that is somewhat indicative of the potency of a drug substance. Consideration of the Minimum Effective Dose (MED) derived from human clinical trials can be useful in calculating an OEL.

Acute Toxicity

The team considers the degree of acute toxicity by all routes. NOELs is Observable Effect Level and LOELs are useful in considering OEB assignments and OEL establishment. Severity of acute (life threatening) effects should also be considered as well as potential for severe skin or respiratory tract damage due to corrosive properties. In addition to other acute effects, it is important to consider effects that can reduce alertness (e.g., certain CNS active compounds) or invoke syncope (e.g., hypoglycemic or hypotensive agents).

Acute Warning Properties (Odor, Irritation, Etc.)

Acute warning properties are of particular importance when a compound has significant potential to harm health. Irritation is a good warning property and is also considered as a toxic effect. When possible, the odor threshold (the concentration at which there is perceptible odor) should be expressed in relation to toxicological properties and NOELs.

Sensitization

Occupational exposure to sensitizers may induce respiratory and/or dermal sensitization. Lack of sensitization after oral and parenteral administration does not necessarily mean that dermal/mucosal or respiratory sensitization will not occur.

For compounds that are sensitizers, it is important to consider the degree and type of sensitization; e.g., whether it is "weak" or "strong" as well as whether it is a skin and/or a pulmonary sensitizer. There is general agreement about the following:

- It is not possible to establish an airborne concentration of a compound that is protective of health for the individual who is already allergic to the material in question.
- Minimizing dermal exposure and lowering the airborne concentration of strong sensitizers reduces the potential of sensitizing employees in the first place.

Genotoxicity/ Mutagenicity

Genotoxic and mutagenic properties per se are considered a toxic effect. Positive effects from in vivo studies are more heavily weighted than in vitro study results. If an expert evaluation results in unequivocal evidence of genotoxicity, the product should be handled with the same safety precautions as a genotoxic carcinogen. If possible, a determination is also made on the likelihood and severity of possible chronic effects. Results of both in vitro and in vivo genotoxicity tests are reviewed and the OEB assignment modified as necessary.

Carcinogens

Carcinogenic effects detected in animals, which cannot be explained by non-genotoxic properties, play a key role in OEB assignment. For non-genotoxic mechanisms of tumor formation (e.g., endocrine dependent tumors, peroxisome proliferators, liver tumors in male mice, etc.), a special hazard assessment is performed in order to consider the lower or lacking sensitivity of humans toward these mechanisms.

Reproductive/Developmental Effects

Effects on male and female fertility are an integral point of the evaluation and the determination of the OEB and OEL. Active pharmaceutical ingredients that can adversely impact any aspect of the human reproductive process (e.g., libido, fertility, conception, spontaneous abortion, fetal development and growth, parturition, and breast feeding) are identified as having reproductive/developmental effects.

Appropriate considerations must be made concerning the dosage, frequency of exposure, route of exposure, etc., or when there is strong cause and effect evidence of reproductive/developmental toxicity in humans or in animal models that are thought to be predictive of human toxicity. The cause and effect relationship is weaker and the outcome is less severe.

The question of embryotoxicity requires special consideration if embryonic effects have been determined in animals. There is evaluation of whether embryotoxic effects are due to systemic maternal effects (which are addressed by the OEL) or whether the embryo/fetus is more sensitive.

Application of Minimum OEB and Maximum OEL

For compounds that possess reproductive, sensitizing, or genotoxic properties, either equivocal or clear, a minimum OEB value (with designation) and/or maximum OEL value should be assigned according to the following table:

Toxicological Properties	Minimum OEB	Maximum OEL (mcg/m³)
Equivocal reprotox and/or sensitizing properties	OEB 2/S1 or R1	1000
Clear reprotox and/or dermal sensitizing properties	OEB 3/S1 or R2	100
Clear respiratory sensitizing properties	OEB 4/S2	10
Equivocal cancer and/or genotox properties	OEB 3	100
Clear cancer and/or genotox properties	OEB 4	10

Interpretation of Reported Adverse Effects

Irreversible adverse effects may be associated with specific compounds. When developing the criteria document for a compound, consideration must be given to "dose-independent" adverse effects of this nature. These effects are classified as occasional, frequent, or very common and must be included in the criteria document and considered in the OEB/OEL determination. The following table, based on pharmacovigilance classification for clinical trials, should be used as a general guide to classify these adverse effects:

Reported Frequency in Clinic	Classification
> 0.1%	Occasional
> 1%	Frequent
> 10%	Very common

Cumulative Effects

Cumulative effects refer to accumulated effects following repeated administration with or without toxicological manifestation. For the extrapolation of animal data to humans, the different kinetic/metabolic behavior is of importance, because the clearance of a chemical in animals is, in general, faster. Therefore, the evaluation of cumulative effects should be based preferably on a comparison of animal and human pharmacokinetic data.

Likelihood of Chronic Effects

These criteria have significant impact on the assignment of the OEB and determination of the OEL. A judgment is made regarding the severity of effects and whether they may have disabling consequences or the potential to cause early death. A very important consideration is whether effects are reversible or irreversible.

Reversibility of Chronic Health Effects

A judgment is made regarding the severity of chronic health effects that can develop from ongoing exposure to a compound and whether they may have disabling consequences.

Effects Are/Are Not Medically Treatable

A judgment is made whether adverse effects are medically treatable and the ultimate impact on the quality of life of an individual. Effects that are trivial and readily medically treatable may be assigned to a lower OEB, depending on other characteristics. However, close consideration must be given when effects are not medically treatable because it may result in the compound being assigned to a higher OEB.

Effects Do/Do Not Require Emergency Medical Intervention

Overexposure to some compounds at levels, that could be encountered in the occupational environment may cause immediate life threatening effects and may require emergency medical intervention. An example is an extremely potent hypotensive agent that, with minor exposure, can induce an immediate and significant decrease in blood pressure.

IH and Occupational Medicine Experience

A judgment is made on the relevance of signs and symptoms experienced by potentially exposed personnel and related exposure levels, workplace conditions, and protection measures.

FINALIZING OCCUPATIONAL EXPOSURE LEVELS

When a compound nears regulatory approval, the results of chronic animal and human pharmacokinetic studies are generally available.

They reassess the OEB assignment that was made at earlier stages of development and modify, if necessary, based on new data and experience that have become available. They also apply all relevant data to discuss and derive an OEL.

Exceptions, where OELs are not derived, are those compounds for which no safe exposure level can be defined (e.g., genotoxic carcinogens).

The derivation of OELs for therapeutic substances, commonly utilized among pharmaceutical companies, is a matter of judgment involving medical, toxicological, and industrial hygiene disciplines represented on the OEB/OEL team. The following is representative of the approach that the team may use, that is generally similar to the process and definitions adopted by international and national bodies that establish OEL for chemicals in the workplace.

Step 1:

Determine the impact of the pharmacological effect on normal, healthy individuals. Identify the appropriate estimated or known NOEL in animal toxicity studies and/or the minimum effective dose from human trials.

Step 2:

Compile the following relevant information that is available about the occupational toxicity of the substance, by any relevant route of exposure:

- Human pharmacology and doses
- Animal pharmacology and doses
- Skin irritation
- Skin penetrability
- Eye irritation
- Pharmacokinetics and metabolism
- Inhalation effects
- Oral toxicity
- Sensitization: Dermal and pulmonary
- Genetic toxicity
- Carcinogenicit: Genotoxic vs. epigenetic
- Reproductive/developmental effects
- Occupational health experience

Step 3:

Collect and consider the following information pertaining to human experience:

- Medical surveillance
- Occupational exposure experience
- Exposure data

Step 4:

Calculate the OEL. An example OEL calculation (expressed in milligrams or micrograms per cubic meter of air) is shown as:

$$\text{OEL} = \frac{(\text{Appropriate dose level in mg/kg-dy} \times \beta) \times (50 \text{ Kg})}{\text{Uncertainty Factor} \times \alpha \times \text{AF} \times 10 \text{ m}^3}$$

In the formula:

- β represents bioavailability by the route of dosing in the relevant bioassay (i.v. is considered 100% or a factor of 1.0 in the calculation).
- represents the percent absorption of the compound via the inhalation route expected in the worker; where no data is available, 100% lung absorption (a factor of 1.0) is assumed
- AF represents the accumulation between workplace exposures, based on the following formula:

$$AF = \frac{1}{(1 - e^{K_{el} \times t})}$$

where K_{el} is the elimination constant equal to the biological half-life divided by 2 ($K_{el} = T^{1/2}/0.693$) and t is the time between exposures; for a conservative estimate of potential workplace exposure, a default value of 16 hours should be used for t.

- The body weight utilized in the calculation is 50 kg
- The volume of air inspired by an average employee during an 8-hour period is 10 m^3

Selection of the Uncertainty Factor is dependent on many variables including NOEL vs. LOEL, inter/intraspecies extrapolation, acute vs. chronic data, the seriousness and irreversibility of effects, the mode of action, the relevance of the observed action/mechanism for humans, half-life and cumulative effects, etc.

Variable	Factor
LOEL to NOEL	10
Subchronic to chronic	10
Interspecies extrapolation:	
• From rodent species	10
• From non-rodent species	5
Intraspecies variability and severity/reversibility of the endpoint	10

If several values are calculated because various NOELs are available, the team applies expert judgment to select the most appropriate. If data exist that lead to a more precise calculation of the OEL, these data should be used in preference to the associated default uncertainty factor. If the calculated value is greater than 5.0 mg/m^3, an OEL of 5 mg/m^3 (8 HR TWA) is utilized.

If clinical data are available, first consideration should be given to the rationale for the minimum effective dose (MED). If the dose is necessary to just affect a physiologic endpoint in the patient (i.e., hypertension) and the product is projected to be used long term (i.e., for the rest of the lifetime), then an OEL can be calculated from this value. Appropriate uncertainty factors for LOEL to NOEL (10 times in lieu of specific data) and, if applicable, for intraspecies variation (e.g., not globally marketed yet) may be applied (again 10 times in lieu of specific data). If the clinical dose has been established to impact an infection or a cancer, it was not set based upon a desired physiologic change in the patient, (i.e., an antibiotic dose is established to have an effect on the microorganism) nor is it meant to be taken long term. Therefore, the MED may not be an appropriate starting point for the OEL calculation unless there are only insignificant side effects noted at this clinical dose. In this case, the OEB matrix should be used, and the OEL at the upper range of the OEB range will be designated.

Step 5:

The team develops a comprehensive Criteria Document that explains the OEL rationale. The Criteria Document includes:

• Physical and chemical properties
• Pertinent toxicological and pharmacological data
• OEB assignment
• Discussion and rationale supporting the OEL including all calculations

The team also provides interpretations and guidance on the OEL in relation to other chemical substances (e.g., raw materials, solvents, reagents, etc.), and where appropriate, adopting criteria definitions and limits published annually by other bodies (i.e., ACGIH-TLV).

CONTAINMENT ISSUES

Understanding the Problem

In defining containment levels, both permissible limits and the actual performance values are expressed in terms of weigh per cubic meter of air over 8 hours or the worst-case shift length. This is based on the normal duration for a shift. However, if an operator worked more than 8 hours, he/she cannot receive a greater dosage; the 8 hours is a convention indicating the period worked in any 24-hour period.

The units of measurement used in potent containment are normally expressed in:

Milligrams	mg	(1/1,000 gram)
Micrograms	µg	(1/1,000,000 gram)
Nanograms	ng	(1/1,000,000,000 gram)

For comparative purposes there are 457 grams to a pound weight, a normal salt crystal weights approximately 3 milligrams. Thus, a product with an OEL of 0.3/µg has a not-to-be-exceed total of approximately 1/10,000 of a sugar crystal in a cubic meter of air in an 8 hour period. Unfortunately this is now a bright line since a result 0.4µg may not produce an effect.

Methods of Ingestion

The above methods of stating performance requirement are all based on the premise that the most effective route of ingestion is through the nasal passage or by breathing

Compound Hazard Assessment/Factors Considered in Assigning OEBs

Category Assignment	Category 1	Category 2	Category 3	Category 4	Category 5
OEL dust mg/m3	1–5	0.1–1	0.01–0.1	0.001–0.01	<0.001
OEL vapor ppm	>1000	100–1000	10–<100	1–<10	<1
Therapeutic daily dose mg/day (pharmacological activity)	$100 \leq TDD$	$10 \leq TDD \leq 100$	$1 \leq TDD < 10$	$0.1 \leq TDD < 1$	$TDD < 0.1$
Acute toxicity	Low	Low/moderate (e.g., R20; R21; R22)	Moderate (e.g., R23; R24; R25)	Moderate/High (e.g., R26; R27; R28)	
LD50 oral route mg/kg	>2000	200–2000	25–200	0.5–25	<0.5
LD50 dermal route mg/kg	>2000	400–2000	50–400	1–50	<1
LC50 inhalation 4H mg/l Aerosols/particles	>5	1–5	0.25–1	0.005–0.25	<0.005
Severity of acute (life-threatening) effects	Negligible	Low/moderate	Moderate/high (e.g., R39/T)	High (e.g., R39/T+)	
Sensitization	Negative	Slight cutaneous allergic reaction	Moderate/strong cutaneous allergic reactions (e.g., R43) Slight respiratory allergic reaction	Prevalent moderate to strong respiratory allergic reactions (e.g., R42; R42/R43)	
Mutagenicity	Negative	Negative	Positive in some in vitro assays, not confirmed in vivo (e.g., R68)	Mutagenic in most relevant in vivo and in vitro assays [e.g., R68 (gr III), R46 (gr I, II)]	
Carcinogenicity	Negative	Negative	Some evidence in animals [e.g., R40 (gr III)]	Confirmed in animals and humans [e.g., R45; R49 (gr I, II)]	OEB 5 may be assigned based on relatively high carcinogenic potency
Developmental/reproductive toxicity	Negative	Inadequate evidence in animals	Evidence of moderate reprotoxic defects in animals (e.g., R62; R63; R64) (OEB 3 may be assigned for human teratogens with relatively	Evidence of strong reprotoxic defects in animals and/or suspected or proved in humans [e.g., R60; R61 (gr I, II)]	

	None	Low (e.g., R33)	Moderate (e.g., R48/Xn)	Moderate/high (e.g., R48/T)	
Cumulative effects (pharmaceutics)	None	Low (e.g., R33)	Moderate (e.g., R48/Xn)	Moderate/high (e.g., R48/T)	
Likelihood of chronic effects (e.g., systemic)	Unlikely	Unlikely	Possible (e.g., R48/Xn)	Possible (e.g., R48/T)	
Adverse effects per oral route (mg/kg-day) (90 day chronic study)			Adverse effects seen ≤ 50 (Xn)	Adverse effects seen ≤ or 5 (T)	
Adverse effects per dermal route(mg/ kg-day) (90 day[a] chronic study)			Adverse effects seen ≤ 100 (Xn)	Adverse effects seen ≤ 10 (T)	
Adverse effects by Inhalation/6H (mg/l-day) Aerosols/particles (90 day chronic study)			Adverse effects seen ≤ 0.25 (Xn)	Adverse effects seen ≤ 0.025 (T)	
Reversibility of chronic health effects	Readily reversible	Readily reversible	Moderately reversible	Slowly reversible	Irreversible
Effects are medically treatable	Yes	Yes	Yes	Usually	Possibly
IH/occupational health experience	No evidence of adverse health effects	Low evidence of adverse health effects	Probable evidence of adverse health effects	High evidence of adverse health effects	High evidence of severe adverse health effects
Acute effects require emergency medical intervention	Not required	Not required	May be required	May require immediate intervention	Requires immediate intervention

[a] For interpretation of shorter studies (as 28 day subchronic studies), indicative values should be multiplied by 3.

through the mouth. For this reason the standard is based on the operator breathing a standard 10 cubic meters of air a day

Inhalation is not the only way of ingestion. There are significant risks from transdermal and mechanical transfer routes. In mechanical transfer, the active is carried on packaging, equipment, clothing to be liberated at another time and place, dosing whoever is unfortunate enough to be present, not necessarily, the operator. There are records of family members who launder the operator's clothes being dosed. Such uncontrolled and unmonitored releases are rarely recorded and the local physician is unlikely to be able to correlate the symptoms with the accidental transfer of an active pharmaceutical ingredient, the drug substance can end up in another drug.

Routes of Exposure

Compounds can enter the body in a number of ways:

- Ocular through the mucous membranes of the eye.
- Inhalation of the active through the nose is the quickest and most common route, but the active can reach the same location orally.
- Oral transmission occurs when breathing through the mouth or swallowing for absorption of the active in the stomach.
- Intravenous transmission through accidental puncture by a sharp object through the skin.
- Transdermal transmission occurs when the active is absorbed through the skin, normally slower in effect than inhalation. However, if the active is in a solution with certain solvents the rate of adsorption can be as great as by inhalation.
- Mechanical where the active is carried on clothing, shoes, packaging, and indeed anything that has come into contact with the active. The active may then be ingested by any of the routes above, by another person, in another place and at another time.
- Cross contamination, by liberating the active to the environment. It is impossible to predict how much will be transmitted to another place and location. The woman who died of anthrax in Connecticut was dosed due to cross contamination in a postal center in another state. Increase signs of activity by the regulators in the area of cross contamination is evident. Allowing potent material out of its containment boundary leads inevitably to cross contamination, even though this may be below the level of detection.

Setting Goals

Once it is understood that there is a problem, ways to quantify the problem must be developed. Before contemplating a solution, it is first necessary to define the containment goals in terms of performance.

APPLYING THE PERFORMANCE REQUIREMENT TO AN ACTUAL PROCESS

The limit value of exposure requirement can be stated as an OEL, PEL or TLV; TLVs, and PEL are not for a typical pharmaceutical compound (only two have been evaluated). Short-term exposures are expressed as an STEL.

Actual performance has to be proven for any system, a wide range of variables makes it impossible for a generic or parametric performance to be stated and case-by-case performance validation and monitoring is therefore required.

Actual performance as opposed to the exposure level (the "not to be exceeded" limit) is expressed as a TWA. It has to take account of the following challenges to the system.

- Material characteristics
    - Specific gravity
    - Particle size distribution
    - Electrostatic properties
    - Flow characteristic
- Equipment issues
    - Late in the maintenance cycle
    - Equipment wear and damage
    - Distortion of high accuracy components
    - Equipment malfunction
    - Operability
    - Ergonomics
- Iterations
    - How many tasks are performed in a shift
    - What type of task is performed at each iteration
- Operators
    - Operator fatigue
    - Operator technique
    - Operator error
- Utility failure

Since each active liberating event is subject to so many factors the actual liberation at each event will vary.

The following graph shows the liberation levels of active material from a containment system over a sequence of repeated events. As can be predicted, the results vary over a range of exposure levels. The control and containment system must consider the worst-case liberation. It also shows how important constant monitoring and proper evaluation is. Most systems are challenged tested with inappropriate materials, with too little iteration, and under ideal circumstances. This cannot truly reflect real, not to be exceeded, performance.

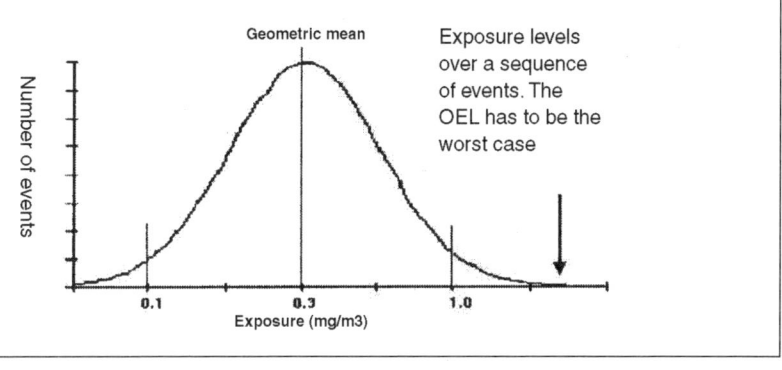

Actual Performance Testing

It is usually unwise to test a system using the active, often the active; is too expensive or does not exist in sufficient quantities for repetitive testing. Surrogate testing has its challenges, too.

The criteria that has to be considered in developing a testing protocol are:

Surrogate Handling

- The test compound has to be loaded into its initiating container without risk of liberating detectable levels.
- The test environment has to be checked for the presence of the compound before any test is performed.
- Personnel handling the target compound can have no part in the operation recovery or testing of the surrogate.
- The surrogate must have similar specific gravity and size distribution to the active. This is to ensure that the dwell time in the air is similar and similar in concentration to the active.
- The surrogate must be easily detected in the concentrations encountered and be in the mid range of detection for the equipment.
- The surrogate must be permitted in the test environment. This is a real issue since the surrogate permitted may be present in the environment (e.g., lactose). Recently a company had intentions of using caffeine; this was prohibited even though coffee was freely available in the plant.

Iterations
- The worst case number of shift iterations must be replicated.

Operators
- The operators should as far as possible try to ensure a reasonable level of poor technique performance. This is best done by giving minimal training to the operators before testing.

Equipment
- Equipment should undergo a number of repetitive uses to represent end of maintenance cycle conditions.
- Where malfunctions can be predicted, they should be induced on some of the cycles.

Cycles
- The whole test sequence has to be repeated a number of times with some cycles being run exactly as events dictate and some identified cycles being run with induced worst case events.
- A range of opertor skill and dexterity models should be applied.

Air Sampling
- Both 8 hr full shift sampling and short term 15 minute samples should be performed, with the short term sampling occurring a potential liberation events.
- The SMEPAC protocol involves particulate monitoring and this may be valuable, but requires a clean environment. ISPE has now published the work of an international ad hoc collaboration formerly known as SMEPAC. It forms an internationally accepted surrogate test protocol.

The results expressed as weight per cubic meters (TWA) should be below the action level set for the active.

Given the list of unit operations and the number of transfers, this could be a challenge. It may be that the number of unit operations in one operator shift has to be reduced. In the options section, some actual performances are quoted; these must be seen as indicative since the actual performance will vary due to:

* Technique
* Equipment condition
* Material characteristics
* Abnormal occurrences
* Energy

In designing the system, it has to be expected that sub-optimal conditions can prevail.

Variance

The OEL is a "guideline" and must reflect the worst case. Because the number of test iterations has to be limited due to cost and time constraints, it is therefore wise to use different and relatively untrained operators in testing so that the greatest challenges occur in the least number of iterations.

Various levels have been set in the past for design, FAT, and action; for instance the action level is not based on scientific evidence, but is more pragmatic. A value of 0.5 of the OEL is normally set but there is really no evidence from actual performance data that excursive events will not occur if this level is adhered to. Far worse is the design exposure level. The author of this document, to set a practical goal for FAT performance, originated this measure. In reality these levels were never challenged because recognized reliable surrogate testing protocols did not exist. Now they do (SMEPAC). It is clear that the 0.2 value that was arbitrarily set is inappropriate. Setting the system performance goal at 0.1 of the OEL is now nearly universal. Dependent on technique, actual results varying from 1:1.1 to 1:100 have been recorded. The culprit here is normally technique and an OEL of 0.1 is inadequate.

REAL-TIME MONITORING

Technology to detect and analyze particulates of specific drug substances does not currently exist in a practical, cost effective, and usable form. IR is the probable future route but is not currently commercially available and, if available, would require detailed work for each substance to establish a spectrographic "finger print." This would make it challenged for a multi-product and R&D facilities. The challenge is to find a parametric indication of performance. By measuring an alarming airflow, pressure, etc. in isolators, fume hoods, etc., many believe that they have an indication of performance. In all the data we have reviewed there is no correlation. Over the past years the use of particulate counters have been seen; typically these systems are good for gross containment systems where the liberation of particulates from the process is significantly greater than the background levels of particulate. When dealing with OELs in single digit micrograms, and nanograms the problem is that a critical liberation is insignificant when compared with the background levels.

Because at very low OELs (10 micrograms and lower) or where a significant number of potential liberations occur in a shift, primary, secondary and tertiary containment boundaries should be considered. Because these boundaries are discrete mini environments the opportunity exists to feed them with ULPA air. By counting a determined critical particle sizes on the exhaust (based on the particle size distribution of the active or active/excipient, mix/blend/granulate), it is possible to compare the particle count profile and containment performance by sampling. A correlation can then be determined so that a particle count exceedance has every chance of indicating a potential liberation of active. Because this detection is in the critical secondary or tertiary zone this liberation is not environmentally available and so corrective measures can be undertaken for an upset condition recovery.

It must be stressed that some false alarms are inevitable and that this is a particle count that cannot distinguish between API, excipient, and environmental particulate. It must also be stressed that the parametrics of isolators or other devices cannot be ignored because they indicate a malfunction that must be corrected but which may not lead to liberation.

The application of primary, secondary, and tertiary boundaries has an Achilles heel. This is not the chamber itself that is of a rugged unitary construction (or should be), nor is it the glazing that should be laminated safety glass or where appropriate, Lexan. The issue is the glove.

There is very little data of full glove failure in the pharmaceutical industry, but a great deal of literature in the nuclear industry is available. Glove inrush protection is widely touted but is not a proven method of containment. In a deliberate breech test 215 nanograms/M^3 were liberated over 26 minutes with an inflow velocity of greater than 90 feet per minute.

Gloves should:

- Be routinely tested and inspected (daily).
- Stored unfolded and stuffed with acid free tissue to avoid creasing.
- Have a 2 year maximum shelf life.
- Be replaced on a regular and administered basis (6 months).
- Be capped when not in use on critical isolators (OEL of 1 microgram or less containing critical processes).
- Have emergency caps available to close off in case of failure.
- The operator must wear protective disposable gloves on an event basis (i.e., they must be donned before glove entry, removed using hygienic technique, and bagged on exit from the gloves to prevent mechanical transfer/dermal contact from pin-holed gloves).
- The glove must be securely fastened.
- The glove fastening system must not cause risk to the glove
- Hot change out glove systems/techniques should be available and all operators fully trained in the gloving-degloving process.

Editor's Note _____

A warning: Many designers have attended courses and felt that containment was a simple subject that was easily mastered, then went out, built a system and saw it consigned to the boneyard. The author has heard many A&Es and vendors extolling the virtues of their designs, when in reality the owner was seeking help to correct the problems with the systems. Always look for the best possible assistance with containment projects and look for independent references. The cost of designing and proving a containment system can be very high when compared to the capital equipment cost. Getting a bargain and failing is more expensive.

Regulatory Issues

Regulators around the world are increasingly interested in "potent compounds," not because of concerns for the operator, but because of the risk of cross contamination and mix up. Generally, regulators have a poor understanding of what a potent compound is and react to cytotoxic, cytostatic, mutagenic, and other phrases that cause concern. Confusing operator protection and cross contamination is one of the greatest dangers; at the time of this writing, a debate is underway to restore some of these issues.

In 1996, the FDA proposed changes to the cGMP regulations to extend the controls applied to penicillin to cover other classes of materials that may have a high potential for cross-contamination: "Such contaminants include, but are not limited to, penicillin, cephafosporins, cytotoxic anti-cancer agents."

The Australian Code of cGMP for Medicinal Products issued in 2002 also recognized the risks associated with certain products. They recommended cross-contamination should be avoided by, for example "production in segregated areas . . . or by campaign (separation in time) followed by appropriate cleaning."

The 2002 proposed guidelines from Health Canada identified similar hazardous classes of compounds. However they proposed that "campaign production (separation in time followed by cleaning) of the above products is not acceptable."

In Argentina cGMP inspections are conducted to a checklist based on 1992 WHO guidance: Areas for preparation of pharmaceutical highly sensitizing products: penicillins, hormones, *cytostatics* or biological preparations have to be independent and autonomous." Some local inspectors are starting from the position that:

- Cytostatics are oncology agents
- Therefore all oncology products must be cytostatic
- Therefore all oncology products must be handled in segregated facilities

The Orange Guide Europe Section 3.6:

In order to minimize the risk of a serious medical hazard due to cross-contamination, dedicated and self contained facilities must be available for the production of particular medicinal products, such as highly sensitizing materials (e.g., penicillins) or biological preparations (e.g., from live microorganisims). The production of certain additional products, such as certain antibiotics, certain hormones, certain cytotoxics, certain highly active drugs, and non-medicinal products should not be conducted in the same facilities. For those products, in exceptional cases, the principle of campaign working in the same facilities can be accepted provided that specific precautions are taken and the necessary validations are made.

Cross contamination definition:

- Contamination of a material or product with another material or product. (ICH Q7A, GMP Guidance for APIs)
- Any substance accidentally or unknowingly introduced into/onto a product. (E. Melendez FDA/ISPE-Conf 9-23-2004)
- cGMP Regulations 1 CFR 211 recognizes 2 classes of drugs
  - Penicillins
  - Non-penicillins
  - Non-penicillin beta-lactarns (health concerns due to similarities to penicillins)
  - Cytotoxics
  - Steroids
  - Hormones
  - Many others with different pharmacological activity

- 211.42 (c) "There shall be separate or defined areas or such other control systems for the firm's separation as are necessary to prevent contamination. . . ."

Manufacturers have the responsibility to identify drugs with risks and set defined areas or controls necessary to eliminate risk of product cross contamination on a case-by-case basis.

The process is evaluated in FDA cGMP inspections and a review of supporting data and analyses for the firm's product introduction decision is reviewed.

Other Regulations Applicable to Cross Contamination

211.28(a):	Personal protective apparel to protect drugs
211.42(b) & (c)	Design/construction to prevent mix-up or contamination of drugs or between drugs
211.46(c)	Where air contamination occurs during production
211.67(a):	Contamination by equipment
211.80(b):	Handling/storage to prevent contamination of components and drug product containers/closures
211.192:	Unexplained loss of yield

Statutory Requirement [FD&C, Sec.501(a)(2)(B)]
". . . all drugs and APIs must be manufactured in conformity with cGMPs. . . ."

ICH Q7A, Section IV.D. Containment (4.4) ICH Q7A (Governs APIs in USA, Europe, Japan and Australia)
"Dedicated production areas . . . should be employed in the production of highly sensitizing materials, such as penicillins or cephalosporins."

Q7A cGMP Guidance, APIs, Containment 4.41
For materials of an infections nature or high pharmacological activity to toxicity, "dedicated production areas should be considered unless validated inactivation and/or cleaning procedures are established and maintained."

ICH Q7A excerpts applicable to cross-contamination

- Personnel Hygiene: 3.21
- Facilities, Design & Construction: 4.10, 4.11, 4.13
- Utilities: 4.21, 4.22, 4.23
- Containment: 4.42
- Sanitation and Maintenance: 4.72
- Equipment, Design & Construction: 5.15
- Maintenance & Cleaning: 5.21, 5.22, 5.24
- Receipt & Quarantine: 7.22
- Storage: 7.40
- Contract Manufacturer/Laboratory: 16.10
- Repackaging/Relabeling/Holding: 17.41
- Cell Culture/Fermentation: 18.38
- Investigational APIs, Equipment & Facilities: 19.31

Real Performance

There is little published data on real performance, and when the results are reviewed, the reasons become clear. The results we have seen show that performance varies widely between each iteration. There is a wide range of causes, but the chief culprits can be clearly identified.

The greatest risk is transactions—events in which materialsl must pass into or out of the contained boundary. These can be gasses, probes, vents, material, tools, or leaks to name a few. The greatest cause of transactional failure is technique or ignorance. If a transaction requires skills to perform it will fail. Technique failures can be minimized by redundancy and training, but all the best plans, reviews, and training can be defeated by failing to identify the weakest link.

Energy is also a vital ingredient in performance—the greater the energy involved, the greater the risk.

COMPARISONS OF ISOLATORS

Not all isolators have the same performance. These two examples passed the standard parametric isolator test of pressure hold and leak rate.

- *Isolator 1:* Test period 15–25 minutes and six repetitions with 20 kg of Naproxen Sodium results of <0.005–<0.007 microgram/M^3.
- *Isolation 2:* Subgram quantity of Naproxen Sodium, 3 iterations, same time period 0.004–.403 microgram/M^3.

Both isolators have lock chambers for pass in and out. In the first the lock chamber surrounded a secondary bagging system, the latter used wipe decontamination on pass out. Because the events were of short duration, some would suggest that the time weighted average (TWA) based on the data for the 0.403-microgram/M^3 event.

$$\frac{0.403 \times 15 \text{ min}}{480 \text{ min}} = 0.012 \text{ micrograms/}M^3 \text{ 8/hr}$$

But this presumes that:

- No emissions occurred during the rest of the day.
- That 0.403 micrograms/M³ was the worst performance this isolator could achieve.
- That the time was 15 minutes or less and that the ACIGH STEL requirement was met <15 minutes >60 minutes between events = <4 events per shift, not more than 3.1 × OEL liberation. However, the rule of thumb for an STEL is 3 to 5 times the OEL.
- That there were no other events or operations that could release active occurring in that operator's shift and to which he may be exposed.

What do these comments infer?

- There will always be some residual material after the sampling material until it has either fallen to a surface or been captured in a filter. The material that is no longer an aerosol is available for energy to make it an aerosol again or for mechanical transfer to make it available to others at another time and place.
- With only 3 iterations it is statistically impossible that the 0.403 is the worst performance. Over only 3 iterations the system showed a range of 100-fold. Given that the DEL typically set is 0.1 of the OEL, this means that if the lower performance figure was used (0.004 microgram/M³) the system would have performed with an exceedence of 10 times. What this really means is that the safety factors that are currently used are very challenged with poorly performing systems.
- All other events have to be taken into account when assessing a TWA.

Take the case of the Isolator 1. Its results were basically flat with only 2 nanograms separating the best and worst in a sequence of five events. (Note the "<"; this means that nothing was detected, but the sensitivity of the analytical process requires the lowest sensitivity to be recorded as the result.) If you take the handled volume of API into consideration, these two isolators that test parametrically equal are separated by a gross weigh manipulated to detected release ration of more than 1,000,000.

$$\left(\frac{20,000 \text{ gram}}{0.007/\text{microgram}} \right) \left(\frac{(1)}{0.403/\text{microgram}} \right) = 2,857,142 \text{ vs. } 2.48$$

The reason for the difference is simple: Isolator 1 uses two not quite perfect systems redundantly, while Isolator 2 uses only one system that is technique driven.

The following illustrate other examples and also highlight a challenging problem; i.e., that the containment valves of whatever type do a reasonable job with aerosols but do a poor job when it comes to contamination of the critical seals. This material can become available by any of the means of ingestion to others at another time and place. It is therefore vital to protect/clean these critical points.

Most importantly the results show the risk of technique dependency.

EXAMPLE 1   Pilot Plant in a Down Flow Booth

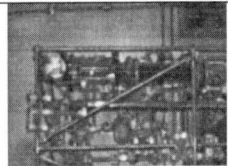
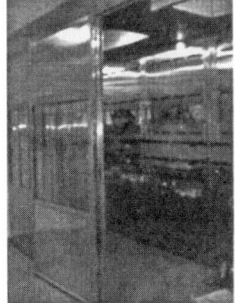
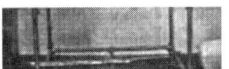

Performance:
Pilot Plant in Unidirectional Flow Hood

Position	µ g/m³	Time	TWA	Comment
Personnel A	115,000	12 min		Open
Personnel B	1.39	13 min		Using sub sash
Personnel A	281,000	13 min		
Inside face	19.9	13 min		
Back wall	185	15 min		
Inside right of door	399	13 min		
Wipes	Wipe µg			
Rear wall	9,360			4″ × 4″10 vertical 10
				Horizontal
Rear floor	72,700			Horizontal
Wipe blank	328			Horizontal

EXAMPLE 2   Containment Results Plotted Against Parametric Performance for Fume
Hoods
The results show that there is no correlation between the two. Fume hoods are totally technique depen-
dent to work and the study shows that they do not work. Data from Eli Lilly reference.

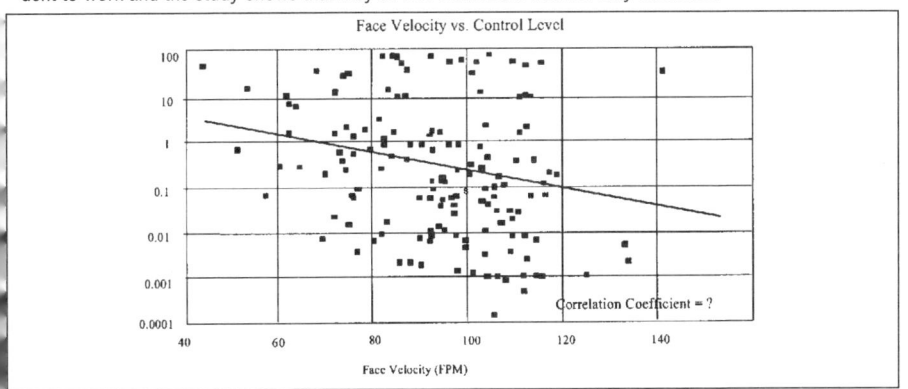

EXAMPLE 3   Isolator Mounted Vacuum Tray Dryer with Stainless Steel Wire Tie Bag Out Technique

Here the results (shown as TWAs with the formula by which they were assessed) shows stellar results, with the bag out by operator 1 first iteration being the worst at 0.014 micrograms/M^3. For the surrogate testing using PharmaConsult U.S. protocols, the operators are not trained so that real world mistakes occur. By placing the bag out bag in in a secondary chamber better figures can be achieved.

Open Filter VDR Isolator

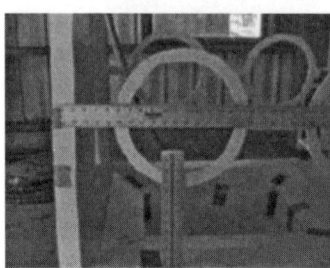
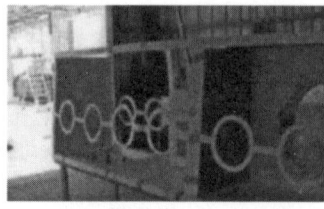
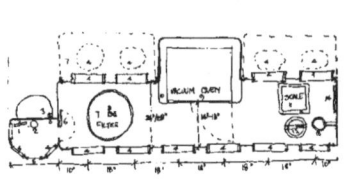
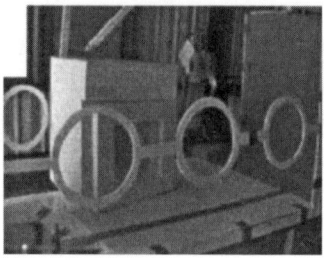

Performance:

Position	µg/m³	Time	TWA	Comment
Personnel manipulate 1	0.137	13 min		
Personnel bag out 1	0.104	20 min	0.0143	PM1+PBO1+WA/480
Personnel manipulate 2	BQL	13 min		
Personnel bag out 2	0.059	20 min	0.01	PM2+PBO2+WA/480
Personnel manipulate 3	0.048	15 min		
Personnel bag out 3	0.033	14.5 min	0.0087	PM3+PBO3+WA/480
Personnel manipulate	BQL			
Personnel bag out	BQL		0.0062	PM4+PBO4+WA/480
Work area	0.014	215 min	0.0062	All above = 0.01616 µm³/8hrs
Corridor	BQL	230 min		
Inside operator A	272.000	14 min		1 Kg to 3 bags
Inside operator B	320.000	14 min		1 Kg to 3 Bags
Blank				3.92 n gram

EXAMPLE 4   Pilot Plant Retrofit

The client with a 0.300-microgram/M³/8 hours product used "shirt sleeve" for all but the reactor charging phase.

Sub Division

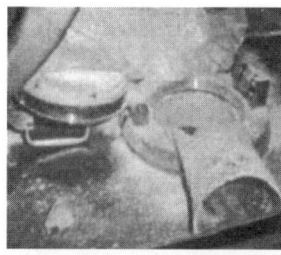
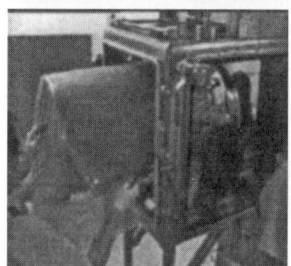
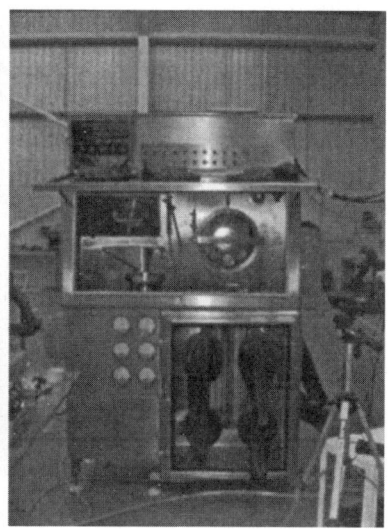

Performance:

Subdivision Isolator

Position	Ng/m³	Time	TWA	Comment
Background	12.7	66	12.7	Target material unopened no activity. No air on
Drum one loading	<5.6	120		Below detection threshold
Deliberate glove breech	215	24	0.471	TWA based on time and presumption of no re-entrainment
Primary operator run 3	63.9	26	0.014	This operator had two samplers on,
Bag out drum out			(3.46)	the second did not record any material
Bag loading				*Drum sleeve fail*
Second operator run 3	<10.6	65		
Third operator run 3	18.4	54	(2.07)	

Wipes per 100 cm² Pass criteria, <1,000 ng/100cm²

A/B canister	5.7–12	
Waste bag	2.3–33	
IBC	31&43	
Seal of A/B Port	60,700	This was with a vendor designed port protector, this was replaced with a correct design unit
	112,000	

EXAMPLE 4   (*Continued*)

Reactor Charging

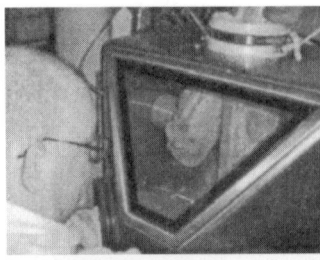
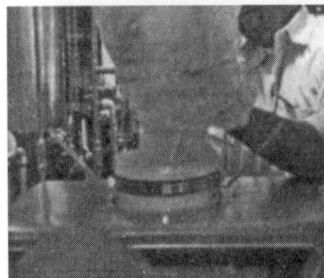
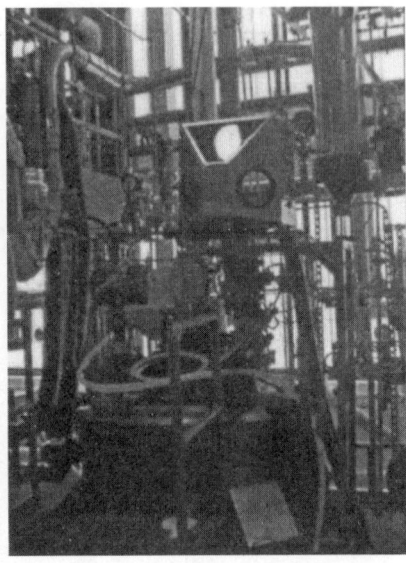

Performance:

Test Results

24 Air samples were taken; 1 recorded detectable amounts of naproxen sodium

The only detection was a background sample when no transfer was undertaken

Issues

• The background level is significant. The client brief excluded in-process issues. Any system is only as good as the weakest link

• Operators were not trained prior to the test to induce upset conditions. At least 3 upsets occurred, the worst being a missed dock of the bag and a bag slip (the loops were too long)

	Ng/m³	Time	TWA	Comment
	431.00	61	54-431	Target material in reactor. No other activity. Lower TWA based on assumption of not emission before or after. Not tenable upper based on constantemission at detected level
Background, 2 charges of 13 KG and transfer locations. Port recovery and waste bagging. Third operator run		16-60		All less than level of detection
	3	18.4	54	

Wipes per 100 cm² Pass criteria, <1,000 ng/100²

A/B seal	114,390	A/B ports are contaminated
A/B canister not seal Compare	21,795	
A/B canister gasket	755,550	With split butterfly valve
Top of reactor changer	46.5	
Deposit base of RTP inside isolator	708,600	

EXAMPLE 4 (*Continued*)

Ported Bag System and alternaties

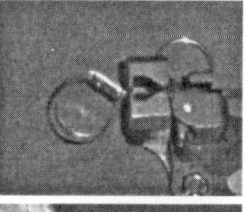
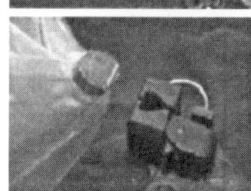
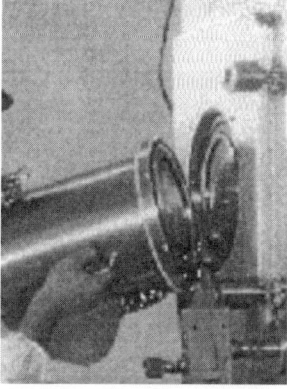
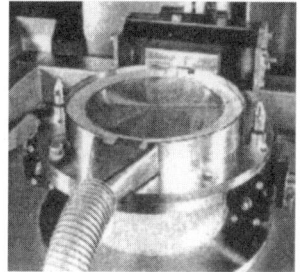
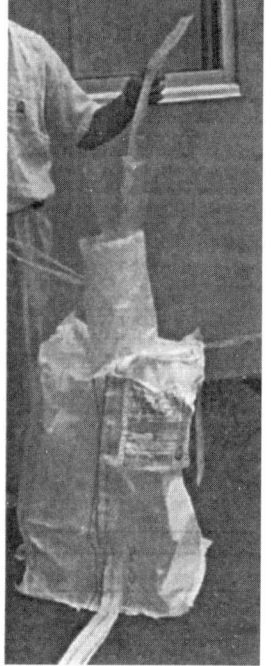

Filter Dryer Offload

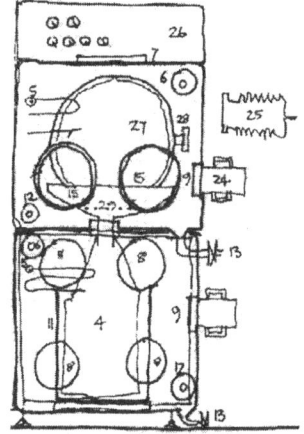
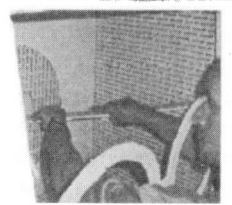
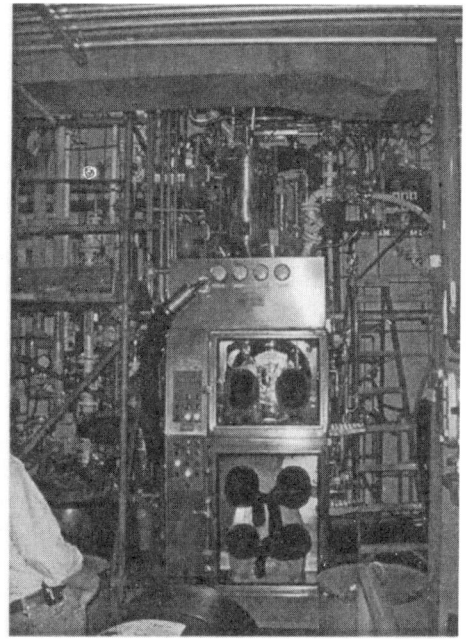

EXAMPLE 4 (*Continued*)

Test Results

14 air samples were taken; 2 recorded detectable amounts of naproxen sodium. Both operators bag out from filter dryer. All A/B ports were rebuilt by operators when the interlocks were found to be defective

• Operators were not trained prior to the test to induce upset conditions. At least 3 upsets occurred, the worst being a missed dock of the bag and a bag slip (the loops were too long).

• The A/B ports were discovered to have been incorrectly assembled by the vendor, discovered when cleaning subdiv insolator.

Performance:

Filter Dryer Isolator Ng/M³ =Filter Volume (*V*) 1000 × wt Time (min) TWA ng/m³/8 hr

Position	Ng/m³	Time	TWA	Comment
Bag out primary operator	12.6	91	2.38 8	Difficulty because the bag was not fully inflated prior to fill
Bagout secondary operator 10 kilo (approx)	11.1	91	2.10 4	

Wipes per 100 cm² Pass criteria, <1,000 ng/100cm²

Bag 1 Port	52,125	Improving technique self taught
Seal	145,950	
Face of FDI above gloves	26.5	
Side by port	74.4	
Seal swab	34,045	

This has to be compared with the FAT of a down flow booth at the factory. The required performance was 10 micrograms/M³ the actual performance over 5 iterations was:

3. 92 micrograms/M³
4. 110 micrograms/M³
5. 140 micrograms/M³
6. 470 micrograms/M³
7. 2,400 micrograms/M³

Time: 16–29 minutes.

WHAT DOES THIS ALL MEAN?
Two redundant but not perfect systems are better than one very good system.

- The best performing valve on the market for a complete system (Alpha part, Beta part, controls, wash ring) costs about $50,000. If it malfunctions, you have a problem.
- Simple split butterfly valve and clamshell with wipe and cap and particle counting. Cost is approximately $25,000. If one system malfunctions, it is statistically improbable the other will fail at the same time.

PERSONNEL PROTECTIVE EQUIPMENT
The following shows the levels of protection afforded.

Effective Protection Factors*

• Half face air purifying respirator	10
• PAPR with loose fitting face piece	25
• PAPR with half face piece	50
• Full face APR	100
• Air line full face pressure demand	1,000
• Self contained breathing apparatus	10,000
Compare to a well-designed isolator:	*1,000,000*

*If worn full time.

Supplied Air and PAPR

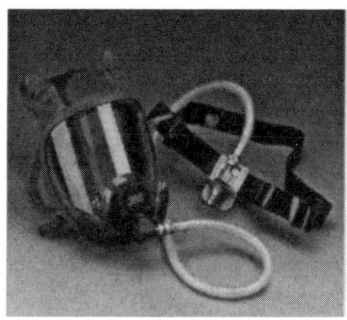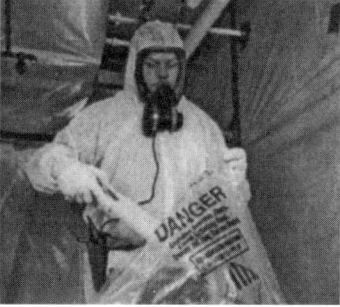

Full Suit Supplied Air
As PPE increases in performance it also hinders the operator's ability to communicate and perform tasks. It is administratively difficult to control and takes up to 1/8th of the operator's day to don and remove correctly. However, it is recommended that all dermal areas be covered so that the operator cannot directly touch skin, the reason being that the gloves may contact the API during transfers and

clean up of the critical seals. If certain solvents are used, transdermal action is as rapid a means of exposure as inhalation.

Editor's Note: _____

CSHA and the European authorities no longer allow PPE as the primary operation protection. A half suit in an isolator has to be seen as the primary line of protection and is therefore PPE and not an engineering control.

TRANSFER SYSTEMS

Without question the most important containment concern is the way in which the actives are connected to the various items of process equipment and are moved around the plant. The key challenge to any containment system is the make-and-breaks that occur as transactions between processes and equipment.

To achieve a successful transfer, material has to be introduced into a container. It is impossible to place powder into a device without contaminating the outside if the inside and outside of the device are in the same environment. In addition, the hands of the operator are contaminated from twisting and tying the bag and from contact with contaminated surfaces. The mere act of expressing the air by twisting and tying the bags ensures that material is liberated to contaminate the environment. The surfaces near the dispensing process are also covered in the product particulate and fine material remains in suspension in the air for a considerable period.

The key to successful containment is to keep the inner product contaminated layer separate to the outer environmental contact layer. This may seem simple, but it is very complex and difficult in reality. This section discusses and reviews the options.

The key elements of a transfer system are that it provides robust containment and is easily handled.

Rigid containers are often used by the pharmaceutical industry because they are robust, can be made of 316L stainless steel and can undergo an elaborate cleaning ritual. Rigid containers can cause bridging and require a secondary device to prevent contamination of the seal where RTP type valves are used.

Rigid Ported Canister   **Ported Bag**

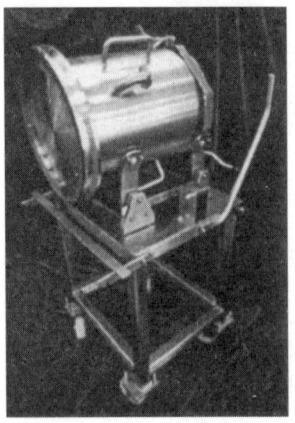
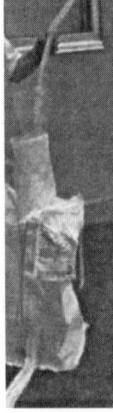

A flexible container does not require such measures because bridging can only occur when the abutments form a rigid foundation; with flexible films this does not occur.

The means by which the active container is attached to the process device is vital to the ability to contain. This subsection examines connection techniques and devices as well as flexible and rigid containers.

Split Valve Connections

There is a range of valves that provide contained transfer. For the purpose of this review they will be categorized as:

- Alpha/beta valves require rotational movement to dock the parts. These valves also require an isolator to allow the valve to be used.
- Split actuated valves do not require rotational docking or isolators and work by two parts clamping together and then acting as a single valve, opening by rotation, leaving the valve in the product path.
- Cone valves have an alpha and beta cone part that interlocks and opens allowing an annular flow.
- Hybrid valves typically have two halves mate and then slide sideways to allow a full bore flow.

A/B Ported Connection

This type of port has been around for over 30 years in the nuclear industry. It works by mating two parts of a door in separate frames together. The diagram illustrates the concept. Both frame and door or port has bayonet lugs, which engage into each other. The lugs are inclined planes so that rotation tightens the faces together. The first part of the rotation engages and pulls the alpha and beta part together. The second part of the rotation causes the Beta door to rotate and be released from the Beta frame, thus allowing the door to be opened. All that is revealed to both the inside and outside is a microscopic area of seal. Because this

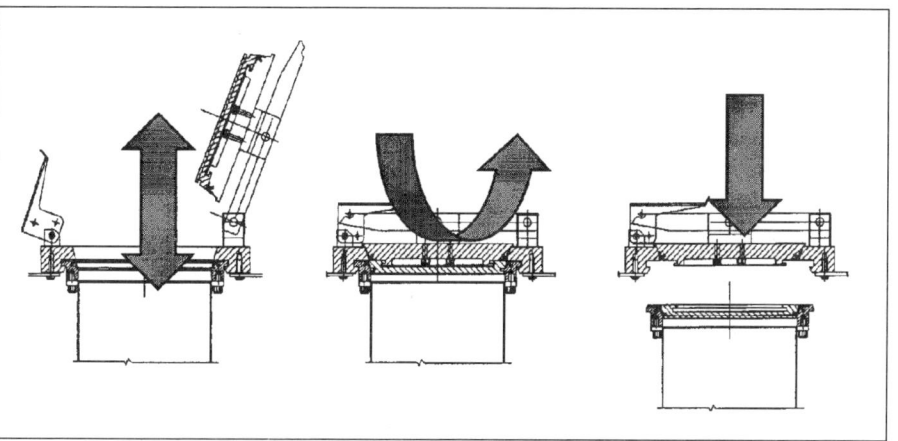

seal is vulnerable, it should be protected from contact with the contaminant. The powder transfer should be separated from the containment door using a chute or tube or other protective device.

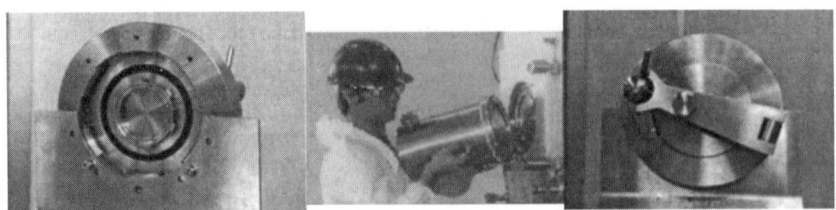

Such ported systems can achieve the highest levels of containment with consistent results in the low nanograms. The issues with such a system are described below.

Interlocks: Most vendors offer a mechanical interlock. The interlock is intended to ensure that the alpha cannot be opened if a beta is not correctly docked. The beta container must be locked so that it cannot be removed while the beta door is connected to the active. It is essential to ensure that the interlock cannot be easily defeated. With some interlocks, it is necessary to defeat the interlock for cleaning and recovery; it is possible to partially rotate the port allowing the port to be opened while unsafe. This is NOT acceptable. Most interlocks are mechanical and the rods or levers have to pass from the contaminated to the uncontaminated areas. During cleaning, solution leakage has been observed through these seals. Careful inspection and maintenance is required.

Contamination of Seals. The seal can be contaminated by transfer from the exposed seal to the unexposed seal. In aseptic transfer this is called the "ring of confidence." Minimizing cross contamination is reliant on reducing the area of cross contamination. However to achieve this, the port becomes very much more complex, is machined to finer tolerances and is more susceptible to damage. A laCalhene port, for instance, uses a simple hinge, while the ACE port is double jointed to allow a parallel rather than radial closing action. The laCalhene port has years of use behind it, while the others are much more recent and have far fewer examples in use. The data given previously show that levels of seal contamination can be very high while the aerosol level is excellent. Protective measures to protect and cover the seals at all times are essential as is constant port maintenance.

Connection of the Product Container to Alpha/Beta Ports

A large array of options has been created for the devices that can be attached to a Beta port. They include:

- Single layer bag for components
- Double layer bag or FIBC with a product transfer chute

- Disposable single use beta ports
- Steam sterilizable beta connection
- Stainless steel canisters
- Liquid path connections
- Sampling systems
- Gamma irradiated delivery systems, ect.

A/B Ported System. The bag consists of two parts, the outer and inner product liner. The outer liner is attached to either a reusable stainless steel or machined plastic bag connector or permanently attached to an injection molded beta port. The bag is connected to the isolator using the beta port and when connected the chute is deployed to charge or discharge the product.

Results using these devices have been as low as "below detection level" with a 2 nanogram M^3 detection limit. These results have been consistently achieved.

Example of a Reusable Beta Connector. The reusable connector can be of machined plastic or stainless steel. The advantage of plastic is that it is lightweight and is unlikely to damage the product liner. The drawback is that plastic is unstable especially when machined and can distort due to memory, machining temperature, and moisture. Stainless steel ports are more robust though they can gall if misused; they are easier to clean, however. Hastelloy ports are available; unfortunately, the elastomers are not as resistant as Hastelloy.

Reusable Connector

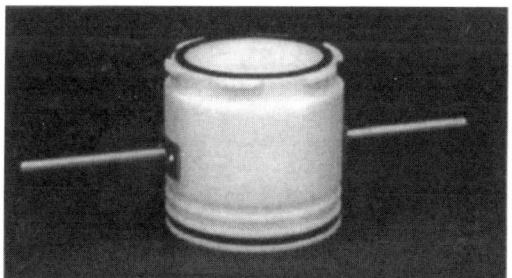

When not closed an Aalpha port should have a protective cap placed on it to protect the seals, occlude alien particulate, and retain any active that remains on the seals. Saran pot covers can be used for this purpose. In the case of the stainless steel beta port, a specially made padded bonnet protects both the product liner and the port from any abrasion or snagging by the stainless steel port.

The size of the port is also a key issue. The larger the port, the greater risk of material crossing the boundary because of the larger exposed seal and greater weight. A/B ports require an isolator and operator manipulation. The ports should be wiped using clean room practice and sterile, pre-wetted clean room wipes.

Saran Pot Covers

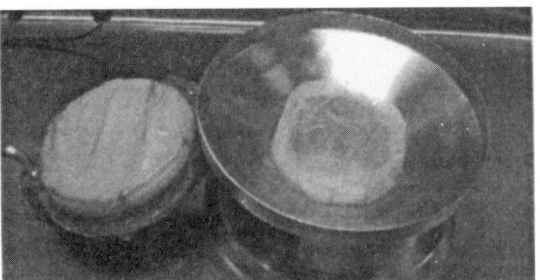

Split Butterfly Valves

During the mid 1990s, these devices began to emerge based upon requirements for Eli Lilly and Glaxo. Most are sold and described as powder free transfer devices. The principle behind this device is that two plates, the mating halves of a butterfly valve, behave as a single butterfly valve and when closed can be de-mated with the two halves forming the containment boundary. This is a very simple idea that is extraordinarily difficult to achieve. Upon examination some are seen as very poor at containment with two metal faces without elastomers forming the occluded faces of the valve. The following diagrams illustrate the principles of this type of valve:

Split Butterfly Valves

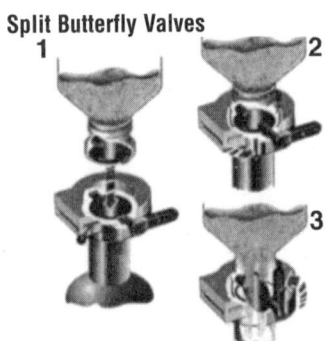

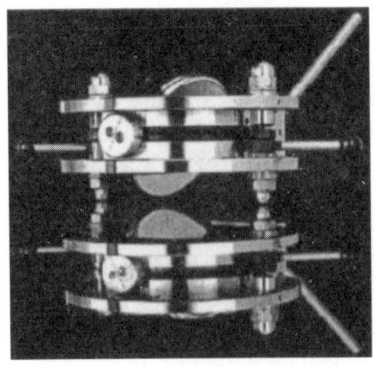

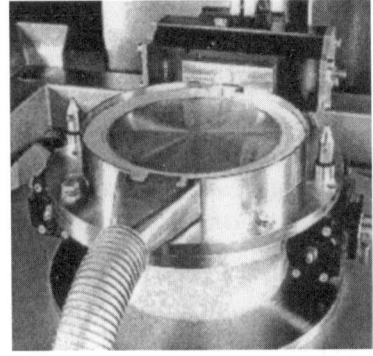

A majority of available valves have seals between the plates and are far better at containment than those without. Unfortunately, it was quickly understood that rotational accuracy and the effect of trapping the active between the seal and the seat meant relatively poor containment. Air sparging was installed on some valves to overcome this problem. These valves have proven to be unreliable in use, where a failure of the valve results in the total discharge of the container. These devices are very expensive. Great strides are being made to produce reliable valves and the leading contenders in this field are listed below.

Buck Valve. The Buck valve has a locator pin and lug assembly to allow the two parts to mate; once mated a cam pulls the two parts together. This means that one part must be able to move to allow for alignment and mating movement. Buck has three versions. The original HC; UHC, which has a ventilated secondary shroud; and the TC version with in-use wash in place (15+ minute cycle time). This valve is equipped with a vacuum wash cycle that cleans then dries the valve. The TC version has shown the best results for both airborne and surface contamination of the valve. The issues with this valve are cost and the drying cycle.

Glatt Valve. The Glatt valve uses a design where the split between the two parts is at an angle rather than tangential to the direction of flow. This allows the valve actuation shaft to be complete with the alpha side driven from the alpha half and the beta from the beta. This has mechanical advantages over valves where the actuation is split in two halves. It also means the valve takes up more space. The 2002 version of the valve replaces the bladder seal of the earlier version with an intelligent seal that withdraws when pressure on the valve is released, combined with an air sparge. The valve is actuated at the end of the cycle but while still closed to dislodge the material that inevitably accumulates on the upstream side of the valve. Because the actuation of the valve is complex, a PLC is normally associated with the valve and this makes the active cumbersome. It also means that it is not recommended to be connected to moving or movable units such as bin blenders or IBCs.

PSL Valve. This is one of the earliest valves and has a metal-to-metal contact rather than an intermediate elastomer. This valve is available in a range of sizes and ratings to suit process use and is of robust construction. While it does not perform as well as the market leaders it is suitable for many applications particularly where it is part of a redundant system with a local secondary containment system.

Cone Valves

The drawback with cone valves is that they form an obstruction to the powder flow in the form of a cone; however, the split valves are not much better since the size of the valve and drive shafts are considerable and provide better areas for the material to accumulate when compared to a cone. The LB Bohle valve can dock at any angle of rotation, a very important feature to be aware of in other valves where they can only make at very specific alignments.

The Matcon Valve. This is the original cone valve. The two parts mate to form a "coolie hat" with the outside of the supply valve being protected by the head of the connection. The valve is lifted allowing annular discharge. If flow promotion is required, the valve can pulse. Typically these valves are of very large diameter. Reasonable test results have been seen for this valve, but it is really a production scale device.

LB Bohle Valve. This valve is similar in concept to a Matcon valve, but at 10 inches is smaller and is pneumatically operated. This makes it a fairly simple valve. The cone can be actuated to promote flow. The performance of this valve was just below that of the highest containment valves; however, the test was conducted over six cycles with no cleaning between cycles.

Hybrid Valves

The two chief hybrid valves are the CORA Tip valve and the Zanchetta. Both valves use magnets in the containment "lids" to bind the two parts together. In the case of the CORA, these two parts are extracted and a leading part on the valve descends to close these parts off before the conventional butterfly valves allow powder transfer. On completion of transfer the valves are closed and the intervening area is air sparged; finally, the magnetic containment covers are returned and magnetically held in place before disconnection. This system was tested over six iterations using lactose air sampling and swabbing and gave excellent results. The Zanchetta is a conventional split butterfly design but the parts are held together magnetically; results appear to be good.

Many of these valves have few installations, while the Buck and Glatt have a greater number.

Comparing Costs

An alpha port RTP is about $6,000 and an isolator to operate it is about $30,000 making for a manually operated contained transfer of about $36,000. It may be ergonomically challenged due to the location of the valve.

A Glatt active split butterfly valve is about $30,000 and is automated. A Buck TC active is about $50,000, but gives the highest currently available performance. An air sparged clamshell is about $15,000 with butterfly valve, about the same price as a CORA Tip valve; the PSL valve comes in at about $10,000.

Other Containment Methodologies

Redundancy and Air Sparged Systems

The main reason why containment systems fail is that they are not provided with redundancy, so if a split butterfly fails in whole or part, whatever is liberated becomes available to the operator. The provision of a redundant system minimizes the risk of this happening.

In aseptic processing redundancy has been a factor for years, one filter providing redundancy to the other. Central to all successful high containment systems is the provision of a separate, redundant containment system.

The clamshell enclosure encloses the primary transfer valve, which opens once the transfer and clean up has taken place and is closed during critical operations provides a redundant system. The clamshell is provided with an exhaust that runs at a velocity of 90 fpm in an open state and provides negative pressure in the enclosure

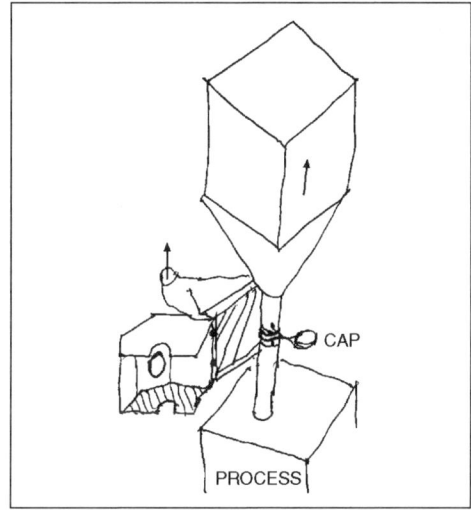

when closed. This is not an isolator in the true sense, but is a barrier enclosure. To minimize particles from becoming dislodged, the base is equipped with a disposable tack mat. Additionally, after a transfer, a wipe down with a wet wipe is advised. As a further feature a bag out for wastes and the ability to provide a cap to both the connecting ends is advised. The unit would be fed ULPA filtered air and particles monitored on exhaust. This allows real time indication of failed transfer event.

An option is to provide a local exhaust at the make and break connects. On its own, an open exhaust, however designed, has a very limited zone of influence. Open exhausts are totally prone to fluctuations due to movement and external conditions as well as the HVAC systems. To enable a typical pharmaceutical particulate to be captured in the air stream and arrested by the filter requires very high velocities. By placing a physical barrier around the transfer external influences are dramatically reduced.

The enclosure is at negative pressure. A decontaminating wipe and clean capping will provide further redundancy so that performance requirements can be met and the valve protected.

Inside such a device any of the following connections systems can be used.

- Bag trick
- Air sparged twin butterfly

- Split butterfly
- Cone valves

Some valves include the secondary and tertiary boundaries in the valve such as the Buck VHC and TC Valves.

The air velocities and pressure differentials required are not great. The HEPA is rated for a 90 fpm velocity at face when the clamshell is open. Because the clamshell will not be fully air tight, make up air will leak into the clamshell. Dependent on the fan type that is used about 1/2: wg can be expected with a velocity through the leak sites at high velocity. Ideal conditions would be–100 pa with a leak velocity of 60 fpm. The whole point of the design is to entrain fluidized particles, but to allow larger particles to drop to the tack mats.

Bag Tricks

Bag tricks were conceived in the mid 1990s emanating from Eli Lilly. The concept was to use tricks with plastic bags to avoid using isolators at all or to make and break transfers while maintaining containment. In the end all of these systems come down to the moment of truth when the liner is cut to leave a product/containment bag and a protective end on the unit from which the bag is disconnected. Bag tricks fall into a number of distinct types:

- Continuous liners, from which containment bags are formed.
- Single units or bags with the ability to remove the residual end from the last transfer
- Composite units, which also have an "isolator" built in.

The tie, taping, and cutting technique is not recommended. Such a technique can be used for product in the 1–10 microgram range dependent on shift iterations.

The challenge is the effective change out from one bag to another. The techniques vary.

Progressive Ring Technique. In this system (ILC Dover), the first bag is connected to the first ring, the second to the second ring and so on. Effectively such a system is limited by the space required for the rings, as well as the problem of cleaning the outside of the annulus.

Slipping Ring Technique. In this method, two rings are used. The first bag is connected to the second ring using an "O" ring and is externally secured using a captive "O" ring to the first "O" ring groove. When fully used the old end is removed as follows: The external "O" ring is removed as is the clamp band used to secure the bag firmly in place. The bag is carefully pushed and folded back until it has been fully folded back over the captive "O" ring and the "O" ring groove is clear. At this point the next bag is secured using the external "O" ring and clamp. Through the second bag the captive "O" ring is forced into the groove while the captive "O" ring on the previous bag is eased out, with careful technique the transfer of "O" rings is continued. The objective is to ensure that no powder passes the first "O" ring position.

Because this is a challenged change out, it is normal to contain this process in an isolation chamber and to design the bag and tubes so that all the transfers required in an operation can be performed without change out. This allows the change out to occur after a full decontamination and clean up.

Using Bags Formed from a Continuous Liner. A continuous tube of lay flat polyethylene is place on a spool in very much the same way as a sausage skin is placed on a sausage-making machine. The bags can be formed in a number of ways.

The material can be twisted and twice tied, and a cut made between the ties, thereby forming the closure of one bag and forming the next bag bottom. This is how links in a sausage are made. The problem is that the polyethylene is electrostatic and so powder fully coats the inner surface; cutting the liner to form the bag allows the powder not trapped to be liberated. Another method is to use a crimp of plastic or metal. The advantage of the crimp is that very high compressive forces are applied. It is also possible to heat seal the bags and to cut through the heat seal. Up to now this has been a challenge due to the environments in which this occurs (explosivity). ILC Dover has developed an anti-static material, with elastic properties and a safe heat sealer process, with a 3″ wide seal. The sealing process develops a central weakening, allowing the bags to be ripped apart. Using such a technique, all the active is encapsulated. These units are very expensive at approximately $60,000 each. Non-rated heat sealers are $6,000 or more compared with the $300 crimping tool and $1 tie.

Bag Ties. There are a number of systems available. A conventional nylon cable tie does not develop sufficient compressive force to be considered.

ILC Dover Tool. ILC Dover has developed a tool that compresses two plastic ratchet lock ties at the same time. The two are then cut apart using a ratchet cutter. The compression forces of the device are not as great as the stainless steel tie device, and pull off failures have been reported. A further feature is a snap on cap to replace the tape that is normally used.

Strap-It/Flanders System

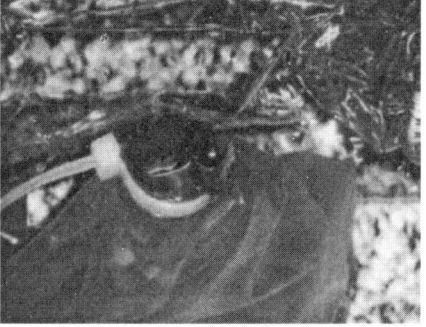

Strap-It/Flanders System. This system uses a stainless steel duct band with a setscrew to secure the band once compressed. The plastic is compressed by hand and held bundled using nylon cable ties. The stainless steel band is placed around the bundled plastic and threaded through clear. A tool is engaged onto the free end of the band and a ratchet used to wind the banding—as the band is wound, the bundle is tightened. Considerable force can be applied. When tight, an allen key is used to place and tighten a set screw. The band is cut using a device on the "strap-it" and the cut end bent back. This procedure is repeated immediately adjacent to the first. A plastic tube cutter is used to cut through the compressed plastic film. When done properly, this is a very effective method since the plastic film is very tightly compressed. If the bands are too far apart, the plastic film exfoliates when cut, releasing trapped powder. This cannot be described as an easy fumble-free technique. This system results in a 1.7—64 nanogram M^3/event (29 minutes) over a number of iterations.

Stainless Steel Ties

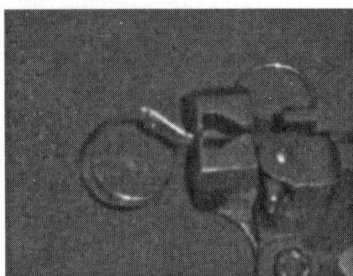 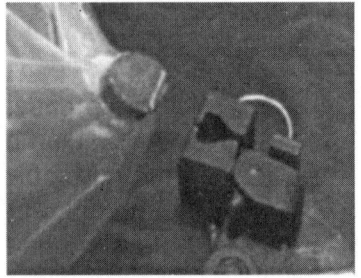

Stainless Steel Ties. For military use, a stainless steel version of the nylon cable tie has been developed. Like the cable tie, the end is threaded through a head, which permits one-way movement only (tightening). A tool is used that progressively pulls the free end of the tie through the head, leading to increasing compression of the plastic bundles. No setscrew is required and the ties are available from a number of suppliers. This is a much simpler process than the one previously described.

In creating a sealed bag, it is important to be able to partially inflate the bag to let the powder in and to evacuate the bag before sealing (effectively the vacuum pack technique used for ground coffee). This method also provides an immediate visual indication if a bag has failed, since it will not be as rigid as vacuum packs normally are. A bag in bag process further reduces the risk of liberated active. In over 30 iterations, all events were below the detection threshold of 1.2 nanograms/M^3.

APPENDIX: GENERAL DEFINITIONS

Active pharmaceutical ingredients and other chemicals are assigned to OEB 1–5 on the basis of their toxicity and pharmacological activity. The OEBs will be called: 1) *Default* (early research compound for which no test data exist: 2) *preliminary* (enough data from development, but not approved by OELC: and 3) *final* once OELC approval is obtained.

Active Pharmaceutical Ingredient (API). This term is synonymous with "drug substance" and is used to describe a pure pharmaceutical compound. Pharmaceutical active ingredient = drug substance = pharmaceutical compound.

Corrosive. Capable of destroying skin tissue or mucous membranes through physical contact. Classification as corrosive (Cor) can be based on the results of validated in vivo or in vitro tests, or may be assumed if the substance pH is < 2.0 or > 11.5. In the event the substance has already been tested, assigned phrases of R34 or R35 would indicate that the substance is corrosive.

Decision Blocks. The drug development timeline is utilized to communicate the stage of development of compounds in the drug pipeline. Decision EDC compounds are new research compounds, while decisions I/IIa, IIb, and III refer to other stages in the development of a product. Decision blocks are also sometimes called "Stages" or "decision points."

Default Occupational Exposure Band. An initial Occupational Exposure Band (OEB) assigned to a compound when no data, save for structure-activity analysis results, are available for determination.

Drug Product. Collective term that includes pharmaceutical intermediates or diluted active material in liquid or solid form. Since these materials are not pure, a drug product is not the same as an active ingredient.

Drug Substance. This term is synonymous with "active ingredient" and is used to describe a pure pharmaceutical compound. Drug substance = active ingredient = pharmaceutical compound.

EHS Personnel. EHS stands for environment, Health, and safety. EHS personnel include those individuals employed in any of the environment, health, or safety disciplines (industrial hygiene, product stewardship, occupational health, occupational medicine, safety, process safety, environmental engineering, etc.).

Highly Active Pharmaceuticals. Active pharmaceutical ingredients that, by virtue of their hazardous properties or pharmacological activity, may have adverse effects on employees and/or the environment. Additionally, upon acute or chronic occupational exposure to employees, these substances may induce severe or irreversible adverse effects. High activity compounds are assigned to OEB 3–5.

Occupational Exposure Bands (OEBs). These are ranges of airborne concentrations of substances as 8-hour time-weighted averages. The OEBs generally observed for level 1–5 compounds are outlined below.

APIs and Other Solids

OEB 1	1000–5000 mcg/m3
OEB 2	100–1000 mcg/m3
OEB 3	10–100 mcg/m3
OEB 4	1–10 mcg/m3
OEB 5	< 1 mcg/m3

Gases and Liquids

V-OEB 1	> 1000 ppm
V-OEB 2	100–1000 ppm
V-OEB 3	10–100 ppm
V-OEB 4	1–10 ppm
V-OEB 5	< 1 ppm

Occupational Exposure Limits (OELs). An Occupational Exposure Limit refers to an airborne limit concentration of a substance. It is usually averaged over a reference period (normally 8 hours) at which, according to current knowledge, there is no evidence that it is likely to be injurious to employees if they are exposed by inhalation, day after day, to that concentration.

OEB 1 Compounds. Compounds that are harmful and/or have low pharmacological activity

OEB 2 Compounds. Compounds that are harmful, and/or have moderate pharmacological activity

OEB 3 Compounds. Compounds that are moderately toxic and/or have high pharmacological activity

OEB 4 Compounds. Compounds that are toxic and/or have very high pharmacological activity

OEB 5 Compounds. Compounds that are extremely toxic and/or have extremely high pharmacological activity

Preliminary Occupational Exposure Level (P-OEL). An airborne concentration of a substance that is a preliminary estimate of the Occupational Exposure Level. Sometimes the P-OEL calculation can be derived during Decision EDC when a compound is assigned a Preliminary OEB. Additional data for the molecule are developed during Decision I/IIa and IIb. Typically, at Decision III sufficient data are available to establish the Occupational Exposure Limit.

Purchased Chemicals. Substances, including raw materials, solvents, and excipients that are not produced by the facility but are purchased from outside vendors.

Reproductive (and/or Developmental) Hazards. Pharmaceutical agents that can adversely impact any aspect of the human reproductive process (e.g., libido, fertility, conception, spontaneous abortion, fetal development and growth, and breast feeding) at doses that are NOT maternally toxic are assigned R1 or R2 designations in addition to OEB 2–5. Generally, R2 is assigned when there is strong cause and effect evidence of reproductive toxicity in humans, or in animal models that are thought to be predictive of human toxicity. R1 is assigned where the cause and effect relationship is weaker and the outcome is less severe.

Sensitizers. Active pharmaceutical compounds known to be human sensitizers are designated as S1 or S2. Substances known to cause dermal sensitization in the occupational or clinical setting are assigned S1. Compounds are assigned S2 if they are known to cause anaphylaxis, or if they are known to cause lower respiratory tract sensitization or occupational asthma. S2 compounds normally have a minimum OEB 4 (OEL < 10 ug/m^3). S1 designations can be given to OEB 2–5 compounds depending on lead effect.

Short Term Exposure Limit. A 15-minute TWA exposure that should not be exceeded at any time during a workday, even if the 8-hour TWA is within the TLV-TWA.

Structure Activity Relationship (SAR). Assessment of the molecular structure of materials to predict the types and degree of pharmacological and toxicological characteristics.

16

Occupational Health and Safety

Authors   George Petroka
Todd Allshouse
Denise Proulx
Joseph Milligan
Dave Kerr

INTRODUCTION

Pharmaceutical manufacturing facilities are required to comply with numerous occupational safety and health regulations, codes, guidelines, and best management practices. Therefore, occupational health and safety management and compliance are important concepts that must be addressed during the design of the facility. Occupational health and safety pertains to all personnel who perform work at pharmaceutical finishing facilities: it covers both company and contract employees working during routine, non-routine, and construction activities. It addresses the chemical, physical, and biological hazards that may be handled and or processed at the facility. It does not address the safety of the products, which are addressed through current Good Manufacturing Practices (cGMPs).

OCCUPATIONAL HEALTH AND SAFETY MANAGEMENT

Health and safety management has the goal of providing guidance and direction in all phases of the safety program, including occupational safety and health, environmental control, fire safety, safety-oriented training programs, and building and equipment design criteria affecting safety codes of standards. Pharmaceutical companies must consider the health and safety of their employees and the protection of the community and the environment to be of primary importance in the design, installation, and maintenance of all equipment, processes, and facilities, as well as during the performance of all operations.

At a minimum, the company should comply with all local, regional, and national health and safety regulations. The primary federal organization in the United States that promulgates and enforces safety and health regulations for general industry, including the pharmaceutical industry, is the Occupational Safety and Health Administration (OSHA). In addition, Section 18 of the Occupational Safety and Health Act of 1970 (the Act) encourages states to develop and operate their own job safety and health programs. OSHA approves and monitors state plans. The following 26 states/territories have approved state plans:

Alaska	Kentucky	New York[a]	Vermont
Arizona	Maryland	North Carolina	Virgin Islands
California	Michigan	Oregon	Virginia
Connecticut[a]	Minnesota	Puerto Rico	Washington
Hawaii	Nevada	South Carolina	Wyoming
Indiana	New Jersey[a]	Tennessee	
Iowa	New Mexico	Utah	

In addition, these agencies address specific areas related to safety and health:

• U.S. Department of Transportation (DOT) addresses the transportation of hazardous materials.
• National Institute for Occupational Safety and Health (NIOSH) is responsible for conducting research and making recommendations for the prevention of work-related injury and illness.

Finally, various organizations exist that publish consensus health and safety standards and guidelines with applicability to the pharmaceutical industry:

• American Conference of Governmental Industrial Hygienists (ACGIH)
• American Industrial Hygiene Association (AIHA)
• American National Standards Institute (ANSI)
• American Society for the Testing of Materials (ASTM)
• American Society of Heating, Refrigeration and Air Conditioning Engineers (ASHRAE)
• Building Officials and Code Administrators International, Inc. (BOCA)
• National Fire Protection Association (NFPA)

WALKING/WORKING SURFACES

Walking and working surfaces in a typical pharmaceutical manufacturing facility refer to any interior or exterior surface that is intended for routine or occasional access by personnel. This may include sidewalks, floors, ramps, stairways, elevated platforms and walkways, fixed and portable ladders, and roof level surfaces. Various building codes and occupational health and safety regulations promulgated throughout the world contain specific specifications for the design and maintenance of walking and working surfaces. These requirements are generally related to the structural design of the surface or the related architectural elements to properly support the required load. This loading must take into consideration personnel, equipment (either permanent or temporary), and materials. Other design requirements include the protection of all open or leading edges where there is a change in elevation usually greater than 3 feet, the degree of incline or slope for

---

[a]The Connecticut, New Jersey, and New York plans cover public sector (state and local government) employment only.

ramps, the elevation transitions between two levels, and the type of floor finishes provided to prevent slippery surfaces. Ice, water, or other liquids, or highly polished or cleanable surfaces can cause walking or working surfaces to become slippery.

The most opportune time to develop strategies to prevent falls and fall-related injuries for both production and maintenance and repair operations is during the design and engineering stages of the project. Key considerations include flooring designs that are sufficient to support the weight of personnel, portable equipment, and materials when elevated. Floor loading should take into consideration the weight of both personnel and any other additional loading that process equipment and materials may add. The capacity of elevated platforms or walkways should be clearly posted to prevent potential overloading.

Providing floor surfaces that offer adequate friction or traction is an important consideration in cGMP or clean environments where smooth or highly polished surfaces may create a hazard when personnel are required to wear gowning or booties over their normal shoes. Special attention should also be given to prevent highly polished surfaces near exterior doors or entranceways. At exterior doors or areas where water or moisture is routinely and normally present, a well-drained or sloped flooring system with increased traction should be provided to prevent water from accumulating.

Even the slightest changes in elevation are potential points for personnel to misjudge footing and increase their potential for slips and falls. Generally, any surface transition greater than 3/8 of an inch can result in a potential tripping hazard. A smooth transition with well-identified changes in elevations should be provided. Standard stair designs are often better navigated than sloped or ramped floor surfaces.

Platforms should be provided for any work requiring material handing or equipment operation. Platforms must be designed in accordance with applicable building codes and be of sufficient capacity for the intended weight loading. Placarding of the platform capacity is required. Any platform intended for personnel access that is 4 or more feet above the surrounding elevation must be protected with an approved standard barrier on all exposed sides. The standard barrier generally consists of three specific elements: the top rail, midrail, and toeboard. The standard railing assembly should be of rigid and durable design capable of withstanding a force of at least 200 pounds in any direction. The midrail should be located halfway between the top railing and the toe board. The toeboard design is normally a 4-inch high plate that is set off the platform elevation by up to $1/4$-inch to allow water to pass beneath.

Industrial stairways should be provided whenever possible for routine access to other elevations and in accordance with applicable building codes. Industrial stairs may be of open or enclosed design. Railings are required and are based on the side or width of the stairs.

Fixed industrial ladders should only be considered when access to elevations is not required on a continuous basis or by all personnel. Furthermore, they are not intended for personnel use if tools and other equipment must be carried and used by personnel. The length and types of vertical ladders fixed to the exterior of buildings or process equipment are governed by various country-specific health and safety standards. Many require the installation of cages or fall-arresting equipment.

Standard Cage for a Fixed Ladder

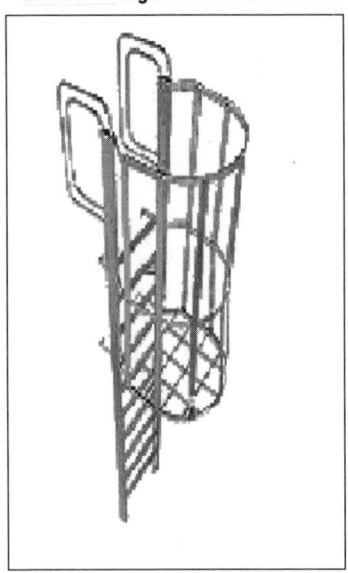

Cages are frequently included on exterior ladderways. They are intended to protect employees from falling away from the ladder or from contact with objects while climbing. However, personnel can still incur a serious fall while contained within the ladder cage. The length of fixed ladders is restricted to allow personnel to take a break from climbing and to limit the height of the potential fall hazard. Fixed ladderways restricted to lengths up to 20 feet generally do not require additional fall protection considerations. Fixed ladders of greater length are often equipped with a vertical guide rail system that allows personnel to use fall arresting equipment. A swing gate that restricts access to the ladderway and only opens outward from the ladderway should protect access to a vertical ladderway from any elevated level.

Any opening in a walking or working surface greater that 6 inches has the increased potential to create a fall hazard and must be barricaded, covered, secured, or otherwise protected. Openings along the edges of platforms should be avoided in the design or must be effectively guarded with a standard railing assembly. Self-closing swinging or overhead gates need to be provided to allow passage of materials without compromising personnel access or safety.

Access to roofs, interstitial spaces, mezzanines, or areas above suspended ceilings in pharmaceutical manufacturing facilities is often required of maintenance personnel to access mechanical or utility equipment. Frequent access to these levels should require the installation of approved walking and working surfaces, as described above. By design, mechanical equipment should be positioned so that access can be obtained from an approved walking or working surface and not within 6 feet of an unprotected edge.

Roofs Often House Mechanical and HVAC Equipment

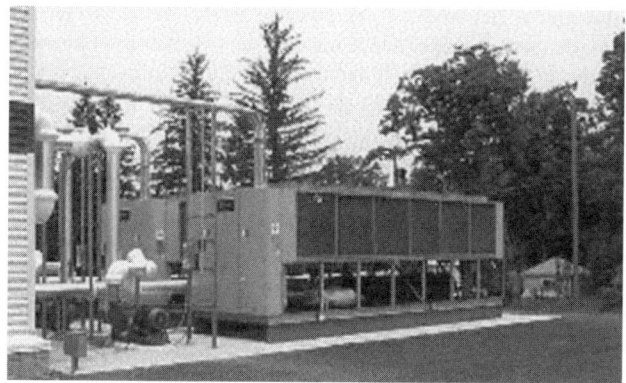

When roofs interstitial spaces, mezzanines, etc. must be accessed, several potential hazards may exist, including exposure to emissions, non-weight bearing surfaces, skylights, unprotected edges, etc. Interstitial spaces present other similar hazards and may require additional features such as lighting and ventilation. Roofs designed for routine access should be of full weight bearing capacity and have perimeter protection provided using a standard railing or an extended exterior parapet wall design. Translucent skylights should also be protected against step-through by physical guarding or the use of a standard perimeter railing.

MEANS OF EGRESS

All facilities must have emergency evacuation paths that lead to safe assembly areas from all buildings and process areas. These paths must be properly designed to accommodate the safe and orderly movement of all personnel without impairing emergency responder access to the site or incident area.

Most countries have regulatory codes detailing the design requirements for emergency evacuation routes. In the United States, NFPA 101: Life Safety Code is the regulatory standard for all industries and jurisdictions. Its requirements should be incorporated into the design and operation of all new and existing facilities. In general, the evacuation routes must ensure that all personnel including visitors are able to reach a safe location, typically known as the assembly area, without incurring any harm from the fire or emergency incident. The following general principles should be incorporated in all emergency egress plans.

- The minimum number of exits from any space or room on any floor, story, or mezzanine should be two, except where the space has an occupant load of less than approximately 30 people and the travel distance to a safe exit is less than 75 feet.

- The number of exits should be increased for higher occupancy loads and when there are increased life safety hazards, such as hazardous materials processing or storage or congested operations.
- Where multiple exits are required, each exit must be capable of being accessed independently of any other exit. Therefore, an occupant must not be required to travel through one exit to reach a second exit.
- Where more than one exit is required for any room or space, the exits must be remotely located from one another. The distance between the two exits must be equal to or greater than 1/3 the diagonal distance of the area served in areas protected with an automatic sprinkler system, and 1/2 the diagonal distance of the area served in areas without an automatic sprinkler system.
- Egress routes should be direct and as short as practical. The route should always direct personnel through less hazardous areas. For example, it is permissible to have occupants from a laboratory egress through an office area. However, an administrative suite should not egress through a chemical processing area.
- Evacuation routes must be designed to accommodate the safe transport of personnel with physical disabilities (e.g., wheelchair access) and any individuals that may have been injured during an incident. Provisions should be made for transporting physically disabled personnel down stairways in a safe and efficient manner. All stairs should be equipped with non-slip treads and handrails. Elevators are typically not permitted to be used as part of an emergency evacuation plan.
- At a minimum, all emergency egress routes should have 1-hour fire resistant construction and automatic sprinkler protection. For high hazard occupancies, a greater fire resistance and damage-limiting construction may be required.
- All emergency evacuation paths must be clearly identified with signs and diagrams indicating the route of travel and the location of the safe assembly area. Doorways along the egress path should be labeled indicating the egress route. Doorways that lead to closed or inaccessible areas should be labeled "No Emergency Exit."
- All emergency evacuation paths must be provided with both primary and emergency lighting of sufficient lumens to allow for the safe movement of personnel. The emergency lighting should not be less than 1 footcandle (10 lux) on average along the egress path. The emergency lighting system must operate for a minimum of 90 minutes once normal electrical power is lost. This can be accomplished using a 1.5-hour UPS or generator back-up power supply.
- For high hazard occupancies such as chemical processing, pilot plants, laboratories using flammable materials, warehouses, and hazardous material storage areas, a secondary evacuation route must be provided. The secondary route shall be provided with the same protective features as the primary egress path.

Exit Doors

The exit door width is determined by the number of occupants expected to utilize the doorway during the emergency but should not be narrower than 32 inches. Where a pair of doors is provided, at least one door leaf must be a minimum of 32 inches. The width must be measured by the projected clear width of the door opening.

All doors located along the evacuation route should open in the exit direction of travel and should be equipped with panic-type latching hardware. Doors should also operate easily with a minimum force of 133 N (30 pound-feet) required for opening. All doors with automated controls should be designed with the capability to be operated manually in the event of an emergency or power failure.

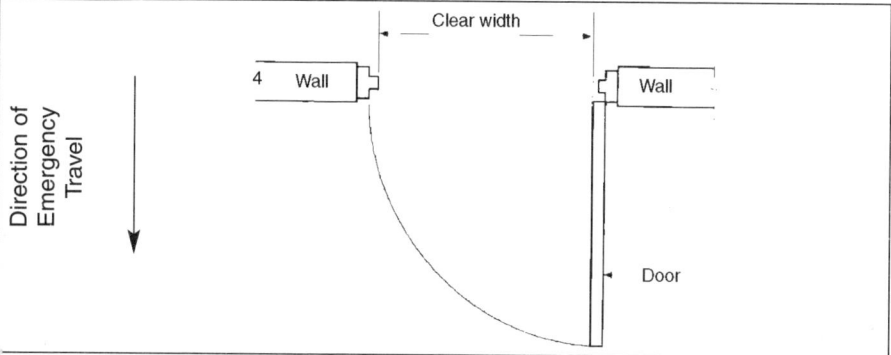

All doors required to be fire rated must have an automatic closing device and must not have glass panels of an area greater than 100 square inches. Fire doors and personnel egress doors should not be blocked open. Fire doors should be approved by a recognized testing agency.

Stairways

The stairway width should be determined by the number of occupants expected to utilize it during an emergency. At a minimum, landings must be the same width as the stairway. A recommended minimum width of 44 inches is suggested for landings. The maximum height between landings is 12 feet.

Stairway risers must be between 4 inches and 7 inches high and treads a minimum of 11 inches deep. Stair treads and landings must be solid, uniform, and slip resistant. Stairs must not vary by more than 3/16 of an inch in the depth of adjacent treads or the height of adjacent risers.

Handrails should be provided at a height of between 34 inches and 38 inches above the surface of the tread. Emergency lighting must be provided in all stairwells.

Corridors and Exit Hallways

The width of any corridor or hallway should be measured by the clear width of the space. The minimum width of the corridor should be no less than 44 inches. Greater corridor widths may be required dependant upon the occupancy load of the area.

Areas of Safe Refuge and Assembly Areas

For some occupancies, including high-rise buildings, it may be advisable to direct personnel to a safe area of refuge rather than an outdoor assembly area. An area of refuge is a room or space enclosed with a minimum of 1-hour rated construction with self-closing fire doors and automatic sprinkler protection. The area of refuge should be adjacent to a stairway and direct egress outside the building. A means of two-way emergency communication with the emergency response team or fire department must be provided.

Stairways and Landings Must Accommodate Persons in Wheelchairs

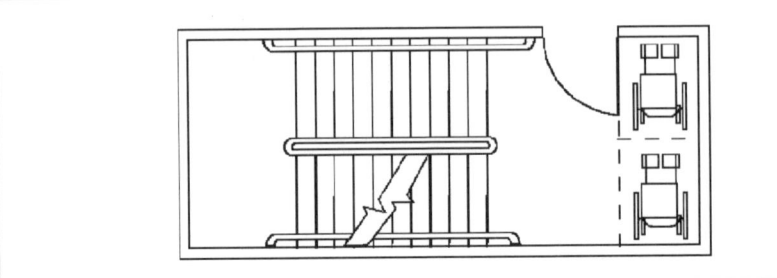

Outdoor safe assembly areas should be located so that personnel are at least 100 feet from the building where an incident has occurred. When identifying safe assembly areas, consider the number of personnel involved, the proximity to other hazards, and the area conditions during inclement weather. Signs should be posted indicating the assembly area.

Emergency Access

Emergency access to the site, buildings, process areas, and internal spaces should be evaluated during the design, construction, and operation of every pharmaceutical facility. The locations of building equipment, utilities, and access paths should not impede access or egress. Utilities such as gas services, electrical systems, and hazardous material transfer systems should be well marked with emergency shutdown valves and switchgear readily accessible. Emergency system alarm annunciator panels should be located in a main fire fighter access or assembly area.

Emergency responder access routes and roads should be provided so that all portions of the facility are within approximately 150 feet of that access road. The access roads should have an unobstructed width of not less than 20 feet and an unobstructed vertical clearance of not less than 13.5 feet. The local emergency response agencies should be consulted to ensure that these recommended road clearances are adequate for the emergency response vehicles typically used on site.

HAZARDOUS MATERIALS

Hazardous materials are defined by their flammability, toxicity, and reactivity characteristics. The handling, use, and storage of hazardous materials in a pharmaceutical manufacturing facility present the potential risk of exposure to personnel, the facility, and the environment. To manage these potential risks, it is critical that facility designers have a thorough understanding of the types of hazardous materials that are planned to be used in the facility as well as the manner in which they will be handled, used, and stored.

NFPA Chemical Hazard Label

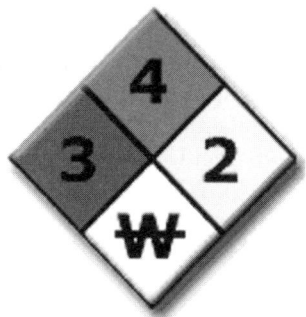

The Occupational Safety and Health Administration (OSHA) regulations contained in 29 CFR 1910 Subpart H address the use and storage of hazardous materials in the United States. However, there are a variety of other of other consensus organizations, including the National Fire Protection Association (NFPA) and the Building Officials and Code Administrators International, Inc. (BOCA), that have developed recommendations for the safe storage and handling of hazardous materials. Although the OSHA requirements apply to workplaces in the United States, the ultimate responsibility for the inspection, permitting, and approval of facilities that handle, use, and store hazardous materials rests with the local authority having jurisdiction, including the local municipality or fire marshal. The local building codes that have been adopted by the approving authority may incorporate different elements of the applicable NFPA standards or BOCA codes. Therefore, it is important that facilities designed to handle hazardous materials meet all of the requirements of the OSHA standards as well as the local codes and other best health and safety practices. In addition to meeting these requirements, some jurisdictions may require prior approval before work activities involving hazardous materials are introduced into a new or renovated facility.

Hazardous Locations

National Electrical Code (NEC) (NFPA 70) defines hazardous locations as areas "where fire or explosion hazards may exist due to flammable gases or vapors, flammable liquids, combustible dust, or ignitable fibers or flyings." Because electrical equipment can be a source of ignition in a hazardous location, the NEC provides detailed recommendations for the construction and installation of electrical equipment and apparatus based on the types of hazards that may be present and the conditions under which those hazards may be present. In the United States, the NEC specifies electrical system hazard classifications in Article 500 Hazardous (Classified) Locations, Classes I, II, III, Divisions 1 and 2.

Class I, Divisions 1 and 2 are those areas where flammable or combustible liquids or gases are used or stored, and where there is the potential for sufficient vapor to form explosive or ignitable mixtures in the air. Division 1 areas contain ignitable concentrations under normal conditions, or are areas where ignitable concentrations frequently exist due to repair or maintenance operations, or where the failure of processing equipment might release concentrations that could be ignited by the simultaneous failure of the electrical equipment. Division 2 areas are those where flammable liquids and gases are used but are normally confined to closed containers and process equipment, or where ignitable concentrations are normally prevented by the use of positive mechanical ventilation. Within each of these divisions there are sub-Group classifications for specific materials and hazard characteristics (see NFPA Standard 70, Article 500.6). Within the pharmaceutical industry, examples of Class I areas are solvent storage, flammable gas storage, process hood areas where flammable liquids are used, and chemical processing areas.

Class II, Divisions 1 and 2 are areas where combustible dusts are present. Class II, Division 1 areas are those where combustible dust is routinely present under normal conditions in sufficient quantity to form an ignitable mixture in air. This would also include those areas where the failure of equipment or process could result in the formation of a dust cloud that could be ignited by the simultaneous failure of electrical apparatus. Dusts that are electrically conductive and are present in hazardous quantities are also included in this classification.

Areas where combustible dust is not normally present in ignitable quantities and where dust accumulations will not interfere with the safe dissipation of heat from electrical equipment are considered Class II, Division 2 locations (see NFPA Standard 70 Article 500.5). As with Class I areas, Class II also has group-specific classifications for highly volatile materials (see NFPA Standard 70, Article 500.6). Typical pharmaceutical Class II operations are micronizing, powder weigh/dispense areas, bulk powder handling, blending, etc.

Class III locations typically do not occur within the pharmaceutical sector. Class III locations are those that are hazardous due to the presence of easily ignitable fibers as would typically be seen in the textile and woodworking industries (see NFPA Standard 70, Article 500.5).

In addition to the applicable electric codes, NFPA 5000, the International Building Code (IC) Building Construction and Safety Code establish classifications for building occupancies based on types of hazardous materials that are being handled. These consensus standards provide facility and equipment design criteria for locations in which flammable and combustible liquids are stored, handled, and used.

Flammable and Combustible Liquids

Many of the common organic solvents that are used during production, laboratory, and cleaning activities in pharmaceutical manufacturing facilities are considered to be flammable or combustible liquids. The primary hazards associated with

DOT Flammable Label

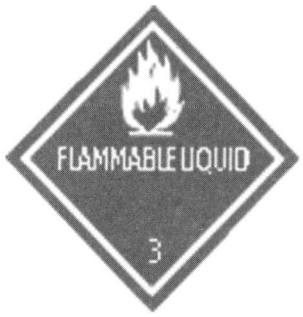

flammable and combustible liquids are fire and explosion. Flammable liquids are defined by NFPA as liquids with flash points below 100°F (37.8°C). Flammable liquids, also referred to as Class I liquids, are subdivided into three categories:

- Class IA liquids have flash points below 73°F (22.8°C) and boiling points below 100°F (37.8°C)
- Class IB liquids have flashpoints below 73°F (22.8°C) and boiling points at or above 100°F (37.8°C)
- Class IC liquids have flash points at or above 73°F (22.8°C) and below 100°F (37.8°C)

Combustible liquids are liquids having a flash point at or above 100°F (37.8°C):

- Class II combustible liquids have flash points at or above 100°F (37.8°C) and below 140°F (60°C)
- Class IIIA liquids have flash points at or above 140°F (60°C) and below 200°F (93.3°C)
- Class IIIB liquids have flash points above 200°F (93.3°C)

OSHA 1910.106 serves as the legal standard for the storage, handling, and use of Class I, II, and IIIA liquids in workplaces in the United States. Much of OSHA 1910.106 is based on NFPA standards, including NFPA 30, Flammable and Combustible Liquids Code. NPFA 30 addresses design and construction, ventilation, ignition sources, and storage issues associated with flammable and combustible liquids under the following storage, handling, and use conditions:

- Bulk storage of liquids in tanks and similar vessels including piping systems
- Storage and handling of flammable and combustible liquids in containers and portable tanks in storage and warehouse areas
- Design and construction of flammable safety cabinets
- Storage and handling of flammable and combustible liquids in manufacturing areas

NFPA 45, Standard on Fire Protection for Laboratories Using Chemicals, also applies to the handling and storage practices of flammable and combustible liquids in laboratory facilities.

Both OSHA and NFPA distinguish between the "storage" of flammable and combustible liquids and "incidental use" where flammable or combustible liquids are handled or used only in unit physical operations such as mixing, drying, evaporating, filtering, distillation, and similar operations that do not involve chemical reaction.

Some of considerations for flammable and combustible liquid storage areas include:

- All inside storage rooms should be designed with a means for containing spills. Options to consider include: non-combustible liquid-tight raised sills or ramps that are at least 4 inches in height; designing the floor of the storage area at least 4 inches below the surrounding floor; or installing an open trench in the room that drains to a safe location.
- All door openings should be equipped with self-closing rated fire doors.
- All inside storage rooms should be equipped with appropriate fire protection equipment, such as sprinkler systems or carbon dioxide systems, pursuant to the requirements of the authority having jurisdiction.
- The construction of the walls and wall openings should meet all applicable code requirements for fire resistance. Where necessary, explosion venting should be provided.
- The quantities of flammable and combustible liquids in any given storage room should not exceed those limits established by OSHA, NFPA, or the local approving authority. OSHA and NFPA have established the following requirements for sprinklered inside storage rooms:
- No more than 10 gallons per square foot of floor area with no more than 500 square feet of floor area in rooms with walls and wall openings having a fire resistance of at least 2 hours.
- No more than 5 gallons per square foot of floor area with no more than 150 square feet of floor area in rooms with walls and wall openings having a fire resistance of at least 1 hour.
- There should be no ignition sources present in the inside storage rooms.
- Electrical wiring, equipment, and apparatus installed and used in inside rooms used for the storage of flammable liquids should be approved for Class I, Division 2 locations.
- All inside storage rooms should be equipped with either gravity or mechanical exhaust ventilation to prevent the build-up and accumulation of vapors. OSHA requires that the ventilation provide a minimum of six air changes per hour.
- The layout of inside storage rooms should maintain aisles that are at least three 3 in width.
- Grounding should be provided for all metal drums, containers, and fixed electrical equipment in storage areas to prevent static electrical discharge. NFPA 77: Recommended Practice on Static Electricity provides information on measures for reducing hazards due to static electrical discharges.
- Class B portable fire extinguishers should be mounted directly outside of each door leading to an inside storage room.
- Reactive materials should not be stored in the same room with flammable and combustible liquids.
- Appropriate eyewash and safety shower equipment should be installed in areas where flammable and combustible liquids are dispensed or in other areas where splashing could occur.
- Climate control should be provided for all storage areas so that flammable and combustible liquids are stored at temperatures below their flash points.

The storage of flammable and combustible liquids should be minimized at the point of use in manufacturing and laboratory areas outside of designated storage rooms. The NFPA limits for quantities of liquids that are located outside of flammable storage cabinets are 600 gallons of Class IA liquids in containers, and 800 gallons of Class I, II, or IIIA liquids in containers. OSHA has established the following limits for quantities of liquids that are located outside of an inside storage room or storage cabinet in a building or in any one fire area of a building:

- 25 gallons of Class IA liquids in containers
- 120 gallons of Class IB, IC, II, or III liquids in containers

The layout of production and laboratory areas in which the incidental use of flammable and combustible liquids is expected to occur should be equipped with an adequate number of suitably sized approved flammable liquid cabinets (both OSHA and NFPA have established limits of not more than 60 gallons of Class I and/or Class II liquids, or not more than 120 gallons of Class III liquids may be stored in any individual flammable liquid cabinet). Furthermore, NFPA recommends that no more than six flammable liquid cabinets be stored in any single fire area.

Toxicity

Laboratory and manufacturing operations associated with pharmaceutical manufacturing activities may require the use of chemicals that may exhibit both acute and chronic toxicity. Many of these chemicals are standard reagents, including acetone and acetonitrile, and may be used in laboratories. In addition, alcohols such as isopropyl alcohol (IPA), ethanol, and methanol may be used in the production process for cleaning or as part of the product blend.

Toxicity indicates there is statistically significant evidence (based on at least one study conducted according to established scientific principles), that acute or chronic health effects may occur in exposed employees, or if it is listed in any of the following:

- OSHA, 29 CFR 1910 Subpart Z: Toxic and Hazardous Substances
- ACGIH *Threshold Limit Values for Chemical Substances and Physical Agents in the Work Environment*
- NIOSH v *The Registry of Toxic Effects of Chemical Substances*

In most cases, the label will indicate if the chemical is hazardous. Key words found on labels such as "caution," "hazardous," "toxic," "dangerous," "corrosive," "irritant," or "carcinogen" can also indicate a chemical's hazard potential. Old containers of hazardous chemicals (pre-1985) may not contain hazard warnings.

Government agencies and professional organizations have established workplace exposure limits for many airborne chemical and physical agents. In addition, many pharmaceutical companies develop exposure limits for their own compounds. (Additional information on this subject can be found in Chapter 18: Potent Compounds.) The most common type of exposure limit is the 8-hour time-weighted average or TWA. Overexposure may occur when 8-hour limits or short-term exposure limits are exceeded.

Compressed Gases

Laboratory and manufacturing operations associated with pharmaceutical activities may require the use of compressed gases. The hazards associated with the storage, handling, and use of compressed gases can be serious: Some gases may be flammable, reactive, or highly toxic; high concentrations of gases released into a work area can create oxygen deficient atmospheres; and, because the gases are under pressure, there is a potential for explosion or a violent release due to the large amount of potential energy contained in the gas cylinder.

Standard Hazard Label for Compressed Gas

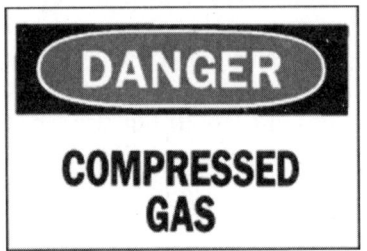

Proper storage is one of the most important design considerations for a facility that will handle compressed gases. Both OSHA (OSHA 1910.101–1910.105, 110, and 111), and NFPA (NFPA 45 and NFPA 55; Standard for the Storage, Use, and Handling of Compressed and Liquefied Gases in Portable Cylinders) have established storage and handling guidelines for compressed gases. Where possible, rooms or areas should be dedicated for compressed gas storage to provide a greater degree of control over potential physical and chemical hazards. All rooms or areas designated for compressed gas storage should be kept free of heat and ignition sources and the storage of combustible materials should be minimized. All storage areas should also be constructed according to applicable building codes, including NEC electric equipment guidelines for class, division, and group, and equipped with appropriate fire suppression systems.

Because of the extreme physical hazards associated with the potential energy stored in compressed gases, the layout of the facility should take into account the movement of compressed gas cylinders and other hazardous materials throughout the facility in order to minimize travel distances as well as minimize the movement of cylinders through or adjacent to areas that are not equipped to handle the hazards (e.g., low hazard areas such as office areas or break rooms). In all cases, cylinders of compressed gases must be securely stored in an upright orientation. Cages or racks are used to store large numbers of cylinders. Cylinders in storage should be equipped with protective safety caps. Straps or bases secured to a wall or other structural member are often used in laboratory areas where single cylinders are used. Cylinder storage should be kept away from high traffic areas and areas where damage due to contact with moving equipment, such as powered industrial trucks is minimized. Flammable gases should be segregated from cylinders containing oxygen and reactive gases. A minimum distance of 25 feet should be maintained between flammable gas and oxygen cylinders. As an alternative, a non-combustible barrier at least 5 feet in height should separate flammable gas and oxygen cylinders. Full cylinders should be stored separately from empty cylinders.

Adequate ventilation should be provided in areas in which toxic and flammable gases are being stored and used. It is desirable to maintain cylinders of highly toxic and pyrophoric gases within walk-in fume hoods or other exhausted enclosures. The uncontrolled release of a compressed gas can cause a hazardous atmosphere, including acutely toxic atmospheres, explosive gas- or vapor-air mixtures, or oxygen deficient (i.e., <19.5% oxygen in air) or oxygen enriched (i.e., >23.5 % oxygen in air) environments. Therefore, it may be necessary to install hard-wired toxic gas, flammable gas (i.e., LEL), and/or oxygen sensors equipped with audible and visual alarms in areas where compressed gases are stored and used. Areas in which the potential for an immediately dangerous to life or health (IDLH) condition could exist due to a release of compressed gases should be equipped with appropriate rescue equipment, including respirators equipped with escape cylinders or self-contained breathing apparatus (SCBA).

All piping systems used for compressed gases should be compatible with the gases that they are designed to hold, and all regulators and outlet connections should be consistent with the guidelines established by the Compressed Gas Association (CGA) to help prevent the mixing of gases. Manual shut-off valves with uninterruptible pressure relief devices should be installed near each point of use of the piping system.

One particular concern among health and safety professionals is the potential for supplied air respirator wearers to connect their breathing air hoses to the outlet connection for another type of gas. Therefore, it is essential that all outlet connections for breathing airlines be designed and installed so that they are unique and wholly incompatible with the outlet connections for all other gas lines. In addition, all lines should be clearly labeled according to the requirements of ANSI A13.1: Scheme for the Identification of Piping Systems.

Cryogenic Liquids

Cryogenic liquids are another class of hazardous material that require careful consideration during facility planning and design. Some of the hazards associated with cryogenic liquids and gases include: severe tissue damage from skin contact with cryogenic liquids and cold equipment surfaces; flammable gas-air or oxygen deficient atmospheres from the vaporization of cryogenic liquids because relatively small amounts of liquid can create large volumes of gas; the rupture of vessels and piping systems from the rapid expansion of gases; and the embrittlement of the structural materials and condensation of atmospheric oxygen from the extremely cold temperatures.

Cyrogenic Liquid Storage Tank

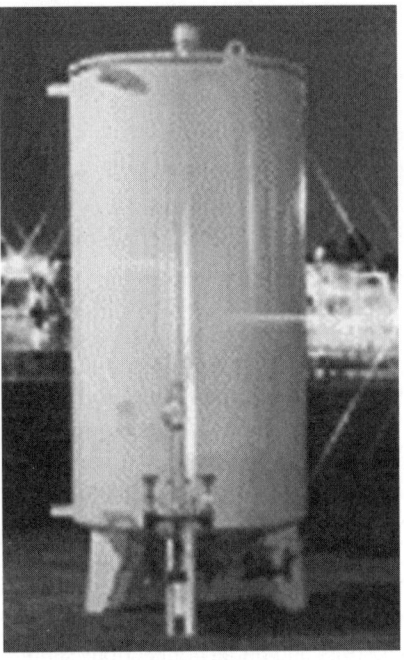

Many of the safe design considerations for the handling, storage, and use of cryogenic liquid use are similar to those for compressed gases including:

- Cryogenic liquids should be kept away from heat, ignition sources, and the unnecessary storage of combustible materials.
- Cryogenic liquids should be stored and transported in such a way that equipment will not become damaged.
- All storage areas should also be constructed according to applicable building codes, including NEC electric equipment guidelines for class, division, and group, and equipped with appropriate fire suppression systems.
- Adequate ventilation should be provided in areas where flammable gas-air or oxygen deficient environments could occur.
- Hard-wired toxic gas, flammable gas (i.e., LEL), and/or oxygen sensors equipped with audible and visual alarms placed in areas where cryogenic liquids are stored and used.

It is critical that all equipment, including tanks, piping systems, and fittings, be specifically designed for use at extreme low temperatures and potentially extreme pressures. All equipment must be equipped with appropriate venting devices and pressure relief valves. All relief devices should be vented to the outside. To prevent tissue damage due to contact with cold surfaces, all fixed equipment should be thermally insulated. When liquid oxygen or flammable liquids are used, all fixed equipment should be properly grounded and appropriate static dissipative devices should be used with portable equipment and personnel. Because liquid oxygen can cause oxygen to become trapped in porous materials in the event of a spill, only hard-surfaced non-porous materials should be used for room finishing surfaces.

Reactive Materials

Reactive materials are those that tend to react spontaneously, react vigorously with air or water, be unstable to shock or heat, generate toxic gases, or explode. There are a variety of different types of reactive materials that can be used in a pharmaceutical manufacturing facility and its associated laboratory spaces, including oxidizers, peroxides and peroxide formers, water reactive materials, and flammable metals. Although many of the hazards associated with the handling and use of reactive materials can be reduced through prudent work practices by the end users, some important design considerations can be incorporated into the facility design.

In particular, it is critical that reactive materials be stored properly. NFPA (NFPA 430: Code for the Storage of Liquid and Solid Oxidizers) and IBA recommend storage and handling guidelines for certain reactive materials and classes of reactive materials. One of the critical issues in storing reactive materials is segregating them from incompatible materials (e.g., oxidizers such as benzoyl peroxide should not be stored with flammable liquids). The storage areas should be constructed according to all applicable building codes, including NEC electric equipment guidelines, and equipped with appropriate fire suppression systems. Because some materials may be water reactive, it may be necessary to design storage areas that are equipped with carbon dioxide or other appropriate fire suppression systems utilizing inert extinguishing agents. In addition, when reactive materials are used, all fixed equipment should be properly grounded and appropriate static dissipative devices should be used with portable equipment and personnel.

Explosive materials should be stored in secured areas that are equipped with appropriate explosion venting devices. Because some reactive materials may be temperature sensitive, refrigerated storage areas may be required. Due to the nature of the materials, the refrigerated areas may need to be equipped with adequate ventila-

Organic Peroxide—A Temperature Sensitive Chemical

tion and hazardous location electrical equipment and apparatus. Other materials that are shock sensitive must be stored in areas where they will not be exposed to damage: They should not be stored above ground level; they should be isolated from vibration-producing equipment; and all rack storage or shelving units should be secured to the foundation and equipped with a means to secure the individual containers to prevent tipping or falling.

The variety of extreme hazards that can exist due to the use of reactive materials underscores our earlier point: Facility designers must have a thorough understanding of the types and nature of the hazardous materials to be used in the pharmaceutical manufacturing facility and its supporting laboratory and storage facilities to identify the safety principles that must be incorporated into a facility design to avoid toxic exposures to personnel and potentially catastrophic events in the facility.

PHYSICAL HAZARDS

Heat

Heat-generating processes and equipment can cause personnel to experience a variety of heat-related injuries or illnesses that range in severity from light-headedness and flushed skin to heat strain and heat stroke. Additionally, personnel can experience thermal burns from skin contact with hot surfaces. In areas where PPE is required to protect employees from physical or chemical hazards, the potential exposure to heat stress can be exacerbated. A variety of consensus standards on heat stress have been adopted, including International Organization for Standardization (ISO) 7243: Hot Environments—Estimation of the Heat Stress on Working Man, Based on the WBGT Index (Wet Bulb Globe Temperature); the American Conference of Governmental Industrial Hygienists (ACGIH) Threshold Limit Value (TLV) for Heat Stress and Heat Strain; and the National Institute for Occupational Safety and Health (NIOSH): Criteria for a Recommended Standard—Occupational Exposure to Hot Environments (Revised).

When designing a facility or process that will utilize heat-generating equipment including drying ovens, high intensity lighting, and high voltage electrical equipment, it is critical to understand the total heat load that will be introduced into each space. This will help to define the heating and cooling needs for the space in order to maintain occupant comfort and product quality during manufacturing operations. All heat-generating equipment should be thermally insulated to reduce the amount of heat that is radiated into the room, to reduce the potential for thermal burns due to skin contact with hot surfaces, and to maximize energy efficiency. Where necessary, local exhaust ventilation (LEV) should be provided for ovens and other equipment that generate hot exhaust streams. Spot cooling can be provided for employee comfort when it is not possible to cool an entire work area. Where radiant heat sources are present, shielding should be used to direct radiant energy away from personnel or critical equipment.

NOISE

Exposure to noise can cause noise-induced hearing loss as well as interfere with critical audible communications, including face-to-face vocal communications, intercom and PA system announcements, and audible alarms. OSHA has established a Permissible Exposure Limit (PEL) of 90 dBA as an 8-hour TWA for noise in 1910.95: Occupational Noise. Other consensus standards, including ACGIH: (ACGIH TLVs and BEIs, TLV for Noise, 2004) and NIOSH (Criteria for a Recommended Standard: Occupational Noise Exposure—Revised Criteria, NIOSH 98-126, 1998) recommend 85 dBA as a criterion level for noise.

Noise is generated from a variety of sources in pharmaceutical manufacturing facilities, including but not limited to: mechanical noise and impacts from motors and other moving equipment; noise due to fluid flow through pipes and valves and from air flow through ducts; air noise at exhaust points; and noise due to the vibration of equipment and surfaces. In designing a facility and selecting equipment, it is important to understand the types and number of pieces of equipment that will be used in any given area to anticipate the total noise that will be generated in an area and, in turn, to identify appropriate noise controls for that area.

Noise control can be achieved by a variety of different methods, including reducing or eliminating noise at the source; enclosing the noise source; and installing sound absorptive room treatments. The most effective means for reducing noise is to select equipment such as fans and motors that are "quiet-by-design" based on manufacturer or supplier sound power data. Additional noise control principles to keep in mind include:

- Ensure that pumps, motors, and other equipment are properly balanced and mounted to eliminate the sources of vibration and minimize the transfer of vibration to adjacent surfaces and the structure of the building itself.
- Minimize noise from pneumatic systems by operating equipment at the lowest pressures that enable proper equipment operation and by installing regulators on pneumatic systems so that supply air pressures to equipment can be easily controlled by the end user.
- Orient exhausts points and other directional noise sources away from areas in which personnel work.
- Provide silencers for equipment with air intakes and mufflers for exhaust points.
- Identify equipment with large unsupported surfaces, such as large sheet metal panels, that may vibrate. Identify ways to stiffen the surfaces by bracing them or reducing the surface areas on which vibration can occur.
- Minimize noise from piping systems by sizing pipes and selecting valves that are appropriate for the anticipated pressure and flow.
- Design and install ventilation systems with properly sized ducts and select proper hoods, fittings, and other system components that will minimize air turbulence.
- Minimize noise from piping systems and air ducts by installing lagging around the pipes and ducts. If pipe and duct lagging is used in GMP areas, the lagging materials must be non-porous and easily cleanable.

If excess noise cannot be controlled at the source, enclosures or dedicated rooms should be considered for the noise-producing equipment. For equipment used in manufacturing areas, identify manufacturer or after-market acoustical enclosures that can be installed around individual pieces of equipment. In these cases, the materials of construction should be non-porous, easily cleanable, and corrosion resistant. In cases where full enclosures are not feasible, it may be possible to install partial enclosures around equipment or insert partitioning walls between the noise source and the exposed personnel.

Vibration

In addition to noise hazards that can be caused by vibrating equipment, personnel who interact with vibrating equipment can be exposed to musculoskeletal disorders (MSDs) due to hand-arm vibration (HAV) and whole-body vibration (WBV). A variety of consensus standards, including ISO 2631-1985: Evaluation of Human Exposure to Whole-Body Vibration; ANSI S3.18-1979: Guide for the Evaluation of Human Exposure to Whole Body Vibration; and the ACGIH TLV for WBV have been developed to address the potential hazards associated with occupational exposure to WBV.

Non-ionizing Radiation

Non-ionizing radiation is defined as electromagnetic energy with a photon energy of 12.4 eV or less that has insufficient energy to ionize matter such as human tissue. The spectrum of non-ionizing electromagnetic energy ranges from optical radiation, which includes ultraviolet (UV), visible, and infrared (IR) radiation with wavelengths of 10 nm to 1 mm, to radiofrequency and microwave radiation (RF/MW) with frequencies of about 300 kHz to 300 GHz and extremely low frequency (ELF) radiation with frequencies of 3 kHz or less. Each of these three classes of non-ionizing radiation is discussed below.

In general, optical radiation can cause adverse health effects to the eyes and skin. Lasers may be used in analytical laboratories for particle sizing or in pharmaceutical packaging areas in which bar coding is used. Various consensus organizations, including ANSI (Safe Use of Lasers, ANSI Z136.1, 2000), have established guidelines for the operation of lasers and the design of facilities in which lasers are operated. In the United States, some states also require the registration of laser equipment. For example, the New York State Department of Labor, Radiological Health Unit licenses certain laser equipment for use in the State of New York. Lasers are classified according to their output power. In general, lasers used for particle sizing and bar coding are low-powered lasers with output powers of less than 5 mW. The use of these lasers requires the implementation of standard precautions to be taken to limit the potential for exposure to laser light. The use of higher-powered lasers with output powers of more than 5 mW requires more rigorous controls. Facility design considerations should be taken into account, including providing non-reflective surface finishing in areas in which lasers will be used to minimize reflection and scattering of laser light, and locating laser equipment so that is limited to responsible personnel only and that potential incidental exposure to bystanders is minimized.

RF/MW radiation-generating equipment in a pharmaceutical manufacturing facility can include equipment that is used for sealing packaging materials and nuclear magnetic resonance (NMR) spectroscopy equipment used in pharmaceutical R&D laboratories. Adverse health effects include heating of the deep tissues, effects on the nervous system, reproductive effects, effects on the eyes, and possible links with cancer. RF/MW equipment is also known to interfere with the function of pacemakers and can cause heating of metal prosthetic devices and other medical implants. Guidelines for exposure to RF/MW radiation have been established by OSHA (29 CFR 1910.97: Non-ionizing Radiation) and a variety of consensus organizations, including the International Commission on Non-Ionizing Radiation Protection (ICNIRP), Institute of Electrical and Electronics Engineers (IEEE) (IEEE Standard for Safety Levels with respect to Human Exposure to Radio Frequency Electromagnetic Fields, 3kHz to 300 GHz, C95.1-1991), and ACGIH.

The two most effective methods protecting personnel from exposure to RF/MW radiation are shielding and distancing personnel from RF/MW sources. When selecting and installing RF/MW radiation-generating equipment, it should be equipped with appropriate shielding materials to prevent radiation leakage and penetration. Once installed, the equipment must be electrically grounded. Because the power density of the radiation emitted by an RF/MW source follows an inverse square relationship with distance (i.e., power density decreases by $1/d^2$), distancing personnel from radiation sources can be an effective control strategy. In particular, care should be taken to distance employees from potential exposures by positioning the equipment away from high foot traffic areas and providing equipment controls that are remote from the radiation sources.

Extremely low frequency (ELF) is generated by the generation, transmission, and use of electrical equipment, including transformers and computer video display terminals (VDTs). In the absence of conclusive data about the potential health effects of exposure to ELF radiation, health and safety professionals have taken the position that all personnel should practice prudent avoidance to limit their exposure to ELF radiation to levels as low as reasonably achievable. Electric fields are generally associated with high voltage electrical equipment, and magnetic fields are associated with high electrical currents. Care should be taken to identify significant sources of electrical transmission and use (e.g., high voltage equipment and high amperage electrical services) and to lay out a facility such that the pieces of equipment are placed in areasthat are not adjacent to personnel work areas. Once installed, all electrical equipment must be properly grounded. Stray ELF magnetic fields associated with equipment carrying high electrical currents can sometimes be effectively controlled through the use of shielding. However, ELF magnetic field shielding can require rigorous design and specialized materials. Therefore, isolating and distancing high voltage electrical equipment is most often the best control.

Confined Spaces

Confined spaces are defined by OSHA as locations that meet the following criteria: They are large enough and so configured that they can be bodily entered; there is a limited means of access and egress; and they are not intended for continuous occupancy. Common examples of confined spaces in a pharmaceutical manufacturing facility include storage tanks, process vessels, tumble blenders, covered mixers, air handlers, and duct work. Other less obvious confined spaces include manholes, vaults, pits, underground storage tanks, and trenches.

Typical Tank Meeting the Definition of a Confined Space

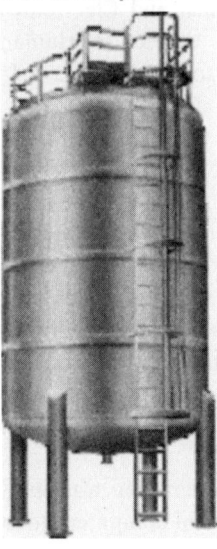

The hazards associated with confined spaces are potentially severe: confined spaces may contain unknown or very high concentrations of airborne contaminants, including gases, vapors, and dusts at levels that are immediately dangerous to life or health; they may contain oxygen-deficient or oxygen-enriched atmospheres; they may contain potentially flammable or explosive atmospheres; they may contain materials such as liquids or powders that could engulf a person; they may have inwardly converging sides or a configuration such that a person could become trapped; and they may contain a variety of other hazards such as electrical, mechanical, thermal, or fall hazards. OSHA 1910.146: Permit-Required Confined Spaces requires employers to develop and implement the means, procedures, and practices necessary to ensure safe operations when employees must bodily enter confined spaces to perform cleaning, maintenance, and servicing activities. The American National Standards Institute (ANSI) Standard Z117.1-2003: Safety Requirements for Confined Spaces and the American Society for Testing and Materials (ASTM) Standard D4276-02: Standard Practice for Confined Area Entry also specify recommended work practices and procedures for safe entry into confined spaces.

Because of the potential hazards associated with confined spaces, it is desirable to design the facility and to select equipment such that the need to enter a confined space is eliminated. Examples of strategies that can be employed to eliminate the need to enter a confined space include:

Process vessels and tanks:
- Design and install clean-in-place (CIP) capabilities to limit the need for entry to perform cleaning.
- Identify equipment with externally mounted features, such as magnetic stirrers, etc., that do not require entry for servicing and maintenance activities.

Manholes, pits, etc.:
- Install sensors and equipment that can be monitored and controlled remotely from outside of the confined space.

Air handlers and ducts:
- Select equipment that will facilitate maintenance and filter changes to be performed externally.
- Provide cleanout openings for ducts.

Standard Confined Space Warning

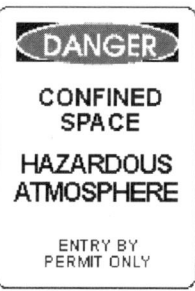

DANGER

CONFINED
SPACE

HAZARDOUS
ATMOSPHERE

ENTRY BY
PERMIT ONLY

CONTROL OF HAZARDOUS ENERGY (LOCKOUT/TAGOUT)

Personnel in a pharmaceutical manufacturing facility may be exposed to a variety of hazardous energy sources during the servicing, maintenance, and cleaning of the various facility and production equipment. These hazardous energy sources include: electrical energy; hydraulic pressure; pneumatic pressure; pressurized gases and steam in process lines and piping systems; chemical energy; potential energy from suspended parts or springs under pressure; kinetic energy from moving parts; thermal energy; and stored electrical charges. It is imperative that all facility, maintenance, and production personnel have the ability to completely isolate equipment from all hazardous energy sources and achieve a "zero energy state" before commencing any servicing, maintenance, or cleaning activities. By rendering the equipment completely inoperative, personnel will be protected from injuries that could result from the unexpected re-energization or start up of the equipment.

Standard Lock and Tag for Equipment Lockout-Target

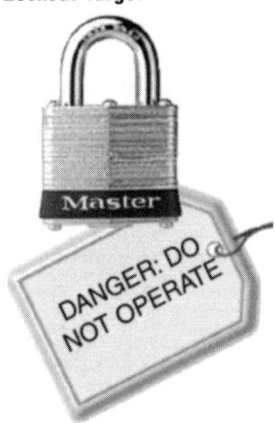

To achieve a "zero energy state," it is necessary to interrupt the transmission of all hazardous energy and physically prevent the restoration of that energy until the required work has been completed. Energy isolation devices, such as circuit breakers, electrical disconnects, and isolation valves, are the primary means for interrupting the transmission of hazardous energy. Locks should then be applied to the energy isolation devices to provide a physical barrier against the accidental restoration of energy (commonly referred to as "lockout").

Hazardous energy control capabilities are an important factor in facility design and the selection of facility and production equipment. When designing and laying out electrical and piping systems, the designers must anticipate the uses of the equipment and the maintenance, cleaning, and servicing needs to ensure that effective hazardous energy control can be designed into the system. Each process or piece of equipment must be equipped with energy isolation devices that are capable of being locked out. In addition, energy isolation capabilities should be provided as close as possible to the individual process or piece of equipment on which work will be performed. In pharmaceutical facilities where potent compounds are being handled and equipment surfaces may be contaminated, it is desirable to provide localized lockout capabilities in each process room to eliminate personnel having to leave the room to implement the hazardous energy control procedures prior to servicing, maintenance, or cleaning.

All energy isolation devices must be readily accessible (e.g., located at ground level near equipment controls) with adequate clearance to accept the application of lockout devices. The design of the facility electrical and piping systems should be such that the application of any one energy isolation device will result in the minimal interruption of service to other downstream equipment or processes. It is particularly important to provide an adequate number of isolation valves in pressurized liquid, gas, and chemical lines to help eliminate need for hot tapping during maintenance activities. It is also important to plan for the ongoing maintenance of equipment and systems, including the changing of in-line filters or the removal and maintenance of in-line pumps. In these cases, the types of appropriate isolation devices, such as isolation valves or flanges, must be installed to limit the potential hazards associated with line breaking. Electrical equipment with capacitors or with the ability to store or build-up an electrical charge must have the capability to be easily grounded and the charge dissipated. Equipment with suspended parts, moving mechanical parts, and springs must have the capability to be physically restrained.

Obviously, there are many possibilities when it comes to hazardous energy control capabilities and "one size" certainly does not fit all. However, in all cases, designers should work closely with the building owners and end users of facility and production equipment and systems to ensure that hazardous energy control capabilities are incorporated into the facility design in order to ensure safe and efficient operations during maintenance, cleaning, and servicing activities.

EMERGENCY EQUIPMENT AND RESPONSE
The most important consideration in emergency planning and response equipment selection is the assessment of the risks of emergency occurrence. Consideration should be made for the types and quantities of hazardous materials handled and stored, and the equipment used in the facility. Response equipment should then be chosen based on the risk assessment.

Emergency Response Equipment
A site must have and maintain an alarm system for personnel. There are different types of alarm systems based on sound or light. Each area should be evaluated to determine the best alarm for the area and ensure adequate coverage of all areas in the facility. (Alarms must comply with the requirements of 29 CFR 10910.165: Employee Alarm Systems). Areas where hazardous materials are used should be equipped with an eye wash and safety shower, spill kits, first aid kit, fire alarm, fire extinguishers rated for the hazard, and a fire suppression system. Typically, a HEPA filter vacuum is provided in a potent compound area to respond to spills of potent powders.

Standard Eyewash-Safety Unit

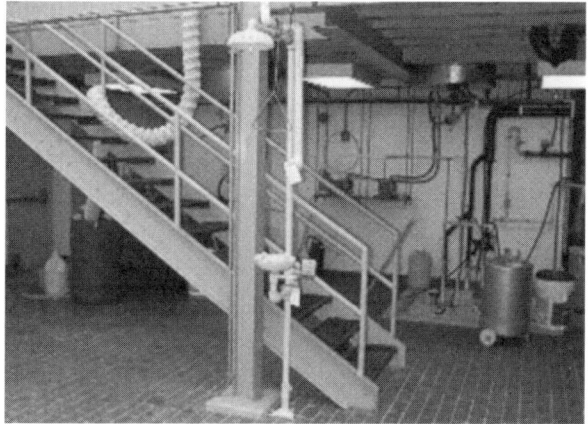

All equipment should be in easily accessible locations that do not block emergency exit routes. In the case of eyewashes and safety showers, quick drenching or flushing of the eyes and body must be provided within the work area at a distance that requires no more than 10 seconds for personnel to reach. In addition, it is must be located on the same level of the hazard and the path of travel must be free of obstructions to allow immediate use of the equipment. Specific details about the placement and design of safety showers and eyewashes are presented in ANSI Standard 358.1.

FIRE PROTECTION

Within the pharmaceutical industry, compliance with cGMP standards and guidelines supports the overall objectives of a fire protection program. Cleanliness requirements, standardized operating procedures, and access control all contribute to the overall safe operation of a pharmaceutical facility.

The following overview of each of the key elements provides an insight into the engineering and management of fire prevention and protection for pharmaceutical manufacturing plants. Engineering criteria are presented in general terms. Detailed design information can only be developed when the specific fire hazards and risks are available. There are many technical resources available to support fire protection engineering efforts. Agencies such as the National Fire Protection Association (NFPA) in the United States, the Health Safety Executive (HSE) in England, FM Global and other organizations produce fire protection reference standards and guidelines for use in the pharmaceutical industry. Many engineering firms also employ fire protection engineers who are well versed in the risks and protection needs of the industry.

Identification and Evaluation of Fire Hazards and Risks

The overall goal of any fire protection program should be to prevent fires from starting and to minimize the loss impact of any fire that does occur. Fire prevention requires constant vigilance supported by protective systems, inspections, and fire-response plans. The early detection of fire, the safe evacuation of personnel, and prompt action to control and extinguish the fire are critical to safeguard employees, emergency responders, and the business.

Fire Triangle

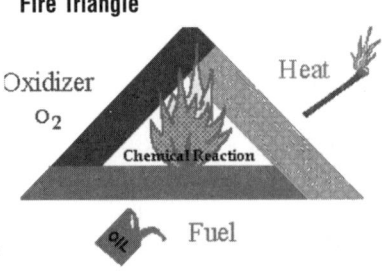

Fire risk assessments must be completed for all sites and operations. The fire hazards must be identified, evaluated, and controlled using a combination of risk elimination, engineering controls, and preventive operating procedures.

Identification and Elimination of Fire Hazards

Whenever possible, fire hazards should be eliminated. This approach must begin during the product and process development stage within R&D. The use of safe and environmentally friendly solvents can play a major role in reducing the combustible loading within a manufacturing plant. Similarly, changing to non-flammable cleaning and decontamination materials eliminates a fire hazard as well.

Installation and Maintenance of Protective Systems

When fire hazards cannot be eliminated, fire safe construction and protective systems should be provided. Most regulatory building and fire codes require the use of fire rated construction for occupancy classes, including pharmaceutical manufacturing and storage. The fire ratings for walls, floor, and ceiling/roof will vary depending upon the level of fire hazard (combustible loading), the size of the building or operation, the number of floors in the building, and the fire exposure to other buildings or occupancies. Fire ratings are typically divided into hour categories ranging from 1 to 4 hours. Building codes and the insurance and underwriting industry specify fire ratings of various construction assemblies. These ratings can be found in code specifications and consensus standards. When a fire rating is specified, it is critical that all components of the wall or ceiling assembly meet the code requirement. For example, the International Building Code specifies 2-hour rated wall construction for laboratories using a moderate volume of flammable liquids. For this occupancy, the wall construction and doors must meet this minimum-rating requirement.

Special consideration must be given to the construction of operations that require Damage Limiting Construction (DLC) such as blast-resistant and pressure-relieving walls and roofs. DLC is typically needed in operations where the potential for an equipment or room explosion hazard exists. Typical examples of these occupancies are pilot plants, chemical processing, flammable liquids and flammable gas processing and storage, combustible powder operations, and larger-scale laboratories. The sizing and design of explosion vents used in combination with pressure resistant walls and roofs must be based on the explosive characteristics of the materials, quantity of the hazardous material, and the hazards of the process. NFP 68: Guide for Venting of Deflagrations and FM Global Data Sheet 1–44 Damage Limiting Construction are both excellent references for these situations.

Process and utility systems should be designed and installed to minimize fire risk. Flammable liquid and gas distribution systems must be installed in accordance with local code and industry best practice. Distribution piping, pump systems, and storage tanks should be provided with remote manual and automatic emergency shut off devices. The materials of construction should also be closely scrutinized to ensure that the potential for accidental releases is minimized. Gaskets, seals, packing glands, and specialty linings should all be evaluated for their resistance to the materials and atmospheres to which they will be exposed. In some instances, welded or double wall piping may be necessary to adequately address the risks. Glass piping and process equipment handling flammable liquids and gases should be avoided. Tempered glass and protective wraps can increase the structural integrity of glass systems; however, the potential for a catastrophic spill or release and subsequent fire outweighs the process benefits of glass systems.

All process equipment (including flammable liquid systems, flammable gas systems, process vessels, packaging equipment, ventilation systems, dryers, etc.) should be electrically bonded and grounded (earthed).

Fire Suppression Systems

Automatic sprinkler protection is the most effective and most economical method of protecting buildings and processes from fire. It is highly recommended that sprinklers be provided throughout all pharmaceutical-manufacturing facilities. Fire loss history within the industry has proven that sprinkler protection is highly reliable and effective at controlling fires in laboratory, warehousing, manufacturing, and support areas. The amount of water damage losses from the accidental discharge or leaking of a sprinkler system is in very low in the pharmaceutical industry. Alternatively, fire damage in non-sprinklered pharmaceutical occupancies is usually catastrophic.

The authority having jurisdiction (e.g., NFPA, local building codes, etc.) and the insurance carrier typically provide sprinkler system design and installation guidelines. Sprinkler densities are determined based upon total combustible loading within the protected area. Sprinkler heads can be installed and maintained so that the cGMP requirements are not compromised. For most installations, the use of a standard chrome plated pendant sprinkler head is the most practical. The ceiling penetrations around the head can be sealed with cGMP compliant caulking material that provides the required level of cleanness. Pendant heads are easily cleaned using a vacuum, compressed air, or a soft brush and present no greater "cleanness" risk than most other room components or pieces of production equipment. Recessed or concealed heads can also be used; however, their escutcheon assemblies may hide contaminants and hinder cleaning. Concealed sprinklers should never have their cover plates caulked. This could prevent operation in the event of a fire.

Control valves for sprinkler systems should be readily accessible and well marked. For large buildings, it is advisable to install floor and/or area isolation valves in addition to system valves. This permits faster system isolation and allows non-affected areas to remain protected during fire incidents or system renovations.

All sites must have on-site fire water systems consisting of fire hydrants, supply mains, and a dedicated water supply capable of providing water at a flow and pressure adequate for the site's automatic sprinkler and fire hose requirements. This system should be sized based on a credible fire scenario considering the occupancy, construction, and design of the sprinkler systems as well as the anticipated hose flow required by firefighters. The firewater flow duration must be considered during the design process. The insurance industry and NFPA provide recommended firewater flow duration periods for administration, manufacturing, and storage occupancies. Typically, a flow duration of 90 to 120 minutes is used within the pharmaceutical industry.

Where sprinkler protection is not practical due to the incompatibility of water with the occupancy, an alternative automatic fire detection and control system should be provided. Several inert gas CFC-free extinguishing systems are now available to the pharmaceutical industry. These systems are typically used within small rooms or equipment where fire suppression is warranted.

Manual Fire Fighting Equipment

Portable fire extinguishers should be provided throughout all manufacturing, storage, and support areas. Extinguishers should be selected based on the fire hazards of the protected area. Considerations should also be given to the potential for non-fire damage that can be caused by some types of extinguishing agents. There are several "clean" agent portable extinguishers currently available that can be used in area where highly hazardous or flammable materials are not present.

Some fire protection codes require the installation of fire hose connections and hose cabinets for special hazard occupancies (laboratories, warehousing, hazardous materials storage, etc.). When required, it is critical that the equipment selected is compatible with the systems and gear used by the local fire department.

Fire Detection and Alarms

Fire detection and alarms are regulatory requirements in the United States and most other countries. In most jurisdictions, all buildings and process areas must be equipped with an automatic fire detection system that is interfaced with a local audible alarm system. Fire detection can be accomplished using smoke or heat detection and/or automatic fire suppression (sprinklers, gase, etc.). Protection must be installed in all occupied areas and in concealed spaces where fire hazards exists either as a result of combustible construction or occupancy. A qualified safety or fire protection engineer should determine the type and number of fire detection systems used for each area. For high value facilities, it is recommended that the automatic fire alarm system be connected to a constantly attended location such as the site security center or maintenance office, a fire and security monitoring service, or the local fire and police department. For alarm systems that are monitored on site, a plan must be in-place for the immediate notification of the site fire brigade and the local fire department.

Fire Alarm Pull Station

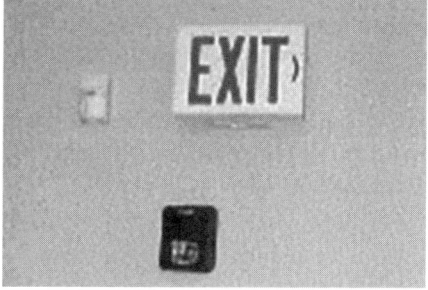

Manual fire alarm activation points should be provided throughout all buildings. The location and number of activation points must be determined based on the local code requirements, hazards of the area, congestion, and location of the egress exits. As a minimum, manual activation points should be located at each egress doorway and within 200 feet (60 meters) of all points within the protected area.

Each site's emergency alarm system should consist of audible and visual notification devices. Alarms should be audible and visible throughout the protected area. To ensure that audible alarms are heard, they should be at least 15 dBA louder that the ambient noise level. Visual alarms such as strobes should also be provided. All alarm systems should be provided with a UPS or back-up generator power supply.

Control of Firewater and Hazardous Material Runoff

Runoff from a fire or hazardous material incident can cause serious property and environmental damage. As a result of several major incidents, many jurisdictions now require emergency containment systems and plans to prevent this type of damage. Firewater runoff must be controlled to prevent environmental impact and the spread of hazardous materials both on site and into the community. A firewater environmental impact assessment should include a determination of the volume of firewater that would be generated by the most credible fire scenario. Total water flow from automatic sprinkler systems, specialized water spray, and fire hose should be included in the evaluation. A firewater flow duration of 30, 60, 90, or 120 minutes (based upon the severity of the fire hazard) should be used to determine the total fire flow. Large quantities of liquids that may be involved in an incident, such as from a ruptured storage tank or process vessel, should be included in the total aggregate volume when calculating the runoff volume. A determination of the water flow path, accumulation, and final deposition point should be made. The impact should include an assessment of the hazards associated with fire debris and hazardous materials that may be entrapped in the run-off as well as the potential for exposure to emergency responders. Where the firewater run-off risk presents a serious safety or environmental risk, a specialized drainage and containment system should be provided.

WAREHOUSE AND MATERIAL HANDLING AND STORAGE

Warehousing operations present a variety of safety and loss prevention considerations in design and operation of a modern pharmaceutical manufacturing facility. These areas are often used for a variety of operations in addition to traditional distribution and logistics. Storage compatibility considerations are particularly important to ensure that a single and credible event occurring in a warehouse facility does not immediately or significantly affect the entire stored inventory or adjoining facilities. Adequate separation by distance and protective separations must be considered in the basic design stage to ensure adequate safety and loss prevention considerations and for future facility flexibility. Commodity classifications and materials requiring adequate segregation include flammable liquids, highly hazardous/reactive chemicals, toxic materials, and high-value finished goods.

Segregation of high-risk materials provides a passive form of protection against a single event affecting the entire inventory. This normally requires flammable liquids to be kept in approved flammable liquid storage rooms or cut-off room, etc. The movement of flammable or hazardous materials throughout warehouse spaces needs to be eliminated or minimized in the design phase to prevent a single spill or upset event from having significant loss impact. Hazardous or highly toxic materials also need to be segregated by hazard classifications. This may require physical segregation with individual spill or firewater containment and security provisions. Provisions should be made for the storage of water reactive compounds in water-resistant lockers to minimize impact due to firewater contact.

Fire protection systems and available water supplies need to be accessed to ensure that automatic sprinkler systems can be designed to effectively suppress/control fire associated with material classifications and pallets, containers, and packaging materials. Several plastics under fire conditions contribute considerably more heat and smoke than ordinary combustible packaging materials. Fire suppression requirements may need to be reenforced or more fire resistance forms of plastics may need to be considered.

Employee safety considerations in warehouse and distribution operations principally include the interface between personnel and material handling equipment. Separate or designated aisle spacing for material transfer and pedestrian traffic should be considered. Pedestrian access and use of the warehousing area as an access route should be eliminated or minimized in the design. Where required, a designated and protected path should be provided that physically keeps pedestrians from encountering material handling equipment. Floor markings, curbing, railing, and fencing are all design considerations when pedestrian and vehicular traffic must share common aisle spaces and contact may be frequent. The use of overhead mirrors and signage, including highly visible tapes, should be used to delineate pedestrian travel routes in warehouse environments. Stationary objects (columns, doorways, storage racks) are frequently contacted and damaged by material handling equipment in warehouse operations. Provisions for protective bollards, railings, and curbs should be provided to protect rack storage and other facility or architectural features.

Operation of forklift equipment at loading docks is a high-risk operation and must be effectively controlled by physical separation, facility layout, and the use of new technology. Separating high-risk loading and unloading areas, including waste handling areas, should be considered.

Adjustable dock boards should be provided to accommodate different size vehicles and to prevent injuries associated while moving or adjusting manual docks boards. Vehicle restraint systems are important features to prevent vehicle movement during the entry and exit of docked vehicles by material handling equipment.

Fueling of material handling equipment with flammable and combustible liquids/gases must take place outside of the main storage area. An outdoor location with adequate space or physical separations, fire protection, and spill containment should be provided. Battery charging should also not take place in the main storage area. Charging areas should be located in areas separate from valuable storage.

Where groups of chargers are required, continuous local room ventilation for removal vapor generation should be provided. Battery charging areas also require the installation of an emergency eyewash and safety shower station to facilitate quick dilution and removal of any spill or electrolyte splashed onto personnel. Removal of batteries also requires lifting and handling equipment; therefore, battery charging and service rooms may need provisions for overhead hoists. Access directly to the exterior is desirable for maintenance and repair requirements.

More advanced automated warehousing systems may include provisions for operators to ride on elevated equipment allowing them to be at the same level as the commodity being handled. These types of systems generally require employees to use an enclosed or captive type cab design, intended to prevent the operator from leaving the controls.

Automated storage and retrieval equipment may strike and pin personnel between or against moving or stationary objects resulting in serious if not fatal injuries. The perimeter of these systems should be well labeled, secured, and supervised by interlocks, motion sensors and other devices designed to prevent the inadvertent entry of personnel while the system is operational. The installation of safe refuge areas in lower or floor level racking systems and emergency stop cords may be required to allow personnel to stop moving equipment when trapped inside the rack storage area.

Order picking operations are more labor-intensive tasks than normal material handling operations, but frequently take place in the warehouse environment. As such, the design of order picking areas must include significant consideration for ergonomic design of the workstations, including illumination levels and design dimensions for reaching racks and for standing at workstations for extended time periods.

Storage racks have a variety of design configurations and capacity requirements. Vendors should be consulted to determine if the intended storage and capacity are suitable. Rack collapse has resulted from both overloading and failure to properly assemble and secure structural members. This is a particular an issue in areas with earthquake or seismic activity. Racks should be subject to an on-going inspection process and capacity should be posted or identified in some manner.

Access to elevated locations in warehouse and distribution facilities is often required. Where access to a fixed platform is required for either personnel or material, an approved interlocked gate arrangement should be provided. This two-gate system allows placement of materials or personnel from the lower level, but provides a continuous railing system around the materials when placed onto the platform. When access is gained to the materials from the platform level, a gate is lifted that encloses the edge along the open platform to provide continuous perimeter protection.

Illumination must be designed in accordance with industry and regulatory guidelines. These levels will vary depending upon the task being conducted. General warehousing operations to order picking at elevated sections of racking all will require different illumination levels. Overhead lighting fixtures need to be installed to prevent contact with material handling equipment and the movement of materials.

Lighting fixtures should also be protected against physical contact and designed to contain broken bulbs and hot discharges that may land on top or in between spaces created by stored materials.

Adequate fire protection is critical for warehouse areas. Automatic fire suppression in addition to fire detection is preferred due to the inherit capabilities to not only detect the fire, but also and simultaneously to begin suppressing the fire. Sprinkler protection in large warehouses operations may require multiple fire systems or zones and dedicated firewater supply and fire pump systems. The type and configuration of storage and the combustible properties of the storage commodity, including shipping and packaging containers, will affect the level of protection required. An in-rack sprinkler may be required for high rack or high volume storage configurations. Other types of ceiling-mounted, fast response, and early suppression fire sprinkler systems are available and allow for storage flexibility, but have limitations on both rack and structural heights. Refrigerated storage enclosures should also be sprinkler protected if the storage commodity is combustible.

Many pharmaceutical finished goods warehouses or distribution facilities may have a potential for a maximum foreseeable loss (MFL) scenario as defined by the company's property insurer. This usually implies that the normal value of the goods in storage is of a significant level and the goods are critical to ensure continuity of product availability in the marketplace. For this reason, an insurance carrier may request additional loss prevention considerations above and beyond normal non-combustible construction, automatic fire detection, and suppression systems. Depending upon the values normally stored and adjacency to other manufacturing operations or other critical product storage areas, MFL separations may be required to protect the storage area from nearby fire exposures. This may involve increased physical spacing between structures on the same site or the construction of 4-hour freestanding firewalls known as MFL walls. These walls must be designed with few openings and must also be able to remain standing even after the collapse of the adjoining sides. Penetrations in these walls are not normally permitted but, where absolutely necessary, they must be protected in extraordinary ways to prevent communication of fire and smoke conditions from one area to another. The construction of these walls is a critical design consideration and requires extensive civil and structural considerations. The location of these walls may also affect materials movement and utility services between areas as well.

Idle pallet and containers/totes storage is a common need in a warehousing and distribution facility. Properly protected areas or adjacent remote storage facilities should be considered when an excessive number of combustible pallets or containers/totes must be stored for future use. When combustible idle pallet storage over 6 feet (2 meters) is needed, it is generally considered to represent a significant fire hazard that may challenge the traditional level of automatic sprinkler protection. Extra hazard sprinkler protection may be required when idle pallet storage must be maintained in the main storage area. Cut-off or separate adjacent rooms with approved and self-closing fire doors are preferred for idle pallet storage.

Architectural features that are passive in design provide the best for containment. These may result in the design of slope floors with diversions at opening or entrances to other adjoining areas. These areas can also be drained to lower elevation areas and depressed loading docks or lower sections of the floors. The elimination floor drains in warehousing facilities is also desirable from a spill containment perspective. In new warehouse facilities, lowering floor slabs a few inches will provide significant containment that can then be directed by gravity through piping to nearby collection basins or exterior loading dock areas.

MACHINE SAFEGUARDING

In any modern pharmaceutical manufacturing facility there are many examples of production, material handing, utility, and mechanical support equipment that requires careful design and installation to ensure safe operation during normal operation, set-up, adjustment, and routine service, maintenance, and repair. Ensuring personnel safety during these different phases of equipment and machinery operation presents many challenges to the facility design and operations teams.

Many vendors who offer stand-alone or packaged equipment have taken the proactive approach of providing machine safeguarding, safety control systems, and labeling as part of their standard product offerings. These systems are usually well designed, but often must be evaluated individually in conjunction with the specific use and application of the machinery and equipment.

As with other project elements, careful design and functional specifications are critical to achieve acceptable machine safeguarding arrangements. Development of specific requirements and confirmation of these requirements during equipment and machinery construction and verification are critical. Machine safeguarding should be a standard and documented portion of any equipment or machinery functional specification and a standard part of the FACTORY ACEPTANCE TESTING conducted at the vendor's facility. Achieving safe equipment and machinery is best achieved while at the vendor's location rather than after installation in the field.

Employee protection during normal operation of equipment and machinery in the work environment is generally addressed by machine safeguarding, safety controls systems, and labeling of hazardous operations.

Machine hazards are generally categorized into two main groups: power transmission and point-of-operation hazards. Power transmission hazards refer to mechanical components that are designed to transfer mechanical energy or power from one location to another. These types of hazards include rotating or reciprocating machine parts, belts, or pulleys in motion. Point-of-operation hazards refer to the point where machinery is actually performing work on the materials placed within the machine or equipment. This includes cutting, shearing, pinching, and bending actions.

Standard machine safeguarding configurations include fixed or secure guards over or around hazardous locations that physically prevent personnel access to the hazardous location. Guarding by distance is another concept that allows materials or supplies to pass through the equipment or machine to perform the required work activity, but is dimensionally, so configured that employee body parts are unable to reach or access the hazard point. Perimeter guarding or hostage guarding is a similar concept extensively used on automated or robotic equipment. Doors are provided around the perimeter of the equipment or access panel that allow the equipment or machine to operate and hold personnel away from or hostage to the actual machine operation. The perimeter guard doors or barriers may consist of interlocked doors or presence-sensing devices, such as light curtains or pressure-sensitive mats that are designed to keep personnel out of a defined area during machine operation. This type of system is common with robotic and automated systems but can present a challenge when service and maintenance work must be performed while some form of hazardous energy being released to the equipment or machine. Access to the equipment should be controlled in a manner that only one guard door or barrier can be removed or opened at a time and the machine comes to an immediate stop upon being opened. If set up work is required while the machine is under power, the addition of exclusive "joggling" or "inching" controls are necessary and must be specifically designed and interfaced with the machine control and logic system.

Pharmaceutical Packaging Line with Safeguard

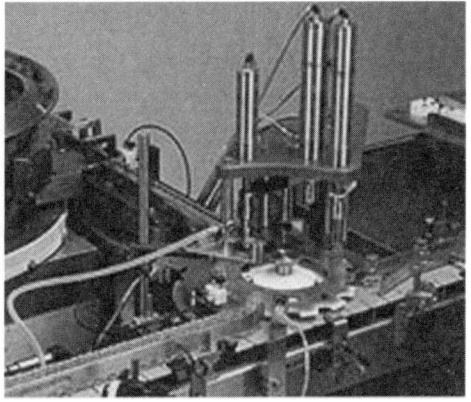

ELECTRICAL SAFETY

Electrical systems should be critiqued at from two perspectives during the design, construction, and operation of pharmaceutical manufacturing facilities: personnel safety and operational safety. Building and electrical codes essentially mandate safe installation criteria and practice; however, it is crucial that the proper operational intent be fully evaluated prior to detailed electrical system design. Designers, engineers, and EHS personnel should try and anticipate future operations and electrical needs to reduce the need for costly infrastructure upgrades. The rapidly changing pharmaceutical manufacturing environment could lead to obsolesce of an electrical system in a few short years, particularly in multi-purpose manufacturing suites and buildings. For example, consider a suite that is constructed for the manufacture of aqueous-based products. Typically, ordinary rated electrical equipment would be installed. However if a flammable solvent is needed for equipment cleaning and decontamination purposes, there may be the need for the installation of hazardous rated electrical devices in certain areas of the suite. Identifying this during the design stage is critical.

In the United States, all electrical installations must conform to the National Electrical Code (NEC). This standard specifies all installation requirements for equipment and wiring of all voltages. Other countries have similar regulatory requirements and electrical standards. Design and installation should only be done by qualified electrical engineers and licensed electricians. A valuable international reference is the International Electrotechnical Commission (IEC). The IEC provides information on identifying and comparing electrical standards and equipment from various countries.

Items that should be considered during the design of electrical systems and the installation of electrical apparatus include the following.

Area Classification

Electrical equipment should be selected based upon the hazards of the occupancy. In the United States, the National Electrical Code (NFPA 70) specifies electrical system hazard classifications in Article 500: Hazardous (Classified) Locations, Classes I, II, III, Divisions 1 and 2. (An explanation of the hazardous locations is described under Hazardous Materials Section of this chapter.) This document and similar regulatory standards in other countries dictate the requirements for electrical equipment and wiring for all voltages where fire or explosion hazards exist due to the use or storage of flammable and combustible liquids, gases, and dusts.

The key is to ensure that electrical systems and apparatus are not potential ignition sources for hazardous materials. Process areas with hazardous-rated electrical equipment should be easily identified with warning signs to ensure that the basis of safety is not compromised.

Static Electricity

Static electricity can occur in all pharmaceutical manufacturing environments. Its presence not only creates safety risks but also can affect product quality and process yield. Static electricity cannot be prevented; therefore, it must be controlled to reduce the risk of fire, explosion, personnel shock, and the effects on material handling. Static is generated any time dissimilar materials move together and are then separated. Typically, the more rapid the movement, the greater the potential for higher static charges. Static charges powerful enough to ignite flammable liquids, gases, and combustible solids can commonly occur in pharmaceutical operations such as liquid and powder transfer, on conveyor equipment, within ventilation systems, and by operators wearing synthetic garments and non-conductive footwear.

NFPA Standard 77: Recommended Practice on Static Electricity is an excellent reference on the fundamentals of static generation and control methodologies. FM

Global's Data Sheet 5–8 Static Electricity also provides sound recommendations and practical guidance for static control. The more common control techniques are:

- Electrically bonding and grounding (earthing) all equipment, walking and working surfaces, hoods, ductwork, and conductive objects to the same electrical potential with a resistance to ground not greater than 10^6 ohms.
- Maintaining relativity humidity between 60% and 70%.
- Installing conductive flooring and footwear, and using clothing that does not create static.
- Installing static eliminators and dissipating devices.
- Avoiding the use of insulating materials such as plastic ducts and piping, plastic drums, and plastic drum liners unless they are specifically designed for static control.

The generation of static can also affect the quality of products and manufacturing process effectiveness. Static accumulations can prevent effective transfer of very fine powders causing the material to cling to containers, weigh scales, and operator's hands and clothing. This can create risks of fire, explosion, and operator exposure as well as loss of product into a process waste stream. With high potency materials and high unit costs for active ingredients, these wastes can be very costly to the operation.

Protecting Employees

Electrical installations that are completed in accordance with a recognized standard such as the NEC in the United States typically result in the proper level of electrical protection for personnel. Additionally, the application of safety standards like OSHA's 29CFR1910.269 Electric Power Generation, Transmission, and Distribution ensures that personnel working with electrical systems are doing so safely. Both of these standards specify that safety devices such as circuit breakers, ground fault circuit interrupters (GFCI), and emergency disconnects are properly sized, installed, tested, and maintained. GFCIs are required for all electrical services in wet or damp locations. This is particularly critical in pharmaceutical manufacturing operations where process areas are washed with water during routine cleaning or decontamination.

Clearances and Space Separation

All electrical systems generate heat. To prevent premature failure of systems and equipment due to overheating, clear spaces must be maintained around the equipment to permit air circulation. Similarly, adequate clearances must be provided to prevent accidental ignition of ordinary combustible materials. Manufacturers and electrical standards provide specific guidance for these distances. These distances are also necessary to allow safe access for routine and emergency service.

APPENDIX: GLOSSARY

ACGIH. American Conference of Governmental Industrial Hygienists is an organization of professional personnel in governmental agencies or educational institutions engaged in occupational safety and health programs. ACGIH establishes recommended occupational exposure limits for chemical substances and physical agents.

ANSI. American National Standards Institute is a privately funded, voluntary membership organization that identifies industrial and public needs for national consensus standards and coordinates development of such standards.

API. Active pharmaceutical ingredient is the compound or medicinal component of the finished solid dosage pharmaceutical.

BOCA. Building Officials and Code Administrators International, Inc.

cGMP-GMP. Current Good Manufacturing Practices and Good Manufacturing Practices are regulations used by pharmaceutical, medical device, and food manufacturers as they produce and test products that people use. In the United States, the U.S. Food and Drug Administration (FDA) has issued these regulations as the minimum requirements.

DOT. U.S. Department of Transportation is the government agency that regulates the transportation of hazardous materials across and over the lands of the United States.

ICNIRP. International Commission on Non-Ionizing Radiation Protection.

IEEE. Institute of Electrical and Electronics Engineers.

IDLH. Immediately Dangerous to Life or Health indicates an atmosphere that poses an immediate threat to life, would cause irreversible adverse health effects, or would impair an individual's ability to escape from a dangerous atmosphere.

MSDS. Manufacturer's Safety Data Sheet is a data sheet that list properties, components, safety procedures and hazards related to the material or mixture of materials.

NEC. National Electrical Code.

NFPA. The National Fire Protection Association is an international membership organization which promotes/improves fire protection and prevention and establishes safeguards against loss of life and property by fire. Best known on the industrial scene are the National Fire codes—16 volumes of codes, standards, recommended practices, and manuals developed (and periodically updated) by NFPA technical committees.

NIOSH. National Institute for Occupational Safety and Health is a part of the U.S. Public Health Service, U.S. Department of Health and Human Services (DHHS). Among other activities, it tests and certifies respiratory protective devices and air sampling detector tubes, recommends occupational exposure limits for various substances, and assists OSHA in occupational safety and health investigations and research.

OSHA. Occupational Safety and Health Administration.

OSHMS. Occupational Safety and Health Management System is a management system that is based on occupational safety and health criteria standards and performance. It aims at providing continual improvement in the prevention of workplace incidents via the effective management of hazards associated with the business of an organization.

TLV. Threshold Limit Value is a term used by ACGIH to express the airborne concentration of material to which nearly all persons can be exposed day after day without adverse effects. ACGIH expresses TLVs in three ways: *TLV-TWA:* The allowable Time-Weighted Average concentration for a normal 8-hour workday or 80-hour workweek.

17
Technology Transfer

Authors: Bruce F. Alexander
                 Charles Sullivan

Advisor: A. J. (Skip) Dyer

INTRODUCTION

Background

During the evolution of a new chemical entity (NCE) from a conceptual molecular structure to the dosage form of an approved active pharmaceutical ingredient (API), a multitude of trials and studies are carefully and systematically undertaken. These studies are necessary to prove that the resulting pharmaceutical product containing the API, when taken appropriately, will be effective and safe. Inherent to these activities and subsequent bulk manufacturing, a series of technology transfers are necessary to prepare the ever-increasing amounts of quality API required to satisfy both research and commercial needs.

Scope

This chapter will focus on technology transfer of API manufacturing processes, although many of the principles will also be applicable to drug product manufacturing. Although the emphasis will be on preparation of the APIs by traditional chemical synthesis, the principles also apply to APIs derived from biotechnology sources, but the specifics will be somewhat different

Definition of Technology Transfer

Technology transfer is:

> The systematic procedure that is followed in order to pass the documented knowledge and experience gained during development and or commercialization to an appropriate, responsible and authorized party. Technology transfer embodies both the transfer of documentation and the demonstrated ability of a receiving unit to effectively perform the critical elements of transferred technology, to the satisfaction of all parties and any, or all, regulatory bodies (1).

Why Is Technology Transfer Important in Facility Design?

As the definition above implies, anything that can be done to facilitate the transfer of process information from one group to another, or enable the receiving unit to effectively execute the process, will improve technology transfer. One thing that can be done is to design the facilities to make it easier to transfer that information. This means that the transferring and or receiving facilities will have features that will minimize ambiguities, misinterpretation of requirements, and unknown consequences of the move. As described in more detail below, these design principles can be applied to either the transferring or receiving facility, but most effectively to both as an integrated system.

KEY CONCEPTS/PRINCIPLES

Technology transfer is primarily a transfer of information from one group of people to another, and therefore the ability to communicate process information effectively is a key success factor.

Types of Technology Transfer

There are five major types of technology transfer that can be envisioned for chemical processes from a business point of view:

- From research to chemical process development
- From process development to manufacturing plant(s)
- One plant to another (internal, within the same company)
- Internal plant to external plant (outsourcing)
- External plant to internal plant (in licensing)

Transfer of processes may also take place within a given plant or during process development, although these are generally not considered to be formal transfers. Those are generally less complicated (although problems certainly do occur). At any rate, the same principles can be applied to transfer between buildings or equipment trains within a site.

The transfer from research to chemical process development is almost always from one bench-scale laboratory to another. As such, it is not of primary interest for the design principles discussed in this chapter.

When transferring from process development (usually from a pilot plant) to manufacturing plant(s), the major considerations usually revolve around scale up issues and the inherent differences between pilot plant and commercial operations. The key principle for technology transfer is that a pilot plant should be able to predict, to the extent possible, what will happen on a manufacturing scale.

When transferring from one manufacturing plant to another, the major consideration is whether a new plant is to be built for the transferred process, or whether an existing plant will be retrofitted. There is generally much more flexibility in a new facility, as discussed in the next section.

User Requirements for Technology Transfer

The following design considerations should be addressed when developing user requirements for facilities that could be involved in technology transfer.

Type of Facility

New vs. Legacy Facility. In new construction, there is the opportunity to optimize the facility for the process that will be transferred. However, there are considerations other than the specific process at hand, such as:

- Requirements of the site/facility master plan
- Whether the facility will be built as a dedicated, multi-product or multi-purpose plant (see below)
- Possible future use of the facility
- Cost and time constraints

Due to the considerable time required to build a facility from scratch (1–3 years depending on size, complexity, infrastructure available, and many other factors), advance planning and an expedited capital approval process are often the key success factors.

In a legacy facility, normally the emphasis is to minimize the interruption to ongoing production, and incremental cost. As the head of R&D for a prominent pharmaceutical company once said at a large gathering, "The purpose of chemical engineers is to make new processes fit into existing equipment." There is something to be said for this approach, since minimizing the changes may greatly reduce the timeframe for the introduction, as well as the cost. However, it is imperative to examine the long-term cost of the production; forcing the process into existing equipment may be cheaper in the short term, but cost more over the lifecycle of the product.

Some factors to consider when examining long-term cost are:

- Economies of scale from using appropriately-sized equipment
- Yield losses due to less than optimum equipment design
- Remaining useful life of existing equipment
- Reduction of operating costs and reproducibility of operations through automation (usually difficult to retrofit)
- Containment issues for hazardous materials (requiring more handling time to incorporate personal protective equipment or non-compliance with industrial hygiene initiatives)
- Increased handling due to poor placement of equipment and other compromised operations
- Lack of space to incorporate more efficient unit operations, such as solids charging
- Location of the existing facility
- GMP considerations, such as segregation of activities

Launch vs. Mature Product Facilities. Launch facilities are generally designed with much more flexibility than those for mature products, and may be operated at much lower utilization of capacity in order to be able to respond quickly to rapidly changing demands. Design considerations are oriented toward keeping the manufacturing facilities from becoming the critical path in time-to-market. By definition, these same considerations facilitate technology transfer, since it is presumed that the easier it is, the faster it could take place. This is particularly true for elements that are largely outside of the control of the company, such as lead time for delivery of new equipment.

Dedicated/Multi-product/Multi-process. There are pros and cons for dedicated facilities, depending on the circumstances. From a strictly technology transfer point of view, a new dedicated facility for a process should give the best results, as it would be designed to optimize the requirements for that process. For an existing facility that was dedicated to a much different product, it can be the worst case, since it may require extensive modifications for the new process. In that case, there are often compromises made to reduce the time and/or cost, which end up making the transfer more difficult because of large potential differences in the equipment from that of the transferring site.

A multi-product facility is generally designed to carry out a number of similar processes, often for a family of pharmaceuticals. Although still somewhat specialized, they have more flexibility than a dedicated plant, and represent, for an existing facility, an intermediate case for technology transfer.

A multi-process plant is designed for a wide variety of chemistries and has the most flexibility. It follows that this type of existing facility would represent the best case among existing facilities for accepting a new process.

Type of Technology

Some technologies are inherently more difficult to transfer than others. These involve unit operations that are sensitive to scale and specific equipment configuration and generally involve critical transport processes. Thus, a slow, homogeneous reaction is usually the easiest operation to transfer, whereas solid phase operations, such as crystallization and drying, may be very difficult. Polymorph issues are particularly prone to subtle differences in equipment and must always be considered.

In addition, certain types of chemistries must be reviewed carefully to ensure the suitability of the site and facility. These may include technologies such as:

- Hazardous reactions (hydrogenation, nitration, phosgenation)
- Solid-phase reactions
- Simulated moving-bed separations
- Those involving water-reactive, noxious or environmentally sensitive materials
- Those using or generating extremely potent products

Type of Process

New Processes. New processes generally have the advantage of a more rigorous process development program. A facility design is no better than its basis, so perhaps the most important factor in designing for technology transfer is a complete understanding of the process. Most pharmaceutical process development groups now create a detailed description of how the major process variables affect product quality through design of experiments, proven acceptable ranges for the parameters, and edge of failure analyses. These create a clear definition of the critical process parameters, and the facility can be designed to ensure that those factors can be controlled within acceptable ranges.

Legacy Processes. Older processes were generally designed with less rigor and often rely on experience in the existing plant to guide design. This can be a very risky undertaking since there are numerous cases where a process has run for years without difficulty in an existing plant but was fraught with difficulties when moved. This often occurs even when moved within an existing site to what appears to be similar equipment. Transfer to other sites or companies only compounds the problem. In these cases, it is highly recommended that skilled practitioners take a critical look at the processing variables and conduct remedial lab work to identify those that are sensitive to change.

Facility Design

Now that we have outlined the user requirements for technology transfer, we will shift our attention to the design principles used to meet those requirements.

Harmonization Between Facilities

Similar Equipment. The case for similar equipment somewhat parallels the regulatory arguments for registering changes with the FDA. One could make the case that designing to minimize the regulatory impact facilitates technology transfer. "Similar equipment" has been well defined for dosage form unit operations in the SUPAC supplement. An equivalent list specifically for APIs does not yet exist, but may not be necessary. As alluded to above, solid-state operations are the most difficult to transfer, and the equipment for many of those are, in fact, covered in the supplement. The equipment in the two facilities involved in the transfer should be as alike as possible, but sometimes the differences are subtle. Considerations include:

- Vessel geometry and materials of construction (MOC)
- Size, so vessels can be filled to a similar percent of working volume, as this affects mixing and heat transfer rates

- Agitation, which can vary significantly between types of agitators and for different scale operations
- Heat transfer characteristics
- Isolation and drying equipment

More details are given in the section on Gap Analysis. There may be an inherent conflict between technology transfer and upgrading of equipment at the receiving facility. Changing the technology during transfer greatly increases the chance for failure, and upgrades ideally should take place prior to the transfer.

Automation Design. Utilizing the same control system design basis (as illustrated in Appendix A: Case Study) can facilitate technology transfer by improving communication. It is much easier to program the process control system at the receiving facility when that site employs the same process control modules. For example, specific modules may be defined to control such things as:

- Transfer in or out of the vessel
- Pressure and venting
- Temperature

This can be taken to the point where the same flow chart of processing modules can be used, although we will probably never be able to transfer the process on a compact disk that contains all of the necessary program elements for the new facility.

Utilization of Pilot Plants. As will be illustrated in the case study, the most important principle here is to design pilot plants that mimic large-scale operations. There has been a tendency in the past to use pilot plants to run lab processes on a larger scale. Often, the top priority in a pilot plant was making clinical supplies; process development or technology transfer considerations were addressed only as time permitted. The perspective should be more on "scaling down" of commercial operations with a goal of duplicating to the extent possible such things as:

- Heat transfer capabilities, including those in reflux condensers
- Mixing characteristics
- Time constants for transfers, temperature changes, and phase separations
- Solid-phase operations such as centrifugation, agitated drying, and crystal sizing, which should be carried out on equipment whose results are scalable

Flexibility for Duplication of Conditions

As indicated above, flexibility is a distinct advantage, particularly to avoid the inevitable compromises that take place when modifications are necessary at either facility to duplicate conditions in the other facility. This principle applies to both the transferring and receiving units, as ideally the pilot work can be done in equipment that is directly scalable to the manufacturing plant. This both minimizes modifications at the larger, more expensive scale, and reduces the probability of surprises during the transfer.

Gap Analyses

Most companies have set up well-defined processes for technology transfer because of the penalties for not doing it right. These may include delayed schedules, increased costs, and regulatory issues. Formal processes generally call for a gap analysis early in the project. These analyses usually address pertinent gaps in the equipment between the two sites and differences in operating procedures between the transferring site and those proposed at the receiving facility.

Equipment. The major considerations for an equipment gap analysis are shown in a template format included in Appendix B.

Implications for Operating Parameters. Although often not specifically addressed in a gap analysis, the interaction of subtle differences in equipment characteristics and operating parameters should also be considered. For example, if the centrifuge at the receiving facility has a larger basket diameter and/or higher speed capability, the effect on cake compression should be considered. Ideally, the compressibility would be studied in the development lab or the receiving equipment would be run at a lower speed to duplicate the G forces.

Another issue involves parameters that may not be well defined in the first place, such as steam flow rate during steam stripping or "full vacuum" during drying. The principle here is to understand what is actually taking place when the material is processed in the transferring facility, and to either duplicate those conditions in the receiving facility or determine that they are not important.

Robust Process/Consistent and Predictable Operation

As mentioned in the introduction, the second benefit from good design is to allow the receiving facility to carry out the process successfully once the transfer of information has taken place.

Critical Process Parameters. Critical process parameters [i.e., "those parameters which, if not controlled, can affect a critical quality attribute of the product," (ICH Q7A Guideline)] must be determined from the development work or historical data in the plant. That information is necessary to ensure that the normal operating range (NOR), which is based on the ability of the equipment to control that parameter, is well within the proven acceptable range (PAR) for each critical parameter.

Polymorph Issues. Horror stories abound on changes in polymorph, or even the appearance of new polymorphs during technology transfer. A key function of the process engineer is to understand how equipment characteristics affect the local environment experienced by the product, since use of exactly the same equipment may not be possible or even desirable at the new location.

Since transfer of a process is sometimes used as an opportunity to "upgrade" the receiving facility, new technology may be difficult to avoid. Equipment improvement may make sense from a business, control, efficiency, and maintenance point of view, but may present technical challenges during the transfer. For example, if the drying equipment is changed from an agitated pan dryer to a paddle dryer, a different polymorph may unexpectedly emerge due to the higher energy input per unit volume.

Regulatory Considerations

As mentioned, in addition to company management, regulatory bodies must be satisfied with the transfer.

Validation. Again, as part of the receiving facility's ability to successfully execute the process, process validation is often required.

Cleanability. Cleaning has become an integral part of the validation process as the requirements continue to become more demanding. This is a result of increased scrutiny as well as the trend to more potent compounds. Those compounds have lower acceptable limits of residue that could potentially be carried over into the next product. It is therefore imperative that new equipment be designed for ease of cleaning. Some of the design considerations, which also go hand-in-hand with clean-in-place (CIP) capabilities, are:

- Minimize the length of pipe runs
- Eliminate dead legs, low spots, and sharp angles
- Equipment and lines must be drainable (this includes auxiliary equipment, such as heat exchangers)
- Vessel nozzles must be "visible" from CIP spray nozzles
- Provisions for handling spent cleaning solution
- Surface finishes, so product does not adhere to the MOC of the equipment
- Crevice-free product contact surfaces
- Provisions for drying equipment
- Sufficient vessel drainage capacity to avoid pooling of CIP solutions

Equipment Qualification. As the primary prerequisite for validation on the equipment side, the facility must be designed for ease of qualification. Essentially, qualification is the proof that the process equipment, when properly installed, can do what it was purported to do. (This issue is discussed at length in Chapter 8.) It cannot be emphasized enough that there must be a thorough understanding of what the equipment really needs to do at the outset of the project. Failure to do this is the one of the biggest causes of problems during the qualification.

Ease of Registration. As mentioned, unless there is a need to modernize the equipment, the receiving facility should have equipment that is similar from both a functional and regulatory point of view to that in the transferring facility. Ideally, these would be exactly the same. As referenced previously, the term "similar" has been defined for much of the solid-state equipment used in manufacture of APIs in the SUPAC supplement.

cGMPs. Facilities that make APIs for human consumption must always be designed to meet cGMPs. (This topic is discussed in detail in Chapter 2.)

Data Gathering

Recording of data is critical at both the transferring and receiving facility. At the former, it is necessary to understand the process to be transferred. and, at the latter, to ensure that the process is being carried out the same way.

Instrumentation Systems. All parameters that could affect product quality, safety, industrial hygiene, or the environment should be measured. Unfortunately, this is an area that may be compromised or unavailable in older facilities. Some areas that may be neglected that are important for technology transfer are:

- Agitator speed
- Liquid levels inside vessels
- Boil up and/or condensate rates
- Steam flow rates for steam stripping
- Vacuum/pressure at all critical points in the system
- Jacket flows and temperatures in and out
- Cooling rates
- Condensate temperatures
- Liquid feed rates
- Centrifuge rpm, feed and wash rates

Sampling Systems. Technology transfer often involves extended sampling programs during process assessment and validation. Sampling is often cumbersome and a safety and or industrial hygiene issue in older facilities, and/or may not accurately represent the composition desired. Systems should be provided that allow representative samples to be taken in a safe manner in conformance with cGMPs.

Data Logging. Equipment should be provided that allows for logging and trending of data during the batches. It has become increasingly important to establish historical data necessary for transfers and to define proven acceptable ranges post development, as well as operating data for equipment qualification.

TRENDS/FUTURE DEVELOPMENTS

Formalized Process

Because of the importance of succeeding at technology transfers, most companies have now developed detailed procedures for carrying them out. These include gap analyses (as outlined in that section). The implication for facility design is to provide a more detailed assessment of what needs to be done at the receiving site.

Future Considerations

Pharmaceutical companies have become increasingly aware that it is difficult to predict what equipment will provide an optimum plant environment more than five or ten years into the future. Therefore, more and more designs are including empty space and utility capacity for future installations, as these seem to be the features that will stand the test of time.

REFERENCES

1. Technology Transfer Guide, Post-industrial Review Draft, September 2002, ISPE.
2. SUPAC Supplement.
3. ICH Q7A Guideline.

APPENDIX A

Case Study—Roche Carolina Inc.

Background

In the late 1980s, Hoffmann–La Roche Pharmaceuticals (Roche) made a decision to move chemical manufacturing of APIs out of their U.S. headquarters site in Nutley, New Jersey. The plan was to build a new facility in the southeast United States that would, in particular, be used for manufacture of new APIs for the company's global needs. The topic of technology transfer actually arose at the very beginning of the project during development of the company's mission statement.

The transfer from the process development group to the first manufacturing facility was considered to be the most challenging in the series of transfers that takes place during the lifecycle of a product. Having those two functions at different sites would only increase that difficulty, so it was decided to also move the process development group from Nutley to the same new site.

After an extensive search, Roche purchased a 1400-acre greenfield site outside of Florence, South Carolina. That location provided a great deal of freedom in design of the facility due to its size, openness, and lack of height restrictions. The project began in 1991 to build a pharmaceutical development center (known as the Pharmaceutical Technical Center or PTC) and multi-purpose API manufacturing facility for new products entering the market. The PTC contained a number of technical elements, but the one of primary interest was the pilot plant facility. In the past, technology transfer from a PTC to manufacturing normally took place based on pilot plant runs.

The project was organized as three sub-projects:

• PTC
• Manufacturing
• Site infrastructure

However, the project team was structured to ensure integration among the three projects at the site. The activities and resources at this site were incorporated as a wholly owned subsidiary of Roche, known as Roche Carolina Inc. (RCI)

Design Principles

One of the fundamental components of the mission for RCI was to facilitate technology transfer. This was necessary at two levels:

• Transfer of processes back and forth from RCI Manufacturing to other Roche manufacturing plants, particularly the largest one in Basel, Switzerland.
• Transfer of processes from the PTC pilot plant to RCI Manufacturing (or secondarily to other manufacturing plants).

The two main design principles used to achieve this ability were harmonization and flexibility. These principles have been outlined in the section on Facility Design and specific examples of how these principles were incorporated in the design are given below.

Harmonization. Standardization is almost synonymous with harmonization from a facilities point of view because, to the degree that it can actually be achieved, all facilities in an organization will, by definition, be similar. This project had a head start in that regard because Roche had in place a high degree of standardization at the Basel site. Because the first objective was to harmonize the new manufacturing plant with the existing Basel plant, the existing standards were incorporated wherever possible.

The first standard to be adopted, in both PTC pilot plant and manufacturing, was vessel train configuration. That standard utilized six vessels in each reactor bay, arranged in two parallel trains with two vessels on each of three floors. The two reactors on the top floor were designated reactor/feeders; the two on the middle floor as reactor/crystallizers, and the two on the lower floor as reactor/distillers. The vessel names were indicative of their intended functions. Each train would normally have a centrifuge on the level below that. The next (bottom) level would house dryers, with each reactor bay having one dryer dedicated to it. Both hard piping and configurable piping were used.

The design was such that any reactor could transfer to/from any other reactor. The centrifuge could be used by any of the reactor bay's reactor/feeders or reactor/crystallizers. Recall that there was no height restriction for this site, so the resulting 145-foot tall building was not an issue. Although this was the standard configuration, many bays did not have six vessels (typically in the pilot plant), because they were not needed for most processes. In those cases there was only one reactor/distiller, but whatever vessels were present were always in the same configuration.

The type of solid state equipment was also standardized, so that the centrifuges and dryers were of the same design.

Another standard was the process control configuration. The basis for this was a six-module (grouping of equipment functions) system for each reactor:

- Agitation
- Temperature control
- Transfer-in, recirculation
- Pressure control, venting, nitrogen padding
- Condensation (reflux, distillation)
- Transfer out (to transfer station)

As it turned out, even the distributed control system (DCS) was the same for all three facilities (Basel, RCI Manufacturing, and RCI Pilot Plant). Roche was actually on the forefront of process control technology in the 1980s. They were not satisfied with what was available to the market at that time, so they developed their own system—PCR-2 (Process Control Roche). Although a number of DCS systems were evaluated in 1992 for use at RCI, third-party systems could not outweigh the desire to harmonize within Roche. Additionally, DCS systems available at the time did not have the advanced recipe capabilities of the PCR-2 system.

Flexibility. This was another key factor for the RCI project. At the beginning of the project, the team looked at 120 process steps that had been carried out at the Nutley and Basel facilities. It was decided to design the PTC and Manufacturing plants at RCI to be able to carry out 90% of those steps without requiring any equipment modifications. This is an extremely high degree of flexibility and certainly qualifies the plants as true multi-purpose facilities. Cryogenic reactions, high-pressure operations, and handling of high-risk chemistry were not part of the scope.

Some of the design features that were incorporated to achieve flexibility were:

- MOCs for all fixed pieces of equipment were either glass-lined, Teflon®-lined or Hastelloy®.
- All reactors (five or six per bay as mentioned above) were full-service vessels with heating, cooling, and agitation.
- All vessel peripherals were designed around the maximum design pressure of the vessels themselves. This was generally 90 psig and full vacuum.
- All vessels had a wide temperature range capability, generally from $-20°C$ to $+160°C$.
- Variable-speed agitators.

The pilot plant had some additional features to ensure flexibility, because it had been observed in the past that conditions used in the pilot plant could not always be duplicated in the manufacturing facilities. Reactors of many different sizes were included, ranging from 10 gallons to 300 gallons. They were graduated so that any size reaction in this range could be carried out with a volume in the reactor that gave good mixing. This allowed running a reaction on one-tenth scale for virtually any size manufacturing plant, to limit the scale up on transfer to no more than an order of magnitude.

The pilot plant also contained a facility for hydrogenations, acetylations, very high pressures, and very wide temperature ranges ($-70°C$ to $+250°C$). These capabilities were not to be incorporated into RCI Manufacturing until needed because of the cost, although space was set aside for them in the building.

On that last note, it was realized that no matter how flexible the facility appeared to be at the time of construction, it was only possible to see five to ten years into the future. The only thing certain beyond that time frame was the need for space in the building, so empty bays were incorporated in both buildings. The utility headers were designed to support the additional equipment in the future bays.

APPENDIX B

Equipment Comparison Template

1.0 General
   1.1 Equipment train configuration/number/type of vessels
2.0 For all equipment
   2.1 Working volume
   2.2 Material of construction
   2.3 Process control capabilities
   2.4 Containment rating
   2.5 CIP equipment
3.0 Specific equipment
   3.1 Reactors/crystallizers
      3.1.1 Temperature range capabilities
      3.1.2 Agitation
         3.1.2.1 Type of agitator (e.g., retreat curve, pitched-blade turbine)
         3.1.2.2 Baffling
         3.1.2.3 RPM range
      3.1.3 Heat transfer/reflux capabilities
      3.1.4 Pressure rating (if applicable)
      3.1.5 Type of sparger (if applicable)
      3.1.6 pH control (if applicable)
   3.2 Distillation vessels
      3.2.1 Temperature range capabilities
      3.2.2 Vacuum capabilities (absolute pressure and flow rate)
      3.2.3 Column (if applicable)
         3.2.3.1 Theoretical stages
         3.2.3.2 Packing
         3.2.3.3 Diameter
   3.3 Filters
      3.3.1 Type of filter
      3.3.2 Filtration area
      3.3.3 Filter media (e.g., cloth, sintered metal)
      3.3.4 Opening in filter media
   3.4 Centrifuges
      3.4.1 Type of centrifuge (e.g., horizontal inverting basket)
      3.4.2 Diameter of basket
      3.4.3 Rotational speed capabilities
   3.5 Dryers
      3.5.1 Type of dryer (e.g., agitated pan, paddle)
      3.5.2 Temperature capabilities/heat transfer surface
      3.5.3 Vacuum capabilities
   3.6 Mills
      3.6.1 Type of mill

3.6.2 Flow rate capabilities
3.7 Transfers
   3.7.1 MOC of piping
   3.7.2 Ability to maintain temperature
   3.7.3 Control

18
Environmental Considerations

Authors: William Kesack
Peter Wilson
Stuart Dearden

Advisors: Ashok Soni
George Petroka

INTRODUCTION

Pharmaceutical manufacturing facilities are required to comply with numerous environmental regulations promulgated by the U.S. Environmental Protection Agency (EPA), state environmental regulatory agencies, and local environmental ordinances. Therefore, environmental management and compliance are important aspects that must be addressed during the design of the facility. In fact, the environmental regulations could even impact site location because the complexity of the environmental regulations is different throughout the country because of the air and water quality conditions of that area.

The environmental regulations regulate the air emissions, wastewater discharges, and waste streams generated by pharmaceutical manufacturing facilities. In fact, many companies are required to obtain preconstruction permits from the appropriate regulatory agency for equipment and sources of air emissions, wastewater discharge, and solid waste processing activities prior to initiating construction activities, including site development and foundation work.

In most cases, the cost impact on the design and construction of a new facility is minimal compared to the overall construction cost of a new facility. However, preparation and approval time for the various permits can take several months to a year, which can severely impact a project schedule. Therefore, environmental permitting is schedule critical and must be considered very early in the project. It is suggested that an evaluation of environmental requirements for the facility be performed during the very early stages of the project and should be included during the basis of design (BOD) phase of the project.

The evaluation should also address design issues for the facility, including structural and facility layout issues. These issues will impact the cost of the project although they may not be applicable in all situations. Questions to be asked include:

- Will the air emissions from my facility be in compliance with the air pollution regulations? If not, what type of air pollution control equipment will be required to meet the requirements?
- Where should the raw material and waste storage areas be located with respect to layout of the facility? Inside or outside? If these areas are located outside, is containment required for the storage and associated loading/unloading area? Is the facility subject to stormwater permitting requirements?
- Where will the wastewater discharge from the new facility go? To a local publicly owned treatment works (POTW) or sewer treatment plant? Does the local POTW have enough capacity to accept and treat the wastewater from my facility? And has the necessary capacity been purchased from the sewer authority? Will the wastewater be discharged to a nearby stream or other type of surface water? Will the facility need to pretreat the wastewater prior to discharge? If so, what type of pretreatment is required?

These are just some of the many environmental issues that must be addressed during the design and construction of a pharmaceutical manufacturing facility.

This chapter addresses the various media regulated by the environmental rules and regulations and provides the reader with "food for thought" when moving forward with the design of a new pharmaceutical manufacturing facility.

KEY CONCEPTS/PRINCIPLES

The major emphasis of this chapter is the requirements associated with the design, construction and operation of a finished product manufacturing facility. Many of these same issues apply to research and development and chemical manufacturing facilities that produce the active pharmaceutical ingredients (APIs). Because of differences in potential environmental impact, the requirements for R&D facilities are typically less stringent, while those for the chemical manufacturing facilities are more stringent.

Although not within the scope of this text, it is important to understand that most pharmaceutical manufacturers have implemented programs to reduce, and in some cases eliminate, the different environmental impacts from their operations. These programs—which come under names such as product stewardship, green chemistry, process review, waste minimization and source reduction are all aimed at reducing the environmental "footprint" of pharmaceutical manufacturing and R&D. The facility designer's workload is often reduced significantly by these programs because they reduce or eliminate the need for designing and permitting the "end of pipe" emissions controls and environmental management facilities described in this chapter.

The three main environmental areas that finished manufacturing facilities are subject to are: 1) air quality (i.e., emissions of air contaminants to atmosphere); 2) wastewater (i.e., discharge of pollutants to surface waters); and 3) waste generation (i.e., the generation, treatment, and disposal of solid waste). Designers and operators must also address other issues, such as storage tanks, risk management/right-to-know requirements, and spill management and response.

Air Emissions

Air emissions at these facilities can be generated by facility equipment (boilers, internal combustion engines/electric generator units, tanks, etc.), process equipment, and R&D operations (pilot plants and bench-top scale work performed or exhausted via fume hoods). During the basis of design (BOD) process, the facility designer needs to develop a projected and detailed emission inventory for specific substances [such as the criteria and hazardous air pollutants (HAPs)] that might be emitted from the facility. After the emission inventory is completed, an evaluation must be performed to determine which rules and regulations will apply to the facility.

Wastewater

Similar to air emissions requirements, there are regulatory and industry standards for operations involving discharge of pollutants that may impact the quality of surface waters. The discharges of concern to a designer or operator of a pharmaceutical facility include stormwater and wastewater from facility processes and operations such as boilers, equipment washing, equipment cooling, and water purification. In addition, construction permits are required to document measures taken to prevent damage to surface waters when more than one acre of land is disturbed during the construction of the facility.

Waste Generation

The pharmaceutical manufacturing industry can generate a wide variety of solid waste streams that may impact the environment. These waste streams typically include product waste and direct by-products from the manufacturing process, and also non-process wastes from supporting activities. Additionally, there may be chemical waste from laboratory operations and other special wastes from support activities.

ENVIRONMENTAL REQUIREMENTS

Air Quality

The EPA protects the air quality of the United States. The Clean Air Act (CAA) is the law or legislative action that governs the EPA and enables them to develop, enact, and enforce the rules and regulations developed in accordance with the CAA and associated amendments. Many states also have a state environmental agency such as a Department of Environmental Protection that develops and enforces state regulations, which must be as stringent as and include all of the requirements of the federal EPA regulations. There are also many states where a local county or city promulgates its own rules and regulations that it enforces. Once again, these local regulations must be at least as stringent as the federal and state regulations.

The EPA has developed ambient air quality standards for various areas of the United States for the following six common air pollutants or "criteria" pollutants: ozone, particulate matter (PM), carbon monoxide (CO), nitrogen dioxide (NO_2 or

NO_x), sulfur dioxide, and lead. The CAA established two types of standards: primary standards that establish levels to protect public health, and secondary standards that establish levels to protect public welfare, including visibility, effects on animals, crops, vegetation, and buildings. Currently, millions of people live in areas of the United States where levels are considered unhealthy for one or more of the criteria pollutants.

The EPA also regulates the emissions of toxic or hazardous air pollutants (HAPs). These are pollutants that are known or suspected to cause cancer or other serious health or adverse environmental effects. At this time, EPA regulates the emission of 188 HAPs.

In order to control or minimize the discharge of air pollutants, the EPA has developed source-specific standards known as New Source Performance Standards (NSPS) and National Emission Standards for Hazardous Air Pollutants (NESHAPs) for Source Categories, which regulate the emissions of criteria pollutants and HAPs, respectively, from specific sources. Both the NSPS and NESHAP requirements can regulate sources located at pharmaceutical manufacturing facilities.

The types of air permits that may be needed must be considered early in the project. The first thing that must be done to accomplish this is to identify all equipment and processes that will discharge any air contaminants into the atmosphere. As mentioned previously, this equipment can include mechanical equipment, process sources, and bench top or research and development activities. After all the equipment is identified, an estimate of the potential and expected actual emissions from the various pieces of equipment and total facility emissions must be determined.

The air regulations require that emission estimates initially be based on the design capacity of the equipment and the assumption that the equipment can operate continuously—i.e. 24 hours per day, 365 days per year, or a total of 8,760 hours per year of operation. This is particularly relevant for boilers and other types of equipment that can operate continuously. However, much of the equipment operated in a final dosage pharmaceutical manufacturing facility is batch equipment such as fluid beds, coaters, and mixers where materials are added to the equipment, the necessary operation is performed, and the material is removed from the equipment prior to transfer to the next piece of equipment. In these situations, the amount of operational down time for cleaning or equipment turnover to prepare for the next batch run can be considered when calculating the potential emissions from the equipment or facility. This is defined as the equipment's or facility's "Potential to Emit" (PTE) and is the basis for determining the applicable permitting and regulatory requirements for the facility.

The PTE is then used to determine how the facility will be classified with respect to the CAA regulations. If the PTE for the facility exceeds certain thresholds for a specific air contaminant, then the facility would be classified as a "Major Source" for that air pollutant and is subject to complicated air quality permitting requirements. The major source limit for areas surrounding major metropolitan areas (such as Philadelphia, New York, Washington, D.C., Los Angeles and San Francisco) is much lower than in other areas of the country. This is because the EPA has determined through actual monitoring that the air quality in these areas is above National Ambient Air Quality Standards (NAAQS) and may adversely impact the health of the exposed residents in these areas. The pollutants of concern in these areas are oxides of nitrogen (NO_x) and VOCs, which are typically emitted from pharmaceutical manufacturing facilities. Major source levels for NO_x and volatile organic compounds (VOCs) in these areas are facilities with a PTE of >25 tons per year, which is typically measured by the regulatory agencies on a 12-month rolling period. Major source levels for pharmaceutical companies in areas of the United States that have air quality in attainment with the NAAQS levels is 100 tons per year. Therefore, the location of the facility will impact the complexity of the air quality permitting requirements.

As discussed previously, many states have their own air quality rules and regulations that the agency also enforces. These agencies also are in charge of the air permitting requirements. Most state agencies require facilities to obtain preapproval or construction permits prior to initiating construction of the operations that emit air contaminants. This allows the regulatory agency to review the proposed process and ensure that the air emissions from the operations will be in compliance with the rules and regulations and minimize health impacts to individuals located near these facilities. After an application has been submitted, the agency will initiate its review process and issue a construction permit that will contain various terms and conditions that must be complied with during the construction and start-up of the source. This review process can take between a month to almost a year depending on the amounts and types of emissions that will be emitted from the new facility. The review time also varies from state to state, but typical review times are a minimum of one month.

Some streamlining of the permitting process has recently taken place within the regulatory agencies. The agencies have recently begun to develop general permits for air emission sources such as boilers, storage tanks, and emergency electric generators among others. A general permit is a permit that applies to a type source that is routinely permitted and conditions do not change for the source. Therefore, a general permit is developed with conditions that apply to any company that is willing to accept and operate its source in accordance with the terms and conditions of the general permit. Approval times with a general permit are less than a month and many times a company can initiate the construction of a source covered by a general permit within days of notifying the appropriate regulatory agency. The availability of general permits varies across the United States and depends upon the regulating agency. Some states that have general permits are Pennsylvania, New Jersey, and Florida and many other states have general permits that are available. It is recommended that the applicable rules for the area that the facility will be located be reviewed to determine if a general permit can be used for the facility.

The EPA has developed specific rules and regulations for the sources listed below that might be installed at pharmaceutical manufacturing facilities. The NSPS regulate the emissions of criteria pollutants, such as NO_x, VOC, CO, PM, and SO_2; contain emission limits that must be met from the source; and also include required monitoring, recordkeeping, and reporting requirements for the type of process being installed. The NESHAPs regulate the emissions of HAPs, such as methylene chloride, hexane, and other organic solvents, as well as metals and other air contaminants that can be emitted from other types of facilities. A list of some of the HAPs that may be used in pharmaceutical manufacturing facilities as of early 2004 is contained in Table

1. A complete listing of the 188 HAPs regulated by the Clean Air Act can be found in Section 112(b) of the Act or the EPA's website www.epa.gov/ttn/atw/188polls.html.

TABLE 1   Some Hazardous Air Pollutants That May Be Emitted from Pharmaceutical Manufacturing

75058	Acetonitrile	75092	Methylene chloride
56235	Carbon tetrachloride	78933	Methyl ethyl ketone
67663	Chlorine	108101	Methyl isobutyl ketone
67663	Chloroform	1634044	Methyl tert butyl ether
107211	Ethylene glycol	91230	Naphthalene
75218	Ethylene oxide	108952	Phenol
50000	Formaldehyde	108883	Toluene
NA	Glycol ethers	79005	1,1,2-Trichloroethane
108952	Phenol	79016	Trichloroethylene
110543	Hexane	121448	Triethylamine
7647010	Hydrochloric acid	1330207	Xylenes (isomers and mixture)
67561	Methanol		

Note: For glycol ethers, the following applies: Includes mono- and di-ethers of ethylene glycol, diethylene glycol, and triethylene glycol R-(OCH2CH2)n -OR' where n = 1, 2, or 3; R = alkyl or aryl groups; R' = R, H, or groups which, when removed, yield glycol ethers with the structure R-(OCH2CH)n-OH. Polymers are excluded from the glycol category.

The NESHAPs are similar to the NSPS standards in that they list emission limits for specific types of sources and also list the monitoring, recordkeeping and reporting requirements for that type of source.

New Source Performance Standards (40 CFR 60)
- Combustion units, i.e., boilers (Subpart Dc)
- Hospital/medical/infectious waste incinerators (HMIWI) (Subpart Ec)
- Fuel oil and solvent storage tanks (Subpart Kb)
- Stationary gas turbines/cogeneration units (Subpart GG)
- Commercial and industrial solid waste incinerators (CISWI) (Subpart CCCC)

National Emission Standards for Hazardous Air Pollutants (40 CFR 63)
- Ethylene oxide emissions from sterilization (Subpart O)
- Pharmaceutical production (Subpart GGG)
- Reciprocating internal combustion engine (RICE) (Subpart ZZZZ)
- Industrial, commercial and institutional boders and process heaters (Subpart DDDD)

Air Pollution Control Equipment
Many times air pollution control equipment must be installed to meet the air quality regulations. This section describes some common air pollutant sources and control methods used in the pharmaceutical industry.

New boilers to be installed at facilities should be equipped with technology that reduces the emissions of NO_x from the unit. Technology is currently available that can reduce emissions of NO_x from boilers fired with natural gas to 30 parts per million, by volume corrected to 3% oxygen content or lower. This technology includes low-NO_x burners and or flue gas recirculation. Many states are also requiring boilers that burn fuel oils to meet certain emission limits. For instance new boilers installed in Pennsylvania that will burn No. 2 distillate fuel oil may have to meet an NO_x emission limit of 90 ppmv correct to 3% oxygen content.

Another air pollutant commonly generated by many pharmaceutical facilities is particulate matter (PM). To control PM emissions, the pharmaceutical industry installs dust collectors and/or high efficiency particulate air (HEPA) filters to minimize the discharge of particulates to the atmosphere. The selection of dust collection and filtration equipment depends upon the nature and concentration of PM from the process and the expected exhaust gas volume of the generating processes. For example, a pharmaceutical facility where significant quantities of powders are dispensed, milled, granulated or blended will usually require installation of a filtered dust collection system. In facilities where high hazard or potent (e.g., cytotoxic drugs) API powders will mostly be handled, HEPA filtration systems are necessary. These systems should be designed where possible to have HEPA filters installed near the particulate source to reduce exhaust duct contamination. The reduced duct contamination will result in lower maintenance, modification, and decommissioning costs. Some pharmaceutical process equipment, including fluid bed coater/driers and coating pans, which may generate PM, include integral filtration capabilities.

There are several different types of air pollution control equipment that can be used at pharmaceutical manufacturing facilities to control and/or minimize the emissions of VOCs and other organic solvents. The choice for the selection of the appropriate technology depends on the type and concentration of the pollutant that needs to be removed from the exhaust gas stream. These technologies include thermal oxidation (combustion), scrubbers (absorbers), condensers (condensation), and carbon adsorbers (adsorption).

A detailed discussion of these technologies is not within the scope of this book, but a brief discussion on these technologies and the advantages and disadvantages is presented. Additional information concerning these technologies can be found in Reference 1. Also, many equipment suppliers have detailed information on the type of equipment that they manufacture for the facilities.

Thermal Oxidation

Thermal oxidation is one of the most common methods used in final dosage pharmaceutical manufacturing facilities to remove organic solvents and/or VOCs from the production equipment exhausts. Thermal oxidation uses temperature to convert the solvents into water and carbon dioxide. Figure 1 is a picture of a typical regenerative thermal oxidizer.

Sometime catalysts are used in conjunction with thermal oxidation, which reduces the temperature and supplemental fuel requirements required to oxidize the

FIGURE 1 Thermal Oxidizer

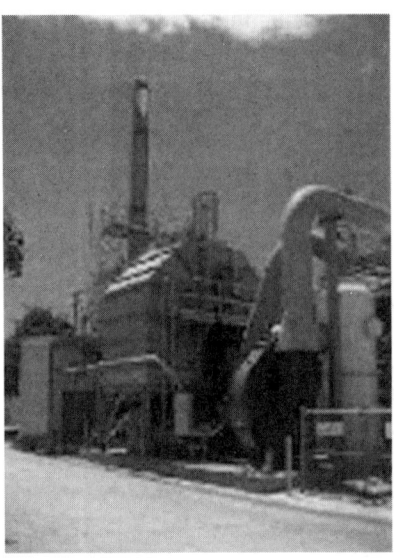

air contaminants. Many times, heat recovery equipment, such as air-to-air heat exchangers, regenerative beds, and/or waste heat boilers are used in conjunction with thermal oxidizers to recover and use some of the energy contained in the hot exhaust gases to either preheat the dirty exhaust gases or make steam for use in the facility. Thermal oxidizers are also very efficient at removing the air contaminants from the exhaust gases, and equipment manufactured today can easily achieve removal efficiencies greater than 95% and up to greater than 99% if designed correctly for the exhaust gas stream.

However, thermal oxidizers can be fairly expensive to operate because of their large energy consumption, particularly if the correct heat recovery is not selected to minimize fuel use. Careful planning is necessary to identify which processes show cost and environmental justification for installation and use of thermal oxidizers. The environmental and regulatory compliance benefits must be weighed against the environmental and cost impact of the energy used in their operation.

Absorption

Scrubbers or gas absorbers are highly effective in removing acids and other compounds that have high solubility with the material that is selected as the scrubbing media. For example, VOCs such as alcohols can be removed by water scrubber systems. Scrubbers can also be designed (e.g., with oxidizing treatment chemicals) to chemically remove some air pollutants. However, scrubbers are typically not used today to remove air contaminants from exhaust gases generated at a pharmaceutical manufacturing facility unless the facility emits acid gasses such as those generated when chlorinated solvents are treated by a thermal oxidizer. The combustion of chlorinated solvents creates hydrochloric acid that must be removed from the exhaust gases before they are discharged to the atmosphere. If these compounds are not removed from the exhaust gases, significant damage to surrounding metal surfaces will occur due to the contact with the acid gases.

Scrubbers are relatively simple to operate and take up minimal space. They are also very effective at removing air contaminants such as hydrogen chloride. Removal efficiencies of greater than 99% can easily be achieved with properly designed scrubbers. However, most scrubbers create a liquid discharge that must be treated and disposed of properly. Pretreatment of the liquid discharge may be required before it can be sent offsite as a wastewater discharge. Scrubbers are also relatively inexpensive to purchase and operate compared to other air pollution control technologies, such as thermal oxidation.

Condensation

Condensation converts gaseous air contaminants to a liquid by either lowering the exhaust gases' temperature or by increasing its pressure. Typically, condensation is used in vacuum systems where the pressure of the exhaust gases can easily be increased at the same time their temperature is reduced. Condensers are not typically used in a final dosage manufacturing facilities because the concentration of the air contaminant in the exhaust gases is not sufficient to make the effective use of a condenser. Condensers are typically found in the pharmaceutical chemical synthesis facilities that are used to make the active pharmaceutical ingredient (API) or in API pilot development facilities that of similar design.

The efficiency of a condenser to remove air contaminants from the exhaust gases is highly dependent on the concentration and vapor pressure of the air contaminant. The higher the concentration and vapor pressure of the air contaminant the more efficient condensation is for removing air contaminants from the exhaust gases.

Adsorption

Adsorption uses solid materials, such as carbon, silica gel, or molecular sieves to attract the gaseous air contaminants and retain these contaminants on the surface of these materials. Eventually, the air contaminants that have been adsorbed on the solid material must be removed to allow the continued removal of the air contaminants from the exhaust gases or the solid material will become saturated with the air contaminant. Once this happens, removal of the air contaminant from the exhaust gas will no longer be achieved.

Adsorption systems are typically made up of two or three beds of solid adsorbent materials. This allows the continued removal of the air contaminant from the exhaust gas streams. In two and three bed systems, one bed is used to remove the air contaminants from the exhaust gases while a different bed is regenerated; i.e., the air contaminants are removed from the solid adsorbent with steam or hot air. If steam is used to remove the air contaminants from the solid adsorbent, wastewater-containing solvent is created that must be treated appropriately. Sometimes, the solvent can be recovered from the steam and reused in the process. The reuse of solvent in a pharmaceutical manufacturing facility is typically not considered because of the strict FDA requirements associated with validation of the manufacturing process. Adsorption systems are typically more expensive to install and operate than the other technologies and are only justified if the solvent can be recovered and reused in the process.

The following factors must be considered when selecting air pollution control equipment to remove air contaminants from the manufacturing equipment exhaust gases:

- Ensure that the controlled emission limits are in compliance with the applicable rules and regulations for permitting including any technology requirements, such as Best Available Control Technology (BACT) or Lowest Achievable Emission Reduction (LAER).
- Is there Operational flexibility? Can the permit be written to use appropriate air pollution control devices only when processes justify their use? This is particularly important when the pollution control device has a secondary environmental impact or high operating costs.
- Effectiveness of the equipment to remove the expected air contaminants.
- Cost effectiveness of the equipment to remove the air contaminants. A cost analysis should be performed based on the initial equipment and installation cost and the annual operating cost. Typically, an annualized cost based on the equipment, installation, and operating costs are developed based on the amount of air contaminant removed. Sometimes this cost, based on the dollars per ton of air contaminant removed is used by regulatory agencies to determine if the installation of air pollution control equipment is justified.
- The creation of an additional environmental discharge that must be treated or disposed of properly. Examples of this are wastewater discharges from scrubbers and the generation of hazardous waste from the regeneration of adsorbers with steam.

Summary

During the design and construction of a final dosage manufacturing facility, a thorough evaluation of the potential air contaminants that will be discharged from the facility for a reasonable future time period must be performed. To do this, consideration must be made of all expected processes, which will occur at the facility. Once the type and amount of air contaminants that will be generated by the facility have been determined, the design team must perform a comprehensive review of the applicable environmental regulations where the facility will be sited and identify appropriate air pollution controls to comply. It is then prudent to arrange a meeting with the local agency to introduce the project and have the regulatory agency review any specific requirements the agency might have for the facility with respect to permit application preparation and submittal, application review time and fees, and technology requirements.

Once the applicable rules and regulations have been identified, the company must then determine if any of the process emissions must be reduced with the installation of air pollution control equipment. If air pollution control equipment is required for the project, it is highly recommended that time and finances be used to perform an independent engineering evaluation of the available control technologies because "one size does not fit all" when it comes to removing air contaminants from the production equipment exhaust gases. The engineering evaluation will ensure that the selected technology is the most viable from a technical and economic impact for the selected application. Once the technology has been decided on, the design and installation of this equipment must be integrated with the facility design to ensure that sufficient space and utilities are available for the selected equipment. The designer must also ensure that appropriate monitoring and recording devices are installed to collect the necessary data required by the regulatory agencies.

It is important that these steps take place early in the project because the regulatory rules do not allow construction of the air emission source, including boilers, emergency electric generator units, and manufacturing processes until the necessary approvals (e.g., construction permits) are obtained from the appropriate regulatory agency. Significant fines and penalties can be assessed for initiating construction of the air emission sources without the appropriate approvals.

WASTEWATER

Wastewater issues must also be considered before initiating the design process of a pharmaceutical facility. It is important to identify the agencies regulating wastewater discharge early in the design process to prevent costly delays and design changes. A decision must be made as part of the facility siting process about whether the local municipal sewage treatment facility or POTW (Publicly Owned Treatment Works) will be used to treat wastewater generated at the proposed facility, or if it will be treated by an on-site wastewater treatment system. Most U.S. pharmaceutical facilities use a local POTW to treat their wastewater. This is because in most cases, it is more costly to design, build, and operate an on-site treatment system than to pay sewage use fees to the local POTW. Figure 2 describes the sources and routes of wastewater from a typical pharmaceutical manufacturing facility.

Typically, only relatively large pharmaceutical facilities will show cost justification for operating their own wastewater treatment facility. However, if there is not an option for the pharmaceutical facility to discharge wastewater to a POTW, or if it shows cost-benefit, the facility designer/builder will need to design, permit, and construct a facility to treat wastewater for direct discharge to a body of water. In addition to being more costly, construction of an on-site wastewater treatment system is a lengthier process because of design and permitting requirements. The permit process may be slowed by concerns from the local community.

If the local POTW option is chosen, arrangements must be made either with the local municipality or directly with the sewer authority to ensure that the POTW has capacity to accept the facility's wastewater. In some cases, a facility will purchase treatment capacity at a POTW in the form of EDUs (Equivalent Discharge Units). The POTW operates under permits from the state or the EPA, which requires them to treat wastewater to specific water quality standards before dis-

FIGURE 2 Typical Pharmaceutical Manufacturing Wastewater Sources and Routes

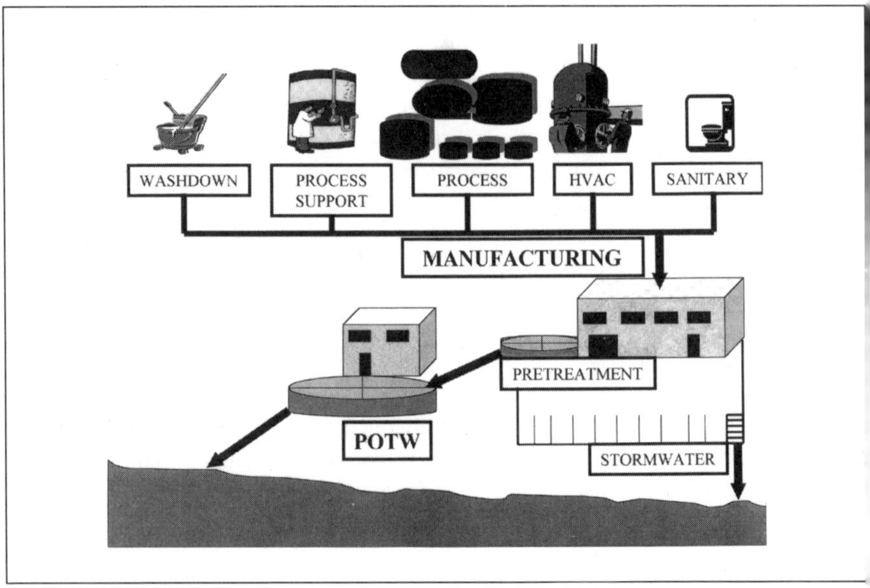

charge. In order to meet the discharge requirements, POTWs require industrial sources which discharge to their plant to meet other specific standards called Pretreatment Standards.

Pharmaceutical manufacturing facilities may also need to sample, collect and possibly treat stormwater according to federal or state stormwater permitting requirements. Careful planning is necessary to reduce or eliminate sources of regulated stormwater since it will affect the construction and operating costs of a facility. Prevention of environmental impact to groundwater must also be considered in facility design and operation. Engineering design and operational options such as double-walled underground piping, separate wastewater collection and treatment systems, and leak containment and detection must be considered.

Wastewater Permitting

The permitting requirements and process for wastewater discharges parallel the air permitting requirements and process. In this case, Federal legislation called the Clean Water Act passed responsibility for regulating wastewater discharges to the USEPA. If a state chooses, they may implement their own wastewater programs that must be at least as stringent as USEPA requirements. State programs are approved by the USEPA.

For facilities that will discharge wastewater to a POTW, participation in a wastewater pretreatment program is usually required. Pretreatment requirements are set by the USEPA and require POTWs that receive wastewater from industrial sources to enforce pretreatment programs. Under pretreatment regulations, POTWs identify and require a pretreatment permit for significant industrial users who discharge into their plant. The issued permit contains discharge limits and monitoring requirements for these individual sources.

A significant industrial user is defined as a facility that 1) is an industrial user subject to categorical standards (described below); 2) discharges more than 25,000 gallons of wastewater per day; 3) will make up 5% or more of the POTW's wastewater treatment capacity; or 4) is determined to present a reasonable potential for either adversely affecting the POTW's operation or for violating a pretreatment standard.

All facilities discharging to a POTW under a pretreatment program are required to prevent discharge of pollutants that will result in damage to the wastewater system, potentially harm sewer workers, interfere with the POTW's ability to treat wastewater, or pass through the POTW in violation of its permit conditions. For example, prohibitions include pollutants that might corrode or cause fire or explosion in the sewage collection or treatment system or that could raise the POTW influent temperature above 104 °F.

Pretreatment permits require wastewater sampling by the permittee to demonstrate that permitted discharge conditions are met. The pretreatment regulations also identify specific wastewater discharge and monitoring standards for industries in certain industrial categories called categorical standards or effluent limit guidelines. Pretreatment categorical standards have been set for four subcategories of pharmaceutical manufacturing: fermentation; extraction products; chemical synthesis; and mixing, compounding, and formulation. The pharmaceutical categorical standards are described in 40 CFR Part 439. The pretreatment categorical standards are tied to Standard Industrial Classification (SIC) codes for pharmaceutical manufacturing (Codes 2833, 2834, and 2836). There are no categorical pretreatment requirements for pharmaceutical R&D activities unless the facility will discharge directly to surface waters from an on-site treatment plant.

Discharge limitations under the categorical pretreatment standards are specific to the type of pharmaceutical manufacturing. For example, discharge requirements for the chemical synthesis subcategory include about 24 parameters, mainly organic solvents, while the mixing, compounding, and formulation subcategory includes only 5 parameters (acetone, n-amyl acetate, ethyl acetate, isopropyl acetate, and methylene chloride).

Regulatory agencies encourage POTWs to require other or more restrictive standards for their industrial users depending on local (e.g., plant-specific) or regional environmental concerns. For example, limits for radioactive materials and certain heavy metals may be included or be lower than EPA limits. Since many of the limits are concentration based, facility planners must prepare a detailed pollutant discharge and water use estimate, which considers both average and peak wastewater discharges at the facility.

If the decision is made to treat wastewater on-site, a permit must be obtained from the USEPA or state environmental agency. If the treated wastewater will be discharged to a river, stream or other body of water, an NPDES permit (National Pollutant Discharge Elimination System) is required. An NPDES permit sets requirements for treatment plant operation, including pollutant discharge criteria.

The pharmaceutical categorical standards (40 CFR Part 439) also describe NPDES effluent limits for the four pharmaceutical manufacturing categories and for pharmaceutical R&D. These limits are abbreviated as BCT, BAT, BPT, and NSPS limits. Whichever discharge option is chosen, the regulatory permit writer must consider the environmental impact of the discharge in setting treatment requirements. For example, a wastewater plant that will discharge to a stream that is designated as environmentally sensitive or is significant for recreational or historical reasons will be subject to more stringent discharge requirements. Often, negotiations are required between the permitting agency and the permittee, particularly in communities where development pressures are high or where there are environmentally sensitive receiving waters.

Facility Design Considerations for Wastewater Management and Groundwater Protection

In order for a permit to be written for discharge of wastewater, the facility designer must identify all potential sources of wastewater and pollutants from the proposed facility and whether the predicted discharge will present a permitting issue. If so, engineering controls to pretreat or treat the wastewater will be necessary. Decisions must be made as to the feasibility of treating multiple pollutant sources in the facility either individually or in a combined stream.

Pharmaceutical manufacturing and some R&D work often involve a batch process that results in short-term high pollutant concentration peaks in wastewater discharges. If these batch discharge peaks could result in exceedance of discharge permit limits, methods to treat or moderate the discharge must be considered. The most common pollutants of regulatory concern found in pharmaceutical facility wastewater include organic solvents, biochemical or chemical oxygen demand (BOD_5 or COD), and pH. Metals are often included in pharmaceutical facility wastewater permitting criteria but are not commonly a discharge issue. Compatibility of the materials of construction with the characteristics of the wastewater must be considered during the design of the facility. For example, copper plumbing should not be used in a drain line for acidic wastewater both because it might fail from corrosion but also may result in wastewater discharge above copper concentration limits.

A relatively simple method to spread out pollutant discharge concentration peaks over time is to install an equalization system. An equalization tank system, which collects a large volume of wastewater and utilizes either passive or active mixing before discharge, can be designed and installed to meet this requirement. Equalization systems can be installed to collect wastewater from a process area, a building, or for an entire site in order to take advantage of the larger wastewater flow for mixing.

Some process wastewater is better treated at its source. Wastewater from chemical API, fermentation, and some pharmaceutical manufacturing processes are well suited for treatment at the point of generation since treatment systems are often more efficient at treating wastewater with higher pollutant concentrations.

Several types of treatment systems are available for wastewater from chemical API and pharmaceutical manufacturing processes. Membrane filtration, ozonization, and ultraviolet (UV) light systems can be considered either alone or in combination to treat effluent from chemical reactor systems (e.g., cleaning, aqueous rinses, and mother liquors) and from aqueous-based pharmaceutical compounding and bottling processes (e.g., tailings and primary cleaning). Treatment efficiency will vary considerably depending upon the physical/chemical properties of the pollutant(s) to be removed. These treated wastewaters can also be discharged to equalization systems to further reduce plant discharge concentrations. Another treatment system for wastewater with highly concentrated pollutants is an evaporation system that uses heat to evaporate water from wastewater, resulting in a sludge waste for disposal.

Pharmaceutical fermentation systems are usually designed with the capability to thermally inactivate the culture organisms as the final step of the batch process. Fermentation processes usually generate wastewater with a high BOD/COD loading that can be moderated by an equalization system.

Wastewater produced by facility support equipment at pharmaceutical plants is also well suited to pretreatment at its source. For example, pH control systems are commonly installed on boiler blowdown and washing equipment discharges where corrosive cleaning chemicals are used. Treatment of discharges from water treatment systems such as RO and ion exchange equipment is usually not necessary, but should be considered depending on local limits. If good work procedures are implemented in a lab facility, pH control is not usually needed for wastewater from laboratories. However, neutralization/equalization systems should be considered as a precaution, particularly for large lab facilities. In some instances, the installation of a pH neutralization system may be a requirement for obtaining a construction permit from local permitting agency to ensure that the discharge of the wastewater from the facility will meet the local requirements and not cause damage to the sewer system.

If on-site wastewater treatment is chosen, a plant must be designed to meet the present and future treatment requirements for the facility's discharge. Discussion of design of wastewater treatment facilities is beyond the scope of this text. Treatment plant designers should consider both sequential batch reactor (SBR) type or membrane type wastewater treatment systems. Both types of treatment systems are well suited to handle the peak load conditions of wastewater discharged from the batch processes typical of many pharmaceutical manufacturing operations.

All systems handling wastewater, including plumbing, tank and treatment systems, must be designed to be capable of reliably containing the physical and chemical constituents they will carry. Consideration should be made to install double-walled systems with leak detection in critical systems, particularly where potential groundwater contamination might result from failure of primary systems. Similarly, oil and process chemical tanks and tank filling areas should be designed with secondary containment, dikes, berms, or other spill- and leak-containment systems.

Stormwater

Water discharges from runoff of rainwater and snowmelt in contact with pharmaceutical manufacturing and construction activities must also be permitted according to USEPA stormwater requirements. Most states have USEPA-approved programs to regulate stormwater. It is particularly important to design manufacturing facilities to reduce or eliminate exposure of stormwater to materials handling and other activities and equipment to minimize operational requirements of stormwater permits.

Similar to the wastewater regulations, stormwater requirements for pharmaceutical facilities are triggered by manufacturing in the 283-SIC codes. Pharmaceutical R&D facilities are exempt from stormwater requirements as long as the facility has not been assigned a 283-SIC code.

A stormwater permit is required if a pharmaceutical manufacturing facility will conduct activities with raw materials, intermediates, products, by-products, or wastes, that will be exposed to stormwater. Stormwater permits require stormwater sampling and a description of methods to prevent pollution resulting from stormwater runoff. The most common method for stormwater pollution prevention is collection and containment and, if necessary, treatment. Collection and containment of stormwater is commonly achieved by installation of dikes, curbs and sloped surfaces that drain into a water-impermeable basin.

There are two types of stormwater permits that can be obtained: a general permit and an individual permit. The general permit is most often used because it includes pre-written operating conditions for multiple types of industrial activities; these are more quickly approved. The individual permit requires specific permit conditions to be written by the permittee, which must be reviewed and approved by the permitting agency.

In order to avoid the operational and most of the permitting requirements of a stormwater permit, the facility can be designed so that no stormwater exposure to industrial materials will occur. In this case, a conditional-no exposure exclusion can be claimed in lieu of a permit. Since most pharmaceutical manufacturing and warehousing activities are conducted indoors, this exclusion is usually accomplished by ensuring that all materials handling operations and equipment such as loading docks are protected from rainfall.

Construction activities where more than one acre will be disturbed also require NPDES stormwater permitting. Construction stormwater permits require two components: erosion and sedimentation (E&S) control and stormwater management.

An E&S control plan is usually also required by the municipality where construction will occur. The E&S plan describes measures that will be taken to prevent environmental damage from unstablized soil from clearing, grading, and excavation activities being washed by water runoff into nonconstruction areas. This can be accomplished by installation of basins to collect stormwater, gravel beds, and "silt fences" that allow water but not soil permeation.

Stormwater management practices incorporated into construction permits include housekeeping, containment, and other management practices to prevent pollutants at construction sites such as fuels, oil, paint and other chemicals and materials used in construction from causing environmental damage after stormwater exposure.

WASTE STORAGE AND WASTE HANDLING ISSUES

All pharmaceutical manufacturing facilities will generate waste materials that must be properly disposed of after the wastes are generated. The wastes from pharmaceutical manufacturing facilities can be categorized into municipal, industrial, hazardous, infectious/medical, and other special types of waste materials. Federal legislation identified as the Resource Conservation and Recovery Act (RCRA) passed responsibility to the EPA for regulating the generation, storage, transportation, treatment, and disposal of hazardous waste. Many states have written their own rules and regulations that have been approved by the EPA that implement these requirements. Figure 3 depicts the sources and disposal methods for waste materials from a typical pharmaceutical manufacturing facility.

FIGURE 3   Sources and Disposal Methods for Waste Materials

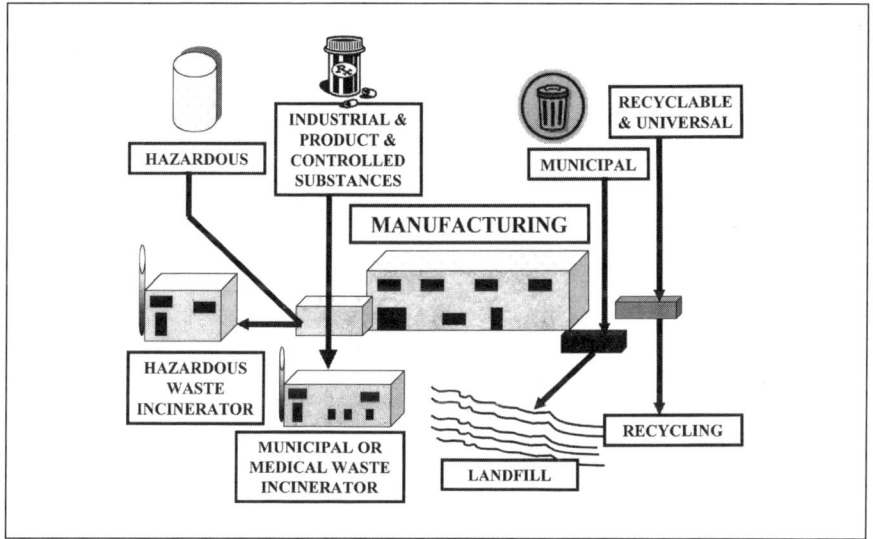

Most pharmaceutical manufacturing facilities only store waste materials that are generated during operation of the facility and hire others to transport, treat, and/or dispose of these waste materials. In this case, most states have specific requirements for the generation and storage of waste materials prior to having others transport the waste materials for disposal. However, in some instances, facilities may treat and dispose of wastes onsite, which requires significantly more oversight and involvement with the regulatory agency than a facility that just generates and stores wastes.

Permitting requirements are minimal for facilities that only generate and store wastes. Therefore, the impact to project schedule is minimal. However, during the design of the facility, careful consideration must be given to how the waste will be handled and stored so that the manufacturing operations of the facility are not impacted. Issues that must be addressed during the design of the facility include:

- How will the waste be moved from the point of generation to storage prior to disposal?
- How will the storage areas be laid out?
- How much room is required for storage?
- How will storage areas be designed for safe storage of incompatible and flammable wastes?
- How is the waste transported from the facility to the disposal facility?
- Do the waste storage areas require secondary containment?
- Do the waste transfer areas require secondary containment?

Figure 4 is a picture of a typical solvent waste storage area.

FIGURE 4   Waste Storage Area

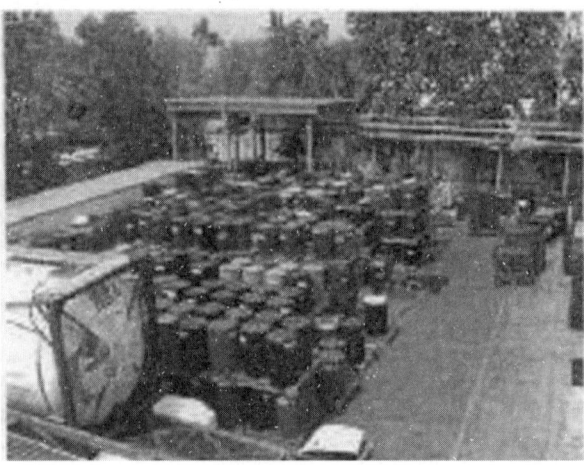

If waste treatment, such as incineration of solvent (hazardous) waste or other waste types is considered, the facility designer should understand the complexity, time, and additional cost that will be required to obtain the necessary construction permits from the appropriate regulatory agencies. Companies typically choose to treat wastes on-site if there is a perceived sensitivity to the waste material, (e.g., biological waste from research and development that the company may not want transported over public highways or disposed of in inappropriate locations). Alternatively, a facility may want to have complete "cradle-to-grave" responsibility of the waste material to ensure proper treatment and disposal of the waste materials generated at the facility.

One of the key components of waste management rules and regulations is pollution prevention. Therefore, it is recommended that a complete analysis of the waste streams that will be generated by the facility be conducted during the design of the facility. The evaluation should include ways that the amount of waste generated at the facility can be minimized in order to reduce the burden associated with the storage, treatment and ultimate disposal of the waste generated at the facility.

The following sections describe the different types of waste materials that can be generated by a pharmaceutical manufacturing facility and discuss some of the environmental issues related to the specific waste types.

Municipal Waste

Municipal waste is the most common form of waste generated at pharmaceutical manufacturing facilities, and is typically composed of office trash, cafeteria waste, and other solid waste streams that are not the result of industrial processes. While special permits are usually not required for disposal of municipal waste, procedures should be established to ensure that other special waste streams are not inadvertently co-mingled with the municipal waste. This is particularly important in states or municipalities where specific requirements exist for industrial waste streams or recyclable materials. Waste containers of all types and sizes must be clearly identified to designate what type of waste they contain, and personnel must be made aware of the different waste streams and their acceptable components.

Waste minimization and reduction requirements may also be an aspect of the local regulations, so that determination and tracking of the amount of municipal waste generated may be required for either reporting reasons or as part of the minimization plan. Regular tracking of the amount of waste generated for all waste streams can be very useful to identify potential areas of waste minimization and reduction, which in turn can generate significant financial savings. Many elements of municipal waste can also be segregated for recycling, further reducing disposal costs.

All waste streams should have designated disposal areas and dedicated containers. Storage areas, collection methods and transport routes should be an important consideration in facility design. These can be important with respect to maintaining GMP compliance and for maintaining acceptable aesthetics.

Recyclables

While paper and glass have traditionally been seen as the primary focus of a recycling program, the type and scope of recyclable materials has been expanding, particularly in the office environment. At a site level, office paper and cardboard are still a key component of any recycling program. Glass, aluminum, and plastic containers, such as those in cafeteria waste, are also traditionally part of a recycling program.

In the office setting, items such as toner cartridges, ink-jet cartridges, and computer electronics have the potential to be recycled. Many of these items contain significant amounts of hazardous metals that can leach out and potentially contaminate the environment when deposited in a landfill. A typical computer monitor, for example, may contain several pounds of lead. Donation programs can be employed to supplement recycling, such as the donation of surplus or outdated computer equipment to institutions within the local community. Many states and municipalities may have specific recycling requirements and may also require periodic reporting of the amount of material recycled. As with municipal waste, a tracking program should be established to identify the type and amount of waste recycled on a regular basis (2).

Industrial Waste

Industrial waste includes waste generated from industrial processes, which, in most cases, must be handled differently from conventional municipal waste. Typical industrial wastes encountered in the pharmaceutical industry may include unused packaging, blister packs and foil, unused gelatin capsules, dusts from air filtration or vacuum systems, off-spec or outdated materials, and unused product containers (3). Secondary materials, such as wood pallets, may also be considered industrial waste.

Some states have placed restrictions on where industrial waste may be sent for disposal. Landfills and incinerators may require special permits in order to be able to accept and process industrial waste streams. This may in turn require the company generating the waste to quantify and report the types of industrial waste sent for disposal, and may also require that waste reduction plans be created and implemented for these types of wastes. Many times approvals are required from the disposal facility prior to accepting wastes from a company. Therefore, companies should make sure contracts are established with the waste disposal company prior to initiating operations at the new facility that generate wastes. Procedures must be put in place to ensure that, like municipal waste, these wastes are not accidentally mixed with other non-industrial wastes. Recycling opportunities may also be identified, such as for cardboard or wood materials, to help reduce the amount of industrial waste sent for disposal.

Product Waste

Off-specification and returned or recalled finished products, including sample returns, may frequently need to be sent for disposal from the facility. These can range in amounts from a few small packages to a trailer load of finished products. Expired bulk materials, including both active ingredients and excipients, may also require disposal. Product waste must be segregated from the other municipal and industrial waste streams, and careful consideration must be given to the components and their chemical characteristics.

Incineration of product waste is the preferred method of destruction for most pharmaceutical manufacturing companies, and waste vendors that offer incineration will require a detailed profile of the constituents of the product waste. Key characteristics that may need to be identified include sulfur and halogen content of the product, and whether the product contains any hazardous components (such as flammable or compressed gases, flammable solvents, metals, or toxic materials) (4). Some product wastes (e.g., waste chemotherapy drugs) may need to be disposed of as a hazardous waste.

Good sources of information to facilitate this profiling include the company's Manufacturer's Safety Data Sheets (MSDSs), the *U.S. Pharmacopoeia,* and internal documents that define the chemical composition and percentages. As with industrial waste, special permits and reporting requirements may be necessary to accept and process product waste. Procedures should also be in place to provide for GMP compliance where necessary, such as logging of lot numbers prior to release for disposal.

Hazardous Waste

Hazardous wastes are wastes that pose specific hazards based on their chemical and physical characteristics. Some of these wastes are specifically listed, while others may exhibit a particular hazardous characteristic. Some of the listed wastes are individual substances, while others are process-specific.

If a solid, liquid, gas, or mixture meets the characteristic definition or appears on one of the lists, it must be handled and disposed of as a hazardous waste. Hazardous characteristics include ignitability, corrosivity, reactivity, and toxicity. Listed process-specific wastes include mixtures of spent solvents from selected activities, as well as other substances that may appear on product lists. Federal regulations under RCRA require these wastes to be disposed of as hazardous waste. Many states also include specific hazardous waste regulations that supplement, but do not replace, the federal regulations.

Within a pharmaceutical final-dosage manufacturing facility, the most common source of hazardous waste is spent flammable solvents and solvent mixtures generated by the QA/QC laboratories. Facilities producing parenterals may also generate expired acids and bases that would normally be used for pH adjustment. Facilities that manufacture the actual API are very chemical intensive and generate significant amounts of solvent-laden waste that would be classified as hazardous waste. In some cases, expired products may also contain hazardous constituents, and some active ingredients may also be hazardous; examples of these include ethanol and benzoyl peroxide.

In all cases, strict storage and handling requirements must be followed and specific RCRA training and detailed emergency plans, i.e., Preparedness, Prevention and Contingency Plans (PPC Plans), are required. All facilities that generate hazardous waste must acquire an EPA identification number. This number is location specific, so that companies with multiple locations must apply for a separate identification number for each facility.

Depending on how much waste they generate on an annual basis, facilities are allowed to store waste for several months without being required to acquire a permit as a hazardous waste storage facility. In most cases, storage of accumulated waste when exempt from permitting requirements is limited to 90 days. While this allows the facility to exempt itself from the storage facility permit requirements, a strict set of regulations still apply to the handling, storage, and disposal of these wastes. Failure to adhere to these regulations can result in significant penalties and monetary fines.

Adequate space must be allocated for dedicated storage of hazardous waste; and specific design requirements pertaining to security, fire protection, ventilation, and spill containment are key considerations when designing these spaces. Storage facilities must be designed to prevent incompatible hazardous wastes (e.g., acid, oxidizer, and flammable wastes) from reacting with each other. Hazardous waste liquids must also be stored in areas capable of containing a spill of the largest container or 10% of total storage capacity, whichever is greater. Disposal of hazardous wastes also carries significant potential for future liability if not handled correctly. Companies that generate and dispose of these wastes retain "strict liability," so that if the waste is improperly handled or disposed of by the selected waste vendor, the generating company can be held responsible for future costs of mitigation or remediation related to the waste. Therefore, selection of a qualified waste vendor is critical to avoiding this potential liability. Many companies choose to perform an initial audit of its selected transportation and disposal companies to ensure that these facilities perform their waste management activities in compliance with the hazardous waste regulations. A periodic audits process should also be instituted to ensure continued compliance with the hazardous waste management rules and regulations. The actual disposal of these wastes also requires adherence to a manifest system that tracks the movement and ultimate disposal of the waste. More than any other type of waste, hazardous waste requires a high level of training, record keeping, and site planning to ensure regulatory compliance (5).

Other Special Wastes

Waste streams that may be less prevalent at a manufacturing site would include biological (i.e., medical or infectious controled substances) or radioactive wastes. Both require special handling and specialized waste vendors. Handling, storage, and disposal are subject to both federal and, in many cases, state and local regulation. In the event that significant amounts of these wastes are generated on a regular basis, care must be taken to provide secure, dedicated areas for storage and accumulation. As with all types of waste streams, transport routes within the facility should be carefully laid out to prevent potential contamination that could occur during collection and transport to the storage area.

CONCLUSION

This chapter provided an overview of the environmental compliance issues that must be addressed during the design, construction, and operation of a final dosage manufacturing facility. The emphasis has been on issues surrounding the discharge of air emissions and wastewater, and the generation of solid waste at these facilities. The cost impact associated with addressing environmental compliance during the design and construction of the manufacturing facility is minimal compared to the overall cost of the project. If pollution control equipment for air emissions and/or wastewater is required or waste processing equipment such as incinerators are desired, the construction costs for the facility will increase, but the cost of this equipment is still minimal compared to the cost for the construction of the rest of the facility.

Compliance with the environmental requirements can impact the design and construction of the facility in other ways. One example is the decision of where to build the new facility. Factors that may impact site location include:

- *Complexity and strictness of the regulations for the desired location.* The U.S. EPA develops regulations must be followed throughout the United States; however, many areas have regional that regulations that are more complex and strict than other areas because of local environmental sensitivity or because the air and water quality in the area cannot be impacted significantly.
- *Available utilities.* It is much easier to locate a facility in an area where sewers and a wastewater treatment plant are available than to choose a location where the facility must design and operate its own wastewater treatment plant and obtain a permit to discharge the wastewater to a nearby stream or river.

Environmental compliance issues can also impact project schedule. As mentioned previously, many regulatory agencies require that environmental permit applications be submitted and approved prior to initiating construction of the facility. Depending on the types of sources that will be operated at the facility, this may even include groundbreaking activities. Review and approval time by many regulatory agencies is 3-months or more and can sometimes take up to 18-months if the facility will emit large amounts of air contaminants. Examples of projects that may require significant review and approval times are facilities located near major metropolitan areas that have the potential to emit more than 25 tons per year of volatile organic compounds and/or oxides of nitrogen from sources like boilers, internal combustion units for electric generators, and manufacturing equipment that uses organic solvents. Facilities in other areas of the United States that emit more than 100 tons per year of these and other pollutants will also require significant review time.

Therefore, it is recommended that a serious evaluation of the environmental requirements be performed during the basis of design (BOD) phase of the project. This will ensure that all of the requirements are identified early in the project and the impact on the project schedule and cost to address the environmental compliance issues can be determined. The evaluation will also help avoid the hidden surprises such as potential violations and monetary penalties for installing and operating equipment that does not meet the necessary requirements. In a worst case situation, the regulatory agency may even require that the installed equipment be shut down and not operated until the necessary approvals have been obtained. Therefore, it is prudent that these requirements be addressed even though it appears that the impact of these requirements is small compared to the rest of the issues surrounding the construction and operation of the final dosage pharmaceutical manufacturing facility.

REFERENCES

1. Buonicore A., Davis, W. (eds.) Air & Waste Management Association, *Air Pollution Engineering Manual.* New York: Van Nostrand Reinhold, 1992.
2. Glysson E.A. Solid Waste. In: Corbitt R.A. *Standard Handbook of Environmental Engineering.* New York: McGraw-Hill, 1990.
3. EPA Office of Compliance Sector Notebook *Project: Profile of the Pharmaceutical Manufacturing Industry.* Washington, D.C.: US Government Printing Office, 1997.
4. Davis M.L. Definition and Classification of Hazardous Waste. In: Freeman H.M. (ed.) *Standard Handbook of Hazardous Waste Treatment and Disposal,* 2nd Ed. New York: McGraw Hill, 1998.
5. Karnofsky B. (ed.) *Hazardous Waste Management Compliance Handbook.* New York: Van Nostrand Reinhold, 1992.

APPENDIX: GLOSSARY

API (Active Pharmaceutical Ingredient). The compound or medicinal component of the finished solid dosage pharmaceutical.

BOD (Basis of Design). A written summary of the design requirements of a facility based on the general requirements for its operational function.

BOD or BOD5 (Biochemical Oxygen Demand). A measure of the concentration of pollutants in wastewater which can be broken down by the oxygen consuming biological organisms (mainly bacteria) in a treatment plant.

Categorical Standard. Industry specific standards for treatment, or control of discharge of pollutants under U.S. Clean Water Act or Clean Air Act.

Clean Air Act. A statute passed by Congress and most recently amended in 1990 that regulates the emission of air contaminants to atmosphere.

Clean Water Act. A statute passed by Congress in 1972 and most recently amended in 1987 that regulates discharge of wastewater to surface waters.

COD (Chemical Oxygen Demand). A measure of the concentration of pollutants in wastewater. The COD test measures reduction of chromic acid, a chemical oxidant when mixed with a wastewater sample. Results are expressed in the oxygen equivalent of the reduction.

Criteria Pollutants. Six common air pollutants: ozone, particulate matter, carbon monoxide, nitrogen dioxide, sulfur dioxide, and lead regulated by EPA to protect public health and welfare.

EDU (Equivalent Discharge Unit). A unit of measure for wastewater discharges that is used to track available capacity at the POTW. Typically it is based on the amount of wastewater that can be discharged from a typical, single family dwelling unit. The value of an EDU is typically in the range of 200 to 300 gallons per day.

EPA. Environmental Protection Agency

HAPs (Hazardous Air Pollutants). 188 compounds defined by the Clean Air Act that are toxic in nature.

MSDS (Manufacturer's Safety Data Sheet). A data sheet that list properties, components, safety procedures, and hazards related to the material or mixture of materials.

HEPA. High efficiency particulate air filter, which removes 99.8% of particles 0.3 microns and larger.

NAICS Code. See SIC Code.

NESHAPs (National Emission Standards for Hazardous Air Pollutants). Air quality standards for specific sources that emit any one of the 188 compounds defined as Hazardous Air Pollutants.

NPDES (National Pollutant Discharge Elimination System). A USEPA term to describe programs, including pre-treatment, treatment, enforcement, and permitting under the Clean Water Act for discharge of wastewater or stormwater to a water body.

NSPS (New Source Performance Standards). Air quality standards for specific sources of conventional pollutants.

Ozone. Ground level air contaminant regulated by EPA that is created through the oxidation of oxygen by volatile organic compounds (VOCs) and oxides of nitrogen. VOCs and oxides of nitrogen are two of the main pollutants emitted by pharmaceutical manufacturing facilities.

PTE (Potential to Emit). Maximum capacity of an emission source or facility to emit any air pollutant under its physical and operational design. Physical or operational limitations on a source, including air pollution control equipment, restrictions on hours of operation, or the type and amount of material processed or used can be considered as part of the sources design limitation.

POTW (Publicly Owned Treatment Works). A municipal or other publicly owned wastewater (sewage) treatment plant.

Pretreatment. Treatment of wastewater (usually industrial) before discharge to a POTW.

RCRA (Resource Conservation and Recovery Act). Federal legislation passed by Congress that authorized the EPA to develop and enforce regulations related to the generation, transportation, treatment, and disposal of hazardous waste.

SIC Code (Standard Industrial Classification Code). A numbering system described by the U.S. Office of Management and Budget that classified American industries into certain groupings and sub-groupings by business activity. The SIC coding is being replaced by a new, more specific system called the NAICS. The SIC or NAICS code that an industry falls under will often determine its environmental permitting, operational, and reporting requirements.

SPDES (State Pollutant Discharge Elimination System). A term used to describe an NPDES program administered under a state environmental agency.

Stormwater. Water runoff from rain, snow melt, surfaces, and drainage

Surface Water. Water in a body open to the air such as a stream, river, or lake.

USEPA. U.S. Environmental Protection Agency.

VOC. Volatile organic compounds including most volatile solvents.

WWTP. Wastewater Treatment Plant.

19

Support Laboratories

Author: Terry Jacobs

Advisor: Robert J. Hoernlein

INTRODUCTION

Research and development laboratories are the engines for the pharmaceutical industry; they are where basic research is conducted, compounds are developed, and initial chemical supplies are produced for testing. In a pharmaceutical manufacturing facility, support laboratories are required for testing of the product, and are typically referred to as quality control (QC) laboratories or quality assurance (QA) laboratories. These support the manufacturing operations. Both types have similarities and differences.

The laboratory environment is a place where creative and practical work is conducted. Functional and safety concerns are of importance to protect both the employee and the product. The design of the laboratory environment must take into account the specific needs of this environment, anticipate what changes must occur in the future, and, in the end, create a work environment that is conducive to supporting the facility's mission.

Laboratories are high-energy users and are expensive to build. The energy costs of a typical support laboratory with 100% outside air can be five times that of a normal laboratory. QA laboratories may have recirculated air, or may be at least 100% exhausted.

The laboratory is a strategic tool for the pharmaceutical company, and it is an expensive environment to create. This chapter discusses how to program and design a pharmaceutical support laboratory and how to identify the key issues in this process for both new facilities and the renovation of existing facilities.

CONCEPTS AND PRINCIPLES

Key concepts and principles in designing a laboratory are:

- Establishing a laboratory module
- Understanding the equipment used in a (QC) laboratory
- Creating a "lab" card
- Understanding linear feet of bench required
- Determining whether to use 100% outside air or recirculated air
- Lab flexibility
- Open vs. discrete laboratories
- Compliance issues
- Location of office/write-up space

PROGRAMMING THE LABORATORY FACILITY

This is the program-seeking phase where the criteria for the design identified. In the design process it is critical to differentiate between problem seeking (programming) and problem solving (design).

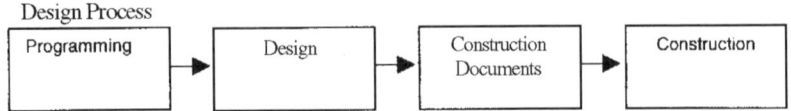

The reason this is important is that there is a natural tendency to begin to solve problems (design) before the design problems (criteria) are defined. The programming phase is where "problem solving" should be identified.

The programming of the facility starts with the mission statement for the project. The mission statement will identify the need for the project, and will help you understand what the business and functional drivers are for the project. Examples would include how much flexibility are you trying to design into your facility or upgrading of existing facilities.

INFORMATION GATHERING: DEFINING THE USERS' NEEDS

The key to information gathering is communication and documentation. The programmer will interview the user to help define their needs, to identify what functions are occurring in their laboratory, and to understand the inter-relationship between their laboratory and other spaces. A "user survey form" is a useful tool to initiate this process.

The following diagram indicates the steps involved in the development of a typical program document.

The following discussion describes and gives examples of the steps presented in the diagram.

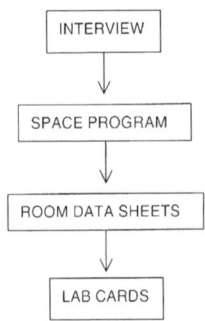

Interview Phase

The interview phase is where the key users are interviewed to define their needs. Issuing questionnaires to complete before interviews is an effective methodology for obtaining information. The scientists and technicians are typically busy; therefore, you must be the editor of the information and assist them in completing the questionnaire. The user should also provide an equipment list of all the present and anticipated future equipment to be utilized.

Typically the following is an example of a typical equipment list for a quality control laboratory. Remember: It is important to gather an equipment list early in the design process.

An Equipment List Is a Basic First Step

Equipment List

No.	Equipment Name	Services Required	Electrical Requirements	UPS Power
001	HPLC	He		
002	HPLC Computer			•
003	HPLC Printer			•
004	Atomic Absorption	CA, Acetylene, N_2O	110v	
005	Dissolution Baths			•
006	FTIR	N_2, Jug Dour, Liquid N_2		•
007	TOC Analyzers		110v	•
008	Milli-Q	DI		
009	UV VIS			•
009	UV VIS Computer			•
010	UV VIS Printer			•
011	Multi-Dose			•
012	Culter Counter		110v	•
013	Light Cabinet			
014	Gas Chromotographs	N_2, Compressed Air	220v	•
015	Gas Chromotographs Computers			•
016	Centrifuge			
017	TPW Table		220v	•
018	Moisture Analyzer			•
019	Nitrogen Generator			•
020	Refrigerator/Freezer		110v	
021	Ovens			
022	Balance Tables			
023	Solvent Storage Cabinets			
024	Book Shelves			
025	Bio-Safety Cabinet			
026	Fume Hood, 12'-0"			
027	Fume Hood, 10'-0"			
028	Fume Hood, 8'-0"			
029	Sink	HCW, DI, EW		
030	Glassware Washer	HCW, DI, CA	480v, 60Hz, 3∅, 30A	
031	Glassware Washer	HCW, DI, CA	480v, 60Hz, 3∅, 30A	
032	Glassware Dryer		208v, 60 Hz, 3∅, 22A	
033	Balance Slab			

Space Program

The space program is a matrix of the required spaces, sizes, and adjacencies, and their projected growth. It is the first step in the programming phase and will establish the first indication of the size of the facility. The space program can be expanded to contain information of lab services, adjacencies, fume hoods and so forth.

A typical QC laboratory will be comprised of the primary laboratory space and the support spaces, which include office space, stability rooms, chemical storage rooms, glass wash and amenities such as a break room.

In establishing a space program for a laboratory, a laboratory-planning module must be established, which will become the planning basis for the facility.

High Pressure Liquid Chromatography (HPLC)
This is used for testing and requires bench top space or racking.

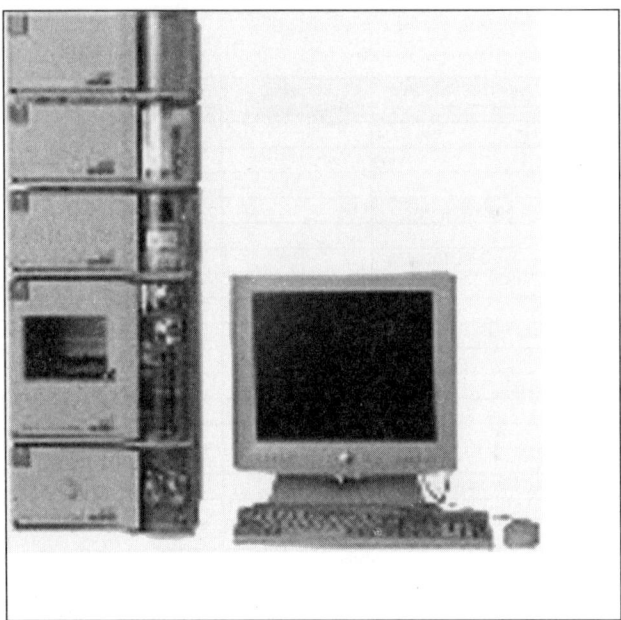

Laboratory Planning Module

The laboratory planning module is the space allocated for each scientist and technician in a facility and should provide a standard amount of space for a typical user. To understand how to generate a laboratory module, it is important to understand how laboratory casework is designed and how it functions. Casework may be *fixed* or *flexible*. The following diagram is a section cut through a typical fixed laboratory bench.

The standard distance between centerline of benches ranges from 10 feet to 11 feet. This space is set by the amount of space needed for two people to work back to back. The standard fume hood is deeper (i.e. 36 inches) and in a 10 foot module will be tight if placed back to back.

Cross-Section of a Fixed Laboratory Bench

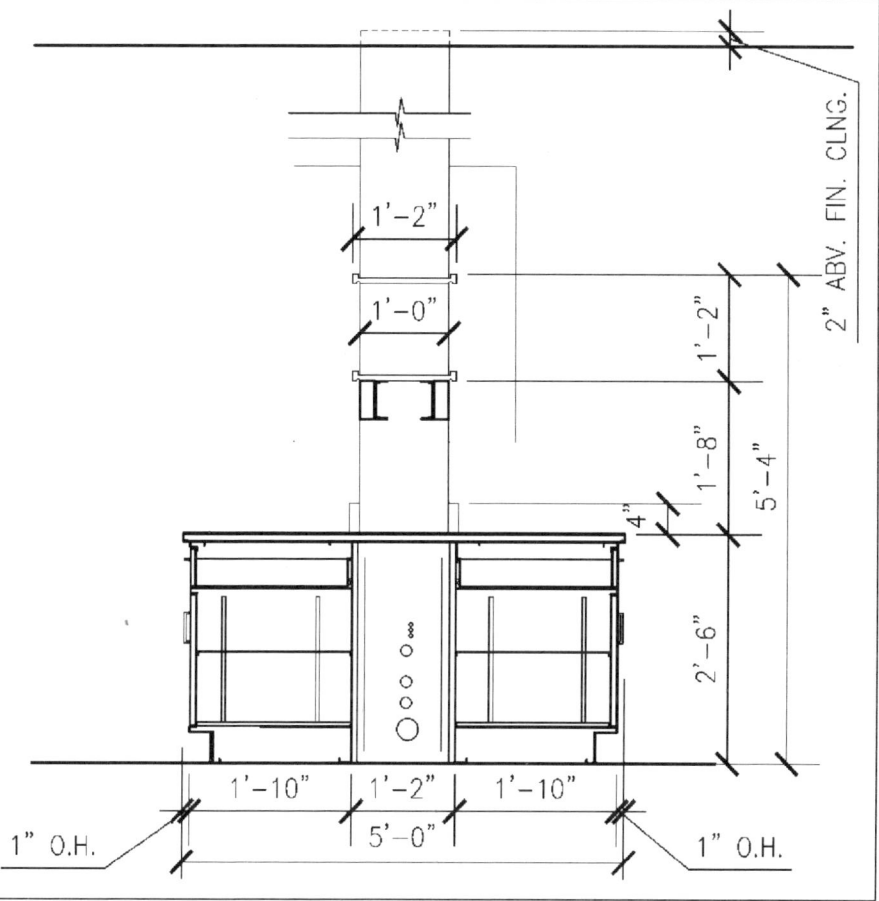

> KEY CONCEPT: Allow for door widths greater than 36 inches wide in rooms that contain fume hoods; otherwise, the fume hood will not fit through the door!

Based on the selection of a planning module of 10 feet to 11 feet, we next will develop a plan for a generic lab module, which will have bench space and office space for the users.

The users will define the ELF (equivalent linear feet) of bench required for each person, and the size and relationship of the office space required.

Rules of thumb indicate that a bench should be no longer than approximately 16 feet. A module is for planning purposes only; the decision to have an "open lab" vs. enclosed rooms may be made at a later date. The result of this exercise is a selection of a planning module for programming.

In addition to the required bench and fume hood spaces, space for equipment and services are required, which can be programmed into the module on a separate space.

Planning Module

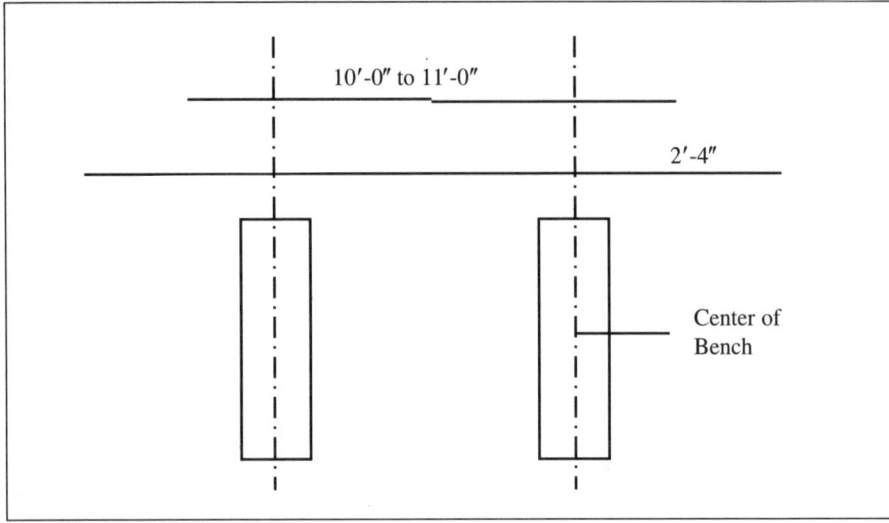

Summary of Space Program

The space program will summarize the total personnel and the total NSF (net square feet) for instance:

Total personnel:	235
Total NSF:	47,000 SF
Total NSF per person:	200 SF

Based on the NSF, a grossing factor that includes walls and circulation can be utilized to determine the range of sizes of this facility. For a laboratory, this factor ranges from 50% to 65%; the calculation is as follows:

$$GSF = \frac{47,000}{.5} = 94,000 \text{ GSF}$$

where GSF is gross square feet. For example, for a facility that is 50% efficient, the total GSF of the facility would be:

$$GSF = \frac{NSF}{\text{Efficiency factor}}$$

KEY CONCEPT: From the GSF we can apply a range of construction costs to determine an initial construction cost. The gross square footage is the actual size of the building or renovated area when complete. A common mistake is not to use the correct grossing factor, "If the space is 30% efficient, I will just add 30% to the net square feet." This is wrong!

Compliance Analysis

As part of the initial programming or Basis of Design Phase (BOD), a compliance analysis of the local and national codes needs to be conducted. Laboratories are potentially hazardous workplaces, that use various solvents and other flammable materials. There also is an increasing trend to use potent compounds, and this will also impact the facility design.

An outline of the relevant codes are as follows:

- International Building Code
- Boca Code
- Local Code Supplements
- The National Codes incorporate by reference other codes such as: National Fire Protection Agency (NFPA) 45 and NFPA 30
- GLPs (Good Laboratory Practices)

Refer to Chapter 15 for complete code information.

KEY CONCEPT: In designing labs to meet the code, remember:

- To understand the quantity of solvents/hazardous materials being used. The code allows for control zones, which govern the amounts of hazardous materials within an area. This is a critical key concept.
- To understand if 100% outside air vs. recirculated air is a requirement. The code will make recommendations for this. Most R&D laboratories are 100% outside air. Many QC laboratories allow for recirculated air. This needs to be discussed with the safety personnel and laboratory director, as well as the design firm.
- Most laboratories are designed as "B" business use.
- To consider pressure requirements for containment. Most laboratories of this nature are designed for negative pressure.

DETAILS/IMPLICATIONS FOR PERFORMANCE

Designing the Laboratory

Creating a "Lab Module" for Planning Purposes

From the programming phase, a laboratory planning module has been established. From the laboratory module, you can begin to organize the laboratory and the concept; i.e., the concept of discrete laboratories or open laboratories. There is a trend (actually, in some companies it is a requirement) to have the office space or write-up space for the technicians and the supervisors located elsewhere and not in the laboratory space.

A discrete lab module is typically a 20 x 30 foot space that has walls on all sides.

In *open laboratories*, walls are eliminated to allow for flexibility and interaction and for sharing of equipment. Except for code issues, there is no limitation on the size of control zones or for the size of open laboratories. The number of control zones is regulated by floor. The control zone determines the quantities of solvents and hazardous materials that may be present.

Discrete Lab Concept

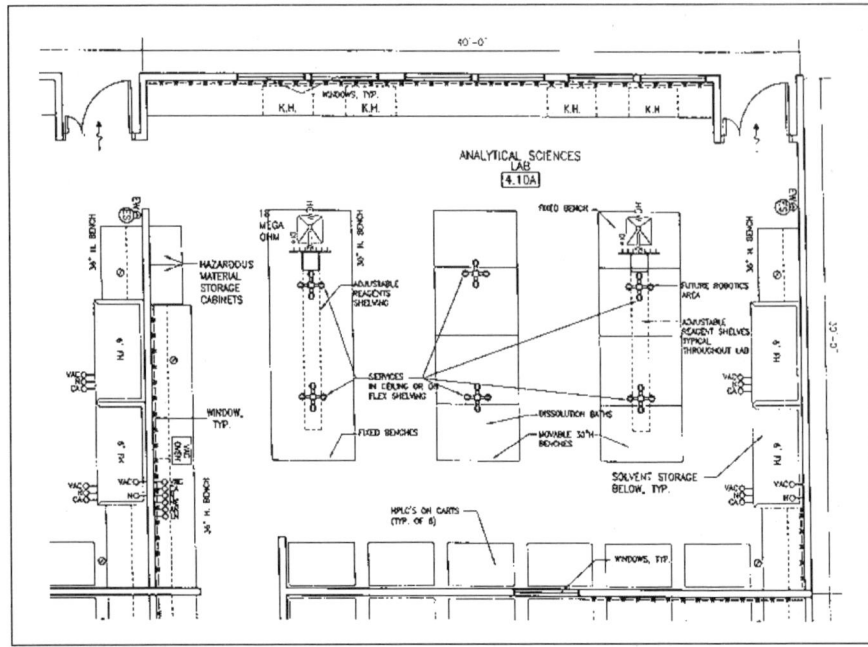

KEY CONCEPTS: Consider what degree of flexibility is desired in the laboratory. This effects the selection of casework and design. For complete flexibility, all the services may be located in the ceiling, with casework on wheels. This is the latest trend in laboratory design.

Movable casework may not be required in QC laboratories where the functions are set up for a period of time to meet the user's needs. There is a range of casework choices that can meet the user's needs and budget.

Open Lab Concept

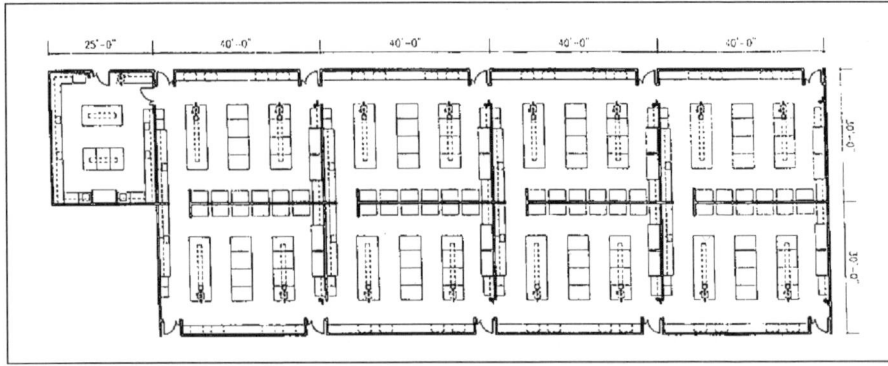

Casework Options

Casework options can vary from fixed benches, systems that are moderately flexible, to completely flexible systems, as the following diagram illustrates.

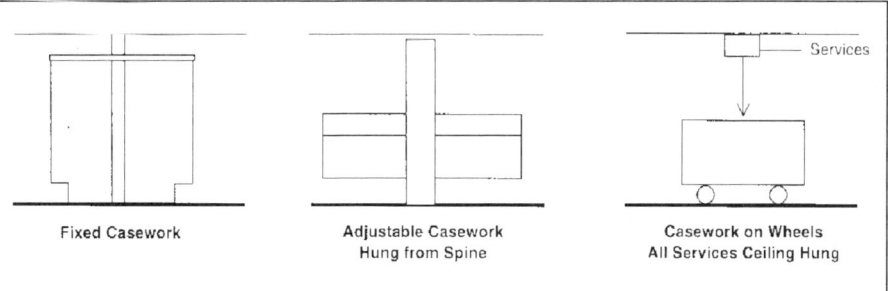

| Fixed Casework | Adjustable Casework Hung from Spine | Casework on Wheels All Services Ceiling Hung |

Many QC laboratories utilize HPLCs, which require bench space and can be stacked. A "low tech" design option is to create a "split bench" that may be lowered to 30 inches instead of the standard 36 inches height.

Providing Space for the Employee

The trend in the design of QC laboratories is to have the employee's workspace located outside the laboratory. This is for health and safety reasons both, as well as practical consideration—the employee can now drink coffee at his/her desk! The following is a sample of a floor plan illustration. key concept: Provide glass between the labs, office space, and exterior (outside) views.

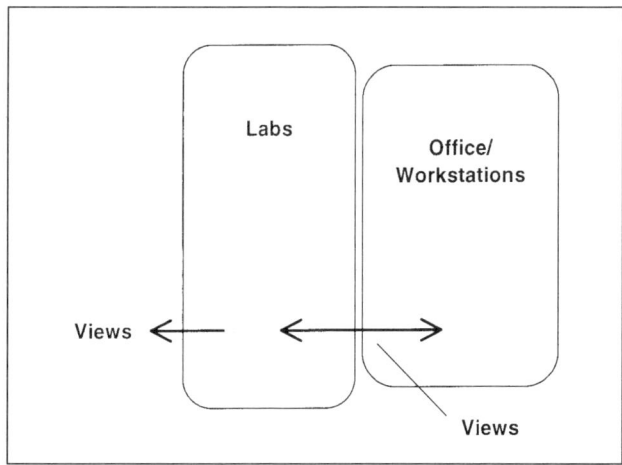

Some laboratories test biologicals. The following is a summary of biosafety levels.

Biosafety Levels

Biosafety Level 1: Lowest Level of Hazard
- Typical laboratories with work done on benchtops or in chemical fume hoods.
- Minimum of 3 to 4 AC/H of outside air.
- Negative pressure to adjacent spaces.

Biosafety Level 2: Moderate Level of Hazard
- Limited access to lab.
- Biosafety cabinets Class I and II are used.
- 100% outside air systems.
- Minimum of 6 to 15 AC/H of outside air.
- Negative pressure to adjacent spaces.
- High equipment loading.

Biosafety Level 3: High Level of Hazard
- Serious or potential lethal hazard as a result of exposure by inhalation.
- Work conducted in Classes I, II and III biosafety cabinets.
- Separate HVAC system
- Negative pressure to adjacent spaces and must be monitored.
- All exhaust must be HEPA filtered.

Biosafety Level 4: Highest Level of Hazard
- All work is conducted in Class III cabinet or pressure suit.
- All vent lines are HEPA filtered.
- Separate HVAC system with monitoring and control of pressurization. Supply fans are interlocked to the exhaust system so that in case of exhaust failure, the space shall not become positively pressured.
- Both supply and exhaust air from space is HEPA filtered with exhaust being bag in/bag out.

Egress

Labs should have two exits from each space where possible with doors swinging out. Fixed elements such as fume hoods and bio-safety cabinets should be located away from doors and traffic. The National Fire Protection Association (NFPA) has recommendations on door swings depending on the lab classification.

Lab Services

Typical services to benches may include compressed air, vacuum, di-ionized water, hot and cold water, and lab gases such as nitrogen, helium, and so forth. These gases may be centralized and piped to the bench, or be located at the bench.

MEP Issues for Laboratories

Heating, Ventilation, and Air Conditioning (HVAC)
The key issue in designing QA/QC laboratories in terms of HVAC is to determine if air can be recirculated with possible terminal HEPA filter on the return air, or if it

must use 100% outside air. The typical air change of a 100% outside air system is 8 to 10 air changes/hour. Temperature and humidity are typically 68° F to 75° F with 50% relative humidity. Generally, the laboratory should be negative with regard to air flow from the corridors. For clean areas such as microbiology, the lab air flow will be positive to the corridor. Point exhausts may need to be provided for specific pieces of equipment.

Fume hood and biosafety cabinets are typical of QC laboratories. Fume hoods typically have face velocities of 60–100 CFM of hood opened at 18 inches, and may have vertical or horizontal siding; the exhaust duct velocity is from 1000–3500 FPM.

Biosafety cabinets are designed in three types depending on the user needs.

Types of Biosafety Cabinets

Classification	Bio-Safety Level	Application
Class I	1, 2, 3	Low to moderate risk biological agent
Class II	1, 2, 3	Low to moderate risk biological agent
Class III	4	High risk biological agent

There are three basic elements of containment in laboratories. These are:

1. Laboratory practices and procedures
2. Safety equipment
3. Facility design

Electrical Issues

During the design phase, equipment requiring special electrical needs should be identified from the equipment list and located on the "lab" cards. Equipment requiring emergency power or uninterrupted power supply (UPS) should be identified.

Materials and Finishes

Materials used for a typical QC laboratory may follow the following matrix.

	Floors	Base	Ceiling	Walls	Comments
Typical labs	VCT	VB	ACT	GWB	
	V	EP		EP	
Microbiology	V	V	ACT	GWB	May have drywall ceilings
			cleanable	EB	

VCT, vinyl composition tile; V sheet vinyl; EP, epoxy; VB, vinyl base; ACT, acoustical tile, cleanable or non-cleanable; GWB, gypsum drywall; EP, epoxy paint.

PROJECT MANAGEMENT ISSUES AND COSTS

The costs for the average renovation or new construction of QC and QA laboratories fall within a range of $200.00 to $400.00 per square foot. Higher and lower costs are possible. Many QC laboratory projects involve renovation within existing facilities, which requires staging and phasing to keep the facilities operational; this will increase costs.

Another consideration is to look at the life cycle cost of the facility, as the following chart illustrates. The facility cost is small, compared to the personnel cost!

TRENDS AND FUTURE DEVELOPMENTS

There is an increasing trend toward automated equipment and robotic laboratories. The issue to consider now are to allow extra space for bench or floor mounted equipment in the future, so that the laboratory may be modified with robotics and more automation in the future.

The design of the workplace outside of the laboratory is also key because increasing time is spent not at the actual bench. The introduction of natural light and expansive use of glass between the laboratories and office/work space will create a positive working environment for the employee.

A summary of trends in the design of QC/OA laboratories are as follows:

- Separate lab space from work up space
- Use of flexible laboratory casework
- Use of split bench
- Use of laboratories vs. metal casework
- Sustainable design (LEED, or Leadership in Energy and Environmental Design)
- Introduction of natural light and glass between laboratories and offices
- Use of robotics for laboratories

Lifetime Science Facility Cost

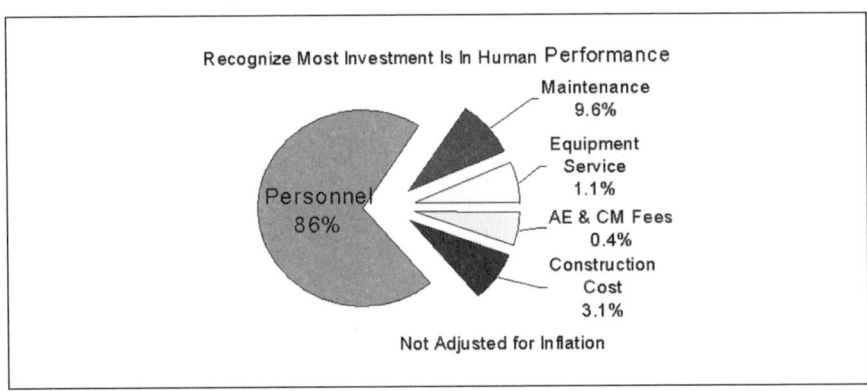

REFERENCES

ANSI/AIHA Z9.5, 1992, Laboratory Ventilation.
ANSI/ASHRAE 110, 1885, Methods of Testing Performance of Laboratory Fume Hoods.
ANSI/NFPA, 1991, Fire Protection for Laboratories Using Chemicals.
ASHRAE, 1991 Applications, Chapter 14, Laboratories.
BOCA and International Building Codes.
NIH/CDC, Biosafety in Microbiological and Biomedical labs.
ISPE Delaware Valley Chapter, Lecture, Bernie Friel, Introduction to R&D, June, 2003.

20
Packaging/Warehousing

Author: Michael Bergey

Advisor: Thomas Jeatran

INTRODUCTION

What Is Packaging?

In its simplest terms, packaging is preparing goods for transport, distribution, storage, retailing, and use. Packaging is essentially a service function that does not exist without something to put inside the package. Packaging has evolved from simple clay pots and woven bags and baskets into the multi-billion dollar market that it is today. Primitive packaging was not concerned with the contain, protect, and transport functions of modern packaging. Back when craftspeople were responsible for selling their own wares, the benefits of the product were divulged to the purchaser verbally on the spot; packaging graphics and other package-specific information was not necessary. As society developed and the idea of a central store was born, the craftsperson was no longer able to provide the information when the wares were purchased. Thus, the need for a fourth packaging function—inform/sell—became apparent. As our society continued to evolve, the study of demographics provided data that helped firms make smart decisions about package designs. These efforts gave way to entire industries focusing on packaging design, graphics, marketing, and converting (those firms that take raw materials and create packaging materials such as paper, paperboard, corrugated cardboard, and plastic.). Packaging science continues to progress at a remarkable pace. With this growth have come additional regulatory and environmental hurdles. Firms are concerned with the four Rs: *Reduce* minimizing the amount of packaging material in any given application without jeopardizing the integrity of the goods within; *Reuse* where possible, creating packaging systems that can be used over and over again; *Recycle* collecting used packaging materials to be re-processed into new material; and *Recover* as in recovering energy from packaging material by incineration rather than sending it to a landfill. Each of these ideals comes with specific political implications.

Why Is Packaging Important?

The Food and Drug Administration (FDA) ensures that drug products are suitable for their intended use by making certain that companies who manufacture drug products follow very specific guidelines during the manufacturing process. The same federal regulations that govern the manufacture of drugs also apply to the packaging of these products for distribution and sale to the end user. From the time the drug product is approved for packaging and distribution until it is prescribed/purchased and used by the consumer, it is the packaging systems that provide the means to ensure that the safety, efficacy, strength, and purity of the drug product are not compromised. For the purposes of this chapter, we will concern ourselves only with packaging for finished pharmaceutical products, medical devices, and other GMP (Good Manufacturing Practice)-industry specific applications. We will use the term "drug product" to collectively describe these applications.

Packaging and Good Design Practices (GDPs)

In the course of packaging operations, preserving the integrity of the drug product and the safety of the patient is of utmost importance.

CONCEPTS AND PRINCIPLES

Packaging Functions

There are four rudimentary package functions to evaluate when determining the design criteria for a packaging system. These functions do not exist independently of each other, and each must be considered with the others in mind during the package design process.

Contain

This function is concerned with providing a receptacle to keep some quantity of product together in a single mass. When programming for the contain function, the package designer must consider the physical attributes of the product (solid, liquid, granular, paste, discreet item); the product's nature (corrosive, volatile, flammable, toxic, pressurized, etc.) and the quantity of material to be packaged.

Protect/Preserve

The protect portion of this function refers to protection of package contents from physical damage, such as vibration, abrasion, and extremes in temperature and humidity. There are several relatively recent elements of the protect function that have become common in GMP industry packaging programs. Child-resistant package opening features are required by law on some drug products. Tamper-evident features have become prevalent since the first Tylenol® tampering incident in 1982. And more recently, anti-theft and anti-counterfeit measures have appeared. The preserve portion pertains to stopping or inhibiting chemical degradation of the package contents. For example, oxygen, water vapor, and light each have potentially detrimental effects to certain drug compounds, and barriers to these elements must be designed into the package to prevent damage to the product. The preserve function is the most critical with respect to preserving the integrity of the drug product.

Transport

The transport function is most applicable to unit loads (skid quantities) of goods; however, proper package design for transportation starts all the way back at the primary package. Transportation of goods is always seen as hazardous in some way to the product being moved, and therefore it is important for the packaging engineer to consider this notion when designing each aspect of the package.

Inform/Sell

In clean industry applications, the inform function gives the consumer specific information about the contents of the package. There are laws and regulatory requirements that dictate what kind of information appears on the drug product package. Some of this information is preprinted (drug name, strength, quantity of doses, and drug manufacturer), and some is printed in real time on the packaging line (lot or batch number and product expiration date). This function tells the consumer what is inside the package. There is usually printed information at all levels of packaging, even on the drug product itself in the case of tablets and capsules. The drug name, the strength of the dose, the total quantity of doses, and the name and address of the drug manufacturer are absolute minimums for pre-printed information. Most printed information appears on the unit of sale, usually the secondary paperboard carton in most applications. In the case of Rx or prescription medications, there is also pre-printed information for the doctor and/or patient in the form of a separate, folded package insert that is placed in the carton with the bottle, pouch, or blister.

When considering the sell function, there are obvious differences between Rx packages and Over-The-Counter (OTC) packages. Typically, Rx medications have minimalistic package decorations, and one or two colors of ink. Doctors prescribe Rx medications, and the consumer usually does not have an opportunity to compare one package to a competitive product. On the other hand, OTC packages must compete directly with other medications side by side on the store shelf, and drug manufacturers go to great lengths to differentiate their products from those of their competitors.

Levels of Packaging

Primary Packaging

The primary package is the first level of containment that is in direct contact with the finished drug product. This could be a blister card or pouch for tablets or capsules; a glass or plastic bottle for tablets, capsules, powders, or liquids; a glass or plastic syringe, ampoule, or vial for injectable drug products; or an aluminum or laminate tube for creams and ointments. This first level is critical with respect to maintaining the safety, efficacy, strength, and purity of the drug product. Primary packaging materials must neither be additive nor subtractive to the chemistry of the drug. Primary packaging is the level most prominent in the stability (shelf life) of a drug. Different drugs pose different packaging challenges with respect to stability. Some are susceptible to water vapor or carbon dioxide; others to oxygen or light.

Certain packaging materials resist these and other potential threats, although there is no universal barrier. Some packaging materials utilize a laminate structure, combining the benefits of two or more materials in a single multi-layer barrier. The dosage form is directly exposed to the packaging room environment at some point in most primary packaging operations, usually after it is removed from its bulk container and prior to its introduction into the primary package. This thereby necessitates the use of strict engineering and environmental controls during the primary packaging process to ensure that the drug product is not compromised in any way.

Secondary Packaging

Secondary packaging typically consists of some quantity of primary package units contained within a secondary container, usually a paperboard carton or tray. It can be as few as one primary unit, or any multiple of units. Any additional supplementary components are usually added at this level, such as patient and physician instructions, and sales and marketing materials. This level of packaging is typically the unit of use, and for OTC products, it is the unit of sale at the retail level. For OTC products, it is the package first seen by the consumer on the store shelf. Secondary packaging tends to be graphics-intensive for this reason.

Tertiary Packaging

Tertiary packaging may or may not exist, depending on the user requirements for a given packaging configuration. It is most commonly employed with OTC formulations, usually reserved for bundling together multiple units of use into units of sale at the wholesale level. Examples are stretch banding, shrink bundling, and overwrapping. Tertiary packaging is more of a logistical packaging component, making it easier to configure distribution loads for shipment, and to break down distribution loads at the point of sale. It is a constraint dictated by wholesale and retail distributors more so than the end user. It is easier to load bundled units of six or ten secondary packages into shipping cases, and unload these bundles for placement on store shelves than to handle individual units.

Distribution

Drug product packaged for sale is usually placed in corrugated shipping containers for distribution. These containers have some kind of information on them, either preprinted or in the form of a printed shipper label. The shipper label is prevalent due to regulatory requirements associated with lot number and expiration dating. Corrugated shippers can be palletized into a unit load or they can be distributed in quantities as small as a single case.

Unit Load

Entire lots of packaged drug product bound for warehouses or distribution centers are usually unitized in pallet quantities. Corrugated cases are stacked and interlocked to provide a stable load and prevent damage to the package contents. These unit loads are stacked and stored in warehouses to await shipment to the consumer. In the case of physician's samples, it is possible that a single drum of tablets or capsules on the primary end of the packaging chain can become an entire trailer load of double-stacked pallets on the shipping dock by the time primary, secondary, and tertiary packaging features are added.

This chapter covers good design practices for primary, secondary, and tertiary packaging spaces for non-sterile applications, with a section that specifically addresses sterile packaging as well. The same hygienic zoning principles (white, gray, black, transition, and proper gowning techniques) that apply to pharmaceutical processing also apply to pharmaceutical packaging.

PACKAGING PLANT DESIGN CONSIDERATIONS

A pharmaceutical packaging plant can be a stand alone, dedicated facility or a part of a larger manufacturing and warehousing operation. Typically, packaging plants are purpose built, but there have been many manufacturing-to-packaging area or warehouse-to-packaging area conversions undertaken in recent years. As a part of a longer term growth plan, it is not unusual for a pharmaceutical company to build a packaging plant and a warehouse, with future plans to allow packaging to expand into the warehouse area and build additional warehouse space as necessary. Careful consideration must be given to this approach, so that maximum utilization of vertical warehouse space can be realized when it is converted to packaging space. Adding mezzanine areas for office space and mechanical equipment such as HVAC systems are typical ways to maximize the old warehouse space overhead.

Packaging Floor Layout

The packaging plant should be laid out with packaging rooms in a grid pattern, with clearly defined paths for personnel, raw materials, and finished goods to flow freely into and out of the packaging space. The intent should be to keep all packaging areas as centralized and equidistant from support areas as possible. Building columns should be designed into walls so that the packaging rooms are free and clear for maximum flexibility with respect to equipment layout. Glass can be utilized to give the plant a wide open feeling and allow supervisors and inspectors to view the work in process, but the cost of this type of construction and its life safety implications must be factored into the final design. Hallways should be large enough to permit the flow of materials and personnel, and also to facilitate the movement of packaging equipment. The lengths and widths of the largest expected machinery must be known, and the means to move this equipment from the receiving dock to any packaging room and back out to the maintenance and storage areas must be designed into the packaging plant layout.

Warehousing

Maximum throughput is realized when there are dedicated raw material and finished goods warehouses, and flow of materials can be linear (i.e. raw materials warehouse to packaging floor to finished goods warehouse). It may appear that these warehouses function in a similar fashion, but they operate quite differently. A raw material warehouse is typically high bay, with large volumes of palletized packaging components stored in racks until requested by the packaging floor. Material pulled from the warehouse can be sent to any number of packaging rooms. There is a great diversity of materials stored in the warehouse—everything from heavy, dense rolls of blister films that can weigh over 1,000 pounds per pallet, to very light pallets of flattened, folded corrugated shipper cases. Components such as bottles and caps take up a great amount of warehouse space, and most firms use a "just in time" component ordering philosophy with their suppliers to minimize the quantities of these materials that must be stored on site.

A finished goods warehouse consists of pallet loads of finished product, in shipping cases and ready for distribution. These loads are typically uniform and are floor stacked as many as 4 pallets high, depending on the stability of the palletized load. Trucks are loaded with pallets 2 units high, so it is efficient to store finished goods 2 high or 4 high to minimize fork truck motions. Finished goods usually remain in the warehouse only as long as it takes for the Quality Assurance department to review the packaging batch record and approve the batch for shipment.

BASIC GMP PACKAGING AREA DESIGN PRINCIPLES

- Packaging facilities should be designed to allow product, packaging components, work in process, finished goods, and waste to move through the plant in sequential order whenever possible. Material flows and storage should be designed with preventing cross contamination in mind.
- Packaging areas should be of sufficient size to allow adequate space for materials, equipment, and personnel. Proper space must be provided for operation, maintenance, and cleaning of packaging equipment.
- Separate areas shall be designated for packaging operations, equipment cleaning, storage of clean equipment and tooling, and storage of dirty equipment and tooling.
- Personnel and materials should not transition from a black zone to a white zone without first passing though a transition zone.
- Restrooms and other personnel convenience areas should not open directly into primary or secondary packaging areas.
- Exposed wood pallets and other wood products should not be used in primary packaging areas where direct product exposure is possible.
- HVAC systems should be designed to prevent cross contamination and infiltration of extraneous matter. Proper filtration must be provided in areas where contamination is a possibility.
- Horizontal surfaces in architectural details should be avoided to minimize the collection of particulate matter. Sloped sills should be utilized.

Packaging Process Assessment

Prior to undertaking a detailed facility design, a thorough study of the current and potential future packaging process parameters must be undertaken. The following outline can be used in this assessment:

- *Product:* Toxicity, sensitivity, drug classification, number of SKUs, stability requirements, dosage form, package format, packaging materials, labeling
- *Production:* Campaign, changeovers, product mix, scale, clinical vs. commercial, batch size, number of lots, throughput speeds, number of lines
- *Quality Assurance:* Standard operating procedures, validation, reject rates, quality inspections, exception handling, pest control, cleaning procedures
- *Equipment:* Dedicated/multiuse, primary, secondary, tertiary, fixed/portable, changeovers, automation, accumulation, back-up, redundancy, tooling and spare parts
- *Personnel:* Accessibility, flow, training, biometrics/passwords, gowning, workstations
- *Logistics:* Fork trucks, battery charging, storage racks, cold storage, quarantine, hazardous materials, controlled substances
- *Environment and Safety:* OSHA, EPA, PPE, SOPs, confined space, environmental monitoring, lighting levels, sound levels, fire safety
- *Support Facilities:* Restrooms, locker rooms, break rooms, cafeteria, nurses station, label storage, retained sample storage
- *Utilities:* Compressed air, electricity, vacuum, specialty gases

Packaging Space Layout

In designing packaging space for pharmaceutical and medical device applications, care must be taken to protect the integrity of the product. There are risks associated with drug product exposure to other drug products, to foreign substances, and, in some instances, to operations personnel from the drug product itself. Care must be taken in providing proper facility design to mitigate or completely eliminate these risks. Packaging areas are typically located adjacent to manufacturing areas, the raw materials warehouse and the finished goods warehouse. Ideally, drug product and packaging components flow into one end of the process, and finished goods flow out of the other end of the process. The waste streams created by the packaging process must also be taken into consideration. Prior to detailed design, a flow diagram of the packaging process should be constructed to show all process inputs and outputs, and all points of operator intervention. During the design stages of a packaging facility project, the design and engineering firm must have access to accurate electronic drawings of the packaging processes, including plan views, equipment elevations, and utility connection points. Packaging suites tend to be relatively clean areas with high levels of activity, noise, and movement. This is the direct opposite to what happens in processing areas where most of the work being performed takes place in closed systems, out of sight from operating personnel. Because of all this activity, most firms want packaging areas to include large viewing windows where automated packaging processes can be viewed by customers or visitors from a black or gray area where gowning is not a requirement. This should be taken into consideration during the design phase of a project.

Spatial Requirements

Packaging areas require adequate floor space for equipment, personnel, and materials. Entrances to packaging areas must be properly sized so that the largest piece of equipment in the given process can be moved into and out of the space without major building modifications or service interruptions. Provisions must be made to move all equipment into or out of an area regardless of its position in the process. A minimum of 5 feet or more should be provided between equipment and packaging area partitions to provide access to equipment power panels, allow for the movement of equipment and materials, and provide safe egress for personnel in the event of an emergency. In a well-designed packaging process, all normal operator intervention should take place from one side of the line. This includes regular adjustments; charging the line with raw materials such as bottles, caps, labels, foil/film, folding cartons and package inserts; and removing finished goods from the line. Dimensionally, packaging spaces should be designed to maximize equipment utility while minimizing space.

Safe Egress

Safe egress must also be considered in packaging area design. Because of the linear nature of automated packaging processes, the complete line layout including a full compliment of skids of packaging components must be factored into life safety plans. Some automated lines can be as long as 150 feet or more, and conveyors or equipment could possibly compromise normal paths to emergency exits. Additional exits may be needed, or as a last resort, line crossovers or swinging conveyor sections can be utilized as necessary.

Ceiling Heights

In most applications, both in primary packaging suites and secondary packaging areas, ceiling height should not be less than 10 feet. In instances where drug product is fed from above the machine, such as vertical pouching and some horizontal applications, a ceiling height of 14 or even 16 feet may be applicable. In every case, the equipment manufacturer and/or packaging line integrator must be consulted to understand the maximum required working height for the equipment in question.

Lighting

Lighting levels of between 60- and 75-foot candles is generally sufficient for most packaging operations. In some localized areas, levels may need to be higher if there is an on-line human inspection task to be performed, or perhaps lower if there is a backlit automatic machine-based inspection to be performed. However, most of these automated inspection areas tend to be shrouded, and adjustment of local lighting levels is not required.

Packaging Space, Packaging Equipment, and Packaging Process Relationships

Packaging processes are typically designed in a linear fashion. Primary packaging operations are followed "in-line" by any number of secondary and tertiary processes. Individual machines are linked to each other by a series of conveyors, and logical process controls and buffer zones provide for an "integrated" packaging operation. On one end of the spectrum, some processes are highly automated, with minimal operator intervention; on the other end, there may be an entirely manual process, with human operators performing all typical machine functions. There are many factors that dictate the degree of automation—equipment costs, operating costs, labor rates, desired throughput, and the duration of the packaging campaign, to name a few.

Packaging lines are usually arranged in either a U shape, with the beginning of the line and the end of the line located in the same general vicinity, or straight through, with the beginning and end of the packaging process located at opposite ends of the packaging area. The design method chosen is impacted by the general plant layout and vice versa. Plant layout not withstanding, there are distinct advantages and disadvantages to each method. In a U-shaped design, the packaging area tends to be operator centric, with the human/machine interface located on the inside of the U. This enables one operator to potentially manage more than one machine station. All staged packaging components such as foil, cartons, and package inserts would also be located on the inside of the U. A supervisor would have a central vantage point to manage the entire operation. In a straight-through configuration, operations are process centric, with multiple operators located at different machine stations along the length of the line. Materials and packaging components are staged on one side of the line. Regardless of the line layout chosen, material and personnel flows must be properly designed to avoid mix-ups.

Utility Requirements: General

HVAC

The packaging facility designer must be familiar with industrial HVAC, as defined in various documents by the American Society of Heating, Refrigerating and Air-Conditioning Engineers (ASHRAE) and the American Conference of Governmental Industrial Hygienists (ACGIH). Knowledge of local construction codes, National Fire Protection Association (NFPA) standards, environmental regulations, and Occupational Safety and Health Administration (OSHA) regulations is also assumed. The HVAC system must comply with these and all applicable building, safety, hygiene and environmental regulations.

Critical Parameters

Temperature, humidity, and airborne particulates are the critical room parameters that may affect product or packaging components. Microbial contamination should also be considered. Air changes and room pressure are usually not critical parameters. However, the relative direction of air flow between spaces may be a critical parameter, if airborne particulates and/or vapors could have a detrimental affect on product or material in another space. Operating ranges for critical parameters need to be considered in establishing design criteria. The concepts of "alert" and "action" points are highly applicable to HVAC control systems.

Temperature

Room temperature may be a critical parameter for both open and closed operations. Most products, materials, and processes can handle a wide range in temperatures. However, the width of this range decreases as the exposure time increases. Product stability and personnel comfort must be considered in establishing room temperature requirements. The USP excursion limits for raw materials and finished product storage are 59°F–86°F (15°C–30°C) with a customary CRT (Controlled Room Temperature) working environment of 68°F–77°F (20°C–25°C). However, individual product and material requirements may differ.

Relative Humidity

Room relative humidity (RH) may affect exposed product or packaging materials that are sensitive to water vapor. Typically, exposed humidity-sensitive products require humidity controlled to 30–50%. If humidification is needed, boiler water additives should not make breathing air unsafe in conformance with ASHRAE IAQ (Indoor Air Quality) guidelines and local codes. If RH control is required, the boundary of the space to be controlled should be designed to minimize the potential of moisture migration. Utilization of construction materials having low moisture permeability should be considered. If dehumidification is to be provided, the system selected should not adversely contaminate the product. Cooling coil type systems generate large amounts of condensate that must be drained properly to avoid microbial contamination. Liquid and dry type desiccant systems should be evaluated for potential carry over of desiccant into the supply air system and its effect on the exposed product.

Airborne Particulates

There are no particulate classification requirements for packaging facilities, such as those that exist for aseptic processing. It is good design practice to design primary packaging areas to Class 100,000 levels. There is no requirement to validate the space to this level of cleanliness, although many firms do. Cross contamination can originate from both the internal environment and from outside the packaging facility. In all air handling systems, the filtration should be evaluated for its ability to trap outdoor particulates. In re-circulation systems, the filtration must be evaluated for cross-contamination of product and general housekeeping particulates. If the facility is multi-product and some of the products have no tolerance for cross contamination with other products, then air should not be returned from these spaces (even if HEPA filtered). In a facility where multiple products are exposed, dedicated air handlers and ductwork are probably more practical and cost-effective than filtration of return air or the use of once-through air. Capital costs will be higher, but on-going operating costs should be lower. The requirements for filtration of supply air depend on the level of protection required but at a minimum should meet ASHRAE IAQ standards.

For Primary and Secondary Packaging Areas. Minimum of 85% efficiency filters are recommended. If air is returned to the HVAC system, a 99.97% HEPA filter in the supply or return duct system generally provides adequate protection against cross-contamination between exposed products or materials. If the HEPA filter is critical to deterring cross contamination, it should be regularly tested for specified efficiency. If a failure of the primary HEPA filter would jeopardize product integrity, a backup HEPA filter should be considered. Class 100,000 cleanliness levels have been successfully achieved with HEPA filter banks installed in the air handling unit. The use of terminal HEPA filters is not a requirement. If HEPA filters or 95% DOP filters are utilized on the supply air system, periodic testing is recommended to confirm proper filter effectiveness. This testing can be of the total air stream type, and therefore scan testing of the entire filter face would not be not required.

Room Relative Pressure

Room relative pressure may be a critical parameter if the product is exposed and:

- If is in a multi-product building, where some or all products are in dry form, exposed to room air without barriers or capture, or can become airborne and migrate by air to other product areas. The same applies for products in vapor form where vapor migration could have a detrimental effect upon other products or materials.
- If airborne concentrations of product, materials, or contaminants are high enough to pose an exposure threat to operating personnel. When this occurs, both personnel and products exposed in the facility could be at risk.
- If adjacent spaces are uncontrolled, such that airborne migration of particles in either direction is possible.

There is no quantified requirement for relative pressurization. The velocity and direction of airflow between spaces should be adequate to prevent counter-flow of airborne particulates or vapor contaminants for spaces where airborne cross contamination is a concern. Relative pressure gradients should be designed to prevent airborne particulates from passing from a given primary packaging space to an adjacent primary packaging space. Conversely, pressurization should be set up to prevent airborne particulates from passing from any other adjacent space into primary packaging spaces. Transition zones and airlocks can be used to separate primary packaging rooms from adjacent secondary rooms and common corridor/staging areas. When doors are closed, pressure should be demonstrably positive or negative. Pressurized air locks may have either positive or negative relative pressure, depending on what is best for the particular situation. Airflow variations from exhaust fans, dust collection systems, and vacuum or process systems should be accounted for in the control logic of the HVAC system.

Air Change Rates

There is no minimum GMP requirement for air changes per hour. Air flow into and out of a space should be based on providing the required cooling, heating, relative humidity, pressurization, particulate control, dilution ventilation, and recovery time from an upset (spill or dust emission). These factors generally result in air change rates of between 4 and 20 per hour.

Monitoring

Regular monitoring of critical points should indicate to the user when requirements exceed pre-set operational limits. If alert points are being utilized, these can indicate when a monitored parameter is beginning to drift out of control.

Worker Comfort

Maximum and minimum room temperatures and humidity should be within OSHA or local health guidelines. See ASHRAE Standard 55 and International Standards Organization (ISO) Standard 7730 for requirements and guidelines. Conditions may need to be adjusted for workers in protective clothing. A range of 25% to 60% RH is recommended for worker comfort where occupancy is continuous. However, since some facilities will have 100% outdoor air systems, the need and cost of comfort dehumidification and humidification where humidity will not affect the product should be assessed.

Ventilation for Hazardous Environments

Recirculation of flammable vapors is not recommended. Areas where flammable materials are stored or exposed will usually be served by once-through air systems. Local spot exhaust is recommended at points of flammable material exposure. Building electrical hazard classification and static grounding should be applied to HVAC components and instrumentation, in accordance with national and local codes. When dilution ventilation is used to control flammable vapors, the Threshold Limit Value (TLV) for the material drives the dilution air volume, not the Lower Explosive Limit (LEL). Air borne flammables can lead to very large air handling volumes, increased operating costs, and worker health problems. Permissible product and constituent airborne concentrations will depend upon material toxicity, as determined by the facility user.

Electrical

Most major pieces of packaging equipment will have a central control panel with a single power connection point. Larger machines are usually three-phase loads. In most cases on primary packaging machines, heat sealers, and shrink tunnels, there is a substantial resistive load associated with heaters and sealing bars. Any sub-systems with different voltage requirements are usually fed from step down transformers within the primary integral panel. There are exceptions to this with add-on auxiliary systems such as vacuums, printers, and other single-phase loads. Care must be taken to quantify the existing packaging equipment load, and estimate all potential future equipment loads that could be added at a later date due to the inherent flexibility of secondary packaging operations. Primary electrical distribution and low voltage wiring for machine controls from machine to machine is usually run in raceways underneath of the framework of the equipment. This can be in conduit or, in the case of integrated bottle packaging lines, custom wire raceways designed and provided by the equipment manufacturer. It is customary to provide convenience outlets as required around the perimeter of packaging spaces. A data port should be located near the supervisor's area if required.

Compressed Air

Some packaging equipment tends to consume large amounts of compressed air. Component orienting equipment such as vibratory bowls and bottle unscramblers use small micro-jets to orient parts or propel parts around rails during the packaging process. Venturi systems use compressed air to generate vacuum for suction cups that are used to pull cartons and inserts from magazines. Bottle cleaners use blasts of compressed air to blow dust and other particles from bottles prior to filling. Collectively, these loads can be substantial. Total compressed air volume, pressure, and peak loads must be understood before properly sized compressed air supply systems can be designed. It may be necessary to provide more than one supply point for a given packaging line and install surge tanks as necessary depending on peak load requirements. Compressed air quality for machine operation should meet or exceed the packing equipment manufacturer's requirements. Compressed air that comes in direct contact with drug product or primary packaging material product contact surfaces should be clean, dry, pharmaceutical-grade air.

Chilled Water

Many packaging operations use arrays of electric cartridge style heaters and sealing tooling to create certain package features. Sealing stations on many machines utilize chilled water to precisely control sealing temperatures and, because some machines are compact by design, to ensure that the heat from the sealing bars does not migrate into other machine stations. In most cases, this chilled water is provided by a local stand-alone chiller located within the packaging area. This heat load must be accounted for.

Other Utility Requirements

- *Dust collection:* Usually required for powder fill and uncoated tablet filling applications. Depending on the level of control required, dust control can be an integral part of a balanced HVAC system, or a localized stand-alone feature at the point of use.
- *Nitrogen and other specialty gases:* Used in several different ways in packaging processes, most notably to displace oxygen in primary packaging for oxygen sensitive products. Depending on the quantity required, the gas can be provided in cylinders, or piped in to the packaging area from a remote source.
- *Vacuum:* Can be provided in three ways: induced by compressed air and venturi, supplied by a vacuum pump that is integral to the packaging system (preferred), or provided by a remote vacuum generating system.

Primary Packaging Suite Details

Primary packaging areas are usually designated as white zones, accessed through a transition zone designed to facilitate proper gowning procedures. Room pressure gradients cascade away from the primary room, through the air lock or transition zone, and into secondary packaging and other support areas to ensure that contaminants are not transferred into the area. Typical primary packaging processes consist of horizontal blister machines, bottle filling equipment, vertical and horizontal pouch filling equipment and other processes where the drug product or medical device is exposed to the general room environment for some period of time. The drug product can be a tablet, capsule, liquid, cream, powder, or other dosage form. Drug product is exposed when bulk drug containers are opened, when the bulk drug product is transferred to the product hoppers or tanks on the filling equipment, and where the drug product has been transferred to the primary package but before the package is completely sealed. This is the case with blister packaging prior to top web seal, horizontal pouch applications before final top seal, and bottling operations prior to capping. Primary packaging rooms should have the same critical design criteria as pharmaceutical manufacturing suites.

Finishes

Finishes in primary packaging areas should be as smooth, durable, and as monolithic as possible to provide maximum cleanability and prevent areas where dirt could accumulate. Ceilings should be seamless with a smooth finish and coated with epoxy paint. Lay in ceiling tiles are acceptable in some instances provided they are washable, non-shedding, and utilize clips and gaskets to hold them in place. Walls should be monolithic, with coves at sills and base to facilitate proper cleaning. Some means of impact resistance should be provided to prevent damage from pallets and material handling equipment in areas susceptible to such damage. Stainless steel panels and corner guards are preferred. Floors should be monolithic—epoxy terrazzo, troweled epoxy, or seamless welded vinyl are examples of monolithic flooring systems.

Equipment

Primary equipment tends to be fixed; i.e., once the packaging process is defined, there will not be any major changes to the primary equipment. There will be tooling changes from lot to lot and put-up to put-up, but in most instances the machine footprint, staging requirements for raw materials, and utility requirements will not change. Auxiliary systems such as chillers, printers, and vacuums should be scrutinized for clean operation.

Utilities

Utility service for packaging equipment in primary areas should stub up through the floor whenever possible to maintain clean uncluttered walls and prevent conduit or pipe drops from the ceiling. Where primary packaging equipment transitions to the secondary process through a dividing wall, it is acceptable to bring utility services to the machine at the point where the primary discharge conveyor passes through the wall.

Materials Staging

Only material quantities for the current lot should be staged in primary packaging areas. This includes drug product and packaging components. Total material staging requirements are usually not more than 2 pallets for each component due to the storage density of the drug product and the rolls of foil in blister forming operations. Bottling operations are a special case. Bottle staging and bottle unscrambling should take place in a secondary area because of the space taken up by unit loads of bottles and caps.

Secondary and Tertiary Packaging Areas
Secondary packaging areas are usually designated as gray zones. The drug product or medical device is contained within the primary package, and the risk of exposure to product or operator is minimal. The space must be configured to support flexible operations. It is not necessary to totally enclose secondary and tertiary areas. Segregation between packaging lines must be maintained, preferably by solid partitions at least 4 feet high. It is acceptable practice to provide air conditioning for an entire secondary packaging gallery with a single air handling system.

Finishes
Finishes in secondary packaging areas should be durable and cleanable. Ceilings at a minimum should be lay-in ceiling tiles that are washable and non-shedding. Walls should have coves at sills and base to facilitate proper cleaning. Epoxy coated CMU is acceptable. Some means of impact resistance should be provided to prevent damage from pallets and material handling equipment in areas susceptible to damage. Stainless steel panels and corner guards are preferred. Floors can be troweled epoxy, vinyl tile or epoxy paint. The level of fork truck traffic is a primary determinant for which floor system to use.

Equipment
Where primary equipment tends to be fixed, secondary and tertiary equipment tends to be more flexible in nature. Typical secondary and tertiary operations consist of checkweighing, cartoning, labeling, hand packing operations, bundling, banding, overwrapping, case-packing and palletizing. There are numerous auxiliary operations that typically take place in secondary areas, such as printing, coding, and package inspection.

Utilities
Because of the flexible nature of most secondary and tertiary packaging operations, stubbing up through the floor is not practical. Packaging equipment should be fed from strategically located stainless steel or extruded aluminum power poles that extend up into the suspended ceiling and can be relocated as necessary as packaging process layouts change. Attempts must be made to minimize individual ceiling drops, and cords and conduit must be kept off of the floor.

Packaging Room Materials Staging
Lot quantities of secondary packaging components can amount to considerable floor space, depending on package complexity and lot size. Typically, when a packaging

process is programmed, space for a single pallet of each packaging component is allotted on the packaging floor. As material is expended, more material is signed into the area. Each process must be assessed on a line-by-line basis, however, because high throughput situations may require more than one pallet of certain components on hand.

Support Areas and Adjacencies

Overflow Materials Staging
For high volume or large lot size packaging operations, it is customary to provide a staging area adjacent to the packaging area for packaging components. In most instances, rack storage is not necessary. Packaging materials are staged in pallet quantities on the floor, usually single stacked so that the material can be easily moved with a pallet jack when it is needed. It is necessary to provide segregated staging for each individual packaging line to prevent mix-ups. These areas should be treated as secondary packaging areas from a facility design standpoint.

Wash Areas
Packaging equipment must be cleaned between lots and especially between products. Most packaging equipment is not designated as clean-in-place; therefore, it is practical to clean equipment and tooling in a centrally located area. In most instances, it is only necessary to clean product contact surfaces such as product hoppers and filler parts in the central wash area. Parts and tooling can be cleaned manually in specially designed wash basins or automatically in commercial parts washers. It is necessary to understand exactly what is to be cleaned so that the appropriate wash basins or automated equipment can be selected. Depending on the cleaning method chosen, proper hot and cold water service, drainage, and electrical service must be provided. Some cleaning procedures require elevated water temperatures and/or a purified water rinse, and this must be taken into consideration during the design phase of the project. A properly designed wash area will have separate, defined staging areas for "dirty" equipment to be cleaned, and for equipment that has been designated as clean and ready for use.

Equipment Storage
It is necessary to provide space for excess equipment in any packaging facility plan. Although it makes good business sense to keep as much equipment as possible fully utilized, there still needs to be equipment storage space available. Storage areas should be located near the maintenance shop. Although most machine maintenance is done in place on the packaging floor, there are instances where major modifications or complete rebuilds are undertaken, and this work typically takes place in the shop. Machines may be staged for a period of time on the way in for service, and possibly on the way back out to the packaging floor as well.

Equipment storage areas should be large enough to handle this modification/rebuild volume, spare machinery, and other equipment as necessary. Due to the weight and size of packaging machinery, floor storage is most appropriate. Some rack storage is appropriate for small auxiliary equipment such as printers, scanners, and other devices. Spare parts, sub assemblies, and smaller equipment can be stored in shelving units.

Tooling Storage

Tooling presents some special storage requirements over and above typical equipment storage parameters. Tooling pertains to the product-specific parts required to permit a packaging machine to run different products or formats. Tooling can be product contact parts on a primary packaging machine (such as slats and funnels on a tablet filling machine), or timing screws on a bottle filling machine. There is also tooling in secondary applications such as the tuckers, plows, and folding rails on a cartoning machine. Regardless of the application, the following special conditions apply to tooling storage:

- Controlled temperature and humidity to minimize corrosion on untreated surfaces.
- Condensed storage; some tooling sets can be quite small.
- Segregated storage; so that a set of parts for a given format can be stored together and not be mixed up with other sets.
- Special protection for sensitive machined tools such as seal tooling, forming dies, and punches to prevent nicks and other marks.

When planning a tooling a storage area, it is important to understand the types of packaging equipment that will be used, and the total numbers of sets of tooling for each packaging machine. It is not unusual for a single blister forming machine to have ten or more individual sets of tooling. As most tooling is quite expensive, it usually goes into storage when a given product run is completed.

Maintenance Shop

Adequate space should be provided for a maintenance and engineering area to support packaging operations. There are various levels of machine maintenance, from minimal daily maintenance checks to manufacturing machine tooling in-house. Firms will make business decisions about how much maintenance to perform using in-house personnel, and how much to perform using contracted or OEM resources. These decisions will have a direct bearing on the size of the maintenance area to be designed. Packaging equipment maintenance can function as a stand-alone support unit, or it can be merged with a manufacturing machinery maintenance unit if these functions are required in a multifunctional plant. Both are GMP functions, but the major difference is that most manufacturing maintenance happens in the field out in the manufacturing plant, while some packaging equipment maintenance occurs in the maintenance area. Care should be taken, however, to keep facilities maintenance and equipment maintenance areas separate for GMP reasons.

Label Room

Labeling is perhaps the most GMP intensive parameter associated with packaging. Printed materials are always present in packaging areas, and the FDA insists that the creation, storage, and use of printed materials be managed in a controlled fashion. There are pre-printed materials such as cartons, blister foils, pouch films, physician/patient inserts, and other high volume (skid quantity) materials that must be managed under GMP guidelines, but these items are typically stored in a warehouse and retrieved as needed. The label components that require an extra level of security are batch or lot specific labels with lot number and/or expiry information, and small unit of use labels that contain detailed product information. Typically, unprinted stock is stored in the warehouse, and lot quantities are brought into the label room for printing. Labels are usually quite dense from a storage perspective, so lot quantities may be a case or two, and maybe as much as an entire skid, but rarely more. Labels are printed as needed, and should be placed in a locked, rolling cart after inspection and approval. Printed labels are transferred to the packaging floor for use via the secure carts. The size of the label room is completely dependent on the size and complexity of the packaging operation. The end user must be consulted about the details of the packaging process to ensure that a properly sized labeling area is designed. Finishes, space conditioning requirements, and light levels should be the same as for secondary packaging. Space must be provided for raw label storage, finished label storage, cart storage, label printers, inspection machines, records, and printing inks. Depending on the chemical composition of the inks, special storage cabinets and ventilation may be required. Additionally, security measures such as card access and security cameras are usually required.

Testing Labs and Other QA/QC Areas

Depending on the type of packaging process, some in-process testing of packages is required. Most tests are concerned with the integrity of the seals on the primary package. Leak testing equipment and pull strength testers are the principle pieces of equipment utilized for in-process testing. Most test equipment is bench top, with a few exceptions. Casework with adequate linear bench top space is required with cabinetry for storage of test materials. A means to temporarily stage packages to be tested is also required.

Office Space

Typically, office space is provided for packaging supervisors and managers in the gray or black areas. Space must be provided for operations personnel such as first line supervisors, area managers, and administrative support. Some firms also want the planners, buyers, and other analysts close to the packaging operations, and if this is the case, space must be provided for them. There are other support functions such as engineering and document control that must be assessed and provided for as necessary. It is also important to understand the proposed hours of operation, as a multiple shift operation will require additional office space or a shared office plan.

Special Design Considerations

Flammable Materials Storage

Some printing inks and other substances used in the packaging process are flammable and require special storage. The design firm needs to understand the nature of the flammable materials as well as the total maximum quantity of materials required to be stored at the facility. If the packaging area is a part of a larger multiuse facility with other flammable material storage requirements, it may be appropriate to use a smaller flammable storage cabinet for lot-sized quantities of materials in the packaging area, and store the larger quantities of flammable materials in a general centralized storage area.

Controlled Substances

There are very specific storage requirements for controlled substances, as defined by the U.S. Drug Enforcement Agency (DEA). The Code of Federal Regulations, Section 1301.72 permits small quantities to be stored in a safe or steel cabinet, and requires larger quantities to be stored in a specially constructed vault with controlled access and alarm capability. The CFR Section provides all of the required construction details for compliance.

Refrigerated/Frozen Storage

Some biologics and other drug formulations need to be stored in a refrigerated or frozen state. Drug products may need to be conditioned as raw materials, finished goods, or both. The maximum quantities of drug product required to be stored as a raw material and as finished goods must be known for proper sizing of the environmentally controlled area. Typically, the required storage area for finished goods is many times that of the same drug product as a raw material due to the different densities of drug product per pallet. There may also be multiple products that need to be stored. Cold storage areas should be properly designed to provide uniform temperature distribution across all levels. There will be major differences in system and supporting facility design to consider depending on whether the requirement is for refrigerated storage (typically 2 to 8°C) or frozen storage (typically–25°C or more). Most applications can utilize prefabricated systems consisting of gasketed sheet metal encased foam panels and doors. A safety allowance of at least 25% should be factored into the square footage calculations for growth.

Some other typical requirements for cold storage areas:

- Temperature monitoring system
- Alarms for over temperature or under temperature
- Redundant mechanical systems for back up in the event of mechanical failure and for defrost cycle allowance

- Emergency generator back-up
- Temperature mapping and validation
- A secondary source of cooling water if the refrigeration system condensers are water cooled
- Pre-action fire suppression system

PROJECT MANAGEMENT ISSUES (COST/SCHEDULE/QUALITY)

Costs

Generally speaking, packaging facilities are typically built to the same standards and finishes as non-sterile manufacturing facilities. Facility construction costs per square foot of packaging space tend to be somewhat lower than manufacturing space, because there are fewer unusual design features. Costs per square foot can be anywhere from $125 to $250 or more, depending on geographical region and level of finish selected. Special environmental conditioning for sensitive products or special construction for hazardous products can greatly increase costs. Specialized HVAC equipment to maintain tight temperature, humidity, and room pressure tolerances adds to the total cost. The cost of ongoing operations can be substantial as well. Packaging equipment notoriously consumes compressed air, and the usage must be understood to accurately determine the total cost of operating the packaging plant.

Packaging equipment can be very expensive, especially for custom built, one-of-a-kind machines. Higher machine output also translates directly to higher machine cost. Prices run from less than $10,000 for a very rudimentary carton erector, to as much as $5 million for a top-of-the-line, highly automated, fully integrated, high speed bottle line. It is important to note that there is no standard budgetary "rule of thumb" to try to compute the cost of packaging equipment. It is incredibly variable, depending on the package format, desired throughput, level of automation, machine flexibility, and other factors. In clean industries, certainly all primary packaging equipment and most secondary packaging equipment purchased is qualified and validated. There is a cost associated with the formal documentation required to specify, purchase, install, qualify and validate packaging equipment. In this case, there is a general "rule of thumb" that can be used for planning purposes. Equipment qualification and validation costs on average are 8–15% of total costs.

Schedule

There is a natural progression to finish packaging areas after manufacturing areas and before warehousing. Construction crews will use the roughed in packaging areas for staging for the finish work in the manufacturing areas, then move staging into the roughed in warehouse to finish the packaging area and so on. Equipment installation and validation activities follow the same natural set of sequences. Packaging equipment lead-time needs to be factored into the master project timeline. Lead-time will

Typical Timeline for Custom Packaging Line

Project Task	Duration (Months)	Cumulative (Months)
Develop user requirements specification	1	1
Develop functional and design specifications	1	2
Prototyping and proof of concept	2	4
Approval to proceed	Milestone	
Detailed design	4	8
Drawing release	Milestone	
Parts and subsystems procurement	4	12
Assembly	3	15
Testing and debugging	1	16
Factory acceptance testing and shipping	1	17
Qualification	0.5	17.5
Validation	0.5	18
Approved for use	Milestone	

vary with the cost and complexity of the equipment; complex, high-speed equipment can take as long as 18 months to deliver. A typical timeline for a custom packaging line might look like this:

TRENDS/FUTURE DEVELOPMENTS

Packaging Trends

Although solid dosage forms are still the obvious volume leader, advances in biotechnology are making parenterals (vials, syringes, cartridges, etc.) more and more common. These products are typically very expensive, and they usually require special temperature considerations. Most have a 2°C to 8°C storage requirement and can be out of refrigeration for a very limited time during labeling, packaging, and shipping operations. Others are actually frozen products at –25°C and below (freeze-safe containers are becoming a very big business). Properly designed refrigeration in close proximity to the packaging lines is critical. The need to ensure sterility throughout the packaging/labeling operation is also extremely important (e.g., container/closure integrity for vials, syringes, cartridges). As advances in biotechnology lead to increased numbers of products gaining FDA approval, these issues will become more and more crucial.

Most new prescription drug products are higher in cost compared with 10 or even 5 years ago. This has led to a changing philosophy by major pharmaceutical firms to spend more on the packaging to protect the product, and to make the packaging more convenient for the physician, pharmacist, nurse, and patient. One of the most visible signs of this is the strong trend to unit dose packaging (blisters for oral solid dosage forms, and syringes or cartridges for parenterals). This trend also addresses the increasing attention to medication errors, most of which can be traced to the repackaging or reconstitution of products. Since many of the biotech products are intended for self-medication by patients, the only way to ensure compliance with dosing regimens is to have a unit dose package that is ready to use. The down side of this for manufacturers and packagers is the tremendous increase in total packaged volume that results from unit packages (e.g., ten syringes vs. one vial). Add to this the fact that most biotechnology companies with home use kits on the market are including alcohol swabs, needles, and reconstitution aids in the package to make administration even simpler and more convenient. All of this increased complexity in packaging is putting renewed emphasis on the proper design of packaging facilities and critical support equipment. This is also creating some divergence of packaging operations toward generics (less expensive, faster) vs. newly approved products (expensive, more complex).

OF SPECIAL NOTE

Radio Frequency Identification (RFID) Technology and Its Implications for Pharmaceutical and Medical Device Packaging

RFID is a technology that been around since the 1940s. It uses radio waves to read information from and write information to special chips or tags that can be embedded in standard label stock or directly applied as self adhesive devices. If you are a regular user of toll roads and you have an "EZ Pass" type transponder in your car, then you are a lot closer to this technology then you might have thought. In the last decade, it has made inroads into the packaging industry. Most recently, Wal-Mart has informed its top suppliers that they must begin using RFID technology at the pallet level by the year 2005. Other concerns such as the Department of Defense, British retailer Tesco, CVS, and the Red Cross are working on pilot RFID applications. The intent is to move the use of the technology even further down the supply chain, all the way to the unit of use. One of the principal benefits of the technology is that no direct "line of sight" scanning is required, as with bar code systems, so entire skid loads can be scanned without unloading the pallet. RFID is also capable of reading and writing anywhere in the supply chain, so information can be upgraded in the field if necessary. The most promising application in packaging is the incorporation of the RFID tag into a label. Many cut label suppliers are looking into ways to incorporate the "smart tag" into their label making processes. There are also several label printer and applicator machine manufacturers who will be offering a unit capable of printing human readable labels and writing data to an embedded chips using RF. At first glance, RFID seems like a can't miss proposition. In the laboratory, the technology performs flawlessly, reading and writing information at incredible speeds in a controlled environment. However, in the field, the performance is hampered by a number of factors.

- *Cost:* There is a cost associated with the tags themselves, and a one-time cost associated with the reading and writing hardware and software. Sophisticated tags can cost up to $1.00 each, although for most applications the cost is currently around 30¢ each. It is anticipated that as demand increases, the cost will drop further to less than 10¢ each. Readers can cost anywhere from $500 to $10,000; and magnified over a multi-unit operation, these costs could be prohibitive. These costs are spread out between manufacturers and converters who will ensure that the tag is present and properly encoded, and the distribution centers, wholesalers and retailers who will interpret information from the tags in a variety of ways.

- *Speed and operational effectiveness:* The best case is when an entire pallet load of individually tagged units could be read at once. There are many factors that prohibit this from happening. The degree of RF penetration to the center of the pallet, the orientation of the tag to the reader, and the packaging materials used to name a few. Metals and foils reflect RF waves, and liquids tend to absorb them.

- *Tag durability:* The tag manufacturing process needs to be properly monitored to ensure that the tags are robust prior to application. In the course of secondary processing and application, the tags need to be handled properly to ensure that they are not damaged. Many secondary operations include embedding the RF tag into label stock, which is sent to the user in roll form. The tag must endure the stresses associated with the radius imparted on the label as it wound onto the roll. In some circles, estimates of the number of tags that do not work right out of the box prior to any additional processing run as high as 10%.

- *Industry standards:* Or more accurately, the *lack* of industry standards. This technology at its current stage of development is reminiscent of bar coding technology when it was in its early stages 25 years ago. There really are no industry standards that dictate how the units should be built, or how information is written or read. Different retailers will have different requirements, and different suppliers will have different capabilities. But just as industry demand led to accelerated development of standards for bar coding, the same forces will have very similar effects on RFID standards development. There is a not for profit organization called EPC global that is spearheading the standards effort. It is a joint venture between the European group EAN International and the Uniform Code Council. Its goal is to develop and commercialize the Electronic Product Code Network, which it hopes will become the global standard for RFID. Developmental shortcomings aside, RFID is really a very promising technology.

It will permit scan free (as compared to current bar coding technology) data acquisition on a grand scale, with expectations approaching 1,000 tags per second. It will play a major role in manufacturing and packaging logistics, point of sale transactions, and inventory control. Full scale implementation of RFID technology for packaging is not a question of if, but rather when.

BIBLIOGRAPHY

Code of Federal Regulations, Section 1301.72.

Cosgrove, J. "How Real Is RFID?" *Packaging Machinery Technology* Magazine, Vol. 1, No. 1.

IPSE Baseline Guide, Packaging, Labeling & Warehousing (DRAFT).

McTigue Pierce, L. RFID Comes of Age PDQ *Food & Drug Packaging,* February 2004.

Merck Engineering Design Standard, GMP Area Design Standard for Non-Sterile Pharmaceutical Dosage Form Facilities.

Walter Soroka W. Fundamentals of Packaging Technology, 2nd Edition.

Index